Food and Beverage Consumption and Health Series

RED WINE AND HEALTH

FOOD AND BEVERAGE CONSUMPTION AND HEALTH SERIES

Handbook of Green Tea and Health Research
Helen McKinley and Mark Jamieson (Editors)
2009. ISBN: 978-1-60741-045-4

Marketing Food to Children and Adolescents
Nicoletta A. Wilks
2009 ISBN: 978-1-60692-913-1

Food Labelling: The FDA's Role in the Selection of Healthy Foods
Ethan C. Lefevre (Editor)
2009. ISBN: 78-1-60692-898-1

Fish Consumption and Health
George P. Gagne and Richard H. Medrano (Editors)
2009 ISBN: 978-1-60741-151-2

Milk Consumption and Health
Ebbe Lange and Felix Vogel (Editors)
2009 ISBN: 978-1-60741-459-9

The Salmonella Outbreak in Peanut Products: The FDA vs. Greed
Benjamin K. Glynn (Editors)
ISBN: 978-1-60741-950-1

Red Wine and Health
Paul O'Byrne (Editor)
2009 ISBN: 978-1-60692-718-2

Food and Beverage Consumption and Health Series

RED WINE AND HEALTH

**PAUL O'BYRNE
EDITOR**

Nova Science Publishers, Inc.
New York

Copyright © 2009 by Nova Science Publishers, Inc.

All rights reserved. No part of this book may be reproduced, stored in a retrieval system or transmitted in any form or by any means: electronic, electrostatic, magnetic, tape, mechanical photocopying, recording or otherwise without the written permission of the Publisher.

For permission to use material from this book please contact us:
Telephone 631-231-7269; Fax 631-231-8175
Web Site: http://www.novapublishers.com

NOTICE TO THE READER

The Publisher has taken reasonable care in the preparation of this book, but makes no expressed or implied warranty of any kind and assumes no responsibility for any errors or omissions. No liability is assumed for incidental or consequential damages in connection with or arising out of information contained in this book. The Publisher shall not be liable for any special, consequential, or exemplary damages resulting, in whole or in part, from the readers' use of, or reliance upon, this material. Any parts of this book based on government reports are so indicated and copyright is claimed for those parts to the extent applicable to compilations of such works.

Independent verification should be sought for any data, advice or recommendations contained in this book. In addition, no responsibility is assumed by the publisher for any injury and/or damage to persons or property arising from any methods, products, instructions, ideas or otherwise contained in this publication.

This publication is designed to provide accurate and authoritative information with regard to the subject matter covered herein. It is sold with the clear understanding that the Publisher is not engaged in rendering legal or any other professional services. If legal or any other expert assistance is required, the services of a competent person should be sought. FROM A DECLARATION OF PARTICIPANTS JOINTLY ADOPTED BY A COMMITTEE OF THE AMERICAN BAR ASSOCIATION AND A COMMITTEE OF PUBLISHERS.

LIBRARY OF CONGRESS CATALOGING-IN-PUBLICATION DATA

Red wine and health / [edited by] Paul O'Byrne.
    p. ; cm.
 Includes bibliographical references and index.
 ISBN 978-1-60692-718-2 (hardcover)
 1. Red wines--Health aspects. I. O'Byrne, Paul.
 [DNLM: 1. Wine--analysis. 2. Antioxidants--pharmacology. 3. Biogenic Amines--physiology. 4. Cardiovascular Diseases--prevention & control. 5. Phenols--pharmacology. 6. Wine--microbiology. WB 444 R312 2009]
 RM256.R43   2009
 615'.321--dc22
                                         2008052429

Published by Nova Science Publishers, Inc. ✢ *New York*

Contents

Preface		vii
Chapter 1	Characterization of Wines through the Compositional Profiles of Biogenic Amines and Related Compounds. Focusing on the Description of Toxicological and Organoleptic Features *Javier Saurina*	1
Chapter 2	Dielectric Properties and Wines *A. García Gorostiaga, J.L. Torres Escribano and M. De Blas Corral*	25
Chapter 3	Red Wine Phenolics: Reasons for Their Variation *Patrícia Valentão, Luís Guerra, David M. Pereira and Paula B. Andrade*	53
Chapter 4	Antioxidants and Antioxidant Activity of Red and White Wines Affected by Winemaking and Other Extrinsic and Intrinsic Factors *Lachman Jaromír and Šulc Miloslav*	91
Chapter 5	Methods for the Determination of Natural Antioxidants in Red Wines *L.M. Ravelo-Pérez, A.V. Herrera-Herrera, J. Hernández-Borges and M.A. Rodríguez-Delgado*	143
Chapter 6	Biogenic Amines in Wines: A Review *Fernanda Galgano, Marisa Caruso and Fabio Favati*	173
Chapter 7	Safety and Healthiness Enhancement of Red Wines by Selected Microbial Starters *A. Caridi and R. Sidari*	205
Chapter 8	Sugars, Organic Acids and Glycerol Metabolism of Lactic Acid Bacteria from Fruits and Fermented Beverages: Influence on the Products Quality *María Cristina Manca de Nadra, Fabiana María Saguir and Ana María Strasser de Saad*	235

Chapter 9	Levels of Pesticide Residues in Red Wine and Health Risk Assessment *José Oliva, Paula Payá and Alberto Barba*	279
Chapter 10	Sulphur Dioxide in Wines: Automated Determination Using Flow Injection Analysis *Constantinos K. Zacharis, Paraskevas D. Tzanavaras, Demetrius G. Themelis and John A. Stratis*	303
Chapter 11	Does Oak Aging Improve the Antioxidant Activity of Red Wines? *Pedro Rodríguez-Rodríguez, Patrick Rabión, Gaspar Ros-Berruezo and Encarna Gómez-Plaza*	323
Chapter 12	Red Wine and the Metabolic Syndrome: Possible Contribution of an Old Remedy for an Emergent Problem *Rosário Monteiro, Marco Assunção and Conceição Calhau*	339
Chapter 13	Red Wine and Vascular Endothelium *Dimitris Tousoulis, Nikos Papageorgiou, Charalambos Antoniades, Costas Tsioufis, Gerasimos Siasos and Christodoulos Stefanadis*	359
Chapter 14	A Prooxidant Mechanism of Red Wine Polyphenols in Chemoprevention of Cancer *S.M. Hadi, M.F. Ullah, Uzma Shamim, Sarmad Hanif, Asfar S. Azmi and Showket H. Bhat*	373
Chapter 15	How Do We Demonstrate that There is a Potential Therapeutic Role for Moderate Wine Consumption? *Creina S. Stockley*	389
Chapter 16	Kidney Protection by Wine through an Enhancement of the Antioxidant Defense System *Ramon Rodrigo and Joaquin Toro*	401
Chapter 17	Keeping the Track of Quality: Authentication and Traceability Studies on Wine *Maurizio Aceto, Massimo Baldizzone and Matteo Oddone*	429
Chapter 18	Human Health Benefits, Antimicrobial Properties and the Future of Phenolic Compounds as Preservatives in the Food Industry *María Cristina Manca de Nadra and María José Rodríguez Vaquero*	467

Short Communication

	Dielectric Properties and Wines Impasses, Developments… *A. García Gorostiaga, J.L. Torres Escribano and M. De Blas Corral*	487

Index 493

PREFACE

The book revises the principal strategies for the characterization of red wines based on compositional profiles of biogenic amines as a source of information. Special attention is paid to toxicological and organoleptic repercussions associated with the presence of these natural components of wines. This book also aims to characterize the red wine through dielectric parameters. An overview of the basics of the dielectric properties of materials, specifically in foods is also presented.

Phenolic compounds in wines, especially in red wines, possess strong antioxidant activity in vitro. Phenolic compounds, obtained in red wine, are natural constituents of grapes and wines. They have the largest effect in decreasing atherosclerosis by both hypolipemic and antioxidant mechanisms. Thus, phenolics show a positive effect on human health and they may cause an increase of antioxidant activity of blood plasma. In this book, the effect of total phenolics [TP], total anthocyanins [TA] on the antioxidant activity [AA] is discussed. Furthermore, the applications of the different analytical methods that have been developed so far for the analysis of natural antioxidants in red wine are discussed, such as high-performance liquid chromotography (HPLC), gas chromatography (GC), and capillary electrophoresis (CE). Also, the agents influencing the phenolic profiles of red wine are overviewed.

Wine safety and healthiness depend on the interactions among various factors, several of which of microbial origin. This book explores scientific knowledge on the microbial role in the healthiness and safety enhancement of red wines, by proposing a specific selection of microbial starters. Furthermore, the growth and metabolism of lactic acid bacteria (LAB), which are essential in the quality of many fermented beverages like cider and wine, are discussed. In addition to malic acid, some other organic acids, sugars and carbon sources may be utilized by LAB modifying the sensory quality of these products. In fruit juice and related product, for example, they are considered spoilage microorganisms.

Sulphur dioxide (SO2) is one of the most debated chemical components used in enology. Its important antioxidant, preservative and antiseptic properties are indispensable for the health, stability and quality of wine. Flow injection analysis offers great potentials on the field of automation in terms of high sampling rate, precision, accuracy and cost effectiveness. This book reviews automated flow injection methods for the determination of sulphur dioxide in wines.

Moderate wine intake could play a protective role in several systems, including cardiovascular, digestive and neuroendocrine ones. Since the description of the French paradox, many beneficial effects of red wine have been described, namely those linked to cardiovascular disease protection. The most recent findings regarding the effects of red wine or its components on the adipose tissue are reviewed. In addition, it has been shown that red wine polyphenolics causes substantial falls in blood pressure, thus improving endothelial function and decreasing oxidative stress. These studies on vascular endothelium are also looked at.

The main component considered responsible for the reduced risk of death in alcoholic beverages is ethanol. This book reviews the data generated to date on the amount of phenolic compounds necessary to elicit certain cardioprotective effects. This data may have implications for national alcohol and dietary guidelines, for medical practitioners who 'prescribe' daily moderate wine consumption, as well as for the wine industry per se redeveloping healthier wine styles and types.

Chapter 1 - This chapter revises the principal strategies for the characterization of red wines based on compositional profiles of biogenic amines as a source of information. Special attention is paid on toxicological and organoleptic repercussions associated to the presence of these natural components of wines.

Biogenic amines occur in a wide variety of food products from the decomposition of protein components by the action of microorganisms. In the case of wines, small amounts of amines are already present in grape juice although they are mainly formed during the vinification. Alcoholic and malolactic fermentations as well as wine aging have been described as the principal processes contributing to the formation of amines. The most abundant amine in wines is putrescine which represents about a 50% of the overall amine contents. In addition, significant amounts of histamine, tyramine and phenylethylamine are often found. The presence of high amounts of amines in wines may be responsible for certain undesirable effects. For instance, amines such as histamine and tyramine may produce adverse effects on the vascular and central nervous systems. Other amines such as putrescine and cadaverine seem to modify negatively the organoleptic properties of wines so that its presence is not recommendable either. Apart from toxicological and organoleptic issues, compositional profiles of amines have been utilized as potential descriptors of wine features and quality. Characterization studies commonly rely on the application of chemometrics to facilitate the extraction of information dealing with the wine properties and winemaking practices.

Chapter 2 - The wine has been extensively described on the basis of chemical composition and sensory considerations. The authors aim to characterize the red wine through dielectric parameters. These studies are carried out on samples of red grape juice and red wine made from red varieties of grapes.

This chapter covers 3 aspects of the study of dielectric properties of wines:

Firstly, an overview is presented of the basics of the dielectric properties of materials, specifically in foods: related concepts of microwaves and radiowaves, parameters used, the measurement systems and factors of influence. Secondly, a review is carried out including comprehensive bibliographies on this subject and its more directly related topics along with, where feasible, quantitative data extracted from the literature. Thirdly, the authors focus on the specific characteristics of the employed materials, both the wines (and, in some cases, the original grape juices they come from) and the measurement system. The authors used the open-ended coaxial probe technique. In certain cases, the authors also measured other parameters such as electric conductivity.

Some of the conclusions the authors reached after carrying out this study are: both must and wine behave as diluted aqueous solutions, highly influencing in the ionic conductivity within the 200 MHz zone. This means that the loss factor is increased by the ionic loss. However, in the study range of high frequencies the relaxation phenomena of free water are dominant. Regarding the temperature, the variation of the dielectric properties showed completely different behavior at 200 MHz and at higher frequencies.

Specific tests carried out were:

Dielectric properties of grape juice and wine after alcoholic fermentation from 200 MHz to 3 GHz. Comparison between water, must and wine. The dielectric properties of wine from 200 MHz to 20 GHz after cold stabilization and filtration are also presented.

Variation of dielectric properties with temperature from 200 MHz to 6 GHz

Chapter 3 - Phenolic compounds are natural constituents of grapes and wines. The determination of polyphenols composition of red wines has long been attracting the attention of scientists, due to its responsibility in the organoleptic characteristics, such as as flavour, colour, bitterness and astringency, which constitute important quality parameters of wine. In addition, beneficial effects on health of this grape product have been described, such as antioxidant, anti-inflammatory, antimicrobial and cardioprotective, for which phenolic compounds exert a determinant role. Wine phenolics belong to several groups: hydroxybenzoic and hydroxycinnamic acids and their derivatives, flavonoids, like anthocyanins, flavan-3-ols and flavonols, stilbens and tannins. The complex phenolics composition of red wine changes until its consumption and is affected by several factors, such as grape variety, environmental conditions, yeasts strains and fermentation, winemaking procedures, oxygenation, aging and storage. In this chapter the agents influencing the phenolic profiles of red wine are overviewed.

Chapter 4 - The French have low coronary heart disease mortality with high fat consumption; this epidemiological anomaly known as the *"French Paradox"* is commonly attributed to the consumption of red wine. Phenolic compounds in wines, especially in red wines, possess strong antioxidant activity *in vitro*. Phenolic compounds obtained in red wine have the largest effect in decreasing atherosclerosis by both hypolipemic and antioxidant mechanisms. Phenolics (esp. catechins, resveratrol, phenolic acids and anthocyanins) show a positive effect on the human health and they may cause an increase of antioxidant activity of blood plasma. The long-term uptake of red wine has a positive impact on antioxidant activity [AA] of blood plasma in rats *in vivo* and increases AA by 15-20% compared to a control group. Major anthocyanins found in red wine are malvidin-3,5-O-diglucoside and 3-O-glucoside, cyanidin-3-O-galactoside, cyanidin-3-O-glucoside and 3,5-O-diglucoside, peonidin-3-O-glucoside, delphinidin-3-O-glucoside, and petunidin-3-O-glucoside. In this article the effect of total phenolics [TP], total anthocyanins [TA], individual anthocyanins, procyanidins and phenolics contained in red grapes, musts, grape seeds and skins and wines on the antioxidant activity [AA] is discussed. The significant impact of varieties, viticultural regions and locations, climate conditions and vintage has been shown. Likewise, the ways and individual stages of the vinification technology process (maceration in red wine production), and storage conditions affect color, TP, TA and AA and health aspects of produced wines. Likewise, resveratrol, another free radical scavenger mainly contained in the skins of grapes, inhibits the risk of cardiovascular diseases. Higher amounts of *trans*-resveratrol have been found in wines from cool and wet climate regions and lesser amounts are typical for warm and dry regions. During an attack with *Botrytis cinerea* the plant forms a resveratrol barrier surrounding the attacked site where the resveratrol concentration is low, but it is four times higher in the neighbor. Changes in the TP content and AA affected by grape variety, vineyard location and winemaking process in white and blue varieties from different vineyards of the Czech Republic were studied. Significant differences in TP among varieties were found. Analysis of variance showed statistically high differences among red and white wines and growing locations. Wines differed significantly in TP content and AA increased significantly during the winemaking process. Statistically significant differences in AA values were found among growing areas, wines and varieties. Significant positive correlations between TP and AA were determined. Total antioxidant status [TAS] of white and blue vine varieties (Czech Republic) revealed significant differences in AA between white and red wines. Moreover, differences were ascertained between individual varieties of red wine. The results obtained supported the assumption that variety plays a considerable role in TAS; the blue vine varieties showed a much higher TAS. Analysis of variance in AA showed statistically high significance between red and white wines. AA increased during the winemaking process, esp. in Zweigeltrebe, St. Laurent and Pinot Noir wines, suggesting thus higher AA of wines compared with grape musts at the beginning of the winemaking process. The highest increase was determined during fermentation and maturation stages of red wine.

Chapter 5 - Wine can be considered one of the most consumed drinks in the world, subjected to strict regulations concerning its quality in regards to truth-to-label and absence of additives. Among the different types of wines available, red wine is particularly important especially for its high antioxidant content. In this sense, research interest in this field has been intensified in the light of recent evidence regarding their important role in human health, particularly, several preventive effects on cancer, coronary heart diseases, neurological degeneration, inflammatory disorders, etc. Analytical methods for the analysis of antioxidants in red wines include mainly high-performance liquid chromatography (HPLC) and, with less applications, gas chromatography (GC). However, in recent years, the popularity of capillary electrophoresis (CE) has also increased the amount of works dealing with this subject. Therefore, the aim of this chapter is to describe the applications of the different analytical methods that have been developed so far for the analysis of natural antioxidants in red wine.

Chapter 6 - Biogenic amines are basic nitrogen compounds that can have toxicological effects on human health when present in foods and beverages at significant levels. These compounds are produced in small amounts in all living organisms and play an important role in cell growth and development, as well as in protecting stressed cells. Their presence at dangerous levels is principally attributed to microbial decarboxylation of the corresponding amino acids, and hence the occurrence of biogenic amines can be related to both food safety and food spoilage, becoming a useful index for the assessment of food quality and of the related manufacturing practices.

Nowadays an increasing attention is given to the presence in wine of biogenic amines, whose level and the possible synergic effect with ethanol may represent a significant risk for some consumers. The major toxicological implications are related to aromatic amines, such as histamine, tyramine, and 2-phenylethylamine; nevertheless, for these amines it is quite difficult to establish the exact threshold of toxicity, which depends on the efficiency of the detoxification mechanisms of different individuals. However, some countries have set limits for histamine in wine ranging from 2 to 10 mg/L, while for tyramine levels exceeding 10 mg/L in beverages should be considered unsafe. Several other amines may be found in wine, among them polyamines, that can enhance the adverse effect of aromatic amines, or cause negative consequences on wine aroma. Moreover, spermine and spermidine, that have secondary group, are involved in nitrosamine formation, compounds with a known cancerous action. Volatile amines, such as methylamine and ethylamine, come from amination of non-nitrogen compounds, such as aldehydes and ketones, and they have not a toxic action, but can exert a negative effect on wine aroma.

Biogenic amines usually found in wine are cadaverine, histamine, 2-phenylethylamine, putrescine and tyramine; agmatine and ethanolamine can be abundant, but they are generally little investigated. Low biogenic amine amounts, as normal constituents of the raw materials, can be released in must from grape and pulp during the winemaking process, and the biogenic amine concentration may increase as consequence of alcoholic fermentation, yeast autolysis, malolactic fermentation and wine aging, usually being red wines richer in amines than white wines.

In this work an overview of the presence of biogenic amines in wine is given, with a focus on the main factors affecting their presence and concentration in this alcoholic beverage.

Chapter 7 - The modern consumer is remarkably health conscious; consequently, he searches for foods and beverages having positive biological properties, such as high contents in antioxidant and anticancer substances and low content in toxic compounds. Wine safety and healthiness depend on the interaction among various factors, several of which of microbial origin. In general, the effects of these factors on wine composition and safety are studied separately. This chapter explores scientific knowledge on the microbial role in the healthiness and safety enhancement of red wines. The following could give a good reason to propose a specific selection of microbial starters: (a) production of wines with low levels of sulphur dioxide using yeasts able to inhibit malolactic fermentation; (b) production of wines with low amounts of acetaldehyde using low-producing yeasts or acetaldehyde-removing lactic acid bacteria; (c) production of wines with low amounts of methanol using low-producing yeasts; (d) production of wines with low amounts of ethyl carbamate using yeasts low-producing urea during arginine degradation or lactic acid bacteria low-producing ethyl carbamate; (e) production of wines with low amounts of biogenic amines using low-producing yeasts or lactic acid bacteria; (f) production of wines with low amounts of medium-chain fatty acids using low-producing yeasts; (g) production of wines with high healthy phenolic compounds content using yeasts producing enzymes, reactive metabolites and/or parietal mannoproteins that interact with phenolic compounds; (h) production of wines with low amounts of ochratoxin A using yeasts or lactic acid bacteria able to remove it; (i) must detoxification by selected yeasts from pesticides, fungicides, and heavy metals originating from vineyard treatments. Genomic strategies could also be used to improve the useful microbial traits.

Chapter 8 - Growth and metabolism of lactic acid bacteria (LAB) are essential in the quality of many fermented beverages like cider and wine. In these cases, they convert L-malic acid into L-lactic acid during the malolactic fermentation (MLF). In addition to malic acid, some other organic acids, sugars and carbon sources as glycerol may be utilized by LAB modifying the sensory quality of these products. In fruits juice and related product, they are considered spoilage microorganisms.

Carbohydrates metabolism by LAB follows the homofermentative or heterofermentative pathways with formation of lactate, or lactate, acetate, ethanol and CO_2, respectively. Studies on tomatoes microflora demonstrate that it is mainly constituted by obligatory heterofermentative LAB. D, L-lactic and acetic acids, CO_2, ethanol and diacetyl formed from glucose and fructose by LAB, affect the sensory properties of tomato purée by producing undesirable buttermilk and fermented flavor. In *Oenococcus oeni* strains from Argentinian wines growing in synthetic medium with acetate, equimolecular amount of D-lactate and ethanol in molar relation higher than 1 are produced from glucose. In deficient nutritional condition, glucose is diverted to the cysteine biosynthesis with decreased D-lactate recovery. In these strains the favorable effect of L-malic acid on the growth in synthetic medium and without essential amino acids is correlated with the energy gain associated with MLF.

Heterofermetative LAB from wine can metabolize citrate mainly to acetate, lactate, and carbon dioxide. Cells of *O. oeni* co-metabolizing citrate-glucose increase rate and molar yield growth. End products from glucose change: ethanol decreases and acetate is formed with ATP production via acetate kinase. It have been also demonstrated in this bacterium that citrate avoid essential amino acids requirement for growth. Fermentation balances indicate that part of citrate is diverted to the amino acids synthesis derived from aspartic acid.

Glycerol, produced during alcoholic fermentation in beverages, brings desirable properties (body, softness). But if it is used by LAB, depending on the pathway involved, the products formed can affect the product quality. Apparently the pathways to degrade glycerol in the species *Pediococcus pentosaceus* are variable. In the wine *Ped. pentosaceus* N_5p strain, glycerol is incorporated by an energy-dependent mechanism. It is degraded by the glycerol kinase (GK) pathway producing D-lactate, acetate and aroma compounds which can alter the flavor balance. *Ped. pentosaceus* CAg from beer degrade glycerol simultaneously by GK and glycerol dehydratase pathways producing high volatile acidity and aroma compounds that confer unacceptable flavors.

Chapter 9 - The control of pests and diseases of the vine (insects, mites, nematodes and fungi) along with pruning and fertilization are the pillars which should underlie a profitable wine production. The emergence of pesticide residues is a direct result of the various treatments with phytosanitary products during the growing period of the vine and especially among the veraison and maturing and their concentration depends on factors such as: active materials, formulations and doses used, time elapsed between application and harvest, pre-harvest interval of the pesticide and environmental factors (sunlight, rain, etc.). The choice of the proper pesticide and application under good agricultural practice criteria (GAP) reduce the presence of residues in grapes and wine to the utmost.

Available data indicate that there are substantial losses of pesticide residues in the transformation of grape to must and this to wine. It is imperative to note the importance of residue dissipation rates in the crop for their possible presence in wine. The oenological processes commonly used in winemaking as crushing, pressing, racking, clarification and filtration are very important in the disappearance of pesticide residues in wine. Lastly, the art of winemaking including or not maceration, adding of tannins, cryomaceration, etc., influence the disappearance of pesticide residues as well. Also, it should be noted that the characteristics of wine preservation (oak age, time in bottle, temperature, etc.) may influence on their disappearance.

This chapter will discuss experimental data on the disappearance and final levels of insecticides, fungicides and herbicides, such as organophosphates, growth regulators, phthalimide, dicarboximide, benzimidazoles, triazoles, dithiocarbamates, strobirulinas, dinitroanilines, urea derivatives, etc., in wine.

The presence of pesticide residues in wine due to the incorrect use of the phytosanitary products on crops and their possible transfer to must and wine greatly concerned the consumer, since there are no maximum residue levels (MRL) for wine established in the European legislation at the moment.

Finally, an approximation of the estimated daily intake (EDI), obtained from the experimental data, will be reported to set comparison with the acceptable daily intake (ADI). In addition, *in vitro* bioavailability trials of some insect growth regulators will be exposed for complementary assessment of health risks due to pesticides residues in red wine.

Chapter 10 - Sulphur dioxide (SO_2) is one of the most debated chemical components used in enology. Its important antioxidant, preservative and antiseptic properties are indispensable for the health, stability and quality of wine. Despite the fact that sulphur dioxide is among the most detested chemical components used in enology, up to now no alternative components were found able to have comparable effective antiseptic and preservative action combined with low toxicity. As sulphur dioxide has toxic effects on humans, the World Health Organization (WHO) has defined the maximum daily intake of sulphur dioxide as 0.7 mg kg^{-1} of body weight, whereas the lethal intake is defined as 1.5 g kg^{-1} of body weight. On this basis, the European Union has established maximum allowed concentrations in wines which are 160 mg L^{-1} for red wines and 210 mg L^{-1} for white and rose wines. It is therefore recommended to limit the use of sulphur dioxide.

Automation is a key demand in modern Analytical Chemistry, especially when it comes to quality control of pharmaceutical, food, and environmental samples which have the most profound effects on human activity and life. In the majority of the cases, a lot of samples have to be analyzed and it is critical to produce reliable analytical information in the minimum of time. Flow injection analysis offers great potentials on the field of automation in terms of high sampling rate, precision, accuracy and cost effectiveness.

The present study reviews automated flow injection methods for the determination of sulphur dioxide in wines, including several detection systems such as UV-Vis spectrophotometry, fluorimetry, chemiluminescence, amperometry, conductivity etc.

Chapter 11 - Antioxidant activity (AOA) is currently considered to be one of the most significant characteristics of red wines. The beneficial influence of the moderate consumption of red wine on human health is generally thought to be due to the AOA of wine polyphenols. An important part of the winemaking process, especially for high quality wines, is aging in oak barrels. Aging affects the chemical characteristics of wines, especially the polyphenol profile and concentration. Some compounds are degraded, new ones are formed. Moreover, some compounds may be incorporated into the wine from the oak wood of the barrels. Some authors claim that younger red wines are more beneficial for health than aged wines but little information exists on the correlation of AOA and wine age.

The authors have studied the evolution of AOA and the total phenol content of wines obtained from different varieties (Cabernet Sauvignon, Petit Verdot and Monastrell) during twelve months of aging in stainless steel tanks or oak barrels to check how this parameter changes with aging and whether it is related with the variety or type of aging.

In general, it was observed that AOA decreases with age. However, the use of oak barrels leads to wines with higher AOA when comparing the results with the control wines stored in tanks for the same period of time.

Chapter 12 - The combination of abdominal obesity with metabolic abnormalities (hyperglycemia, hyperinsulinemia, dyslipidemia, hypertension), collectively termed metabolic syndrome, is increasingly common and largely associated with the risk of developing cardiovascular disease, diabetes and cancer. If traditionally alcoholic beverages were strongly discouraged in the patients presenting these dysfunctions, mounting evidence is now showing that generalization of the deleterious effects of ethanol consumption to all alcoholic beverages is reductive. Since the description of the French paradox, many beneficial effects of red wine have been described, namely those linked to cardiovascular disease protection. Initially, this protective ability was attributed to ethanol. Later on, the relationship has been shown stronger for red wine, and its non-alcoholic components have come into scene, with a special relevance to flavonoids (catechins, procyanidins and anthocyanins) and resveratrol. Conclusive studies revealed that red wine has qualities further than alcohol as de-alcoholized red wine has also been related with health promotion. Considering the central role of visceral obesity and metabolic dysfunction in the metabolic syndrome, the authors will review the most recent findings regarding the effects of red wine or its components on the adipose tissue. Experimental results on the effects of red wine intake upon body weight and adipose tissue in the rat, from which a new possible red wine mechanism of action is advanced, will also be presented. Often forgotten, and probably making most of the difference for the effects exerted, the amount of beverage consumed as well as the pattern and context of drinking, will also be brought to this discussion.

Chapter 13 - Light to moderate alcohol consumption may have a beneficial effect on cardiovascular morbidity and mortality. Red wine has been shown to improve endothelial function and decrease oxidative stress. Consumption of red wine induces significant increases in plasma total antioxidant status and significant decreases in plasma malondialdehyde and glutathione in both young and old subjects. Red wine consumption for 2 weeks markedly attenuates insulin-resistance in type 2 diabetic patients, without affecting vascular reactivity and nitric oxide production. In vitro and in animal models, red wine polyphenolics cause substantial falls in blood pressure, mainly by increasing nitric oxide production. Although red wine has beneficial effects on vascular endothelium, more studies are necessary to evaluate these effects on cardiovascular risk.

Chapter 14 - Moderate consumption of red wine is considered to have a preventive effect against cardiovascular disease and cancer. The effect is attributed to the presence of polyphenols in red wine such as resveratrol, delphinidin, quercetin and gallic acid. Plant derived polyphenols are recognized as naturally occurring antioxidants but also act as prooxidants catalyzing DNA degradation in the presence of transition metal ions such as copper. The mechanism of pharmacological action of polyphenols present in red wine has been the subject of considerable interest as the identification of such mechanisms may lead to the development of novel anticancer and other drugs. Of particular interest is the observation that several polyphenols in red wine such as resveratrol and gallic acid have been found to induce internucleosomal DNA fragmentation in cancer cell lines but not in normal human cells. Some data in the literature suggests that the antioxidant properties of polyphenols may not fully account for their chemopreventive effect against cancer. Studies in their laboratory have shown that quercetin, resveratrol and delphinidin are able to bind Cu(II) leading to its reduction to Cu(I), whose reoxidation in the presence of molecular oxygen leads to the generation of a variety of reactive oxygen species (ROS). Copper is an important metal ion present in chromatin and is closely associated with DNA bases particularly guanine. Based on their own studies and those of others the authors have proposed that the prooxidant action (i.e. generation of ROS) may be an important mechanism of anticancer properties of plant polyphenols. The authors have shown that resveratrol, delphinidin, quercetin and gallic acid in the presence of copper ions are capable of causing DNA degradation in cells such as lymphocytes. The authors have further shown that these polyphenols alone are also capable of causing DNA breakage in cells. Neocuproine (a Cu(I) specific sequestering agent) inhibits such DNA degradation. Bathocuproine, which is unable to permeate through the cell membrane, did not cause such inhibition. The authors have also shown that delphinidin and resveratrol are able to degrade DNA in cell nuclei and that such DNA degradation is also inhibited by neocuproine, suggesting that nuclear copper is mobilized in this reaction. Neocuproine was also shown to inhibit the oxidative stress generated in lymphocytes indicating that the cellular DNA breakage involves the formation of ROS. These results indicate that the generation of ROS occurs through mobilization of endogenous copper ions. It is well established that tissue, cellular and serum copper levels are considerably elevated in various malignancies. Therefore, cancer cells may be more subject to electron transfer between copper ions and polyphenols to generate ROS. Thus, their results are in support of their hypothesis that anticancer mechanism of plant polyphenols involves mobilization of endogenous copper possibly chromatin bound copper and the consequent prooxidant action.

Chapter 15 - The light to moderate consumption of alcoholic beverages has been observed to reduce the risk of, and death from, cardiovascular disease (CVD) by potentially 20-50% compared to abstention and excessive consumption. The main component considered responsible for the reduced risk is ethanol. One of the alcoholic beverages, wine, additionally contains phenolic compounds, that are also observed in fruits and vegetables, the consumption of which is associated with a similar reduced risk of CVD. It has thus been proposed that consumers of wine have a greater reduction in the risk of CVD than do consumers of beer and spirits, but potential confounders include the drinking pattern and associated diet and lifestyle of consumers.

What is perplexing scientists, however, is the amount of phenolic compound that is necessary to elicit a cardioprotective effect e.g. on platelet aggregation or coagulation. In *in vitro* studies effects are generally elicited with a 10- or 100-fold greater concentration of phenolic compounds than is present in blood and at cellular sites of action following moderate consumption. This suggests that the metabolites of phenolic compounds may also be bioactive.

This paper reviews the data generated to date on the amount of phenolic compounds necessary to elicit certain cardioprotective effects, and whether isolated individual phenolic compounds are as effective as those administered in a wine medium. The data suggests that although the phenolic compounds are absorbed into the blood stream in measurable amounts, the metabolite is more likely to be the biologically active compound *in vitro*. Furthermore, when seed-derived phenolic compounds are together with the skin and flesh-derived phenolic compounds in wine, they exhibit greater cardioprotective effects than when present individually in a non-wine medium and are potentially equi-potent to certain conventional pharmaceutical products at reducing the risk of CVD.

This data may have implications for national alcohol and dietary guidelines, for medical practitioners who 'prescribe' daily moderate wine consumption, as well as for the wine industry per se redeveloping healthier wine styles and types.

Chapter 16 - Over the last decade the favorable consequence of moderate alcohol beverages consumption, especially wine, has been widely studied in rodents and humans. As opposed to what the authors might think at first sight, the results of those experiences have supported the view that moderate wine intake could play a protective role in several systems, including cardiovascular, digestive and neuroendocrine ones. Moreover, wine might be helpful for the prevention of pandemical diseases and its complications. The latter is remarkable, considering the fact that chronic pathologies increase every year because of the worldwide lifespan rise and non healthy lifestyle.

Chapter 17 - The quality of a wine is one of the most valuable features in the consumer's view. This is a consequence of a higher level of knowledge and culinary education among consumers: most people are now definitely ready to spend some more money to yield a higher quality product. At present, though, this feature seems not to be a matter of strict control from governments. In so many times laws have been violated that it is impossible not to see how inefficiently the present regulations on wine are working. The number of sophistication procedures is increasing constantly and becoming sophisticated and hard to recognize. More strict analytical controls should be developed and routinely used. An important concept in this field is *traceability*. In commodity economics this concept means "monitoring of goods fluxes from raw materials to the consumers' table" but this process is only based on production of documentation, easily subjected to falsification. Here traceability is expressed in a different way than before: in the chemical sense, *traceability* means to individuate chemical markers to find a link among the geographical zone where a wine is made and the final product of winemaking process, i.e. wine itself. It is mandatory that analytical techniques should be used to fulfill this task. The condition for this to happen is that wines grown on different zones should carry with them a fingerprint from soil to the bottle to be expressed in chemical terms, be it isotope ratios or elemental distributions. As long as this fingerprint is not altered along the whole winemaking process, its recognition could allow one to check whether a wine had been effectively produced in a certain area.

Another key feature in wine research is *authentication*, a concept expressing the possibility to identify and discriminate true samples from false samples. This concept, though not being a synonym of traceability, points to the same direction, i.e. quality.

Among the different techniques available for wine analysis and control, two seem to be highly promising for fingerprint recognition and authentication: isotope ratio – MS for determination of light and heavy elements and ICP-MS for determination of trace and ultra-trace concentrations of elements acting as markers, with particular focus devoted to lanthanides. An increasing amount of publications is being devoted in the last years to the application of these techniques to wine authentication and traceability, a review of state-of-the-art of which is the task of the present work.

Chapter 18 - Phenolic compounds are found in fruit, vegetables, nuts, seeds, stems and flowers as well as tea, wine, propolis and honey, and represent a common constituent of the human diet. Dietary flavonoids have attracted interest because they have a variety of beneficial biological properties, which may play an important role in the maintenance of human health. Flavonoids are potent antioxidants, free radical scavengers and metal chelators; they inhibit lipid peroxidation and exhibit various physiological activities including anti-inflammatory, antiallergic, anticarcinogenic, antihypertensive, antiarthritic and antimicrobial activities. Consumption of phenol-rich beverages, fruit and vegetables has commonly been associated to a reduction of the risk of cardiovascular diseases in epidemiological studies and the regular consumption, during several weeks or months, was shown to reduce cholesterolemia, and oxidative stress. The total polyphenols amounts determined from the same plant and their corresponding antioxidant and antimicrobial activities may vary widely, depending on extraction conditions applied.

Food contamination and spoilage by microorganisms are a serious problem because they have not yet been brought under adequate control despite the news preservation techniques available. Food-borne illness resulting from consumption of food contaminated with pathogenic bacteria has been of vital concern to public health. Unfortunately there is a dramatic increase throughout the world in the number of reported cases of food-borne illness. To reduce the incidence of food poisoning and spoilage by pathogenic microorganisms many synthetic chemicals were utilized. The exploration of natural antimicrobials for food preservation receives increased attention due to consumer awareness of natural food products and a growing concern of microbial resistance towards conventional preservatives. The use of phenolic compounds as antimicrobial agents would provide an additional benefits, including dual-function effects of both preservation and delivery health benefits. Knowing the antimicrobial effect of the phenolic compounds from vegetables on the principal pathogenic microorganisms from the different foods, it is possible to search strategies to combine the synergic antimicrobial effects of phenolic compounds with their natural biological properties. The results will permit to formulate new products to be used as food preservatives or to be included in the human diet.

Short Communication - The wine has been extensively described on the basis of chemical composition and sensory considerations. The authors aimed to characterize the grape juice and red wine through dielectric parameters. These studies were carried out on samples of red grape juice and red wine made from red varieties of grapes and the said dielectric parameters were used in order to find out a possible correlation among these values and the variety or the area where the samples were collected from. The frequency range was from 200 MHz to 3 GHz. Obtained results were not decisive enough.

Another problem the authors found with the open-ended coaxial probe measurement system was the undesirable results the authors obtained during the alcoholic fermentation process. During malolactic fermentation similar problems arose.

Regarding the study of dielectric properties in red wine before and after cold stabilisation, no significant differences could be detected, in the range under analysis from 200 MHz to 20 GHz.

In: Red Wine and Health
Editor: Paul O'Byrne

ISBN 978-1-60692-718-2
© 2009 Nova Science Publishers, Inc.

Chapter 1

CHARACTERIZATION OF WINES THROUGH THE COMPOSITIONAL PROFILES OF BIOGENIC AMINES AND RELATED COMPOUNDS. FOCUSING ON THE DESCRIPTION OF TOXICOLOGICAL AND ORGANOLEPTIC FEATURES

Javier Saurina[*]

Department of Analytical Chemistry, University of Barcelona, Barcelona, Spain.

ABSTRACT

This chapter revises the principal strategies for the characterization of red wines based on compositional profiles of biogenic amines as a source of information. Special attention is paid on toxicological and organoleptic repercussions associated to the presence of these natural components of wines.

Biogenic amines occur in a wide variety of food products from the decomposition of protein components by the action of microorganisms. In the case of wines, small amounts of amines are already present in grape juice although they are mainly formed during the vinification. Alcoholic and malolactic fermentations as well as wine aging have been described as the principal processes contributing to the formation of amines. The most abundant amine in wines is putrescine which represents about a 50% of the overall amine contents. In addition, significant amounts of histamine, tyramine and phenylethylamine are often found. The presence of high amounts of amines in wines may be responsible for certain undesirable effects. For instance, amines such as histamine and tyramine may produce adverse effects on the vascular and central nervous systems. Other amines such as putrescine and cadaverine seem to modify negatively the organoleptic properties of wines so that its presence is not recommendable either. Apart from toxicological and organoleptic issues, compositional profiles of amines have been utilized as potential descriptors of wine features and quality. Characterization studies commonly rely on the

[*] University of Barcelona, Diagonal 647, 08028-Barcelona, Spain. Phone: +(34)934039778, fax: +(34)934021233, e-mail: xavi.saurina@ub.edu

application of chemometrics to facilitate the extraction of information dealing with the wine properties and winemaking practices.

1. INTRODUCTION

Biogenic amines are low molecular weight compounds of basic nature which participate in the normal metabolism of animals, plans and microorganisms. Biogenic amines can be classified according to the number of amino groups they contain in monoamines (eg., histamine, tyramine, serotonin, phenylethylamine, ethanolamine and tryptamine), diamines (putrescine and cadaverine) and polyamines (spermine and spemidine). Another classification relies on the chemical structure of the hydrocarbon skeleton of the molecule that can be aliphatic, aromatic or heterocyclic (see structures in Fig. 1).

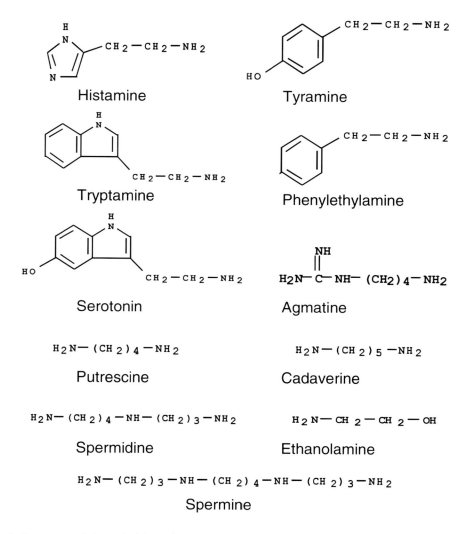

Figure 1. Structures of the main biogenic amines occurring in wines.

Biogenic amines are biologically active compounds responsible for multiple cellular functions. For example, monoamines such as histamine, serotonin, tryptamine and tyramine are involved in physiological tasks of the central nervous system, in the regulation of the blood pressure and body temperature, etc. Also, di- and polyamines are essential in the synthesis of DNA, RNA and proteins, thus, participating in cellular proliferation and differentiation processes (1,2).

The occurrence of biogenic amines is often associated to the degradation of the amino acid precursors by the action of decarboxylase enzymes according to the general scheme of Fig. 2. Also, these compounds are formed in metabolic pathways of transamination of aldehydes and ketones. As excessively high levels of amines may cause problems to the biological systems, living beings have developed catabolic mechanisms of detoxification as schematized in Fig 3a. As a result, biogenic amines are removed mainly via oxidation processes catalyzed by monoaminooxidase (MAO), diaminooxidase (DAO) and polyaminooxidase (PAO) (1,2).

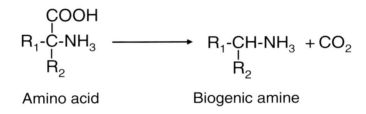

Figure 2. Scheme of the decarboxylation reaction of amino acids.

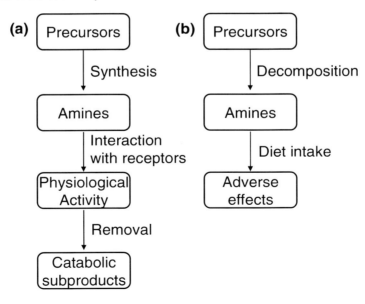

Figure 3. Biogenic amine activity in leaving beings (a) and food products (b).

In the food field, biogenic amines occur in a wide variety of protein-rich foods, including fish, meat, vegetables, fruits and fermented foodstuffs such as dairy products, beer and wine (3,4). Also, spoiled food or products obtained under deficient sanitary conditions may contain high levels of biogenic amines, especially histamine, putrescine and cadaverine. Note that the absence of general mechanisms of elimination in foods leads to a continuous rise in the amine contents due to uncontrolled microbial activity (Fig 3b). Hence, these compounds are sometimes used as indicators of the spoilage of foods due to alteration and putrefaction processes.

2. GENERAL CONSIDERATIONS ON THE EFFECTS AND TOXICITY OF DIETARY BIOGENIC AMINES

Nowadays, it is well known that the biological activity of these compounds may turn into toxicity when they are ingested in high amounts (5,6). This section summarizes the principal considerations dealing with physiological effects and toxicity of amines from dietary sources.

Histamine, which is mainly formed from the decarboxilation of the amino acid histidine, exerts its effects through the interaction with membrane receptors located in several organs and tissues of the body such as brain, stomach, skin, etc (6, 7). This fact explains why histamine is responsible for psychoactive (headache, palpitations and itching), vasoactive (hypotension), cutaneous (rash) and gastrointestinal (nausea, vomiting and diarrhea) effects. Histamine is metabolized in the human body primarily by methylation, oxidation and acetylation.

Histamine poisoning may occur few minutes to several hours following the ingestion of foods that contain unusually high levels of histamine. The toxicological threshold of the oral histamine intake is about 10 mg and amounts higher than 40 mg may cause slight symptoms of intoxication. However these reference values are merely tentative since they depend on the susceptibility of each individual. This toxicity is probably enhanced in combination with other components of the diet such other biogenic amines, alcohol, etc. (8). The interaction with monoamine oxidase inhibitor (IMAO) drugs, which are currently used for the treatment of depression and hypertension, potentiate dramatically the adverse effects of histamine. Hence, clinical signs mentioned above become much more severe in people taking IMAO medications. The toxicological repercussions of histamine on human health as well as the possibility of using its content as an indicator of freshness or spoilage of food, make histamine quantification increasingly demanded.

Tyramine is another important monoamine derived from the amino acid tyrosine. The physiological activity of this amine is related to the release of catecholamine neurotransmitters. Then, the ingestion of tyramine may result in an increase in the blood pressure and cardiac frequency. Tyramine is found especially in aged or fermented foods such as cheese, alcoholic beverages and chocolate (2). The cardiovascular effects of tyramine from dietary sources are likely negligible as the MAO system is highly efficient for its removal. However, sudden and dangerous hypertensive crises may occur in those individuals taking IMAO drugs. For instance, it has been described that oral ingestion of 500 mg of tyramine are apparently asymptomatic in healthy adults while a hypertensive reaction may be induced in people medicated with IMAO with as little as 10 mg. Another toxicological aspect that has been documented is the activity of tyramine as a trigger of migraine episodes in sensitive individuals (9).

Phenylethylamine (PEA) is a naturally occurring trace amine in the nervous system which acts as a neuromodulator of catecholaminergic transmission. PEA, which resembles a natural amphetamine, seems to activate dopamine and endorphins release. As a result, PEA may stimulate feelings such as attraction, excitement and euphoria while it seems to relieve depression. PEA really is abundant in foods like chocolate which has been recognized as a natural antidepressant product (2). However, in sensitive individuals, PEA is thought to be another powerful migraine inductor.

To date, other monoamines such as dopamine and serotonin occurring in food, and particularly in wines, have not been recognized as dangerous components of the diet. Dopamine, serotonin and related amines have crucial effects on mental and physical functions of living beings. Dopamine, which is synthesized in the various areas of the central and peripheral nervous system, displays cardiovascular, renal, hormonal, and nervous activities. Serotonin is another neurotransmitter synthesized in serotonergic neurons from tryptophan. Recent studies suggest that foods rich in these amines (e.g., mushrooms, fruits and vegetables) might affect the emotional response and mood.

Natural polyamines such as spermine and spermidine are involved in growth and cell proliferation since they participate in the synthesis of nucleic acids and proteins (10). The human body, and specially the digestive tract, requires polyamines for the continuous renewal of cells, growth and metabolism. Although cells can synthesize polyamines to some extent, these substances are semi-essential and external supply from the diet is required. DAO and PAO enzymes participate in their metabolism as part of the normal removal processes. Beyond the mentioned physiological functions, polyamines are involved in cancer growth so that recommendations on limits of dietary polyamine intake may be given (11, 12). A different aspect of polyamines, and especially diamines putrescine and cadaverine, concerns their influence on the organoleptic properties of foods. Some studies have been carried out by spiking amines to food and tasting the organoleptic features of the resulting products. In the particular case of wines, it has been evidenced that putrescine and cadaverine modify negatively the flavor (13). In the tasting assays, both professional testers and consumers have concluded that putrescine generates rancid and dirty aromas of putrefaction. Cadaverine has been identified to cause meaty and vinegary odors.

3. BIOGENIC AMINES IN WINES

First studies reporting the detection of histamine in wines were published in the 1950s. In the following decades, other amines such as tyramine, putrescine and cadaverine were progressively found. To date, more than 20 different amines have been identified in wines. Although the significance of these findings initially escaped notice, some researchers postulated that dietary amines might cause some adverse effects. Nowadays, as pointed out in the previous section, the toxicological implications of these compounds seem to be clear and rich-amine products may be harmful, especially for sensitive individuals (5).

Concentrations of biogenic amines in wines depend on multiple factors including the varieties and maturation of grapes and the vinification practices (14). Fig. 4 shows the average contents and variability ranges of several biogenic amines in red wines. Data have been obtained from several studies on more than 50 Spanish wines of different origins.

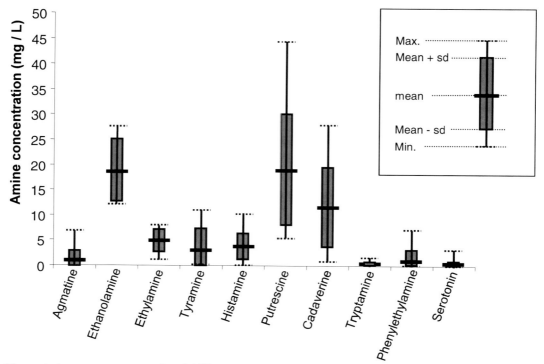

Figure 4. Average contents and variability ranges of amines in a set of Spanish wines.

Although these results cannot be generalized to a wider set of samples or other countries, they are a good reference of typical amine contents (15-17). Furthermore, conclusions extracted are in agreement with other studies which have recognized that putrescine, ethanolamine, cadaverine, ethylamine, histamine, tyramine are most abundant amines (18). These compounds are present at concentrations in the order of magnitude of 1 – 10 mg / L although higher values can eventually be found. Other trace amounts such as tryptamine, agmatine, spermine, spermidine and serotonin are sometimes detected in red wines with concentrations around 0.1 mg / L or lower. It is also well known that, in general, levels found in red wines are significantly higher that those occurring in white wines (a 50% higher or more), probably due to the differences in fermentation and ageing conditions (14). In some cases, too high levels of biogenic amines may evidence deficiencies in the hygienic conditions of the winemaking process. Besides, high amine concentrations are well correlated with other components typically associated to wine spoilage such as butyric, lactic and acetic acids, ethylacetate and diethyl succinate (19). In the following paragraphs, a more detailed description of the relevance of each vinification step on the formation of amines is given. Although many factors influence on the final amine amounts, experts agree that malolactic fermentation and ageing are the most important steps contributing to their occurrence.

Amines such as putrescine and histamine are already present in small quantities in grapes and musts (20). Some authors have suggested that levels in the fruits may depend on certain agricultural issues. For instance, a low potassium concentration in the soil might be responsible for an increase in the putrescine levels in the berries (21). Also, intensive fertilization practices with nitrogen nutrients may contribute to a rise in the concentration of amines (22). Woller et al. concluded that certain grape varieties produced amounts significantly higher of some amines than other stocks (23). For instance, it was found that "Pinot noir" leaded to remarkable quantities of putrescine, histamine, phenylethylamine and serotonin while cadaverine and espermidine were more abundant in "Cabernet sauvignon" (24). Similar studies have been carried out with other grape varieties (25, 26). The formation of amines may also be influenced by the climate of the producing region since warmer areas seem to lead to higher amine levels (27). Anyway, the relevance of amines already present in the grapes with respect to the total amounts in the wines is actually low and, as commented below, other winemaking operations are more important (14,28-30).

Alcoholic fermentation contributes to the formation of small amounts of certain compounds such as tyramine while the appearance of histamine during this step is almost irrelevant. The strains of yeasts and their concentrations during alcoholic fermentation may affect the formation of amines. Then, the use of selected yeasts and the careful control of the fermentation may reduce the occurrence of amines (31-33). As the concentration of yeasts is affected by physicochemical factors such as pH, temperature and SO_2 addition, these operating parameters can be adjusted conveniently to minimize the amine production (34-36). For instance, the addition of small amounts of SO_2 as a bacteriostatic agent hinders the formation of too high levels of amines. Also, auxiliary pre- and post-fermentation operations such as maceration with skins and racking protocols may increase the level of amines (37).

Malolactic fermentation is, by far, the most important step contributing to the formation of amines during winemaking (38). A marked increase in the levels of biogenic amines is usually observed towards the end of the malolactic fermentation, being *Oenococcus*, *Lactobacillus* and *Pediococcus* the principal bacteria responsible for these processes (39, 40). At this point, the control of hygienic conditions and the election of clean microorganisms are fundamental for preventing an excessive production of amines (41-43). For example, certain strains of *Leuconostoc oenos* seem to be highly recomendable for minimizing the production of biogenic amines during this stage (44).

The maturation of wine is also important in the production of amines (45-47). Martín-Álvarez *et al.* noticed that some enological practices widely used to enhance wine quality, such as the ageing of wine on lees, strongly increased the biogenic amine concentration. It has been also observed that amounts of some compounds such as cadaverine, putrescine may rise over this period. In contrast, contents of tyramine and other phenolic components may decrease when wines age. The behavior of histamine seems to be more complex as it increases initially during the first months of maturation while decreases in older wines (see Fig. 5). In this period, again, hygienic conditions of the cellars are very important, and contaminations due to uncontrolled growth of bacteria affect negatively to the quality of wines.

There is an emerging interest in the wine industry in the elaboration of healthier and better products so that lowering the overall amine contents results in a fundamental objective [31, 48, 49]. In the last years, various strategies have successfully been applied to the vinification practices and, as a result, the levels of biogenic amines have decreased progressively. For instance, some years ago, wines containing more that 10 mg L^{-1} histamine were quite common while current levels are lower. Actions for maintaining carefully the hygienic conditions over the whole winemaking process are fundamental for avoiding too high concentrations. Cleaner and more controlled fermentations are carried out in stainless steel tanks as an alternative to traditional wooden barrels.

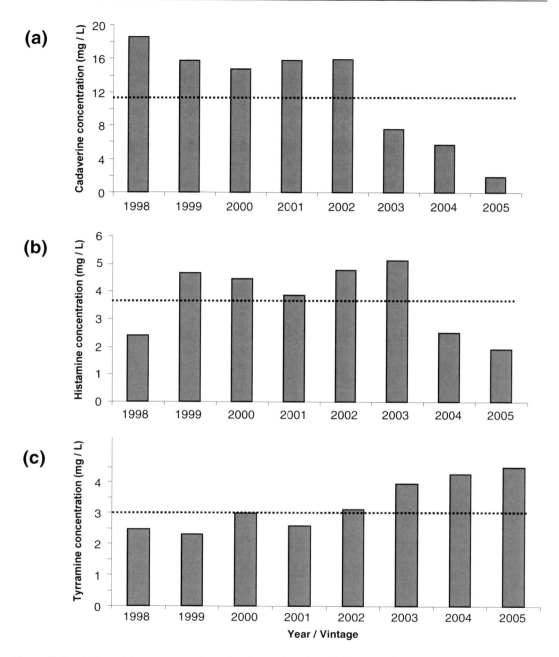

Figure 5. Evolution of the concentration of amines a function of the year of vintage. (a) Cadaverine; (b) Histamine; (c) Tyramine.

Also, suppressing spontaneous microbial processes, especially during malolactic fermentation, and using selected strains of microorganisms have contributed greatly to enhance the wine quality (40). The control of fermentation conditions including pH and temperature is highly recommendable to avoid excessive growth of undesired bacteria. Some studies propose the addition of chemical agents such as lyzozyme to increase the acidity, thus, limiting the microbial activity. Similarly, the addition of sulfite at the end of the fermentation process is a satisfactory operation for reducing the bacterial activity as well. The use of clarifying agents such as bentonite has been checked and a certain diminution of some amines have been reported (23).

Despite the relevance of the toxicological and quality issues derived from the presence of amines, to date, there is no specific legislation in wines. Experts in this field conclude that some regulations are necessary. Then, on the basis of studies on scombroid fish by the U.S. Food and Drug Administration (FDA) (50), more strict restrictions on upper limits will be implemented following in the near future. Some countries, however, have established recommendations concerning upper limits of certain amines. For histamine, the maximum tolerable amounts in various European countries range between 2 mg/L in Germany to 10 mg/L in Switzerland (40).

4. DETERMINATION OF BIOGENIC AMINES IN WINES

The establishment of accurate methods to determine amines in wines is of special interest for satisfying the increasing demand of controls in clinical and food analysis. Various revision papers have been published on this topic (51-53). Typically, the quantification of biogenic amines in food matrices, including wines, relies on liquid chromatography. Other separation techniques such as capillary electrophoresis (CE) are being used increasingly to establish faster and cheaper analytical methods (54). An alternative approach consists of the development of simpler methods focus on the analysis of a single component such as those based on flow-injection analysis (FIA) using conventional labeling reagents (55). Also, enzymatic and immunoreactions have been exploited for implementing rapid assays of selected analytes such as histamine or tyramine. Some commercial kits based on these principles are already available for routine controls of winemaking processes (56). Apart from the individual quantification of one or various amines of interest, a generic biogenic amine index (BAI) has been proposed as an indicator of food freshness, spoilage or degradation. This index is based on the fact that the amount of biogenic amines increases continuously due to bacterial action on amino acids. BAI is certainly important in seafood while its relevance in wines is lower (57).

In general, sample pretreatment procedures proposed for the determination of amines in wines may be simpler that those required for other food matrices (58). Solid phase extraction (SPE) is widely used for amine pre-concentration and clean-up (59-61). Amines can be retained efficiently by anion-exchange in commercial cartridges owing to they are charged positively at the wine pH values. Subsequently, the target compounds can be eluted easily to be further analyzed chromatographic or electrophoretically. Complementarily, reverse-phase C_{18} and polymeric cartridges can be used for additional removal of interferences from polyphenolic and other organic species. Liquid-liquid extraction is, in general, rather inefficient for recovering raw (unlabeled) biogenic amines due to the high polarity of the analytes. This drawback is circumvented in combination with a previous labeling steps (see below), yielding derivatives that can be quantitatively extracted with organic solvents. This is the case of the method proposed by García-Villar *et al.* in which amines are derivatized with 1,2-naphthoquinone-4-sulfonate (NQS) and the resulting products are extracted with CH_2Cl_2 (15).

Since most of biogenic amines display low UV-vis absorption or poor native fluorescence properties, HPLC and CE methods often include a labeling step to attain a sensitive detection. Nowadays, around 80% of the separation methods proposed in the literature rely on derivatization for enhancing sensitivity. From the vast list of probes of the amino group, o-phthaldialdehyde (OPA), 9-fluorenylmethyl chloroformate (FMOC), dabsyl chloride and dansyl chloride are among the most popular (62-66). The labeling reaction is commonly carried out in pre-column mode and the resulting derivatives are separated by reversed-phase HPLC. For instance, the OPA / 3-mercaptopropionic reaction for fluorescence detection of amino compound was readapted by Kutlan for the analysis of amines in wines and other food matrices (67). In certain cases, pre-column labeling can be implemented on a continuous-flow manifold coupled on-line to the chromatographic system (68). Post-column derivatization has been proposed for circumventing drawbacks of the pre-column modes dealing with the completeness of the reaction and stability of reagent and derivatives. The experimental post-column set-up requires on-line connection of the chromatographic effluent with the derivatization system prior to detection. As an example, Hlabangana et al. have proposed a method based on post-column derivatization of amines with NQS (69). A comparison of strategies for the derivatization of amines with NQS is given in Fig. 6 (adapted from to refs. 15, 68 and 69). In another paper, Vidal-Carou and coworkers have reported an ion-pair HPLC method for the determination of mono- and polyamines with post-column derivatization using OPA (70). Apart from pre- and post-column strategies, Busto et al. have developed an on-column derivatization method with fluorescence detection in which OPA reagent is contained in the mobile phase. Then, both separation and labeling processes occur simultaneously inside the analytical column (71). In the last years, however, the number of methods relaying on underivatized amines is increasing. In this approximation, the separation is currently performed by ion-pair or micellar reversed-phase HPLC. UV detection at 220 nm has been utilized as a straightforward possibility which provides sufficient sensitivity for most of the applications concerning dietary amines in wines. Recent progresses on hyphenation between HPLC and mass spectrometry (MS) have facilitated enormously the application of these techniques to wine analysis (72). Hence, amines may be determined directly by HPLC-MS. However, for practical reasons, HPLC-MS methods often include a derivatization step focused on facilitating the separation by conventional reversed-phase mode while improving detection features (73).

As mentioned, the application of CE to the quantification of common dietary amines in wines is gaining popularity due to advantages of this technique on the decrease of sample and reagent consumption and analysis time (74, 75). Most of those labeling agents utilized in HPLC have been readapted to CE analysis. It is well known that typical arguments against the use of CE deal with the low sensitivity and poor detection limits in comparison with HPLC which may hinder its applicability to real samples. However, in the case of wines, the levels of biogenic amines are clearly compatible with the detection limits currently reached with this technique. Furthermore, recent advances in derivatization strategies and innovative on-line pre-concentration methods have contributed to overcome this weakness and, nowadays, limits of detection are close to those achieved by HPLC (76, 77). In one of the applications, García-Villar and coworkers have combined field-amplified sample stacking and in-capillary derivatization in a CE method for the determination of histamine, tryptamine, phenylethylamine, tyramine, ethanolamine, agmatine, serotonin, putrescine and cadaverine (16).

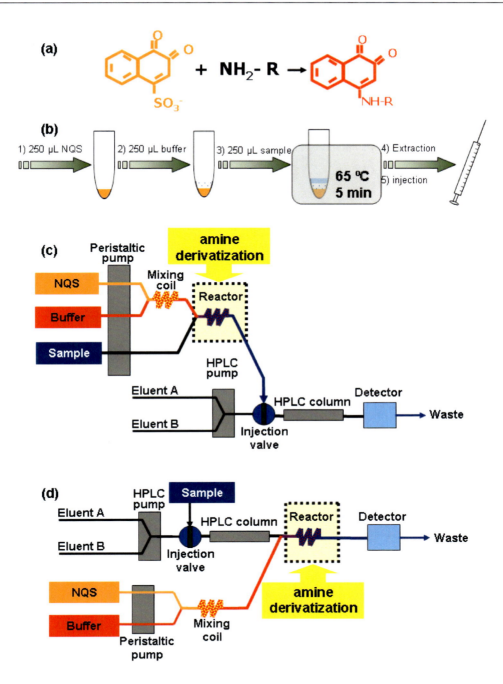

Figure 6. Strategies for the derivatization of amines with 1,2-naphthoquinone-4-sulfonate (NQS). (a) Scheme of the reaction; (b) Off-line (batch) precolumn derivatization; (c) On-line precolumn derivatization; (d) On-line postcolumn derivatization.

The electrokinetic injection contributes to the analyte preconcentration while minimizing the presence of interfering components in the electrophoretic runs. A scheme of the simultaneous preconcentration / derivatization strategy is shown in Fig. 7. In another example, micellar electrokinetic capillary chromatography (MECK) with off-line precapillary derivatization of amines with aminoquinolyl-*N*-hydroxysuccinimidyl carbamate has been applied to wine analysis. Sodium dodecyl sulfate (SDS) has been added as a surfactant for the separation of the resulting derivatives. L. Arce and coworkers have developed an on-line continuous flow clean-up procedure based on SPE to be coupled to the CE system with indirect detection of analytes (78). Modern portable CE microchips have also been designed for the determination of various dietary amines, especially tyramine and histamine, in wines. The target molecules are labeled with fluorescamine and samples are injected into a microfabricated glass CE device. Electropherograms can be obtained in only 2 min (79).

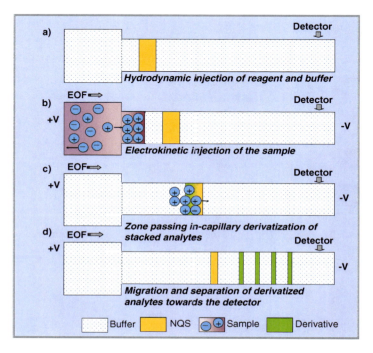

Figure 7. Scheme of field-amplified sample stacking and in-capillary derivatization strategy for the electrophoretic determination of biogenic amines in wines.

Colorimetric and fluorescence reagents utilized in HPLC and CE methods can be adapted to the development of flow-injection methods for a rapid and simple determination of a given target compound. For instance, histamine has been quantified by FIA via OPA reaction and fluorescence detection, using an anion-exchange column to eliminate sample matrix interferences (80).

Among the immunological methods, enzyme-linked immunosorbent assays (ELISA) have been exploited commercially for the determination of biogenic amines (56). In general, they are suitable for routine analysis and work with a small sample amount. Beyond the apparent simplicity, in practice unspecific absorptions may occur. Then, in order to avoid potential interferences, careful washing and separation steps for removing free antigen and unspecific interactions are needed. The accuracy of commercial ELISA for the detection of histamine has been compared with the RP-HPLC method using pre-column derivatization with OPA. Results obtained have shown a good agreement for histamine analysis of wines (81).

In the case of enzymatic methods, various types of enzymes including deshydrogenases, transaminases, decarboxilases, oxidases or peroxidases can be exploited for determining biogenic amines (82). The corresponding enzymatic reactions currently release some small molecules from the degradation of the substrate (e.g., NH_3 and H_2O_2) which are further monitored with a wide range of detection techniques such as spectrophotometry, fluorimetry, chemiluminescence, amperometry and potentiometry. New trends aim at investigating the possibilities of combining various sensors or biosensors in array devices. The resulting so-called electronic tongues and electronic noses are extremely powerful for characterizing complex sample properties dealing with color, taste, aroma and so on. Sensor arrays generate multivariate data to be handled with chemometric methods which facilitate the recovery of information and the simultaneous determination of several analytes while minimizing interference problems (see section 5). For instance, Lange and Wittmann have developed an enzyme sensor array for the simultaneous determination of histamine, tyramine and putrescine in food samples using artificial neuronal networks (ANN) for calibration and pattern recognition tasks. In this application, monoamine oxidase, tyramine oxidase and diamine oxidase are immobilized separately on screen-printed thick-film electrodes integrated in the sensor array. The sample treatment is reduced to extraction and subsequent neutralization prior to amperometic measurement (83).

5. CHARACTERIZATION OF WINES THROUGH THE STUDY OF BIOGENIC AMINE CONTENTS

Contents of low molecular organic acids, polyphenols, amino acids, biogenic amines and inorganic species in wines are strongly dependent on climatic, agricultural and winemaking issues. Reasonably, then, compositional profiles of these families of natural wine components can provide relevant information about wine features. In particular, apart from amines, the elemental and isotopic composition (84), the terpenoid profiles (85), polyphenolic contents (86, 87) and global volatile fingerprints (88) have already been utilized for successful studies of classification and correlation of wines as a function of vintage, origins or other features.

Data Analysis

The type of data handled in these characterization studies is, in general, of multivariate nature. Such multivariate data consist of discrete values of concentrations of selected substances or instrumental sensor measurements. Data are folded, as shown in the scheme of Fig. 8, resulting in arrays of values, the so-called first order data according to the chemometric terminology. The data arrays from each wine can be then analyzed simultaneously in order to gain overall information from the set of samples through a data matrix arrangement. Dimensions of the corresponding matrix D is, thus, $m \times n$, being m the number of samples and n the number of sensor measurements or quantified components per sample.

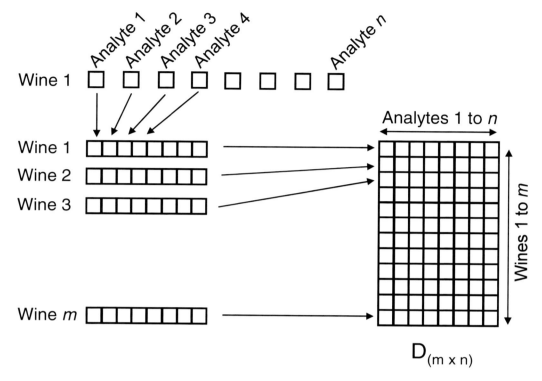

Figure 8. Generation of data sets to be used in wine characterization with chemometric techniques.

Recent trends in food characterization involve the use of complex instrumental fingerprints as multivariate data. For instance, instrumental signals consisting of chromatographic and electrophoretic profiles over time (17), UV-Vis (89), near-infrared (90), fluorescence (91) and mass spectra (92, 93) have been utilized as a source of analytical information in wine characterization. Also, electronic tongues, noses and other kinds of sensor array devices have been introduced as a novel approach for describing certain complex wine properties related to organoleptic characteristics (94-96). In fingerprint analysis, identification and full separation of all components occurring in the samples are not necessary (and often difficult or impossible to achieve). However, the overall structure of instrumental profiles is a reflex of the sample composition of the corresponding samples. For simplicity reasons, this approach is gaining popularity since those time-consuming steps devoted to separate and quantify the desired analytes can be avoided. An example of a red wine fingerprinting from CE is depicted in Fig. 9. In this electropherogram, although various components can be separated, identified and quantified, overlapping peak systems consisting of comigrations of analytes (here, amines, amino acids and polyphenols), matrix components and reagent interferences can be used to enrich the data set. Hence, in general, the occurrence of overlapping systems is not considered as a serious drawback but they result in an additional source of valuable information to be exploited in descriptive tasks.

Principal component analysis (PCA) is the chemometric method most widely used for a preliminary study of the properties of the sample from the mathematical treatment of the corresponding data matrix.

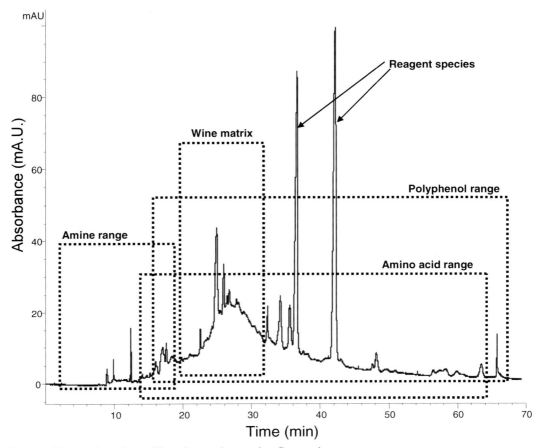

Figure 9. Electrophoretic profile to be used as a wine fingerprint.

Briefly, PCA is based on the concentration of the relevant data variance into a small number of new variables called principal components (PC) by means of a suitable mathematical transformation. The experimental matrix of responses is decomposed into score and loading components. The first principal component (PC1) is that which describes the maximum amount of information from the data; PC2 describes the maximum amount of the residual variance and is orthogonal to PC1, and so on. As PCA retains most of the relevant data variance in the first PCs, the information can be plotted effieicely in a graph of reduced dimensions. For instance, the scatter plot of scores of two or more PCs, commonly PC1 versus PC2, is often used to characterize and classify samples from the variance contained in the corresponding compositional or instrumental data. The distribution of samples on this graph may reveal patterns and other features that might be correlated to the general characteristics of the samples. In parallel, the study of the distribution of variables (loadings' plot) provides information dealing with correlations and relationships with sample properties. Additionally, the simultaneous study of scores and loadings (bi-plot) can be used to explore the interdependences between samples and variables.

Apart from PCA, other chemometric method such as cluster analysis (CA), linear discriminant analysis (LDA), artificial neural networks (ANN) and partial least square regression (PLS) are sometimes used for most specific classification, modeling and correlation purposes. A more detailed description of PCA, CA, LDA, ANN and PLS methods is given elsewhere (97)

Wine Studies

Despite the complexity of factors influencing on the formation of amines, several authors have proposed the use of dietary amines as potential descriptors of wine characteristics and quality. The influence of technological practices on biogenic amine contents has been investigated by several research groups. However, extracting information may result in a difficult task due to the multiple sources of variation commented above. At this stage, the application of chemometric techniques may facilitate the recovery of reliable conclusions.

The type of wine and the content of amines are corelated since both are strongly dependent on the vinification process. As an example, Romero *et al.* have evaluated the possibilities of discriminating among red, white and rose wines using principal component analysis (PCA), cluster analysis (CA) and linear discriminant analysis (LDA) (98). Authors conclude that putrescine, histamine and tyramine are the main descriptors contributing to group samples according to wine type. In another study, Csomos and coworkers have utilized the concentrations of amines and polyphenols for evaluating Hungarian wines from the same producing area and elaborated in the same year (99). PCA plots clearly reveal that red and white wines can be distinguished reasonably as they are located in separated zones.

Apart from wine type, other wine features have also been correlated with the amine composition. In an extended study on Hungarian wines, amines and amino acids have been determined by liquid chromatography with post-column derivatization with ninhydrin (100). From these data, PCA and LDA methods have shown a certain differentiation according to the wine-making technology and, in lesser extension, as a function of the geographic origin, grape variety and year of vintage.

The evaluation of wine origin, and specially the recognition of the authenticity of certain quality specialities, is one of the objectives of some papers published by Kiss and co-workers (101, 102). Amine and organic acid compositional profiles have been used to distinguish among botrytized Tokaji Aszu, foreign botrytized and non-botrytized wines. PCA and LDA graphs can classify successfully these wines according to the origins.

García-Villar *et al.* have studied the possibility of using the biogenic amine composition for describing some wine features (17). 36 samples from 6 Spanish producing regions are included in the analysis. Amine contents have been determined by liquid chromatography with a pre-column derivatization with NQS. Correlations between amines as well as possible relationships with some wine features, such as pH, aging period and producing region have been evaluated using PCA and other chemometric techniques. Regarding the dependence of contents of selected amines with respect to the origin region, the lowest histamine amounts have been found in Penedès wines. Quite low (or non-detectable) levels of serotonin are also characteristic of Penedès wines. Phenylethylamine also allows a certain distinction of wines from various regions into two groups: Penedès, La Mancha and Valdepeñas with low and Navarra, Rioja and Ribera de Duero with high concentrations.

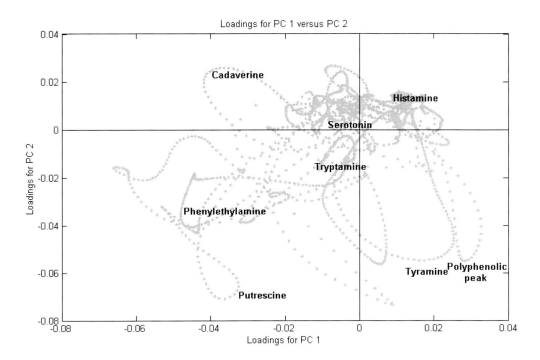

Figure 10. PCA characterization of Spanish wines using chromatographic profiles as analytical data. (a) Scores and (b) loadings of PC1 *versus* PC2. Sample codes: Y = young wine; C =*crianza* wine; R = *reserva* wine; 1 = Navarra; 2 = Penedès; 3 = La Mancha; 4 = Valdepeñas; 5 = Rioja; 6 = Ribera del Duero.

The use of the whole chromatogram as a wine fingerprint has been investigated by PCA and PLS (see results in Fig 10). In this case, the wine age is clearly described by PC1 as young wines are distributed to the bottom right side of the scores' plot, *crianza* wines appears, in general, in intermediate regions and oldest *reserva* samples are mainly placed to the top left part of the graph. Differences among young and aged wines are noticeable although less marked distinction is observed among *reserva* and *crianza*. The loadings' plot provides information dealing with chromatographic variables (i.e., retention time) which can be correlated the main peaks of amines. The wine aging is related with a decrease in the levels of polyphenolic species and younger wines are especially rich in tyramine and polyphenols. Wines to the left part are characterized by high putrescine and phenylethylamine concentrations while wines situated at the top of PC2 contain high histamine and cadaverine levels. As a conclusion, younger wines can be reasonably distinguished from aged ones on the basis of the amine contents. Besides the study of raw chromatographic profiles is proven to be also effective and patterns dealing with aging processes have also been found. Results from these chemometric analysis may contribute to improve the overall knowledge on wine characteristics and to facilitate the extraction of relevant information.

CONCLUSIONS

Although amine contents in red wines are dependent on a wide variety of agricultural and enological factors, there is a general consensus in the fact that too high levels are an evident sign of deficient vinification practices. It has also been found that too high levels of amines have unpleasant organoleptic repercussions as they have been associated to dirty and rancid flavors. Regarding toxicity, the consumption of reasonable amounts of wines is generally asymptomatic for healthy people although they may cause poisoning episodes on susceptible individuals. Symptoms are then similar to allergic reactions, including cutaneuos, gastrointestinal, cardiac and nervous effects.

Winemaking technologies for obtaining low-amine products are one of the new challenges for modern wine industry. Practices for controlling carefully the fermentation and ageing process are fundamental for preserving the quality of wines. Among them, the selection of proper strains of yeasts and bacteria seems to be fundamental for minimizing the amine generation.

The establishment of accurate and robust analytical methods to determine amines in wines is of special interest for satisfying the increasing demand of controls during vinification. Besides, the potential utility of amines as descriptors of wine characteristics has been pointed out by several authors. For this purpose, chemometric methods for data analysis have proved to be suitable to describe efficiently the sample characteristics and to establish relationships with winemaking practices. As a result, important correlations between compositional profiles and wine features can be established. The information gained from these characterization studies could further be exploited to obtain healthier and better wines.

REFERENCES

[1] C. White Tabor, H. Tabor, Polyamines, Ann. Rev. Biochem., 53 (1984) 749-790.
[2] M.H. Silla-Santos, Biogenic amines: their importance in foods, Int. J.Food Microbiol., 29 (1996) 213-231.
[3] S. Bodmer, C. Imark, M. Kneubühl, Biogenic amines in food: Histamine and food processing, Inflammation Res., 48 (1999) 296-300.
[4] A. Halász, Á. Baráth, L. Simon-Sarkadi, W. Holzapfel, Biogenic amines and their production by microorganisms in food, Trends Food Sci. Technol., 5 (1994) 42-49.
[5] C. Jansen, M. van Dusseldorp, K.C. Bottema, A.E.J. Dubois, Intolerance to dietary biogenic amines: a review, Annals of Allergy, Asthma & Immonology, 91 (2003) 233-241.
[6] R.C. Peatfield, G. Fletcher, K. Rhodes, I.M. Gardiner, J. de Belleroche, Pharmacological analysis of red-wine-induced migrainous headaches, J. Headache Pain, 4 (2003) 18-23.
[7] S. Oguri, Y. Yoneya, Assay of biological relevance of endogenous histamine and its metabolites: application of microseparation techniques, J. Chromatogr. B, 781 (2002) 165-179.

[8]   E. Diel, N. Bayas, A. Stibbe, S. Müller, A. Bott, D. Schrimpf, F. Diel, Histamine containing food: Establishment of a german food intolerance databank (NFID), Inflammation Res., 46 (1997) 87-88.
[9]   W. L. Forsythe, A. Redmond, Two controlled trials of tyramine in children with migraine, Rev. Med. Child. Neurol., 16 (1974) 794-799.
[10] S. Bardócz, Polyamines in food and their consequences for food quality and human health, Trends Food Sci. Technol., 6 (1995) 341-346.
[11] A. Manni, R. Grove, S. Kunselman, M. Aldaz, Involvement of the polyamine pathway in breast cancer progression, Cancer Lett., 92 (1995) 49-57.
[12] M.Y. Khuhawar, G.A. Qureshi, Polyamines as cancer markers: applicable separation methods, J. Chromatogr. B, 764 (2001) 385-407.
[13] A. Palacios, C. Suárez, S. Krieger, D. Theodore, L. Otaño, A. Laucirica, F. Peña, Influencia organoléptica de las aminas biógenas producidas durante la fermentación maloláctica del vino, Revista de Enología, 54 (2005) (http://www.acenologia.com/ciencia70_3.htm).
[14] M.C. Vidal-Carou, A. Ambatlle-Espunyes, M.C. Ulla-Ulla, A. Mariné-Font, Histamine and tyramine in Spanish wines: Their formation during the winemaking process, Am. J Enol. Vitic., 41 (1990) 160-167.
[15] N. Garcia-Villar, J. Saurina, S. Hernández-Cassou, High-performance liquid chromatographic determination of biogenic amines in wines with an experimental optimization procedure, Anal. Chim. Acta, 575 (2006) 97 – 105.
[16] N. Garcia-Villar, J. Saurina, S. Hernández-Cassou, Capillary electrophoresis determination of biogenic amines by field-amplified sample stacking and in-capillary derivatization, Electrophoresis, 27 (2006) 474 - 483.
[17] N. Garcia-Villar, S. Hernández-Cassou, J. Saurina, Characterization of wines through the biogenic amine contents using chromatographic techniques and chemometric data analysis, J. Agric. Food Chem., 55 (2007) 7453-7461.
[18] L. Zhijun, W. Yongning, Z. Gong, Z. Yunfeng, X. Changhu, A survey of biogenic amines in Chinese red wines, Food Chem., 105 (2007) 1530-1535.
[19] E. Soufleros, M.L. Barrios, A. Bertrand, Correlation between the content of biogenic amines and other wine compounds, Am. J. Enol. Vitic., 49 (1998) 266-278.
[20] I. Mato, S. Suarez-Luque, J.F. Huidobro, A review of the analytical methods to determine organic acids in grape juices and wines, Food Res. Int., 38 (2005) 1175-1188.
[21] D. O. Adams, Accumulation of putrescine in grapevine leaves showing symptoms of potassium deficiency or spring fever. In Proceedings of the International Symposium on Nitrogen in Grapes and Wine; J. Rantz, Ed.; American Society for Enology and Viticulture: Davis, CA, (1991) 126-131.
[22] S.E. Spayd, E.L. Wample, R.G. Evans, B.J. Seymour, C.W. Nagel, Nitrogen fertilization of white Riesling grapes in Washington must and wine composition, Am. J. Enol. Vitic., 45 (1994) 34-42.
[23] R. Woller, Aminas biógenas: presencia en el vino y efectos en el organismo, Revista de Enología, 54 (2005) (http://www.acenologia.com/ciencia70_2.htm).
[24] M.B.A. Glória, B.T. Watson, L. Simon-Sarkadi, M.A. Daeschel, A survey of biogenic amines in Oregon Pinot noir and Cabernet Sauvignon wines, Am. J. Enol. Vitic., 49 (1998) 279-232.

[25] G.J. Soleas, G.J. Pickering, Influence of variety, wine style, vintage and viticultural area on selected chemical parameters of Canadian Icewine, J. Food Agric. Env., 5 (2007) 97-101.

[26] P. Hernández-Orte, A. Pena-Gallego, M.J. Ibarz, J. Cacho, V. Ferreira, Determination of the biogenic amines in musts and wines before and after malolactic fermentation using 6-aminoquinolyl-N-hydroxysuccinimidyl carbamate as the derivatizing agent, J. Chromatogr. A, 1129 (2006) 160-164.

[27] J. M. Huggett, Geology and wine: a review, Proc. Geol. Assoc., 117 (2006) 239-247.

[28] M.C. Leitao, A.P. Marques, M.V. San Romao, A survey of biogenic amines in commercial Portuguese wines, Food Control, 16 (2005) 199-204.

[29] R.E. Anli, N.Vural, S.Yilmaz, Y.H. Vural, The determination of biogenic amines in Turkish red wines, J. Food Comp. Anal., 17 (2004) 53-62.

[30] T. Bauza, A. Blaise, P.l. Teissedre, J.P. Mestres, F. Daumas, J.C. Cabanis, Changes in biogenic amines content in musts and wines during the winemaking process, Sci. Alim., 15 (1995) 559-570.

[31] M. Caruso, C. Fiore, M. Contursi, G. Salzano, A. Paparella, P. Romano, Formation of biogenic amines as criteria for the selection of wine yeasts, World J. Microbiol. Biotechnol. 18 (2002) 159-163.

[32] D. Torrea Goñi, C. Ancín Azpilicueta, Influence of yeast strain on biogenic amines content in wines: relationship with the utilization of amino acids during fermentation, Am. J. Enol. Viticult. USA, 52 (2001) 185-190.

[33] J.M. Landete, S. Ferrer, I. Pardo, Which lactic acid bacteria are responsible for histamine production in wine?, J. Appl. Microbiol., 99 (2005) 580-586.

[34] T.L. Baucom, M.H. Tabacchi, T.H.E. Cottrell, B.S. Richmond, Biogenic amine content of New York state wines, J. Food Sci., 51 (1996) 1376-1377.

[35] S.C. Souza, K.H. Theodoro, E.R. Souza, S. da Motta, M. Beatriz, A. Gloria, Bioactive amines in Brazilian wines: Types, levels and correlation with physico-chemical parameters, Braz. Arch. Biol. Technol., 48 (2005) 53-62.

[36] T.J. Britz, R.P. Tracey, The combination effect of pH, SO_2, ethanol and temperature on the growth of *Leuconostoc oenos*, J. Appl. Bacteriol., 68 (1990) 23-31.

[37] J.A. Zee, R.E. Simard, L. L'Heureux, J. Tremblay, Biogenic amines in wines, Am. J. Enol. Vitic., 34 (1983) 6-9.

[38] S.Q. Liu, Malolactic fermentation in wine-beyond deacidification, J. Appl. Microbiol., (2002) 589-601.

[39] A. Lonvaud-Funel, Biogenic amines in wine: role of lactic acid bacteria, FEMS Microbiol. Lett., 199 (2001) 9-13.

[40] J.M. Landete, S. Ferrer, L. Polo, I. Pardo, Biogenic amines in wines from three Spanish regions, J. Agric. Food Chem., 53 (2005) 1119-1124.

[41] A. Marcobal, P.J. Martín-Álvarez, M. C. Polo, R. Muñoz, M. V. Moreno-Arribas, Formation of biogenic amines throughout the industrial manufacture of red wine, J. Food Protection, 69 (2006) 397-404.

[42] A. Marcobal, P.J. Martín-Álvarez, M.V. Moreno-Arribas, R. Muñoz, A multifactorial design for studying factors influencing growth and tyramine production of the lactic acid bacteria Lactobacillus brevis CECT 4669 and Enterococcus faecium BIFI-58, Res. Microbiol., 157 (2006) 417-424.

[43] D. Torrea, C. Ancin, Content of biogenic Amines in a Chardonnay wine obtained through spontaneous and inoculated fermentations, J. Agric. Food Chem., 50 (2002) 4895-4899.

[44] S. Guerrini, S. Mangani, L. Granchi, M. Vincenzini, Biogenic amine production by *Oenococcus oeni*, Curr. Microbiol., 44 (2002) 374-378.

[45] N. Jiménez-Moreno, D. Torrea-Goñi, C. Anzín-Azpilicueta, Changes in amine concentrations during aging of red wine in oak barrels, J. Agric. Food Chem., 51 (2003) 5732-5737.

[46] P.J. Martín-Álvarez, A. Marcobal, C. Polo, M.V. Moreno-Arribas, Influence of technological practices on biogenic amine contents in red wines, Eur. Food Res. Technol., 222 (2006) 420-424.

[47] N. Jiménez-Moreno, DC. Anzín-Azpilicueta, Influence of wine turbidity on the accumulation of biogenic amines during aging, J. Sci. Food Agric., 84 (2004) 1571-1576.

[48] A. Costantini, M. Cersosimo, V. Del Prete, E. Garcia-Moruno, Production of biogenic amines by lactic acid bacteria: Screening by PCR, thin-layer chromatography, and high-performance liquid chromatography of strains isolated from wine and must, J. Food Protect., 69 (2006) 391-396.

[49] M.V. Moreno-Arribas, M.C. Polo, Winemaking biochemistry and microbiology: Current knowledge and future trends, Crit. Rev. Food Sci. Nutr., 45 (2005) 265-286.

[50] Processing parameters needed to control pathogens in cold smoked fish, U. S. Food and Drug Administration, Chapter 4 (2001).

[51] A. Onal, A review: Current analytical methods for the determination of biogenic amines in foods, Food Chem., 103 (2007) 1475-1486.

[52] [P. Lehtonen, Determination of amines and amino acids in wine-A review, Am. J. Enol. Vitic., 47 (1996) 127-133.

[53] A. Bouchereau, P. Guenot, F. Lather, Analysis of amines in plant materials, J. Chromatogr. B Anal. Tecnol. Biomed. Life Sci., 747 (2000) 49-67.

[54] A. Kovacs, L. Simon-Sarkadi, K. Ganzler, Determination of biogenic amines by capillary electrophoresis, J. Chromatogr. A, 836 (1999) 305-313.

[55] L. Hlabangana, S. Hernandez-Cassou, J. Saurina, Multicomponent determination of drugs using flow-injection analysis, Curr. Pharm. Anal., 2 (1997) 127-140.

[56] L. Simon-Sarkadi, E. Gelencser, A. Vida, Immunoassay method for detection of histamine in foods, Acta Alimentaria, 32 (2003) 89-93.

[57] J. Kirschbaum, I. Busch, H. Brückner, Determination of biogenic amines in food by automated pre-column derivatization with 2-naphthyloxycarbonyl chloride (NOC-Cl), Chromatographia, 45 (1997) 263-268.

[58] S. Moret, L.S. Conte, High-performance liquid chromatographic evaluation of biogenic amines in foods. An analysis of different methods of sample preparation in relation to food characteristics, J. Chromatogr. A, 729 (1996) 363-369.

[59] O. Busto, M. Mestres, J. Guasch, F. Borrull, Determination of biogenic amines in wine after cleanup by solid-phase extraction, Chromatographia, 40 (1995) 404-410.

[60] Z. Loukou, A. Zotou, A comparative survey of the simultaneous ultraviolet and fluorescence detection in the RP-HPLC determination of dansylated biogenic amines in alcoholic beverages, Chromatographia, 58 (2003) 579-585.

[61] S. Oguri, M. Enami, N. Soga, Selective analysis of histamine in food by means of solid-phase extraction cleanup and chromatographic separation, J. Chromatogr. A, 1139 (2007) 70-74.

[62] P. Herbert, L. Santos, A. Alves, Simultaneous quantification of primary, secondary amino acids, and biogenic amines in musts and wines using OPA/3-MPA/FMOC-Cl fluorescent derivatives, J. Food Sci., 66 (2001) 1319-1325.

[63] M.R. Alberto, M.E. Arena, M.C.M. de Nadra, A comparative survey of two analytical methods for identification and quantification of biogenic amines, Food Control, 13 (2002) 125-129.

[64] R. Romero, J.A. Jonsson, D. Gázquez, M.G. Bagur, M. Sánchez-Viñas, Multivariate optimization of supported liquid membrane extraction of biogenic amines from wine samples prior to liquid chromatography determination as dabsyl derivatives, J. Sep. Sci., 25 (2002) 584-592.

[65] P.R. Beljaars, R. Van Dijk, K.M. Jonker, L.J. Schout, Liquid chromatographic determination of histamine in fish, sauerkraut, and wine: Interlaboratory study, J. AOAC Int., 81 (1998) 991-998.

[66] G. mo Dugo, F. Vilasi, G.L. la Torre, T.M. Pellicanò, Reverse phase HPLC/DAD determination of biogenic amines as dansyl derivatives in experimental red wines, Food Chem., 95 (2006) 672-676.

[67] D. Kutlan, I. Molnar-Perl, New aspects of the simultaneous analysis of amino acids and amines as their o-phthaldialdehyde derivatives by high-performance liquid chromatography. Analysis of wine, bear and vinegar, J. Chromatogr. A, 987 (2003) 311-322.

[68] N. García-Villar, J. Saurina, S. Hernández-Cassou, Determination of histamine in wines with an on-line pre-column flow derivatization system coupled to high performance liquid chromatography, Analyst, 130 (2005) 1286-1290.

[69] L. Hlabangana, S. Hernández-Cassou, J. Saurina, Determination of biogenic amines in wines by ion-pair liquid chromatography and post-column derivatization with 1,2-naphthoquinone-4-sulphonate, J. Chromatogr. A, 1130 (2006) 130-136.

[70] M.C. Vidal-Carou, F. Lahoz-Portolés, S. Bover-Cid, A. Mariné-Font, Ion-pair high-performance liquid chromatographic determination of biogenic amines and polyamines in wine and other alcoholic beverages, J. Chromatogr. A, 998 (2003) 235-241.

[71] O. Busto, M. Miracle, J. Guasch, F. Borrull, Determination of biogenic amines in wines by high-performance liquid chromatography with on-column fluorescence derivatization, J. Chromatogr. A, 757 (1997) 311-318.

[72] Y. Song, Z. Quan, J.L. Evans, E.A. Byrd, Y.M. Liu, Enhancing capillary LC MS/MS of biogenic amines by pre-column derivatization with 7-fluoro-nitrobenzoxadiazole, Rapid Commun. Mass Spectrom., 18 (2004) 989-994.

[73] Z. Loukou, A. Zotou, Determination of biogenic amines as dansyl derivatives in alcoholic beverages by high-performance liquid chromatography with fluorimetric detection and characterization of the dansylated amines by liquid chromatography-atmospheric pressure chemical ionization mass spectrometry, J. Chromatogr. A, 996 (2003) 103-113.

[74] T.C. Chiu, Y.W. Lin, Y.F. Huang, H.T. Chang, Analysis of biologically active amines by CE, Electrophoresis, 27 (2006) 4792-4807.

[75] A. Cifuentes, Recent advances in the application of capillary electromigration methods for food analysis, Electrophoresis, 27 (2006) 283-303.
[76] W.J.M. Underberg, J.C.M Waterval, Derivatization trends in capillary electrophoresis. An update, Electrophoresis, 23 (2002) 3922-3933.
[77] C.H. Lin, T. Kaneta, On-line sample concentration techniques in capillary electrophoresis: Velocity gradient techniques and sample concentration techniques for biomolecules, Electrophoresis, 25 (2004) 4058-4073.
[78] L. Arce, A. Ríos, M. Valcárcel, Direct determination of biogenic amines in wine by integrating continuous flow clean-up and capillary electrophoresis with indirect UV detection, J. Chromatogr. A, 803 (1998) 249-260.
[79] C.N. Jayarajah, A.M. Skelley, A.D. Fortner, R.A, Mathies, Analysis of neuroactive amines in fermented beverages using a portable microchip capillary electrophoresis system, Anal. Chem., 79 (2007) 8162-8169.
[80] G. del Campo, B. Gallego, I. Berregi, Fluorimetric determination of histamine in wine and cider by using an anion-exchange column-FIA system and factorial design study, Talanta, 68 (2006) 1126-1134.
[81] A. Marcobal, M.C. Polo, P.J. Martin-Alvarez, M.V. Moreno-Arribas, Biogenic amine content of red Spanish wines: Comparison of a direct ELISA and an HPLC method for the determination of histamine in wines, Food Res. Int. 38 (2005) 387-394.
[82] J.M. Landete, S. Ferrer, I. Pardo, Improved enzymatic method for the rapid determination of histamine in wine, Food Add. Cont., 21 (2004) 1149-1154.
[83] J. Lange, C. Wittmann, Enzyme sensor array for the determination of biogenic amines in food samples, Anal. Bioanal. Chem., 372 (2002) 276-283.
[84] M. Suhaj, M. Korenovska, Application of elemental analysis for identification of wine origin - A review, Acta Alimentaria, 34 (2005) 393-401.
[85] J.S. Camara, M.A. Alves, J.C. Marques, Classification of Boal, Malvazia, Sercial and Verdelho wines based on terpenoid patterns, Food Chem., 101 (2007) 475-484.
[86] S. Kallithraka, E. Tsoutsouras, E. Tzourou, P. Lanaridis, Principal phenolic compounds in Greek red wines, Food Chem., 99 (2006) 784-793.
[87] M.S.P. Nikfardjam, L. Mark, P. Avar, M. Figler, R. Ohmacht, Polyphenols, anthocyanins, and trans-resveratrol in red wines from the Hungarian Villany region, Food Chem., 98 (2006) 453-462.
[88] S.M. Rocha, P. Coutinho, A. Barros, I. Delgadillo, M.A. Coimbra, Rapid tool for distinction of wines based on the global volatile signature. J. Chromatogr. A, 1114 (2006) 188-197.
[89] M. Urbano, M.D. Luque de Castro, P.M. Pérez, J. García-Olmo, M.A. Gómez-Nieto, Ultraviolet-visible spectroscopy and pattern recognition methods for differentiation and classification of wines, Food Chem., 97 (2006) 166-175.
[90] L. Liu, D. Cozzolino, W.U. Cynkar, M. Gishen, C.B. Colby, Geographic classification of Spanish and Australian tempranillo red wines by visible and near-infrared spectroscopy combined with multivariate analysis, J. Agric. Food Chem., 54 (2006) 6754-6759.
[91] E. Dufour, A. Letort, A. Laguet, A. Lebecque, J.N. Serra, Investigation of variety, typicality and vintage of French and German wines using front-face fluorescence spectroscopy, Anal. Chim. Acta, 563 (2006) 292-299.

[92] E. Boscaini, T. Mikoviny, A. Wisthaler, E. von Hartungen, T.D. Mark, Characterization of wine with PTR-MS, Int. J. Mass Spectrom., 239 (2004) 215-219.

[93] M.P. Martí, O. Busto, J. Guasch, Application of a headspace mass spectrometry system to the differentiation and classification of wines according to their origin, variety and ageing, J. Chromatogr. A, 1057 (2004) 211-217.

[94] V.Parra, A.A. Arrieta, J.A. Fernández-Escudero, M. Iñiguez, J.A. de Saja, M.L. Rodríguez-Méndez, Monitoring of the ageing of red wines in oak barrels by means of an hybrid electronic tongue, Anal. Chim. Acta, 563 (2006) 229-237.

[95] M. P. Martí, J. Pino, R. Boqué, O. Busto, J. Guasch, Determination of ageing time of spirits in oak barrels using a headspace-mass spectrometry (HS-MS) electronic nose system and multivariate calibration, Anal. Bioanal. Chem., 382 (2005) 440-443.

[96] M. Penza, G. Cassano, Chemometric characterization of Italian wines by thin-film multisensors array and artificial neural networks, Food Chem., 86 (2004) 283-296.

[97] D.L. Massart, B.G.M. Vandeginste, L.M.C. Buydens, S. de Jong, P.J. Lewi, J. Smeyers-Verbeke, Handbook of Chemometrics and Qualimetrics; Elsevier, Amsterdam, 1997.

[98] R. Romero, M. Sánchez-Viñas, D. Gázquez, M.G. Bagur, Characterization of selected Spanish table wine samples according to their biogenic amine content from liquid chromatographic determination, J. Agric. Food Chem., 50 (2002) 4713-4717.

[99] E. Csomos, K. Heberger, L. Simon-Sarkadi, Principal component analysis of biogenic amines and polyphenols in Hungarian wines, J. Agric. Food Chem., 50 (2002) 3768-3774.

[100] K. Heberger, E. Csomos, L. Simon-Sarkadi, Principal component and linear discriminant analyses of free amino acids and biogenic amines in Hungarian wines, J. Agric. Food Chem., 51 (2003) 8055-8060.

[101] J. Kiss, A. Sass-Kiss, Protection of originality of Tokaji Aszú: Amines and organic acid in botrytized wines by high-performance liquid chromatography, J. Agric. Food Chem., 53 (2005) 10042-10050.

[102] A. Sass-Kiss, J. Kiss, B. Havadi, N. Adányi, Multivariate statistical analysis of botrytised wines of different origin, Food Chem., 110 (2008) 742-750

Chapter 2

DIELECTRIC PROPERTIES AND WINES

A. García Gorostiaga[*], J.L. Torres Escribano and M. De Blas Corral
Department of Projects and Rural Engineering,
Universidad Pública de Navarra, Pamplona, Spain

ABSTRACT

The wine has been extensively described on the basis of chemical composition and sensory considerations. We aim to characterize the red wine through dielectric parameters. These studies are carried out on samples of red grape juice and red wine made from red varieties of grapes.

This chapter covers 3 aspects of the study of dielectric properties of wines:

Firstly, an overview is presented of the basics of the dielectric properties of materials, specifically in foods: related concepts of microwaves and radiowaves, parameters used, the measurement systems and factors of influence. Secondly, a review is carried out including comprehensive bibliographies on this subject and its more directly related topics along with, where feasible, quantitative data extracted from the literature. Thirdly, we focus on the specific characteristics of the employed materials, both the wines (and, in some cases, the original grape juices they come from) and the measurement system. We used the open-ended coaxial probe technique. In certain cases, we also measured other parameters such as electric conductivity.

Some of the conclusions we reached after carrying out this study are: both must and wine behave as diluted aqueous solutions, highly influencing in the ionic conductivity within the 200 MHz zone. This means that the loss factor is increased by the ionic loss. However, in the study range of high frequencies the relaxation phenomena of free water are dominant. Regarding the temperature, the variation of the dielectric properties showed completely different behavior at 200 MHz and at higher frequencies.

Specific tests carried out were:

- Dielectric properties of grape juice and wine after alcoholic fermentation from 200 MHz to 3 GHz. Comparison between water, must and wine. The dielectric properties

---

[*] Universidad Pública de Navarra, 31006 Pamplona, Spain, e-mail of corresponding author: almudena@unavarra.es, Tel.: +34-948-16-91-58; fax: +34-948-16-91-48

of wine from 200 MHz to 20 GHz after cold stabilization and filtration are also presented.
- Variation of dielectric properties with temperature from 200 MHz to 6 GHz

1. INTRODUCTION

Many authors during several decades have emphasized the importance of knowing the complex permittivity of materials subjected to an electromagnetic field in the range of the radiofrequencies with the goal of applying that energy in fields such as chemistry, engineering, industry, or medicine, given its nature of non-ionizing radiation, besides its use in quality control of semisolid products including foods (Grant *et al*, 1989). In the realm of fruits and vegetables specifically, Tran *et al* (1984) considered important to know these properties when trying to determine the absorption of electromagnetic energy during dielectric heating as well as when interpreting some important biophysical properties such as the nature of water binding forces and the amount of bound water in a product.

In the area of agrarian and food products we can find applications of nearly each region of the electromagnetic spectrum in the text by Mohsenin (1984). Specifically, in the radiofrequency and microwave ranges, some potential or real applications are reviewed by Nelson (1987) and include the drying of products (Williams, 1966; Galeano, 1971; Jones *et al*, 1974; Tulasidas *et al*, 1995), the treatment of seeds (Stone *et al*, 1973), insect control (Nelson and Stetson, 1974), the measurement of water content (Kraszewski, 1973; Kraszewski and Kulinski, 1976; Nelson, 1984; Tran *et al*, 1984), the processing of products (Handat & Hayashi, 1978), or quality assessment (Fritsch *et al*, 1979; El-Shami *et al*, 1992; Harker & Dunlop, 1994).

This chapter has focused on the lower portion of the microwave range, the so called radiofrequencies. The use of this electromagnetic radiation would have some advantages such as being an easy, clean and fast operation, in addition to the non-destructive character. It also offers the possibility of monitoring the process by using continuous variable measurements

The quality and quantity of wines have improved significantly during the last decades as well as the percentage of grapes destined to aging wines. This trend is due partly to the existence of wide analytical capabilities to measure the various major and minor components of the wine. Quality of must (grape juice) and wine analyses is increasing, and these analyses are being accomplished using more and more advanced analytical techniques.

2. BASICS OF DIELECTRIC PROPERTIES

Electromagnetic radiation plays an important role in many human activities as it is one of the basic physical processes by which transfer of energy takes place. Applications for food and products of agricultural origin have been discovered in several regions of the electromagnetic spectrum. Fig. 1 shows a representation of the electromagnetic spectrum, although the limits are not clear and there is some confusion in the designation of its different intervals. The *Institute of Electrical and Electronics Engineers* states in its Standard Dictionary of Electric and Electronic Terms (IEEE, 1997) that "microwaves" is used in a rather loose way to refer to the range of frequencies above 1 GHz. On the other hand, it defines radiofrequency as «the frequency in the portion of the electromagnetic spectrum that is between the audio-frequency portion and the infrared portion», while it notes that it is roughly considered the interval between 10 kHz and 100 GHz.

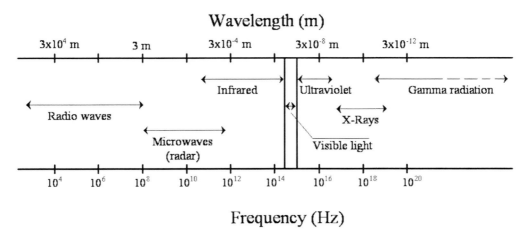

Figure 1.- Electromagnetic spectrum

The electrical properties of materials cover the range from direct current to an unclear limit area of optical properties, at the end of the radiofrequency spectrum. They can be classified as (Nelson, 1973):

> Active: they include the properties characterized by the existence of some energy source in the material that can cause a voltage, as for example bioelectric potential in biological systems.
> Passive: properties that influence the distribution of electromagnetic fields. These are intrinsic properties of the material, determined by its chemical composition and its molecular structure.

Next we will do a brief theoretical review of dielectrics and their passive properties, as these are the ones that have the most interest for us. Out of these passive properties we will focus on the relative complex permittivity. We chose the range of frequencies from few hundreds MHz to few GHz because we can observe between these ranges the presence of different mechanisms affecting the dielectric properties such as ionic conductivity in both bound water and free water.

A time-varying electric field induces a time-varying magnetic field. Maxwell field equations describe the relationship between time-varying electric and magnetic fields. As both fields may involve storage or dissipation of energy in the material, two pairs of parameters are required to characterize a dielectric property of a material. In the frequency range of interest, reference is made to the complex permittivity ε^* and permeability μ^* as the fundamental parameters for the macroscopic description of the dielectric property exposed to sinusoidal fields.

In practice, except for ferromagnetic materials, magnetic polarization is generally very weak, such that the complex permeability μ^* can be replaced by the magnetic permeability of free space μ_0. For the case of interest, most biological and agricultural products are diamagnetic materials with a very low response to magnetic fields (Nelson, 1973).

Energy can be stored or dissipated by the matter within the field. A group of interrelated parameters describe these effects (von Hippel, 1995). The complex permittivity is one of these parameters.

We have studied the relative complex permittivity ε_r^* of musts and wines, which is a function of the relative dielectric constant ε_r' (the real part) and the relative loss factor ε_r'' (the imaginary part).

$$\varepsilon_r^* = \varepsilon_r' - j\,\varepsilon_r''$$

For a given dielectric material, the relative complex permittivity ε_r^* is defined as

$$\varepsilon_r^* \equiv \frac{\varepsilon^*}{\varepsilon_0}$$

These terms refer to the permittivity of free space and, consequently, are dimensionless. The real part is a measure of the material property to store energy whereas the imaginary part refers to the dissipation of energy in the form of losses; i.e. a material property to absorb energy from a electromagnetic field and to convert it in the form of heat (von Hippel, 1995; Engelder & Buffler, 1991; Nelson, 1989; Tinga & Nelson, 1973). At microwave frequencies, the relative dielectric constant ε_r' is large when the dipole moment can orientate itself with an alternating electric field (Roebuck & Goldblith, 1972).

The loss factor ε_r'' actually refers to an effective factor as it is the one that measuring systems provide, and besides the losses associated to the orientation with the applied field of the dipoles it also includes the effect associated to conductivity in direct current. Total measured energy dissipation $\varepsilon_r''(total)$ consists of a dipolar component ($\varepsilon_r''(dipolar)$) and the ionic losses ($\varepsilon_r''(ionic)$) due to the conductivity of component salts (de Loor & Meijboom, 1966; Engelder & Buffler, 1991; Fernández-Martín & Sanz, 1980; Fernández-Martín & Sanz, 1985; Henry & Berteaud, 1980; Hewlett-Packard Co., 1992; Mosig, Besson, Gex-Fabry & Gardiol, 1981; Mudgett, 1974; Mudgett, Smith, Wang & Goldblith 1974; Stuchly & Stuchly, 1980a; To, Mudgett, Wang, Goldblith & Decareau, 1974; Tulasidas et al., 1995).

$$\varepsilon_r''(total) = \varepsilon_r''(dipolar) + \varepsilon_r''(ionic)$$

Ionic losses are given by (de Loor & Meijboom, 1966; de Loor, 1968; Hasted et al., 1948; Haggis et al., 1952; To et al., 1974; Böttcher, 1980):

$$\varepsilon_{ion}'' = \frac{\sigma}{\omega\,\varepsilon_0} \simeq 60\,\lambda\,\sigma$$

where σ is the ionic, d.c. electric or ohmic conductivity of dissolved salts, ω the angular frequency ($\omega=2\pi f$) the dielectric constant of the free space ($\varepsilon_0 \approx 8.854.10^{-12}$ F/m), and λ the wavelength at frequency f ($\lambda=c/f$ being c the velocity of light in vacuum, $c = 2.9979\times10^8$ m/s).

De Loor (1968) points out how it is in the frequency range between 10^7 and 10^9 Hz where the conductivity phenomena play the most important role. This conductivity only contributes losses to the material, which are inversely proportional to the frequency.

The measurement of this ionic conductivity σ, as pointed out by Montoya *et al* (1994) among others, turned out to be highly unstable and cause an increased scattering of the data at frequencies close to zero, i.e. in direct current, what according to these authors was evidence of the existence of a polarization impedance. Therefore, they suggested the measurement of σ in biological media, when $f > 1$ kHz. McPhillips and Snow (1958) studied the evolution of conductivity in milk and water-lactic acid solutions. For that purpose, they measured the conductivity at a frequency of approximately 7 kHz. Mudgett *et al* (1974a) used the conductivity measured at 1 kHz for the calculation of the losses in skimmed milk. Fernández Martín and Sanz (1985) corroborated with their studies that the electric conductivity of milk is independent of the frequency, at least in the 50 Hz to 10 KHz range. Hasted *et al* (1948) established that, with the purpose of making corrections due to electric conductivity, it can be assumed that conductivity does not change with frequency (for low enough frequencies).

The dielectric constant is an interesting parameter only if the material is exposed to an electrical field of an electromagnetic wave. The effect of the electrical field can be twofold:

1. It induces electrical dipoles in the material and tries to align them in the field direction.
2. It tries to align dipoles that are already present in the material if the material contains electric dipoles even without a field.

We also may have a combination of both effects: The electrical field may change the distribution of existing dipoles while trying to align them, and it may generate new dipoles in addition. The total effect of an electrical field on a dielectric material is called the polarization of the material.

3. MEASUREMENT SYSTEM

There are many possible methods and sets of experiments, being one of the most popular for materials with losses in the radiofrequency and microwave range that of open-ended coaxial probe (Grant *et al*, 1989).

The bases in which systems for dielectric measurement in the frequency domain operate (Engelder & Buffler, 1991; Yun *et al*, 1995) are:

1. Generate a signal at the frequencies of interest
2. Direct the signal through the material being probed by means of a measuring mechanism that allows the connection with the source of the signal. This mechanism will depend on the measuring technique and the physical properties of the material.
3. Detect and measure the changes in magnitude and phase for that frequency (S_{11} parameter or reflection coefficient) in the signal reflected by the surface of the sample.

4. The associated software will process these changes in magnitude and phase and convert them to permittivity.

The first three points constitute the essence of a network analyzer together with a set of testing samples of dielectric properties that allows the connection to the measuring instrument and so that it applies the electromagnetic fields in a predictable way, while the fourth point is provided by software that is specific for the analyzer. After this sequence, the source generates the next frequency step and again it provides the reflection parameter for the new frequency.

The functional set used in this chapter for measuring dielectric properties ranging from 200 MHz to 3, 6 or 20 GHz is a dielectric probe measurement system (Fig. 2). It is based on an open-ended coaxial probe and consists of

- Vectorial network analyzers
- Dielectric probe kit
- Others: personal computer, conductivity meter and immersion thermostat units.

The measurement bases are well documented in the literature and some of the references can be found in the bibliography (Engelder & Buffler, 1991; Grant, Clarke, Symm & Spyrou, 1989; Jenkins, Hodgetts, Clarke & Preece, 1990b; Kraszewski, Stuchly & Stuchly, 1983; Marsland & Evans, 1987; Nelson, Forbus & Lawrence, 1994a; Nelson, Forbus & Lawrence, 1994b; Nelson, Forbus & Lawrence, 1995a; Nurul, Birch & Clarke, 1986; Stuchly & Stuchly, 1980b; Tran, Stuchly & Kraszewski, 1984; Tulasidas et al., 1995).

Authors such as Marsland & Evans (1987), Mosig *et al* (1981), Stuchly & Stuchly (1980b), mention some of its advantages:

- It covers a rather broad range of frequencies
- Easy control of the temperature
- It covers a broad range of $\varepsilon_r''/\varepsilon_r'$
- The sample size needed is relatively small
- Very little or no sample preparation is required
- Non-destructive measuring procedure
- It can be applied to measurements *in vivo*

It has also been confirmed that this technique offers high reliability and efficiency in a broad range of frequencies (Nelson *et al*, 1986; Nelson *et al*, 1995b).

Calibrations were made to eliminate the measurement errors caused by the inaccuracy of the system. These calibrations were performed at the beginning of the daily work hours and also when any parameter of the samples changed, mainly with regard to the temperature of the samples. The system was calibrated by using 3 different types of loads: open circuit, short-circuit and deionized water. In order to ensure high accuracy in the measurements, the reference liquid for calibration should be electrically similar to the test material (Misra, Chabbra, Epstein, Mirotznik, & Foster, 1990), and that happens between deionized water and grape juice (high water content). Once the calibration was made, a test was performed using a standard liquid of known permittivity: the deionized water used in the calibration.

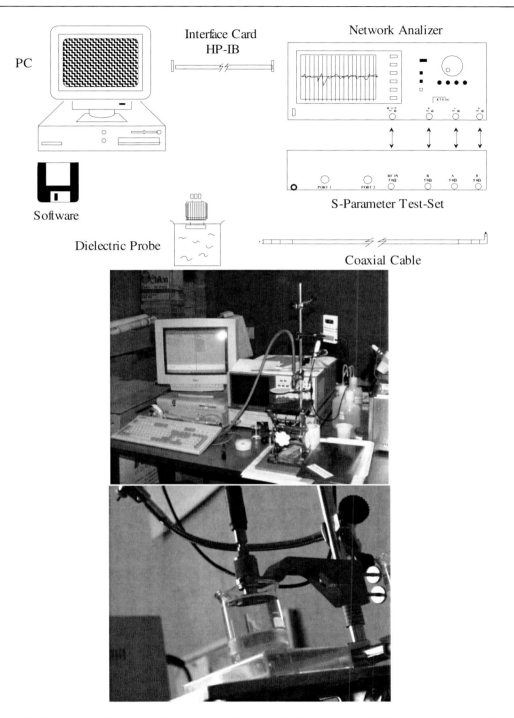

Figure 2. Dielectric probe system for measuring the permittivity complex with the open-ended coaxial probe technique

As recommended by the manufacturer, random errors due to the surrounding environment (variations in temperature, humidity, pressure) or displacements were minimized, and proper working practice was used, such as visual checking of the connectors and eliminating any movement of the cables of the test port after the calibration.

4. NATURE OF DIELECTRIC PROPERTIES VARIATION

Generally, the dielectric characteristics of food products are influenced by the inherent characteristics of the substance, including water content, composition and temperature. On the other hand, Tinga and Nelson (1973) considered frequency of the applied field to be the most dominant. Torres *et al.* (1998) briefly reviewed the dielectric properties of fruits. Their studies related the density, water content, dielectric properties of the products and variations with frequency of the applied field to a quality index of the product and, in addition, these studies suggested equations for predicting dielectric properties.

4.1. Frequency Dependence

Dielectric properties of materials are dependent on the permanent dipole moment associated with any molecules in the materials. With the exception of some materials that essentially absorb no energy from RF and microwave fields, the dielectric properties vary considerably with the frequency of the applied electric fields.
An important phenomenon contributing to the frequency dependence of dielectric properties is the polarization arising from the orientation with the imposed electric field of molecules which have permanent dipole moments.
The mathematical formulation developed by Debye (1929) to describe this process for pure polar materials (e.g. water) can be expressed as

$$\varepsilon^* = \varepsilon_\infty + \frac{\varepsilon_s - \varepsilon_\infty}{1 + i\omega\tau}$$

where ε_∞, represents the dielectric constant at frequencies so high that molecular orientation does not have time to contribute to the polarization; ε_s represents the static dielectric constant, i.e., the value at zero frequency (dc value); and τ is the relaxation time, the period associated with the time the dipoles take to revert to random orientation when the electric field is removed.
The relationships defined by these equations are illustrated in Fig. 3, called simple relaxation spectrum.
In mixtures of materials, or in complicated materials with several different dipoles and several different relaxation times, things get more complicated. The smooth curves shown above may be no longer smooth, because they now result from a superposition of several smooth curves.

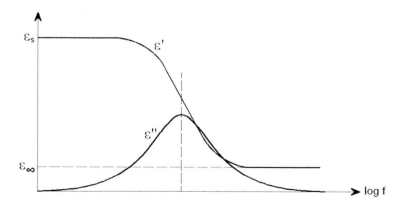

Figure 3. Dispersion and absorption curves representing the Debye model for a polar substance with a single relaxation time

Jordan et al (1978) studied ε'_r and ε''_r as a function of the frequency of formamide, ethanediol, and methanol. They considered the static permittivity that measured at 10 MHz.

Roebuck y Goldblith (1972), studying a 0.5 N sodium chloride aqueous solution observed that ionic losses were predominant under 1 GHz, but over that value dipolar losses dominated.

Ohlsson *et al* (1974) studied the variation of ε'_r and ε''_r at 450, 900, and 2800 MHz frequencies in water, sauce, potatoes and other foodstuffs, noticing that ε'_r decreased slightly as frequency increased, although this decrease was more noticeable in meats and seafood. On the other hand, while the water ε''_r increased at higher frequencies, the opposite trend was observed for foods with high water content, decreasing at higher frequencies as losses due to conductivity increase at lower frequencies. This fact is particularly pronounced in foods with a certain content of salts, such as sauces.

According to Tinga and Nelson (1973), when in a food mixture one of the media is a polar substance such as water, the dielectric behavior of the mixture is considerably different from that of its components. Dipolar relaxation phenomenon in the mixture will not take place at one single frequency, but at a wider range. This broadening of the relaxation curve is due to the interactions between the medium and the materials included.

Seaman and Seals (1991) measured dielectric properties of various fruits at frequencies between 150 MHz and 6 GHz, and observed that when the loss factor of the pulp of those fruits was plotted against the logarithm of the frequency used, the resulting curves were U-shaped, reaching minimum values within the frequency range studied. From approximately 2 GHz on, the ε'_r of the water started decreasing while the ε''_r increased substantially, a behavior of simple dispersion that they also found in the fruits measured using frequencies higher than 1 GHz.

There is a large amount of data available on dielectric properties of agrifoods or products that are directly related with musts and wines, such as saline solutions, alcohols… (Table 1). Our goal here is to offer a brief review of some of the materials that have been published.

More comprehensive reviews can be found in Kent (1987), Nelson (1973) or Datta *et al* (1995). They all cover a wide range of products of plant origin, animal origin, foods, grains, seeds, wood, textiles, and others. Stuchly and Stuchly (1980a) collect data from several authors of biological materials such as albumin, bacteria, blood, bone, brain, eye, muscle, skin, yeasts and others at frequencies between 10 kHz and 10 GHz. Tinga and Nelson (1973) provide also a large amount of tabulated dielectric data of substances classified as agricultural (grains, seeds, beans, corn, cotton, rice ...), biological (albumin, bacteria, blood, bone, fat...), foods (beef stew, raw beef, frozen beef, bacon, eggs, butter, olive oil, fish, milk, potatoes, pears ...), forest products, rubbers, and soils and minerals (clay, sand...).

Nelson et al (1994a, 1994b) provide data obtained from Vitis amurensis grapes, Chilean 'Thompson Seedless' cultivar, that at 23 °C are the following (Table 2):

Table 2. Dielectric constant and loss factor values in grapes at frequencies between 200 MHz and 20 GHz according to Nelson et al (1994a, 1994b

Frequency	200 MHz	500 MHz	1.3 GHz	3.2 GHz	8 GHz	20 GHz
Relative dielectric constant	72	70.8	68.4	63.5	49.6	26.1
Relative Loss Factor	36.4	19.1	13.7	18	28.3	28.6

Dielectric Properties Variation of Grape Juice and Wine at Frequencies from 200 Mhz to 3, 6 and 20 Ghz

All the grape juice analyzed is from the species *Vitis vinifera*, particularly red wine grapes. The most common red wine grapes for aging are from the varieties *cabernet sauvignon*, *tempranillo*, and *merlot*. Besides these, a few samples of *garnacha* (grenache), *mazuelo*, and *pinot noir* were taken.

The variation of the dielectric constant and the loss factor are shown in *Fig. 4* on a logarithmic scale of frequency. The vertical axis represents the dielectric constant or the total loss. These presentations were for water, one sample of grape juice and one sample of red wine, but the same tendencies were observed also for other samples of both grape juice and wine.

The following analysis pertains to both juices and wine. In most cases, for each juice sample there is a must-obtained wine resulting from the alcoholic fermentation. All are analyzed at 200 MHz and 3 GHz frequencies. They belong to different varieties but our goal is to differentiate between must and wine, not between varieties.

The results of the analysis are summarized in Table 3. The mean of the dielectric constant at 200 MHz is greater in grape juices than in wines, whereas the opposite is true at 3 GHz. As for the loss factor at 200 MHz, the mean value of the grape juice is greater than the mean value of the wine. The mean values are practically the same at the higher frequency of 3 GHz.

Table 1.- Values of dielectric properties of food products, alcohols and aqueous solutions at different frequencies and temperatures according to different authors

AUTHORS	YEAR	PRODUCT	FREQUENCY	TEMPERATURE
Roberts and von Hippel	1946	Glycerin and others	5 GHz	28 °C
Haggis et al	1952	Solutions at different concentrations of several alcohols, proteins and salts	3, 9 and 24 GHz	
Lane and Saxton	1952	Water and ethanol	9.35, 24.19 and 48.4 GHz	20 °C
Hasted and Roderick	1958	Aqueous solutions of NaCl and other ionic compounds	582 MHz to 24 GHz	Various
		Solutions of salts in methanol and ethanol	9.375 GHz	20 °C
Garg and Smyth	1965	Some pure primary alcohols	1 to 136.4 GHz	
Buck	1965	Mixtures of water and ethanol at different concentrations	0.3, 1, 3 and 8.5 GHz	5, 15, 25, 35, 50 °C
Risman and Bengtsson	1971	Methanol, ethanol, glycerol, ethanediol, NaCl solutions…	2.8 GHz	20 °C
Roebuck and Goldblith	1972	Potato starch (powdered and gelatinized), aqueous mixtures of potato starch, glucose, sucrose, and glycerol	1 and 3 GHz	25 °C
Ohlsson et al	1974	Beef, fish, potato, sauces, water and aqueous solutions of NaCl	450 and 900 MHz	-20 °C to 60 °C
Ohlsson et al	1975	Beef, fish, potato, sauces, water and aqueous solutions of NaCl	450, 900 and 2800 MHz	+40 °C to 140 °C
Ohlsson et al	1975	Beef, fish, sauces, water, mashed potatoes, boiled peas, and boiled carrots	450, 900 and 2800 MHz	
		Peanut butter, orange juice concentrate, macaroni, chicken, shellfish, pizza, pineapple…	2800 MHz	
Bengtsson	1976	Water, mashed potatoes, boiled carrots, corn oil, and strawberry juice concentrate	2.450 MHz	20 °C
		Grape juice and apple juice at different concentrations	27 MHz	
Jordan et al	1978	Formamide, ethanediol and methanol	10 MHz to 70 GHz	
Grant et al	1989	Ethanol	$\varepsilon_s, \varepsilon_\infty$ and f_R	25 °C
Jenkins et al	1990b	Ethanol	$\varepsilon_s, \varepsilon_\infty$ and f_R	25 °C
Puranik et al	1991	Honey and water solutions in concentrations 0 to 100%	10, 100, 500 and 1000 MHz	
Tulasidas et al	1995	Grapes and sugar solutions at different concentrations	2450 MHz	25-80 °C

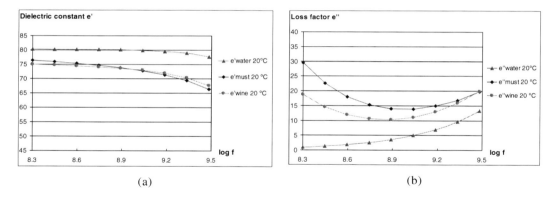

Figure 4. Frequency dependence of the dielectric constant e' (a) and loss factor (b) for typical measurements on water, grape juice and wine samples at 20 °C from 200 MHz to 3 GHz

Table 3. Statistics of dispersion of the dielectric constant ε'_r and loss factor ε''_r at 200 MHz (subscript, 02), at 3 GHz (subscript, 3G), at 6 GHz (subscript, 6G) and at 20 GHz (subscript, 20G) of juices and wines at 20 °C

Variable	Mean	Standard deviation	Range	Minimum	Maximum
Grape juice					
$\varepsilon'_{r,02}$	76.015	0.674	2.532	74.448	76.98
$\varepsilon'_{r,3G}$	65.358	0.722	2.571	64.134	66.705
$\varepsilon''_{r,02}$	28.337	5.892	17.154	20.56	37.714
$\varepsilon''_{r,3G}$	19.976	0.483	1.529	19.402	20.931
Wine*					
$\varepsilon'_{r,02}$	74.587	0.748	2.458	73.279	75.737
$\varepsilon'_{r,3G}$	66.631	0.593	1.835	65.487	67.322
$\varepsilon'_{r,6G}$	55.244	0.497	0.990	54.725	55.715
$\varepsilon'_{r,20G}$	19.520	0.102	0.201	19.408	19.609
$\varepsilon''_{r,02}$	26.598	5.278	17.133	19.927	37.06
$\varepsilon''_{r,3G}$	19.867	0.48	1.328	19.28	20.608
$\varepsilon''_{r,6G}$	30.900	0.505	0.903	30.318	31.221
$\varepsilon''_{r,20G}$	37.876	1.199	2.098	36.492	38.590

* Dielectric parameters at 6 and 20 GHZ were measured on different wine samples from those used at 3 GHz, specifically cold-stabilized and filtered wines.

4.2. Water Content Dependence

Roebuck & Goldblith (1972) defined foodstuffs as complex biological systems in which the major component is generally water. Most studies in dielectric properties of foods have also studied the properties relative to water (Grant, Buchanan, & Cook, 1957; Hasted, 1961; Schwan, 1965; Kaatze & Uhlendorf, 1981; Kaatze, 1989).

Kaatze and Uhlendorf (1981) mention in their work that the first measurements of complex permittivity of water in the microwave range date from 1937 and it was Esau and Bäz as well as Knen who provided these data.

Water has been the object of study with regards to its dielectric behavior for many and varied reasons. The two basic reasons are firstly that it is the main constituent of agrifood products in general, and of musts and wines in particular. Secondly, it is the most active component dielectrically, given that it has a permanent dipole moment, besides its polarizability induced by an electric field. As Nelson (1994a) points out, both the loss factor and the dielectric constant are highly correlated with water content, as water's permittivity largely exceeds that of the dry materials that constitute most agricultural products.

De Loor (1964) pointed out that relaxation frequencies in very complex mixtures such as foodstuffs can be due to different reasons depending on the different ways in which water appears: as a crystal, bound water, free water, etc. De Loor and Meijboom (1966) cite how in materials with high water content, such as blood, skin, milk, and potato, at high frequencies (in the order of GHz) losses are basically determined by the dipolar losses of the free water but at lower frequencies the conductivity in direct current also plays a role. According to these authors, foods with high water content are essentially linear dielectrics with simple relaxation at microwave frequencies, and the relaxation of bound water and other dipolar components at sub-microwave frequencies can be neglected in predictive models of dielectric behavior.

Comparing the values in Table 3 with those obtained for deionised water at 200 MHz (Table 4), we can observe that the mean value of the dielectric constant of wine is lower than that of grape juice and the dielectric constant of grape juice is lower than that of water. At 3 GHz, the loss factors of grape juice and wine are still higher than that of water, but the difference is not large when compared to that of the loss factor at 200 MHz.

Table 4. Relative dielectric constant ε'_r and loss factor ε''_r of deionised water at 20°C, at 200 MHz and 3 GHz

Frequency	ε'_r	ε''_r
200 MHz	80.361	0.718
3 GHz	78.186	13.341

4.3. Chemical Composition Dependence

In chemical terms, foodstuffs consist of water, ash, lipids, proteins and carbohydrates (Mudgett, Goldblith, Wang, & Westphal, 1977). Although water is the major component in foods, its dielectric behavior is modified by the other components in their different saturation and suspension states (Mudgett *et al*, 1974). Dielectric activity of those constituents is given by:

- Salts, represented by ashes, are dielectrically active at high frequencies. They have an effect on dielectric properties due to the relaxation of free water at frequencies in the order of GHz and the ionic conductivity at lower frequencies (in the order of MHz).
- Lipids are generally inert except phospholipids, so it can be expected that their presence lowers dielectric activity.
- Proteins seem to show two levels of activity:

    - High dielectric activity as a result of charging effects at the surface, due to binding effects of water through hydrogen bonds and binding interactions with salts.
    - Dielectrically inert state.

- Carbohydrates can also be present in dielectrically active or inert states:

    - Dielectrically active: dissolved sugars.
    - Inert: starch or cellulose.

Table 5. Must composition from various sources

	MUSTS (g/100 mL)				
	(I)	(II)	(III)	(IV)	(V)
Water	70-85				70-80
Carbohydrates					
Glucose	8-13			Σ=15-25	5-15
Fructose	7-12				5-15
Pectin			0.05-0.2		
Gums	0.07-0.43		0.03-0.4		
Organic Acids					
Tartaric	0.2-1		0.2-0.8	0.7-0.8	0.2-0.5
Malic	0.1-0.8	0.1-0.8		0.2-0.4	0-0.5
Pigments					
Anthocyanins	0.05				
Nitrogenated comp.					
Total Nitrogen	0.03-0.17	0.039			
Mineral Comp.					
Potassium	0.15-0.25		0.04-0.2		
Magnesium	0.01-0.025		0.003-0.015		
Phosphate	0.02-0.05		0.03		

(I) Amerine, 1982; (II) Peynaud, 1996; (III) Ough, 1992; (IV) Lafuente, 1979; (V) Noguera Pujol, 1973.

Kent & Jason (1975) considered that dielectric properties of foods of animal or plant origin are similar in nature at frequencies higher than audio, which IEEE (1997) defines as the band approximately between 15 Hz and 20 kHz, and depend primarily on their water content and the ionic conductivity of the solutions found in their cellular structure. Ohlsson *et al* (1974) stated that dielectric properties would depend not only on the influence of the water and salts or the ash content, but on the way in which the movement of each of its constituents is bound or restricted by the others, making it difficult to predict said properties of mixtures from their individual components. Roebuck & Goldblith (1972) proved that in diluted solutions of ions and organic solutes the dispersion curve moved toward lower frequencies.

Must, obtained mechanically by pressing the grapes, is cloudy because it contains particles in suspension.

In must, the major components are water, sugars, organic acids and mineral salts (Table 5). All are dielectrically active at high frequencies. Minor components are pectic materials, vitamins, enzymes, pigments, nitrogen compounds and others (Ough, 1996; Peynaud, 1996). Besides water, the main components of must are sugars, and within these the most abundant are glucose and fructose, that are present in similar proportion in ripe grapes. The total amount of reducing sugars in grapes is generally no higher than 250 g/l (Ough, 1992).

In wine, the major components are water, ethanol, organic acids, glycerine and mineral salts (Table 6).

Table 6. Wine composition from various sources

	WINES (g/100 mL)					
	(I)	(II)	(III)	(IV)	(V)	(VI)
Water	80-90	85-90%		86-90	75-90	
Carbohydrates						
Glucose	0.5-0.1			} Σ=0.12-0.28		
Fructose	0.05-0.1					
Alcohols						
Ethanol*	8-15	7.2-12	10-14		9-14	10-15
Glycerin	0.3-1.4	0.5-1	0.11-2.3		0.2-2	0.5-1.5
Organic Acids						
Tartaric	0.1-0.6		0.2-0.8	0.2-0.4	0.1-0.2	0.15-0.4
Malic	0-0.6		0-0.5		0.005-0.5	0-0.3
Pigments						
Anthocyanins	0.05	0.02-0.05	0.02-0.05			
Nitrogenated comp.						
Total Nitrogen	0.01-0.09	0.035	0.007-0.098			
Mineral comp.						
Potassium	0.045-0.175	0.1	0.009-0.204			0.1
Magnesium	0.01-0.02	0.01	0.0021-0.0245			0.015
Phosphate	0.003-0.09		0.0025-0.085			0.01-0.1
Sulfate	0.003-0.035		0.007-0.3			0.05-0.1

* Percentage in volume
(I) Amerine, 1982; (II) Peynaud, 1996; (III) Ough, 1992; (IV) Lafuente, 1979; (V) Amerine and Roessler, 1983; (VI) Mareca Cortés, 1983.

Many authors have studied the dielectric properties of aqueous solutions and carbohydrates (Hasted et al, 1948; Malmberg & Maryott, 1950; Haggis et al, 1952; de Loor, 1964; de Loor & Meijboom, 1966; de Loor, 1968; Stogryn, 1971; Roebuck & Goldblith, 1972; Suggett & Clark, 1976; Puranik et al, 1991; Tsoubeli et al, 1995; Tulasidas et al, 1995).

Malmberg & Maryott (1950) studied the dielectric constant of aqueous solutions of glucose and sucrose at 20, 25 and 30 °C for different concentrations and observed that as the percentage of glucose and sucrose increased ε'_r decreased. Hasted (1961) cited the water-sucrose system as the typical example of a system in which interactions between molecules are such that a simple relaxation time replaces both relaxations, that is, the one due to the water and the one due to the sucrose, which happen in very different regions. This author, in the same study, cites Higasi and Nukasawa to indicate that they reached the conclusion that the average relaxation time increased as concentration increased. In those circumstances the concept of bound water with no possibility of rotation no longer makes sense, as water and sucrose affect each other. Later, Suggett and Clark (1976) concluded in their studies on aqueous solutions of sugars that in these, a certain amount of water has its rotation mobility impaired by its interaction with the sugar. Besides, this amount of water with reduced mobility varies from one type of sugar to another, in monosaccharide as well as in disaccharide. According to Rajnish *et al* (1995), given that sugar molecules are relatively large and do not dissociate when dissolved, they inhibit orientational polarization. Therefore, an increase in the content of sugar decreases the dielectric constant.

Nelson (1980) measured the dielectric properties of peaches at different levels of ripeness at 2.45 GHz and 23 °C and did not find useful correlations between these properties and the sugar content, which is generally associated with ripeness in many fruits. Later, the same author took measurements in fresh fruits at 2.45, 11.7 and 22 GHz and did not find correlations either (1983, 1992). In a study of 23 fruits and vegetables, Nelson *et al* (1994a, 1994b) did not find either any evident correlation of the dielectric properties of the materials they measured and the data of soluble solids, which are considered to be made up mostly of sugars.

Mudgett (1987) worked with interactive mixtures, i.e. those in which there are interactions between the different components, and observed that the interesting wavelengths moved to values that were intermediate to those of the pure components. These effects are likely in liquid systems that contain alcohol or high concentrations of dissolved sugars, as is the case in wines and fruit syrups. At the lowest frequencies of the electromagnetic spectrum we can observe the Maxwell-Wagner effect in the case of non-homogeneous materials or heterogeneous materials constituted by two or more phases. It results in the depression of the dielectric constant at those frequencies.

Tulasidas *et al* (1995) worked with aqueous sucrose solutions in distilled water at 2.45 GHz and 25 °C and observed that when the concentration of sugar increased from 15 to 80%, ε'_r dropped considerably. They attributed it to the exclusion of free water by carbohydrates and the stabilization of the hydrogen bonds by the hydroxyl groups. With regard to the loss factor, as water content increased, so did such factor until it reached a maximum around 50%. Past that point, as water content continued to increase, the loss factor started to decrease. Similar observations were made on grapes with water content over 28%. No observations could be made for lower water content samples because the material could not be prepared.

Roebuck & Goldblith (1972) measured the ε'_r and ε''_r of aqueous solutions of glucose, fructose, ethanol, and glycerol at 1 and 3 GHz and 25 °C at various concentrations. In all cases ε'_r decreased as water content decreased, while ε''_r increased with concentration until it reached a maximum that was different for each frequency. At 1 GHz the glucose and sucrose solutions seemed to reach a maximum at a concentration around 70% (no more solutions could be prepared from this point because sugars crystallized). At 3 GHz the maximum was reached at a concentration of approximately 50% and dropped rapidly as the percentage of solids continued to increase. With regard to the glycerol solutions, they showed ε_r'' maxima at each frequency at similar concentrations as the glucose and sucrose solutions, although the maximum ε_r'' for the glycerol solution was much higher than those of the sugar solutions. The ethanol solutions behaved in a similar manner. In aqueous solutions of carbohydrates at microwave frequencies, ε_r'' decreased with lower water content because carbohydrates do not show a considerable dipolar polarization at microwave frequencies and as concentration increases in the solutions, less water is available for dielectric polarization. In carbohydrate solutions, dipolar relaxation takes place at much lower frequencies than in water. As concentration increases, ε_r'' increases also due to the stabilization of hydrogen bonds by the –OH groups of the carbohydrates, which translates in a displacement of the dispersion curve toward lower frequencies than that of water, so ε_r'' at 1 and 3 GHz will be higher in these solutions than in water. Simultaneously, part of the water is bound to the carbohydrates and cannot follow the changes of the applied field, that is, ε_r'' decreases as the content of carbohydrates increases. In short, part of the water is excluded by carbohydrates while part remains bound and cannot follow the field, although this will only happen as long as ionic conductivity is low.

With regard to alcohols, Mudgett *et al* (1974) measured ε_r' and ε_r'' in aqueous mixtures of ethanol at 25 °C and 3 GHz at concentrations varying from 0 to 100%, and observed that as water content increased, ε_r' experienced a rapid increase, while ε_r'' increased to reach a maximum at concentrations of approximately 50%, decreasing from there. Dielectric losses of the mixtures were considerably higher than those of their components in pure form, an effect that was attributed to the interactions between water and the hydroxyl groups that stabilized the structure of the liquid with hydrogen bonds between the hydroxyl groups of the alcohols or carbohydrates and the free water molecules.

The variation of the dielectric constant, ionic loss factor and dipolar loss factor for typical measurements on a stabilized and filteres wine are shown in Fig. 5.

The dielectric constant starts decreasing slowly and then remains almost constant as frequency increases until about 2 GHz. From there, it decreases much faster as we could expect from the results obtained previously.

The ionic loss factor goes from a value close to 20 at 200 MHz to practically cancel itself at a frequency of 5 GHz. These losses due to ionic conductivity have less influence at higher frequencies, from 5 GHz on.

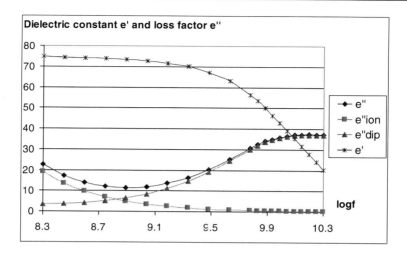

Figure 5. Variation of the relative dielectric constant, total loss factor, ionic loss factor, and dipolar loss factor in stabilized and filtered wines with the logarithm of the frequency in the 200 MHz to 20 GHz range and at 20 °C

The dipolar loss factor is attributable to the molecular friction and collisions produced by the rotation of the dipoles of the polar substances that constitute the wine, particularly the water. This factor, unlike ionic losses, has very low values at low frequencies (approximately 3 at 200 MHz) and as frequencies go up, it suffers a very rapid increase, while the ionic loss factor cancels itself. From frequencies close to 10 GHz the increase of dipolar losses slows down as the frequency increases up to 20 GHz.

With regard to the total dielectric loss factor, from 200 MHz to approximately 1.5 GHz it decreases together with the ionic losses. From that frequency on, it increases together with the dipolar losses, and close to 20 GHz both values are almost equal, as ionic losses are almost nil at that frequency. Given the frequency limitation in the measuring system, we could not find the maximum loss factor nor the frequency at which it happens (relaxation frequency) at 20 °C. But from the shape of the curve, it must be at a frequency slightly higher than 20 GHz.

4.4. Temperature Dependence

Dielectric properties of materials are dependent on temperature (Nelson, 1973). As a general rule, Rajnish *et al* (1995) pointed out that the rate at which ε'_r and ε''_r vary with temperature depends on the frequency, free water and bound water content, and the ionic conductivity of the material.

In polar materials, relaxation time decreases with increasing temperatures, that is, the dipolar loss factor maximum moves toward higher frequencies, as is the case with water (Roebuck y Goldblith, 1972). In the dispersion region or region of dielectric losses, ε'_r increases with temperature, whereas in the absence of dielectric losses, as temperature increases ε'_r decreases. The same author (Nelson, 1989) extended this temperature dependency to materials from agricultural origin, being this dependency a function of dielectric relaxation processes. From his conclusions:

As T increases $\begin{cases} \bullet \text{ Relaxation time decreases} \\ \bullet \text{ Maximum loss factor moves toward higher frequencies} \end{cases}$

As T increases $\begin{cases} f > f_{\text{relax}} \Rightarrow \begin{cases} \bullet \varepsilon'_r \text{ increases} \\ \bullet \varepsilon''_r \text{ increases} \end{cases} \\ f < f_{\text{relax}} \Rightarrow \begin{cases} \bullet \varepsilon'_r \text{ decreases} \\ \bullet \varepsilon''_r \text{ decreases} \end{cases} \end{cases}$

where T is the absolute temperature, f the frequency at which the measurement is being made, f_{relax} the frequency at which the ε''_r maximum was obtained in the area of orientational polarization (relaxation frequency).

When we consider the effects of dissolved salts, it is important not to forget that ionic conductivity has a positive dependency with temperature, that is, it increases as temperature increases, while the water loss factor at frequencies lower than the critical or relaxation frequency has a negative dependency. Therefore, in aqueous ionic solutions the concentration of salts has a very marked effect: on the one hand the dipolar component of ε''_r has a negative dependency with temperature, while for the ionic component this dependency is positive. This means that dielectric losses can decrease initially as temperature increases, to a point in which this tendency reverses, and ε''_r starts increasing as temperature increases. This pivoting point where the trend reverses varies with the concentration of the dissolved salts (Mudgett, 1987).

Furthermore, Hasted (1961) pointed out that for electrolytic solutions, the shifts of the relaxation frequency were larger at the lower temperatures, meaning those a few degrees over 0 °C.

Bengtsson & Risman (1971) found out that in substances with high water content such as peas or meats, at 2.8 GHz, as temperature increased, ε'_r and ε''_r decreased, a behavior similar to that of the water, although the rate at which ε''_r decreased was lower than the water's. These authors agreed with what de Loor described (1968), based on measurements taken on water, potato, and solutions of water and starch in the rate of GHz: when total losses had a dipolar component and another one due to conductivity, the negative temperature coefficient was lower than if those losses due to conductivity did not happen, as conductivity increases with temperature.

Jordan et al (1978) plotted ε'_r and ε''_r as a function of frequency for formamide, ethanediol, and methanol. At 6 GHz they observed that as temperature rose (from 10 to 40 °C) ε'_r increased in all three products.

Henry & Berteaud (1980) studied the effect of temperature in dielectric parameters ε'_r and ε''_r at 5.048 GHz on saline solutions of NaCl, LiCl and KCl at different concentrations, revealing that at low concentrations, as temperature increased ε''_r decreased, that is, the variation $d\varepsilon_r''/dT$ was negative, while at higher concentrations $d\varepsilon_r''/dT$ was positive. The concentration at which this reversal took place varied according to the kind of ionic compound, but at low concentrations ε'_r and ε''_r decreased with temperature the same way the ε'_r and ε''_r of water did. Therefore, (always at 5.048 GHz):

ε'_r (water) > ε'_r (ion)
ε''_r (water) < ε''_r (ion)

Kent & Meyer (1983) measured the dielectric properties of hydrated microcrystalline cellulose. At 2, 6 and 18 GHz, as temperature increased, so did ε'_r and ε''_r.

We will determine the variation with temperature and frequency of the relative dielectric constant and the relative loss factor at frequencies from 200 MHz to 6 GHz of must and wine from black grapes at temperatures ranging from 10 to 30 ºC. We will observe the similarities and differences they present with regards to the variations exhibited by water in the same range of frequencies and temperatures.

The curves that show the variation with frequency between 200 MHz and 6 GHz of deionized water, must and wine at temperatures of 10, 15, 20, 25 and 30 ºC can be observed in Fig. 6.

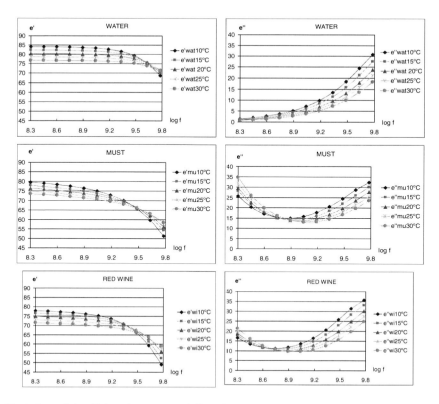

Figure 6. Variation of the dielectric constant (e') and loss factor (e") with frequency at 10, 15, 20, 25 and 30 ºC in deionized water (wat), must (mu) and wine (wi), from 200 MHz to 6 GHz

The variation curves of the dielectric constant with frequency at different temperatures obtained for musts and wines are similar to those obtained for deionized water. Regarding the curves of variation of loss factor, at 6 GHz musts and wines present the same variation with temperature and have values that are comparable to those of water, but at 200 MHz it is noticeable a strong component of electric conductivity due to the components of ionic nature that constitute musts and wines.

5. CONCLUSION

Both in musts and in wines, the variation of the dielectric constant and the total loss factor with frequencies ranging from 0.2 to 20 GHz turned out to be similar to those obtained by other authors for various fruits. While the dielectric constant showed a monotonic and decreasing trend for increasing frequencies, the total loss factor decreased to reach a minimum and then increased. In the area of the lowest frequencies measured, we could observe an important contribution of the ionic conductivity to the value of the total losses.

The dielectric constant ε'_r and the loss factor ε''_r of grape juice at 200 MHz are greater than those for wine. There is a high variability in the loss factor at 200 MHz. At 3 GHz, the dielectric constant ε'_r of grape juice is slightly lower than that of wine, whereas the loss factor ε''_r at 3 GHz is practically the same for grape juice and wine.

The mean values from 200 MHz up to 3 GHz of the dielectric constant of both wine and must are lower than that for water. At 3 GHz, the loss factors of grape juice and wine are still higher than that for water, but the difference is not large as compared to the loss factor at 200 MHz. The bigger difference is due to the ionic conductivity of both grape juices and wines at 200 MHz.

With regard to the variation with temperature, the dielectric constant curves from 200 MHz to 6 GHz for both musts and wines showed the same trends as that of water. The results obtained for the loss factor at 6 GHz showed also the same trend as the water, whereas at 200 MHz, where for water values are very close to zero, in the case of musts and wine the loss factor increased when temperature rose.

ACKNOWLEDGEMENTS

The authors wish to thank the following for permission to reproduce copyright material:

Journal of Food Engineering for pp. 206-209, from García, A., Torres, J.L., Prieto, E. & De Blas, M. (2001). Dielectric properties of grape juice at 0.2 and 3 GHz. *Journal of Food Engineering, 48*, 203-211

Biosystems Engineering for pp. 346-349, from García, A., Torres, J.L., De Blas, M., De Francisco, A. & Illanes, R. (2004). Dielectric characteristics of grape juice and wine. *Biosystems Engineering, 88(3)*, 343-349

Likewise the authors thank Bodegas Nekeas, Bodegas Fernández de Arcaya, Bodegas Irache, Bodegas Castillo de Monjardín and Bodegas Señorío de Sarría (Navarre, Spain) for donating the samples used in the tests.

REFERENCES

Amerine, M. A., Berg, H. W., Kunkee, R. E., Ough, C. S., Singleton, V. L. & Webb, A. D. (1982). *Technology of wine wine making*. 4th edition. Westport, Connecticut: AVI Publishing Company, Inc.

Amerine, M.A. & Roessler, E.B. (1983). *Wines: Their sensory evaluation.* Chapter 4: Composition of wines. New York: Ed. W.H. Freeman.

Bengtsson, N.E. (1976). Dielectric heating as a unit operation in food processing- Heating fundamentals and applications of radio frequency and microwaves. *Confructa, 21(1/2),* 7-23

Bengtsson, N.E. & Risman, P.O. (1971). Dielectric properties of foods at 3 GHz as determined by a cavity perturbation technique, (II) Measurements of food materials. *J. Microwave Power, 6(2),* 107-123

Böttcher, C.J.F. & Bordewijk, P. (1980). *Theory of electric polarization: Dielectrics in time-dependent fields (Volume II).* The Netherlands: Elsevier Scientific Publishing Company.

Buck, D.E. (1965). *The dielectric spectra of ethanol-water mixtures in the microwave region,* Ph.D. thesis, MIT, Cambridge, Mass

Calay, R.K., Newborough, M., Propert, D. & Calay, P.S. (1995) Predictive equations for the dielectric properties of food. International *Journal of Food Science and Technology, 29,* 699-713

Datta, A. K., Sun, E. & Solis, A. (1995). *Engineering properties of foods. Chapter 9: Food dielectric property data and their composition-based prediction.* 2nd edition, rev. and expanded. New York: Edited by Rao, M. A. and Rizvi, S.S.H. Marcel Dekker, Inc.,

De Loor, G.P. (1964). Dielectric properties of heterogeneous mixtures with a polar constituent. *Applied Scientific Research, section B, 11,* 310-320

De Loor, G.P. (1968). Dielectric properties of heterogeneous mixtures containing water. *The Journal of Microwave Power, 3(2),* 67-73

De Loor, G.P. & Meijboom, F.W. (1966). The dielectric constant of foods and other materials with high water contents at microwave frequencies. *J. Fd. Technol, 1,* 313-322

Debye, P. (1929). *Polar molecules.* New York: Chemical Catalog Company

El-Shami, S.M., Zaki Selim, I., El-Anwar, I.M. & Hassan El-Mallah, M. (1992). Dielectric properties for monitoring the quality of heated oils. *JAOCS, 69(9)*

Engelder D. S. & Buffler, C. R. (1991) Measuring dielectric properties of food products at microwave frequencies. *Microwave World, 12(2),* 6-15

Fernández-Martín F. & Sanz P.D. (1980). Electrical conductivity of skim concentrates. Proc. *2nd Intern. Conference Physical Properties Agricultural Materials,* 3/97/1-6

Fernández-Martín F. & Sanz P.D. (1985) Influence of temperature and composition on some physical properties of milk concentrates: V. electrical conductivity. *International Agrophysics, 1(1),* 41-53

Fritsch, C.W., Egberg, D.C. & Magnuson, J.S. (1979). Changes in dielectric constant as a measure of frying oil deterioration. *Journal of the American Oil Chemists' Society, 56,* 746-750

Galeano S. F. (1971). The application of electromagnetic radiation in the drying of paper. *Journal of Microwave Power, 6(2),* 131-140

García Gorostiaga, A. (2001). *Permitividad compleja de mostos y vinos tintos de Navarra medida mediante la técnica de sonda coaxial: caracterización e influencia de componentes mayoritarios.* Ph. D. Thesis. Universidad Pública de Navarra, Spain.

García, A., Torres, J.L., Prieto, E. & De Blas, M. (2001). Dielectric properties of grape juice at 0.2 and 3 GHz. *Journal of Food Engineering, 48*, 203-211

García, A., Torres, J.L., De Blas, M., De Francisco, A. & Illanes, R. (2004). Dielectric characteristics of grape juice and wine. *Biosystems Engineering, 88(3)*, 343-349

Garg, S. K. & Smyth, C. P. (1965). Microwave absorption and molecular structure in liquids. LXII. The three dielectric dispersion regions of the normal primary alcohols. *The Journal of Physical Chemistry, 69(4)*, 1294-1301

Grant, E. H., Buchanan, T. J. & Cook, H. F. (1957). Dielectric behavior of water at microwave frequencies. *Jnl. Of Chemical Physics, 26*, 156-161

Grant, J. P., Clarke, R. N., Symm, G. T. & Spyrou, N. M. (1989). A critical study of the open-ended coaxial line sensor technique for RF and microwave complex permittivity measurements. *Jnl. of Phys. E: Scientific Instruments. 22(9)*, 757-770

Haggis, G. H., Hasted, J. B. & Buchanan, T.J. (1952). The dielectric properties of water in solutions. *Journal of Chemical Physics. 20(9)*, 1452-1465

Handat, M., Sato, I. & Hayashi, H. (1978). Salt content of butter detected by electrical conductivity. *XX International Dairy Congress*, E:411-412

Harker, F. R. & Dunlop, J. H. (1994). Electrical impedance estudies of nectarines during coolstorage and fruit ripening. *Postharvest Biology and Technology, 4*, 125-134

Harker, F. R. & Maindonald, J. H. (1994). Ripening of nectarine fruit (Changes in the cell wall, vacuole, and membranes detected using electrical impedance measurements), *Plant Physiol, 106*, 165-171

Hasted, J. B. (1961). The dielectric properties of water. *Progress in dielectric, 3*, 101-149

Hasted, J. B. & Roderick, G. W. (1958). Dielectric properties of aqueous and alcoholic electrolytic solutions. *The Journal of Chemical Physics, 29(1)*, 17-26

Hasted, J. B., Ritson, D.M. & Collie, C.H. (1948). Dielectric properties of aqueous ionic solutions. Parts I and II. *The Journal of Chemical Physics, 16*, 1-11

Henry, F. & Berteaud, A.J. (1980). New measurement technique for the dielectric study of solutions and suspensions. *J. Microwave Power, 15*, 235-42

Hewlett-Packard Co. (February 1992). Basics of measuring the dielectric properties of materials. HP Application Note 1217-1, HP Literature Number 5091-3300E.

IEEE (Institute of Electrical and Electronics Engineers) (1997). *New IEEE Standard Dictionary of Electrical and Electronics Terms*. Standards Coordinating Committee 10, Terms and Definitions; Jane Radatz, chair. New York, 6th ed.

Jenkins S., Hodgetts T.E., Clarke R.N. & Preece A.W. (1990b). Dielectric measurements on reference liquids using automatic network analysers and calculable geometries. *Meas. Sci. Technol., 1*, 691-702

Jones P.L., Lawton J. & Parker I.M. (1974). High frequency paper drying. Part I- Paper dryind in radio and microwave frequency fields *Trans. Instn. Chem. Engrs., 52*, 121-131

Jordan, B.P., Sheppard, R.J. & Szwarnowski, S. (1978). The dielectric properties of formamide, ethanediol and methanol. *J. Phys. D: Appl. Phys., 11*, 695-701

Kaatze, U. (1989). Complex permittivity of water as a function of frequency and temperature. *J. Chem. Eng. Data, 34(4)*, 371-374

Kaatze, U. & Uhlendorf, V. (1981). The dielectric properties of water at microwave frequencies. *Zeitschrift für Physikalische Chemie Neue Folge, Bd. 126*, S. 151-165

Kent, M. (1987). *Electrical and dielectric properties of food materials*. London: Science and Technology Publishers Ltd

Kent, M. & Jason, A.C. (1975). Dielectric properties of foods in relation to interactions between water and the substrate. *Water relations in foo*. London: R.B. Duckworth (D.E.), Academic Press

Kent, M. & Meyer, W. (1983). Dielectric relaxation of absorbed water in microcrystalline cellulose, *J. Phys. D: Appl. Phys.,16*, 915-25

Kraszewski, A. (1973). Microwave instrumentation for moisture content measurement. *J. Microwave Power, 8*, 323-35

Kraszewski, A., Stuchly M. A. & Stuchly S. S. (1983). ANA calibration method for measurement of dielectric properties. *IEEE Transactions on Instrumentation and Measurement. Vol. IM-32, No. 2*, 385-387

Kraszewski, A.& Kulinski, S. (1976). An improved microwave method on moisture content measurement and control. *IEEE Transactions of Industrial Electronics and Control Instrumentation, Vol. IECI-23, No. 4, November*, 364-370

Lafuente, B. (1979). *Química agrícola III: Alimentos*. Cap. 5: La uva y sus derivados. Reimpresión 1987. Madrid: Ed. Alhambra

Lane, J. & Saxton, J. (1952). Dielectric dispersion in pure polar liquids at very high radio-frequencies. I. Measurements on water, methyl and ethyl alcohols. *Proceedings of the Royal Soc. of London, Vol. A 213*, 531-545

Malmberg, Cyrus, G. & Maryott, Arthur A. (1950). Dielectric constants of aqueous solutions of dextrose and sucrose. *Journal of Research of the National Bureau of Standards, 45(4)*, 299-303

Mareca Cortés, I. (1983). *Origen, composición y evolución del vino*, 1ª ed. Madrid: Ed. Alhambra

Marsland, T. P. & Evans, S. (1987). Dielectric measurements with an open-ended coaxial probe. *IEEE Proceedings, 134, Pt. H(4)*, 341-349

McPhillips J. & Snow N. (1958). Studies on milk with a new type of conductivity cell. *The Australian Journal of Dairy Technology, October-December 1958*, 192-196

Misra, D., Chabbra, M., Epstein, B.R., Mirotznik, M. & Foster, K.R.(1990). Noninvasive electrical characterization of materials at microwave frequencies using an open-ended coaxial line: test of an improved calibration technique. *IEEE Transactions on Microwave theory and Techniques, 38(1)*, 8-14

Mohsenin, N. N. (1984). *Electromagnetic radiation properties of foods and agricultural products*. New York: Gordon and Breach Science Publishers

Montoya, M. M. & López-Rodríguez, J. (1994). An improved technique for measuring the electrical conductivity of intact fruits. *Lebensmittel-Wissenschaft und-Technologie, 27(1)*, 29-33

Mosig, J. R., Besson, J.E., Gex-Fabry, M. & Gardiol, F.E. (1981). Reflection of an open-ended coaxial line and application to nondestructive measurement of materials. *IEEE Transactions on Instrumentation and Measurement, Vol. IM-30, No. 1*, 46-51

Mudgett, R. E. (1974). *A physical-chemical basis for prediction of dielectric properties in liquid and solid foods at ultrahigh and microwave frequencies*. Ph.D. thesis, MIT, Cambridge, Mass

Mudgett, R. E. (1987). *Electrical properties of foods: A general review. Final Seminar Proceedings: Physical properties of foods-2. COST 90bis.* London: Elsevier Applied Science Publishers Ltd., Essex

Mudgett, R.E, Goldblith, S.A., Wang, D.I.C. & Westphal, W.B. (1977). Prediction of dielectric properties in solid foods of high moisture content at ultrahigh and microwave frequencies. *Journal of Food Processing and Preservation, 1,* 119-151

Mudgett, R.E. (1982). Electrical properties of foods in microwave processing. *Food Technol., 36,* 109-115

Mudgett, R.E., Smith, A.C., Wang, D.I.C., & Goldblith S.A. (1974a). Prediction of dielectric properties in nonfat milk at frequencies and temperatures of interest in microwave processing. *Journal of Food Science, 39,* 52-54

Mudgett, R.E., Wang, D.I.C. & Goldblith, S.A. (1974b). Prediction of dielectric properties in oil-water and alcohol-water mixtures at 3,000 Mhz, 25°C based on pure component properties. *Journal of Food Science, 39,* 632-635

Nelson S. O. & Stetson L.E. (1974) Possibilities for controlling insects with microwaves and lower frequency RF energy. *IEEE Transactions On Microwave Theory And Techniques. Paper 3790, Journal Series, Nebraska Agricultural Experiment Station,* 1303-1305

Nelson, S.O. (1973). Electrical properties of agricultural products. A critical review. *Trans. of the A.S.A.E., 16,* 384-400

Nelson, S.O. (1980). Microwave dielectric properties of fresh fruits and vegetables. *Transactions of the ASAE, 23(5),* 1314-1317

Nelson, S.O. (1983). Dielectric properties of some fresh fruits and vegetables at frecuencies of 2.45 to 22 GHz. *Transactions of the ASAE, 26 (2),* 613-616

Nelson, S.O. (1984). Moisture, frequency and density dependence of the dielectric constant of shelled, yellow-dent field corn. *Trans. of the A.S.A.E, 27,* 1573-1578

Nelson, S.O. (1987). Potential agricultural applications for RF and microwave energy. *Trans. of the ASAE, 30,* 818-822

Nelson, S.O. (1989). Dielectric properties of agricultural materials and their use in agricultural engineering and technology. *4th International Conference Physical Properties of Agricultural Materials and their influence on Technological Processes,* 560-565

Nelson, S.O. (1992). Microwave dielectric properties of fresh onions. *Transactions of the ASAE, 35(3),* 963-966

Nelson, S.O., Forbus W.R. & Lawrence, K.C. (1994a). Microwave permittivities of fresh fruits and vegetables from 0.2 to 20 GHz. *Transactions of the ASAE, 37(1),* 183-189

Nelson, S.O., Forbus W.R. & Lawrence, K.C. (1994b). Permittivities of fresh fruits and vegetables at 0.2 to 20 GHz. *Journal of Microwave Power and Electromagnetic Energy, 29(2),* 81-93

Nelson, S.O., Forbus W.R. & Lawrence, K.C. (1995a). Assessment of microwave permittivity for sensing peach maturity. *Transactions of the ASAE, 38 (2),* 579-585

Nelson, S.O., Forbus W.R. & Lawrence, K.C. (1995b). Microwave dielectric properties of fruits and vegetables and possible use for maturity sensing. *ASAE Publication 1-95,* 497-504

Noguera Pujol, J. (1973). *Enotecnia industrial.* Lérida, Spain: Dilagro

Nurul Afsar M., R. Birch J. & Clarke R.N. (1986). The measurement of the properties of materials. *Proceedings of the IEEE, 74(1),* 183-199

Ohlsson, T. & Bengtsson, N.E. (1975). Dielectric food data for microwave sterilization processing. *Journal of Microwave Power, 10(1),* 93-108

Ohlsson, T., Bengtsson, N.E. & Risman, P.O. (1974). The frequency and temperature dependence of dielectric food data as determined by a cavity perturbation technique. *J. Microwave Power, 9(2),* 129-45

Ough, C.S. (1992). *Tratado Básico de Enología.* (Original: Winemaking Basics, Food Products Press, 1992). Zaragoza: Editorial Acribia

Peynaud, E. (1996). *Enología Práctica, Conocimiento y Elaboración del Vino.* (Original: Connaissance et Travail du Vin, 1981). Madrid : Mundi-Prensa

Puranik, S., Kumbharkhane, A. & Mehrotra, S. (1991). Dielectric properties of honey-water mixtures between 10 MHz to 10 GHz using time domain technique. *Journal of Microwave Power and Electromagnetic Energy, 26(4),* 196-201

Risman, P.O. & Bengtsson, N.E., (1971). Dielectric properties of food at 3 GHz as determined by a cavity perturbation technique, (I) Measuring technique. *J. Microwave Power, 6(2),* 101-106

Roberts, S. & Von Hippel, A. (1946). A new method for measuring dielectric constant and loss in the range of centimeter waves. *Journal of Applied Physics, 17(july),* 610-617

Roebuck, B.D., & Goldblith, S.A. (1972). Dielectric properties of carbohydrate-water mixtures at microwave frequencies, *J. Food Sci., 37,* 199-204

Schwan, H. P. (1965). Electrical properties of bound water. *Annals of the New York Academy of Sciences, 125(2),* 344-354

Seaman R. & Seals J. (1991). Fruit pulp and skin dielectric properties for 150 MHz to 6400 MHz. *Journal of Microwave Power and Electromagnetic Energy, 26(2),* 72-81

Stogryn, A. (1971). Equations for calculating the dielectric constant of saline water. *IEEE Transactions On Microwave Theory And Techniques, 19,* 733-736

Stone R. B., Christiansen M. N., Nelson S. O., Webb J. C., Goodenough J. L. and Stetson L E. (1973). Induction of germination of impermeable cottonseed by electrical treatment. *Crop Science,13(2),* 159-161

Stuchly M. A. & Stuchly S. S. (1980a). Dielectric properties of biological substances-Tabulated. *Journal of Microwave Power, 15(1),* 19-26

Stuchly M. A. & Stuchly S. S. (1980b). Coaxial line reflection methods for measuring dielectric properties of biological substances at radio microwave frequencies- A review. *IEEE Transactions on Instrumentation and Measurement, Vol. IM-29(3),* 176-183

Suggett, A. & Clark, A.H. (1976). Molecular motions and interactions in aqueous carbohydrate solutions. 1: Dielectric relaxation studies. *J. Solution Chem., 5(1),* 1-15

Tinga, W.R. & Nelson, S.O. (1973). Dielectric properties of materials for microwave processing- tabulated. *Journal of Microwave Power, 8 (1),* 23-65

To, E.C., Mudgett, R.E., Wang, D.I.C., Goldblith, S.A. & Decareau, R.V. (1974). Dielectric properties of food materials. *Journal of Microwave Power, 9(4),* 303-315

Torres, J.L., De Blas, M., García, A. & Prieto, E. (1998). Propiedades eléctricas de frutas y verduras: una revisión. *Alimentaria, Revista de Tecnología e Higiene de los Alimentos, 295,* 25-29

Tran, V. N., Stuchly, S. S. & Kraszewski, A. (1984). Dielectric properties of selected vegetables and fruits 0.1-10.0 GHz. *Journal of Microwave Power, 19(4),* 251-258

Tsoubeli, M.N., Davis, E.A. & Gordon, J. (1995). Dielectric properties and water mobility for heated mixtures of starch, milk protein and water. *Cereal Chemistry, 72(1),* 64-69

Tulasidas T.N., Raghavan G.S.V., Van De Voort F. & Girard R. (1995). Dielectric properties of grapes and sugar solutions at 2.45 GHz. *Journal of Microwave Power and Electromagnetic Energy, 30(2),* 117-123

Von Hippel, A.R. (1995). *Dielectrics and waves.* New York: MIT Press, Cambridge, Mass, New York. New ed., originally published:: Wiley, 1954

Williams N. H. (1966). Moisture leveling in paper, wood, textiles and other mixed dielectric sheets. *The Journal of Microwave Power, 1,* 73-80

Yun, J. J., Datta, A. K., Lobo, S. & Sapru, A. (1995). Microstructure and dielectric properties of process cheese with varying fat contents. *Proceedings of Scanning 95.* Scanning Vol. 17, supplement V, V.143-V.144

Chapter 3

RED WINE PHENOLICS: REASONS FOR THEIR VARIATION

Patrícia Valentão, Luís Guerra, David M. Pereira, and Paula B. Andrade[1]

REQUIMTE/Serviço de Farmacognosia, Faculdade de Farmácia,
Universidade do Porto, R. Aníbal Cunha, 164, 4050-047 Porto, Portugal

ABSTRACT

Phenolic compounds are natural constituents of grapes and wines. The determination of polyphenols composition of red wines has long been attracting the attention of scientists, due to its responsibility in the organoleptic characteristics, such as as flavour, colour, bitterness and astringency, which constitute important quality parameters of wine. In addition, beneficial effects on health of this grape product have been described, such as antioxidant, anti-inflammatory, antimicrobial and cardioprotective, for which phenolic compounds exert a determinant role. Wine phenolics belong to several groups: hydroxybenzoic and hydroxycinnamic acids and their derivatives, flavonoids, like anthocyanins, flavan-3-ols and flavonols, stilbens and tannins. The complex phenolics composition of red wine changes until its consumption and is affected by several factors, such as grape variety, environmental conditions, yeasts strains and fermentation, winemaking procedures, oxygenation, aging and storage. In this chapter the agents influencing the phenolic profiles of red wine are overviewed.

1. INTRODUCTION

Vitis vinifera is the most important source of grape berries used for wines' production. The selection of specific varieties and its propagation made possible to obtain both delicate

---

[1] Corresponding author: Paula B. Andrade, Phone: + 351 222078935, Fax: + 351 222003977
E-mail: pandrade@ff.up.pt

white wines and deeply coloured astringent red ones. These features are a result of phenolics content and profile and deeply affect the organoleptic characteristics of this product. Hence, they constitute a valuable tool in winemaking industry, especially for red wines, contributing to a definition of quality and style of a particular wine (Somers & Ziemelis, 1985).

Red wine phenolics (**Table 1**) consist primarily of anthocyanins and flavan-3-ols along with minor compounds, such as pyranoanthocyanins and its *p*-coumaric, acetaldehyde and pyruvic acid adducts, whose identification is recent, due to the use of new analytical methods, such as high pressure liquid chromatography coupled to mass spectrometry (HPLC-MS).

Table 1. Main phenolic compounds found in red wine.

	Compound	Reference
Anthocyanins	pelargonidin	Valentão *et al.*, 2007
	delphinidin	Kallithraka *et al.*, 2006; Valentão *et al.*, 2007
	delphinidin-3-glucoside	Spranger *et al.*, 2004; Lorenzo *et al.*, 2005; Revilla *et al.*, 2001
	delphinidin-3-glucoside-pyruvate	Revilla *et al.*, 1999; Atanasova *et al.*, 2002
	delphinidin-3-glucoside-acetate	Monagas *et al.*, 2007; Kelebeck *et al.*, 2007; Atanasova *et al.*, 2002
	delphinidin-3-(*p*-coumaroyl)glucoside	Revilla *et al.*, 1999; Kelebeck *et al.*, 2007; Atanasova *et al.*, 2002
	petunidin	Kallithraka *et al.*, 2006
	petunidin-3-glucose-pyruvate	Revilla *et al.*, 1999; Atanasova *et al.*, 2002
	petunidin-3-glucoside	Spranger *et al.*, 2004; Lorenzo *et al.*, 2005; Revilla *et al.*, 2001
	petunidin-3-glucoside-acetate	Monagas *et al.*, 2007; Revilla *et al.*, 1999; Kelebeck *et al.*, 2007
	petunidin-3-(*p*-coumarate)glucoside	Spranger *et al.*, 2004; Monagas *et al.*, 2007; Revilla *et al.*, 1999
	malvidin	Kallithraka *et al.*, 2006; Valentão *et al.*, 2007
	malvinidin-3-glucoside	Valentão *et al.*, 2007; Lorenzo *et al.*, 2005; Fischer *et al.*, 2000
	malvinidin-3-glucose-pyruvate	Spranger *et al.*, 2004; Monagas *et al.*, 2007; Atanasova *et al.*, 2002
	malvinidin-3-glucoside-acetate	Kallithraka *et al.*, 2006; Revilla *et al.*, 2001; Makris *et al.*, 2006
	malvinidin-3-(*p*-coumaroyl)glucoside	Kallithraka *et al.*, 2006; Revilla *et al.*, 2001; Makris *et al.*, 2006
	malvidin-3-(*p*-coumaroyl)glucoside-pyruvate	Spranger *et al.*, 2004; Monagas *et al.*, 2007; Revilla *et al.*, 1999
	malvidin-3-(caffoyl)glucoside	Monagas *et al.*, 2007; Revilla *et al.*, 1999
	malvidin-3,5-diglucoside	Valentão *et al.*, 2007
	peonidin	Kallithraka *et al.*, 2006; Lorenzo *et al.*, 2005
	peonidin-3-glucoside	Spranger *et al.*, 2004; Valentão *et al.*, 2007; Revilla *et al.*, 2001
	peonidin-3-glucoside-acetate	Revilla *et al.*, 2001; Revilla *et al.*, 1999; Kelebeck *et al.*, 2007
	peonidin-3-(*p*-coumaroyl)glucoside	Spranger *et al.*, 2004; Revilla *et al.*, 2001; Monagas *et al.*, 2007
	cyanidin	Kallithraka *et al.*, 2006; Valentão *et al.*, 2007
	cyanidin-3-galactoside	Valentão *et al.*, 2007; Makris *et al.*, 2006
	cyanidin-3-glucoside	Spranger *et al.*, 2004; Lorenzo *et al.*, 2005; Valentão *et al.*, 2007
	cyanidin-3-glucoside-acetate	Revilla *et al.*, 1999; Atanasova *et al.*, 2002; Kelebek *et al.*, 2006
	cyanidin-3-(*p*-coumaroyl)glucoside	Revilla *et al.*, 1999; Atanasova *et al.*, 2002

Table 1. Continued

	Compound	Reference
Procyanidins	procyanidin A2	Kallithraka et al., 2006
	procyanidin B1	Spranger et al., 2004; Makris et al., 2006; Monagas et al., 2007
	procyanidin B2	Spranger et al., 2004; Teszlák et al., 2005; Makris et al., 2006
	procyanidin B3	Spranger et al., 2004; Ritchey & Waterhouse. 1999; García-Falcón et al., 2007
	procyanidin B4	Spranger et al., 2004; García-Falcón et al., 2007
Flavan-3-ols	(+)-catechin	Spranger et al., 2004; Ritchey & Waterhouse, 1999; Russo et al., 2008
	(-)-epicatechin	Spranger et al., 2004; Ritchey & Waterhouse, 1999; Russo et al., 2008
	(-)-epicatechin-3-gallate	Teszlák et al., 2005
Flavonols	quercetin	Ritchey & Waterhouse et al., 1999; Kallithraka et al., 2006; Tarola et al., 2007
	quercetin-3-rutinoside	Russo et al., 2008; Kallithraka et al., 2006; Makris et al., 2006
	quercetin-3-glucoside	Fischer et al., 2000; Tao et al., 2007; Zafrilla et al., 2003; Ritchey & Waterhouse, 1999
	quercetin-3-galactoside	Hernández et al., 2006
	quercetin-3-glucoronoside	Hernández et al., 2007b; Hernández et al., 2006; Makris et al., 2006
	myricetin	Kallithraka et al., 2006; Makris et al., 2006; Bautista-Ortín et al., 2007a
	myricetin-3-galactoside	Hernández et al., 2007b; Hernández et al., 2006; Simón et al., 2003
	myricetin-3-rhamnoside	Simón et al., 2003
	myricetin-3-glucoside	Zafrilla et al., 2003; Makris et al., 2006
	kaempferol	Russo et al., 2008; Kallithraka et al., 2006; Makris et al., 2006
	kaempferol-3-glucoside	Zafrilla et al., 2003
	kaempferol-3-rutinoside	Hernández et al., 2006
	isokaempferol	Kallithraka et al., 2006
	isorhamnetin	Makris et al., 2006
	isorhamnetin-3-rutinoside	Hernández et al., 2006
Hydroxybenzoic acids	ellagic	Hernández et al., 2007b; Simón et al., 2003
	gallic	Karagiannis et al., 2000; Russo et al., 2008; Tarola et al., 2007
	protocatechic	Russo et al., 2008; Hernández et al., 2007b; Bautista-Ortín et al., 2007a
	vanillic	Russo et al., 2008; Hernández et al., 2007b; Lorenzo et al., 2005
	syringic	Ritchey & Waterhouse, 1999; Russo et al., 2008; Hernández et al., 2007b
	3,4-dihydroxybenzoic	Andrade et al., 1998; Garcia-Viguera & Bridle, 1995
	p-hydroxybenzoic	Russo et al., 2008; Hernandez et al., 2007a; García-Falcón et al., 2007
Hydroxycinnamic acids	cis-feruloyltartaric	Teszlák et al., 2005
	ferulic	Lorenzo et al., 2005; Bautista-Ortín et al., 2007a; Cabrita et al., 2008
	chlorogenic	Tarola et al., 2007
	p-coumaric	Karagiannis et al., 2000; Quirós et al., 2007, Lorenzo et al., 2005
	caffeic	Karagiannis et al., 2000; Tarola et al., 2007, Quirós et al., 2007
	trans-feruloyltartaric	Waterhouse et al., 2002
	trans-coumaroyltartaric	Waterhouse et al., 2002; Hernández et al., 2007b; Hernandez et al., 2007a
	cis-coumaroyltartaric	Hernández et al., 2007b; Makris et al., 2006; Hernandez et al., 2007a
	2,5-di-S-Glutationil-caffeoyltartaric	Gambelli & Santaroni 2004
	trans-caffeoyltartaric	Waterhouse et al., 2002; Hernández et al., 2007b; Hernandez et al., 2007a
	cis-caffeoyltartaric	Hernández et al., 2007b; Fischer et al., 2000; Makris et al., 2006
Stilbenes	cis-resveratrol	Tarola et al., 2007; Quirós et al., 2007; Hernández et al., 2007b
	cis-piceid	Quirós et al., 2007; Hernández et al., 2007b
	trans-resveratrol	Russo et al., 2008; Tarola et al., 2007, Quirós et al., 2007
	trans-piceid	Quirós et al., 2007, Hernández et al., 2007b

The first studies regarding phenolic compounds in wine were undertaken by Ribéreau-Gayon (1964) and, since then, structural determination of a variety of minor compounds and products arising from reactions involving anthocyanins and procyanidins has been achieved.

The wide consumption of red wine is probably the explanation for the so called French paradox (Renaud & de Lorgeril, 1992), which consists in diminished coronary heart disease mortality despite high intake of saturated fat. Several studies have been conducted on the beneficial effects of wine phenolics in human health. Although all major types of flavonoids present in wine have shown beneficial effects in disease incidence and progression, anthocyanins from red wines appear to be one of the most important groups.

Oxidative stress can account for the development of several diseases, such as atherosclerosis or diabetes. Due to its structural characteristics, phenolic compounds scavenging ability against oxidative species is high. Moreover, non-coloured phenolics have also been shown to inhibit lipooxygenase and to present ion chelating activity (Morel et al., 1994). Wine polyphenols are able to inhibit LDL oxidation and many flavonoids, such as quercetin, epicatechin and catechin, strongly inhibit platelet aggregation (Keli et al., 1994), thus interfering in the pathophysiology of atherosclerosis and other cardiovascular diseases (Cabornneau et al., 1998). Therefore, a moderate consumption of wine, especially red wine, has been associated with lower risk of cardiovascular disease.

Red wine phenolics are also related with cancer preventive actions: quercetin is a potent anticarcinogenic in whole-animal models (Fazal et al., 1990) and resveratrol can inhibit cyclooxygenase-2 and cytochrome P450 1A1 enzymes, thought to be important in carcinogenesis (Subbaramaiah et al., 1998, Kanazawa et al., 1998).

As referred above, research on organoleptic characteristics of wine has concluded that polyphenols play an important role in wine colour and astringency. Moreover, it has been shown that complex, yet minor, compounds, previously regarded as not important, are responsible for much of the organoleptic properties observed.

The changes in phenolic composition can arise from a diverse number of causes, mainly related with grape berry, winemaking procedures and aging technologies. A deeper insight shows how cultivar type, grape ripeness stage, geographical origin of grapes, maceration, yeast and malolactic bacteria strains, fermentation and clarification techniques, aging and storage conditions affect red wine phenolics.

Attending to the numerous studies regarding polyphenols variation in red wines, mainly due to its beneficial effects on human health, in this chapter recent findings on these matters are overviewed. The initial part of this chapter constitutes a chemical approach to red wine's main phenolic constituents, followed by a description of factors influencing their profile.

2. PHENOLIC COMPOUNDS IN RED WINES

The main phenolics classes occurring in grapes and wines are anthocyanins, flavonols, flavan-3-ols and proanthocyanidins. Among non-flavonoids, hydroxycinnamic and hydroxybenzoic acids derivatives and stilbens are also important to red wine chemical characterization (**Figure 1**).

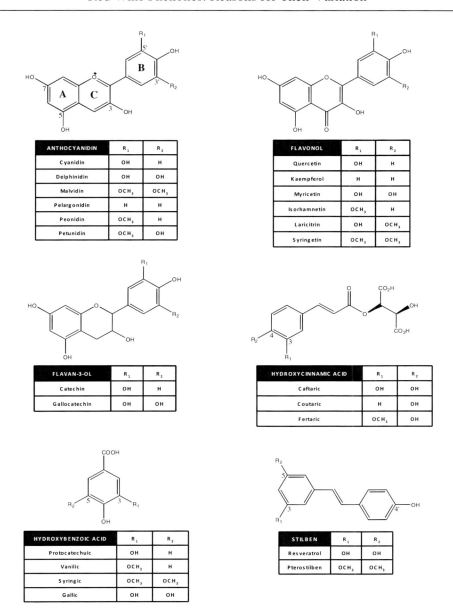

Figure 1. Some of the main phenolics classes in wine.

Anthocyanins

Anthocyanins are water soluble plant pigments responsible for the blue, purple and red color of many plant tissues, usually with molecular weights ranging from 400 to 1200 (Prior & Wu, 2006). These compounds are glycosilated polyhydroxi and polymethoxy derivatives of 2-phenyl-benzopyrylium (flavylium) salts. The most common sugars are glucose, galactose, rhamnose and arabinose. These sugars are usually linked at the 3 position of the C ring or at the 5 and 7 position of the B ring, occurring as mono-, di- or tri-saccharide forms. Although very rare, glycosylation at the 3', 4', or 5' positions of the B ring is also possible (Wu & Prior, 2005). Despite the knowledge of about 17 anthocyanidins (anthocyanins' aglycones), only six of them are ubiquitously distributed in nature: cyanidin, delphinidin, petunidin, peonidin, pelargonidin and malvidin (**Figures 1 and 2**).

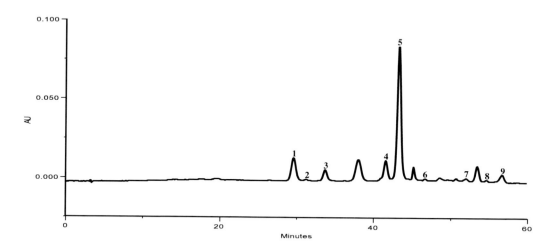

Figure 2. HPLC anthocyanins profile of wine samples inoculated with *Dekkera bruxellensis*. Detection at 500 nm. (1) malvidin-3,5-diglucoside; (2) cyanidin-3-galactoside; (3) cyanidin-3-glucoside; (4) peonidin-3-glucoside; (5) malvidin-3-glucoside; (6) delphinidin; (7) cyanidin; (8) pelargonidin; (9) malvidin (adapted from Valentão *et al.*, 2007).

With the exceptions of 3-deoxyanthocyanidins and their derivatives (Nip *et al.*, 1969; Hipskind *et al.*, 1990; Lo *et al.*, 1996), there is always a glycosyl group in C-3, which means that aglycones are rarely found in nature. The sugar moiety may be acylated by aromatic acids, mostly hydroxycinnamic acids (caffeic, ferulic, *p*-coumaric or sinapic acids) and sometimes by aliphatic acids, namely malonic and acetic acids. These acyl moieties are usually linked to the sugar at C-3 (Harborne, 1964).

The multiple possibilities regarding the identity and position of sugars and acyl moieties, as well as the position and number of hydroxyl and methoxyl groups on the anthocyanidin skeleton, gives rise to a great number of compounds, with over 600 anthocyanins being known today (Andersen, 2002).

In solution, anthocyanins are highly affected by pH, presenting different forms that will be reflected in the compound's color (**Figure 3**). The relative amounts of these four conformations contribute to wine's final color and can be affected by pH, temperature, light, presence of metals and the anthocyanidin itself (Brouillard & Delaporte, 1977; Brouillard, 1982; Strack & Wray, 1993).

Among the several analytical methodologies available for the detection, identification and quantification of these compounds, HPLC is universally applied as a reference technique, mostly using C18 columns. Due to the effect of pH in the structural conformation of anthocyanins, with flavylium cation accounting for about 95% of the equilibrium composition to pH 1.5 (da Costa *et al.*, 2000), highly acidic solvents are required. As so, the use of methanol/water and acetonitrile/water at different proportions and acidified at pH 1.5 with formic, perchloric or phosphoric acid is a common practice.

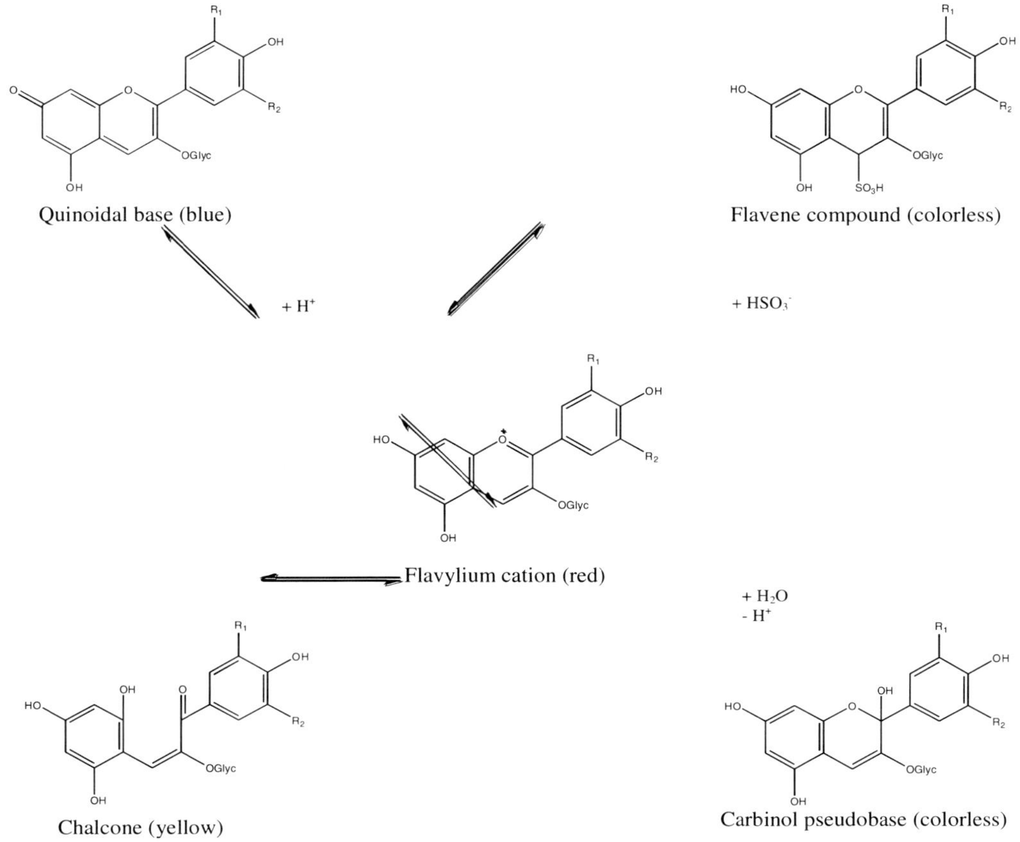

Figure 3. Variations on anthocyanidin structures (adapted from Cooke *et al.*, 2005).

The occurrence of these compounds in wine arises from their presence in grapes. They appear mainly localized in skins, particularly in the first external layers of the hypodermal tissue, exclusively in vacuoles (Ros Barcelo *et al.*, 1994). This is very important, as the type of technique used for wine preparation will strongly affect the final anthocyanins content. As referred, winemaking techniques that involve contact with grape skin yield wines with much higher content in these compounds comparatively with removal of skin in the early stages of the process. Additionally, the time of contact with the skin plays a major role, as there is an optimum time that origins maximum anthocyanins extraction.

Recently, much attention has been given to anthocyanin derivatives, which are, themselves, wine pigments, identified by using more sensible techniques. These derivatives arise from the reaction of anthocyanins with distinct compounds, belonging to different chemical classes (Atanasova *et al.*, 2002) (**Figure 4**).

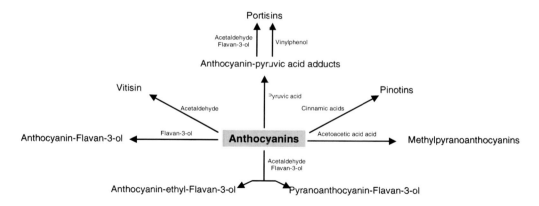

Figure 4. Main anthocyanin-derived pigments found in red wine.

Flavonols

Flavonols (**Figure 1**) can be found in grape skins, although in much smaller quantities than anthocyanins. For this reason, they are only present in wines obtained by techniques that involve contact with grape skin.

During many years these compounds were thought to be found only in the glycosilated form. However, the development of analytical techniques revealed that aglycones could also be present in wine, although in trace amounts. Flavonols in grapes exist only as 3-glycosides, while the corresponding aglycones can be found in wines, together with the glycosilated form, as result of acid hydrolysis that occurs during winemaking and aging. The four aglycones usually present are quercetin, kaempferol, isorhamnetin and myricetin. The most common sugar involved is glucose, although galactose and glucuronic acid can also be found (Castillo-Muñoz et al., 2007). Some of the flavonols described in *Vitis vinifera* include 3-glucosides and 3-glucuronides of kaempferol, quercetin and myricetin, as well as the 3-glucosides of isorhamnetin and 3-galactoside of kaempferol (Castillo-Muñoz et al., 2007).

Recently, syringetin, syringetin-3-glucoside, syringetin-3-glucoside-acetate, laricitrin, and laricitrin-3-glucoside have been reported for the first time (Wang et al., 2003; Amico et al., 2004).

Some studies showed that flavonol content increases as a consequence of solar exposure of the berry skin. This results are in line with the fact that flavonols absorb UV light strongly in UV-A (325-400 nm) and UV-B (280-325 nm) regions, which could mean that the plant produces these compounds to act as a natural sunscreen, protecting from radiation damage (Price et al., 1995; Haselgrove et al., 2000). This is important as wines produced from grapes submitted to greater levels of radiation will present higher flavonol contents.

Flavonols act in wine as copigments, stabilizing the color that result from anthocyanins' presence, by protecting the flavylium ion against water attack that would disrupt the C ring conjugation, resulting in a loss of color (**Figure 3**) (Brouillard, 1982).

Flavan-3-ols

Flavanols are a very abundant class of flavonoids present in grapes (mostly in skins and seeds) and, consequently, in wine (Waterhouse, 2002). These are often called flavan-3-ols to identify the location of alcohol group in C ring.

Flavan-3-ols occur in grapes as monomers, oligomers and polymers, being (+)-cathechin and (-)-epicatechin the major monomers. These two compounds are isomers as result of the saturation in positions 2 and 3 of C ring, with (+)-cathechin corresponding to the *trans* form (2R, 3S) and (-)-epicathechin to the *cis* one (2R, 3R), both with 3', 4' catechol substitution in B ring. Apart from these compounds, another substitution pattern can be found in B ring, which is the result of 3', 4', 5' hydroxylation.

When condensation of flavan-3-ol units takes place, proanthocyanidins (condensed tannins) are formed. Condensation results from covalent bonds established between flavan-3-ol units, being 4→8 and 4→6 the most common linkages (Waterhouse, 2002).

Tannins

Tannins, with molecular weight varying from 1500 to 8000, are responsible for many of the organoleptic properties of red wine, such as body, bitterness and astringency (Noble, 1990; Vidal *et al.*, 2004), and contribute to others, like color, through their interactions with anthocyanins.

The designation of tannin includes compounds of two distinct chemical groups: hydrolyzable tannins (polymers of ellagic acid, or of gallic and ellagic acids, with glucose, Bruneton, 1993) and condensed tannins, which result from the condensation of monomers of flavan-3-ol units (Waterhouse, 2002).

Without a doubt, the most well known property of tannins is their capacity to precipitate proteins. Obviously, this will also affect the enzymatic and apoenzimatic content of wine, which is particularly important when oxidative enzymes are considered (Mira & Chozas, 1993). This is one of the main reasons of red wine's improved resistance against oxidation when compared with white ones.

These polymers tend to grow constantly over aging, reaching a point at which they are no longer soluble, forming precipitates, very common in older wines.

Hydroxycinnamic Acids

Hydroxycinnamic acids are the major non-flavonoids in grapes and wines, being the main class of phenolics in white wine.

Derivatives of *p*-coumaric, caffeic and ferulic acids are the most common compounds. The free acids do not exist in grapes. Instead, they occur as esters of tartaric acid: *p*-coutaric, caftaric and fertaric acids respectively, are found in all grape juices and, consequently, in all wines (**Figure 1**).

Nevertheless, these naturally occurring compounds are extensively hydrolyzed in wine's aqueous acid solution, yielding the free acids, which may further react with ethanol from wine by sterification (Waterhouse, 2002).

Also, these compounds can be decarboxylated by microbial species. The products of these decarboxylations are ethylphenols that give rise to strong smoky and aromatic odours and flavours, like horsy smell (Silva *et al.*, 2005).

Oxidations and complexations are also described. For instance, in the case of hydroxycinnamic derivatives, one-third are found unchanged in wine, one-third are oxidized and linked to sulfhydryl compounds and the rest are found as complexes with nucleic acids (Macheix *et al.*, 1990). Any of these transformations can be caused by enzymes, which may be native to grapes or have their origin in microorganisms (Macheix *et al.*, 1990).

Hydroxybenzoic Acids

Hydroxybenzoic acids have a C6–C1 general structure, deriving directly from benzoic acid and differing in accordance with hydroxylations and methoxylations of the aromatic ring (**Figure 1**). This group represents includes minor compounds in new wines, while matured ones, like those kept in oak barrels, possess elevated levels of hydroxybenzoic acid derivatives, mainly ellagic acid (a dilactone formed by the reaction between two molecules of gallic acid). Ellagic acid arises from the breakdown of hydrolyzable tannins (Budic-Leto & Lovric, 2002).

Some other compounds included in this group are gallic, vanillic, syringic and gentisic acids, which can be involved in white wine browning (Barón *et al.*, 1997).

These compounds have been described as normal components of wine aroma. Depending on their concentration levels and aromatic properties, some of them contribute positively to wine aroma, but others are responsible for wine off-flavours (Martorell *et al.*, 2002).

Stilbenes

Stilbenes constitute a minor class of compounds, with resveratrol (3,5,4'-trihydroxystilbene) (**Figure 1**) being the most representative compound. These compounds can be found in grapes, as they are produced as result of *Botrytis* infection, among other fungal attacks (Langcake & Pryce, 1976; Langcake & Pryce, 1977). For this reason, this kind of compounds is regarded as phytoalexins, being also synthethized as a result of abiotic stresses caused by, for example, UV light (Langcake & Pryce, 1977) or aluminium chloride (Adrian *et al.*, 1996).

Resveratrol can exist both as *cis* or *trans* isomer, as well as the glycosides of each one of them. This compound is the main responsible for the beneficial effects associated with red wine consumption: several epidemiological studies strongly suggest a cardioprotective and anticancer action (Hung *et al.*, 2000; Jang *et al.*, 1997), among many others.

Taking into account that this compound is synthesized by grape skin cells, it has been suggested that resveratrol requires a relatively long maceration time to be extracted and, consequently, to be present in high amounts in wine (Siemann & Creasy, 1992).

In addition to the classes of compounds referred above, there are many others that play a relevant role in wine composition. This is important as these compounds contribute to wine's total phenol levels, which highly influences its organoleptic characteristics as well as antioxidant activity (Tommaso *et al.*, 1998).

For instance, tyrosol is a by-product that arises from shikimic acid pathway that occurs in grapes and leads to eugenol formation (Ough & Amerine, 1998). Apart from grape origin, tyrosol is especially relevant as it can result from yeast metabolism during wine maturation and, in this case, it is derived from acetic acid.

Although HPLC coupled to diode array detection (HPLC-DAD) is, nowadays, the main analytical technique for the analysis of phenolics in wine, other methodologies are very important to wine science.

The development of new analytical methods, in HPLC-MS, has revealed the presence of many minor compounds, both naturally occurring constituents and reaction products. In addition, capillary electrophoresis (CE) has also been successfully used for the analysis of these secondary metabolites in wine: comparisons of CE and HPLC analysis of phenolic compounds in wines, as well as in grape seeds and pulps, have been reported (García-Viguera & Bridle, 1995; Bridle & Gárcia-Viguera, 1996) and CE techniques are today a valuable tool in wine analysis (Andrade *et al.* 1998) (**Figure 5**).

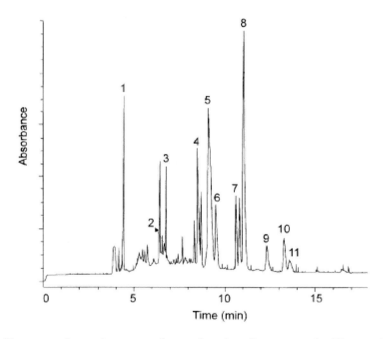

Figure 5. Capillary zone electropherogram of port wine phenolic compounds. (1) tyrosol, (2) (-)-epicatechin, (3) (+)-catechin, (4) syringic acid, (5) unidentified compound, (6) *p*-coumaric acid, (7) caffeic acid, (8) gallic acid, (9) 3,4-dihydroxybenzoic acid, (10) *cis*-coumaroyl tartaric acid, (11) *trans*-coumaroyl tartaric acid (adapted from Andrade *et al.*, 1998).

Wine science is still, nowadays, a very active area. There are some reactions and compounds just described in recent papers, such as direct anthocyanin-flavanol adducts and adducts in which the anthocyanin and flavan-3-ol moieties are linked through a methylmethine bridge, also called ethyl bridge (Remy *et al.*, 2000; Salas *et al.*, 2004) (**Figure 4**).

The development of more sensible techniques has lead to a deeper understanding of the multiple factors that affect wine composition, as today is possible to detect compounds in very low concentration that were, in the past, not instrumentally detectable.

The main reasons for wine's phenolics variation will be referred below.

3. FACTORS AFFECTING PHENOLIC COMPOSITION

3.1. Grape Variety and Geographical Origin

It has long been known that flavonoids production is highly stimulated by sunlight. In fact, Spayd *et al.* (2002) verified this when comparing grape cluster under the sun or in the shade. Therefore, vineyards location must take into account such aspects. In fact, the use of south facing slopes and partial deleafing of vines during grape ripening is a common practice.

Wine composition is a reflection of the grapes used to produce it. Polyphenols production is strictly controlled by the genes of the enzymes involved in their biosynthetic pathways; therefore, the polyphenols profile of a given cultivar is a direct consequence of its genetic potential.

Andrade *et al.* (2001) described that, in what concerns to port wine grapes, no qualitative differences between cultivars were found, but (-)-epicatechin was the major compound in Rufete and Tinta Cão varieties. Additionally, kampferol 3-glucoside and isorhamnetin 3-glucoside were important compounds in all samples, except in Rufete variety.

Dopico-García *et al.* (2008), when comparing *Vinho Verde* grapes cultivars (Azal Tinto, Borraçal, Brancelho, Doçal, Espadeiro, Padeiro de Basto, Pedral, Rabo de Ovelha, Verdelho and Vinhão), found that samples were distinguished by anthocyanin, *p*-coumaroyl derivatives and flavan-3-ols (**Figure 6**).

Makris *et al.* (2006a), studying wines from different prefectures of Greece, described that procyanidin B1 and B2, most anthocyanins and some free hydroxycinnamic acids where highly influenced by cultivar and geographic origin, while flavonols were mainly assigned by geographical origin-based differentiation. Similarly, caftaric acid was significantly affected by both factors, while the remaining hydroxycinnamate derivatives were less influenced.

In the study of Zafrilla *et al.* (2003), anthocyanins determination showed that major compounds, such as malvidin and its acetate derivative, are more important in origin differentiation. The environmental influences were responsible for changes in the principal polyphenolic constituents. Additionally, the effect of the level of ripening of grape berries, along with differences in geographic regions, modulated even more the phenolic profiles or their total content.

Gambelli & Santaroni (2004) studied southern Italian red wines produced in Puglia and Molise regions. These vineyard locations vary on average temperature and rainfall, so that the vintage season is delayed in Molise. Gallic, caffeic and caffeoyltartaric acids were cultivar dependent, while anthocyanins were mainly dependent on the geographical origin of vineyards. In this study, non-coloured phenolics were not affected by those factors.

Andrade *et al.* (1998) showed that port wines produced with several grape varieties from Douro region exhibited different composition (**Figure 7**).

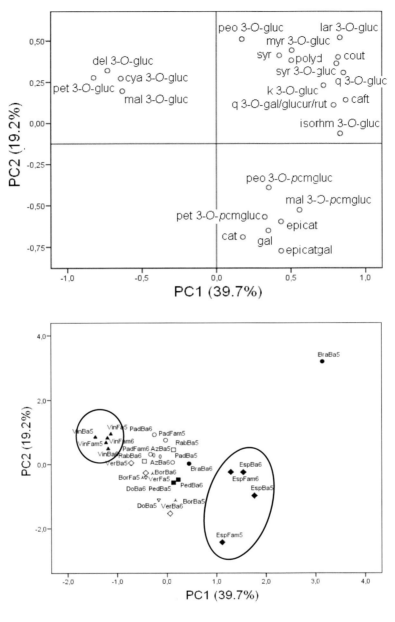

Figure 6. Principal component analysis of all analysed phenolic compounds in red *Vinho Verde* grapes: loadings and scores plots. Sample code is composed of grape variety (Espadeiro [Esp], Padeiro de Basto [Pad], Vinhão [Vin], Azal Tinto [Az], Borraçal [Bor], Brancelho [Bra], Doçar [Do], Pedral [Ped], Rabo de Ovelha [Rab] and Verdelho [Ver]), origin (Famalicão [Fam], Quinta Barreiros [Ba] and Quinta Facha [Fa]) and vintage year (2005 vintage [5] and 2006 vintage [6]); compound abbreviation: delphinidin (del), cyaninidin (cya), petunidin (pet), peonidin (peo), malvidin (mal), glucoside (glc), *p*-coumaroy (pcm), gallic acid (gal), caftaric acid (caft), coutaric acid (cout), catechin (cat), syringic acid (syr), epicatechin (epicat), epicatechin gallate (epigal), myricetin-3-glucoside (myr-glucose), polydatin (polyd), quercetin-3-galactoside/ quercetin-3-glucuronide (q 3-O- gal/glucur/rut), quercetin-3-glucoside (q 3-O-gluc), laricitrin-3-glucoside (lar 3-O-gluc),: kaempferol-3-glucoside (kaemp 3-gluc), isorhamnetin-3-glucoside (isorhm 3-gluc); syringetin-3-O-glucoside (syr 3-O-gluc) (adapted from Dopico-García *et al.*, 2008).

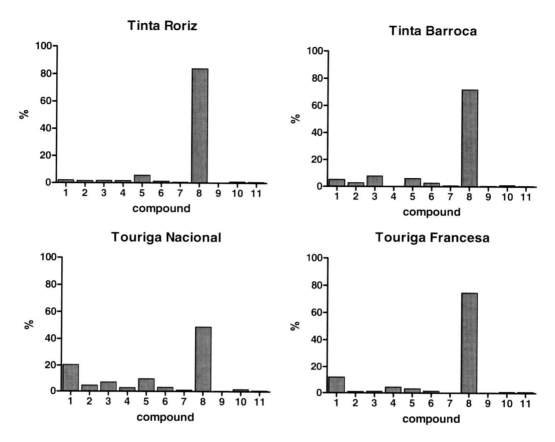

Figure 7. Phenolic compounds profile in experimental wines of four distinct Douro grape varieties. Identity of compounds as in figure 5 (adapted from Andrade *et al.*, 1998).

Touriga (Nacional and Francesa) wines contained more than twice total phenolics than those from Tinta (Barroca and Roriz) ones, being the major differences due to tyrosol. Wine from Touriga Francesa presented higher amounts of gallic acid. In addition, Tinta Roriz wine contained less of all identified compounds, excepting for gallic acid.

Analysis conducted on Greek varietal wines, produced under the same environmental conditions and by the same enological methodology, showed that French cultivars, such as Syrah and Cabernet Sauvignon, exhibited lower amounts of polyphenols than native varieties (Kallithraka *et al.*, 2006). It was also suggested that Vertzami variety, rich in polyphenols, could be combined with poorer grape varieties in co-winemaking procedures, to produce a balanced wine, both in taste and colour.

3.2. Maturity Stage

Changes taking place during the ripening of grape berries do not occur simultaneously, being influenced by genetic, climatic and geographical factors and culture practices. Therefore, the moment of harvest will determine, according to the stage of ripening, the quantitative and qualitative profile of grapes and hence, of wine. Traditional indicators of grape maturity include the physiological, industrial and technological criteria. The industrial criteria, based fundamentally on the increase of must density accompanied by a decrease in total acidity and increase in sugars, is relatively recent, but is now being abandoned in favour of new parameters, such as "phenol maturity". This happens because the increase in polyphenol content of grapes does not follow the increase in sugars, for their peaks do not coincide. In fact, the evolution of phenols in grapes is dependent on the nature of the phenol, family of compounds and other factors, such as climate and soil (Pérez-Magariño et al. 2006). Nevertheless, Bautista-Ortín et al., (2007a) showed that berries with a larger size and less mature (lower sugar content) exhibited low anthocyanin levels.

In the study of de Simón et al. (1992), hydroxycinnamic acid derivatives, especially *p*-coumaric and caffeic acids decreased during berry growth and ripening, although such reduction was less marked near the end of maturation. Variation in the concentration of phenolic compounds was found to be constituted by two phases. The first coincided with the *veraison* (initial phase) and the second one with the full maturity. In the first phase, caffeoyl and *p*-coumaroyl esters of tartaric acid and flavan-3-ols suffer a strong decrease, while benzoic acids show a slight increase. On the second phase, caffeoyl and *p*-coumaroyl esters and flavan-3-ols suffer a slight decrease, while benzoic acids increase noticeably (de Simón *et al.*, 1992).

The stage of grape ripeness is regarded as an important factor in the availability of anthocyanins, as the degradation of the berry skin facilitates anthocyanins extraction. The time of maceration is also critical to obtain wines with good colour intensity and stability since short periods lead to poor anthocyanin extraction and longer periods result in unstable colour. The use of macerating enzymes helps to degrade the cell walls that are the limiting barrier that prevent the release of polyphenols into the must during fermentation (Bautista-Ortín *et al.*, 2006; Bautista-Ortín *et al.*, 2007a).

Revilla *et al.* (2001) has also studied the anthocyanins composition of several grape varieties and its evolution during ripening. Tempranillo grapes revealed a slight increase of malvidin derivatives (3-glucoside, 3-glucoside-acetate and 3-(*p*-coumaryl)glucoside) during maturation, while other non acylated anthocyanins suffered a slight decrease over the same period. However, the anthocyanins fingerprint of a wine not always corresponds to that of grapes of origin. This means that additional changes occur, probably during alcoholic fermentation, and several causes have been presented, such as rate of anthocyanins extraction, degradation or polymerisation during alcoholic fermentation or even different capacity to adsorb to yeast walls (Revilla *et al.*, 2001).

3.3. Yeast

Alcoholic fermentation is conducted by yeasts, namely *Sacharomices cerevisiae*, and consists in the fermentation of sugars to yield alcohol (Jackson, 2000). *S. cerevisiae* is particularly adapted to this metabolism, since it can withstand moderately high ethanol concentrations. The continuous increase in ethanol during this process was shown to enhance the extraction of grape compounds (Jensen *et al.*, 2008).

The choice of a yeast strain is an important factor that affects wine colour, once these microorganisms have different capacities to retain or adsorb phenolic compounds. The use of different yeast strains is a valuable tool, during both fermentation and wine aging, to obtain a stable and highly coloured wine (Bautista-Ortín *et al.*, 2007b). Caridi *et al.* (2004) observed differences in wine colour, total polyphenols, monomeric anthocyanins, flavonoids, total anthocyanins, flavan-3-ols and proanthocyanidins according to the yeast strain used in wine fermentation.

Secondary metabolites produced during yeast fermentation are involved in the formation of anthocyanin derived pigments. One of the major products of yeast metabolism is acetaldehyde, which mediates the reaction between anthocyanin-derived pigments. Metabolites that present keto-enol tautomerism, such as pyruvic acid, acetoacetic acid and acetaldehyde, participate in the cycloaddition in C-4 and C-5 of anthocyanins, producing pyranoanthocyanins (**Figure 4**). Monagas *et al.* (2007) described anthocyanins to be the most affected compounds by the yeast strain, independently of the grape variety, while hydroxycinnamic acids and derivatives and the remaining non-anthocyanic phenolic compounds were less influenced by the yeast strain. Pyranoanthocyanins and metabolites resultant from alcoholic fermentation, such as methyl and ethyl gallates and tyrosol, were more influenced by must composition and pH and less influenced by yeast strain (Monagas *et al.*, 2007).

Yeasts not only affect the extraction of grape polyphenols during maceration and fermentation, but can also interact and favour the formation of more stable anthocyanin forms during maturation and aging. *S. cerevisiae* possesses pectinases (polygalacturonases) that are able to hydrolyse skin pectin, hence favouring the extraction of anthocyanins (Sanchez-Torres et al., 1998). β-Glucosidase activity of certain *S. cerevisae* strains is responsible for the breakdown of the glucosidic bond in anthocyanidin-3-glucosides originating the less stable free anthocyanidins (Monagas *et al.*, 2007; Bakker & Timberlake, 1985). Moreover, it appears that the hydrolysis of tartatic esters of *trans*-caffeic and *trans*-coumaric acids is also dependent on the yeast strain (Monagas *et al.*, 2007).

Yeasts may also adsorb anthocyanins into their cell wall. The wall of yeast cells is composed of glucans and mannans, presenting chitin in lower amounts. Mannoproteins located on the outer layer of the yeast cell wall determine most of the surface properties, including its ability to adsorb wine molecules, like anthocyanins. This behaviour has also been observed with rehydrated active dried yeasts and purified polyphenolic compounds (Monagas *et al.*, 2007).

Essays conducted with wine inoculated with *S. cerevisiae* have shown interactions with a large fraction of coloured polyphenols, clearly biphasic, starting with a rapid adsorption and evolving into a slow, constant and saturating fixation, reaching a maximum at around one week. Moreover, the extent of polyphenols interactions varies according to the chemical family of polyphenols: hydroxycinnamic acids interacted quicker than the majority of all other compounds. Anthocyanins were slightly adsorbed, with malvidin-3-glucoside being the most affected glycoside. The polarity of the compounds does not seem to be related with the adsorbance efficiency, although contradictory results have been found. It is still not clear whether the real mechanism by which anthocyanins interact with yeast walls is dependent on hydrogen bonds or is, on the contrary, limited by anthocyanins' own reactivity or by adsorption sites on the cell surface (Mazauric & Salmon, 2005). Additionally, the amount of anthocyanins, namely of malvidine derivatives, adsorbed by fragments of yeast walls are slightly lower, suggesting that minor differences might exist between cell wall fragments, live yeast and yeast lees (Mazauric & Salmon, 2005).

As referred, yeasts mannoproteins interact with polyphenols, sometimes causing their precipitation and consequent decrease in wines. The enrichment of wine must with polysaccharides, like commercial mannoproteins, lead to different results in several studies. Some argue that polysaccharides may act as protective colloids that slow or prevent anthocyanins decrease. On the other hand, reports have described the formation of mannoprotein polyphenol colloidal complexes that could be unstable in face of alcohol accumulation. Although both sources of mannoproteins show the same type of effect, differences can be observed in what concerns the changes caused, once these mannoproteins differ in reactivity, structural composition and are introduced in the wine at different pace and moment. Yeast selection should consider the mannoproteins by these microorganism, since some strands overexpress these compounds (Guadalupe et al., 2007).

Contaminating yeasts of the genus *Dekkera/Brettanomyces*, especially *Dekkera bruxellensis*, are mainly responsible for phenolic acids decarboxylation into the corresponding vinylphenol and reduction by a vinylphenol reductase, which transforms the vinyl into the corresponding ethylphenol. The most studied by-products of *Dekkera* metabolism are 4-ethylphenol and 4-ethylguaiacol, originated from *p*-coumaric and ferulic acids, respectively, despite lactic acid bacteria may also undertake this pathway (Cabrita et al., 2008; Edlin et al., 1995). Silva et al. (2005) reported the changes in the non-coloured phenolics profile (**Figures 8 and 9**) of varietal wines from the Dão region inoculated with *Dekkera bruxellensis* yeast.

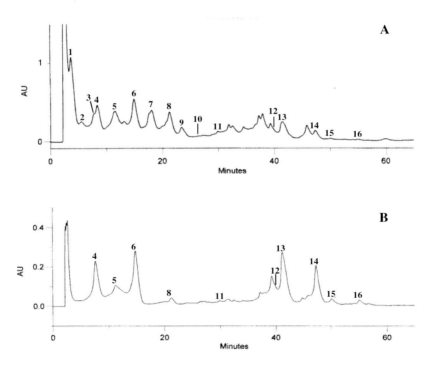

Figure 8. HPLC profile of non-coloured phenolics in Dão wine samples inoculated with *Dekkera bruxellensis*. Detection at (A) 280 and (B) 350 nm. (1) gallic acid; (2) 3,4-di-hydroxybenzoic acid; (3) tyrosol; (4) *trans*-caffeoyltartaric acid; (5) *trans-p*-coumaroyltartaric acid; (6) caffeic acid; (7) syringic acid; (8) *p*-coumaric acid; (9) epicatechin; (10) ferulic acid; (11) sinapic acid; (12) ellagic acid; (13) myricetin; (14) quercetin; (15) kaempferol; (16) isorhamnetin (adapted from Silva et al., 2005).

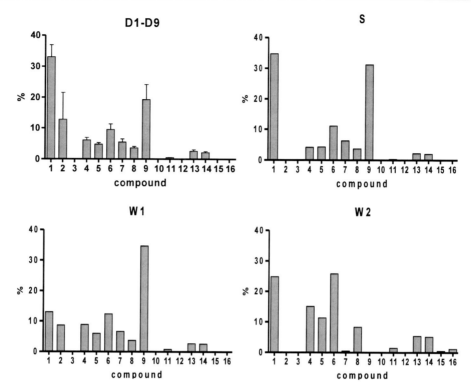

Figure 9. Phenolic compounds content in Dão wine samples: witness samples with refrigeration (W1), witness sample (W2), samples inoculated with 9 strains of *Dekkera bruxellensis* (D1-D9) and inoculated with *Saccharomyces cereviseae* (S). Identity of compounds as in Figure 8 (adapted from Silva *et al.*, 2005).

Increased levels of epicatechin were observed, compared to witness samples under the same conditions, which may be explained by the use of tannins as substrate by yeast enzymes. Decreased amounts of quercetin were observed, as well as of *trans*-caffeoyltartaric and *trans*-coumaroyltartarid acids, although not followed by the accumulation of correspondent free acids, caffeic and *p*-coumaric acids, respectively, due to its rapid metabolisation. In addition, there appeared to be some variability in yeast strains, for some caused an increase in 3,4-dihydroxybenzoic acid (Figure 9). However, the inoculation with *D. bruxellensis* did not affect the anthocyanin composition (**Table 2**).

The deterioration of red wine by *D. bruxeliensis* is ascribed to the horsy smell from 4-ethylphenol and the smoky or spice flavour from 4-ethylguaiacol (Valentão *et al.*, 2007). The production of ethylphenols and vinylphenols is now a common parameter in wine quality control. Valentão *et al.* (2007) observed that all samples inoculated with *D. bruxellensis* exhibited higher content of 4-ethylphenol than of 4-ethylguaiacol. This could be important once the interaction of vinylphenols, the intermediary compounds, with anthocyanin-pyruvic acid adducts yields portisins, recently discovered in Port wine samples (Mateus *et al.*, 2004).

Lees are composed of yeast cells produced in the alcoholic fermentation, tartaric salts, bacteria and plant cell fragments, being found at the bottom of fermentation tanks.

Table 2. Anthocyanins content in Dão wine samples (mg/l)[a] (adapted from Valentão et al., 2007)

Sample[b]	Malvidin-3,5-diglucoside (Rt 29.6 min)	Cyanidin-3-galactoside (Rt 30.6 min)	Cyanidin-3-glucoside (Rt 33.7 min)	Peonidin-3-glucoside (Rt 41.5 min)	Malvidin-3-glucoside (Rt 43.2 min)	Delphinidin (Rt 46.7 min)	Cyanidin (Rt 51.9 min)	Pelargonidin (Rt 54.6 min)	Malvidin (Rt 56.7 min)	Total
W1	70.5 (12.0)	nq	nq	14.7 (2.9)	179.1 (33.6)	2.0 (0.2)	3.1 (0.2)	2.3 (0.5)	10.0 (2.8)	281.5
W2	73.0 (0.6)	nq	nq	15.0 (0.0)	189.5 (1.4)	nq	4.7 (0.2)	nq	8.0 (4.9)	290.3
D1	63.5 (1.3)	nq	nq	14.8 (0.2)	168.4 (3.2)	1.6 (0.3)	3.7 (0.0)	nq	11.1 (5.2)	263.2
D2	67.1 (0.0)	nq	nq	14.0 (0.7)	168.9 (0.5)	1.3 (0.1)	4.0 (1.2)	nq	8.4 (0.2)	263.8
D3	54.9 (2.3)	nq	nq	11.7 (0.5)	155.6 (7.1)	1.2 (0.5)	3.5 (0.0)	1.5 (0.1)	6.5 (0.6)	234.8
D4	57.9 (1.1)	nq	nq	13.3 (0.3)	150.6 (1.5)	2.0 (0.5)	3.3 (0.0)	3.2 (0.8)	6.7 (0.9)	237.1
D5	69.6 (0.4)	nq	2.7 (0.1)	14.3 (0.3)	165.6 (3.0)	1.6 (0.1)	3.7 (0.2)	2.6 (1.2)	8.4 (0.1)	268.5
D6	55.5 (0.2)	nq	1.4 (0.5)	13.5 (0.1)	159.4 (0.7)	2.3 (0.4)	2.9 (0.2)	nq	7.9 (0.5)	242.8
D7	65.4 (1.9)	nq	2.1 (0.6)	14.0 (0.5)	178.3 (5.6)	1.9 (0.0)	4.6 (0.4)	2.1 (0.6)	8.6 (0.6)	277.0
D8	66.4 (2.3)	nq	nq	12.9 (0.1)	163.2 (1.2)	2.1 (0.3)	3.4 (0.1)	1.6 (0.2)	8.8 (0.1)	258.4
D9	59.0 (1.9)	nq	nq	12.0 (0.7)	158.4 (5.6)	2.1 (0.0)	2.8 (0.2)	1.4 (0.4)	9.0 (0.0)	244.8
S	62.8 (4.7)	nq	nq	13.2 (0.5)	158.8 (7.4)	1.5 (0.2)	3.1 (0.1)	1.6 (0.4)	5.2 (1.2)	246.2

[a] Values are expressed as mean (standard deviation) of three determinations; nq: not quantified. [b] Identity of samples as in Figure 9.

Their use in enological practice for the manufacture of red wines is now a more frequent methodology to improve wine quality than before, when its use was restricted to *grand crus* white wines made by the *champenoise* method (Mazauric & Salmon, 2006), for it allows a distinctive yeast aroma (Hernández *et al.*, 2006).

Yeast lees partial desorption by protein denaturation treatments shows that pyranoanthocyanins, formed during fermentation, are adsorbed, justifying its decrease in wines throughout aging on lees (Mazauric & Salmon, 2006).

Periodic stirring of the lees, *batônnage*, is a common practice in many regions in order to enrich the wine (Hernández *et al.*, 2006). However, in what concerns phenolics, it was shown that this practice in aging containers produced wines with the same *cis*-resveratrol, (+)-catechin, *cis-p*-coumaric, vanillic and *trans*-caffeic acids contents than those without stirring (Hernández *et al.*, 2006).

3.4. Malolactic Fermentation

Alcoholic fermentation, conducted by yeasts, can be followed by malolactic fermentation, that consists on the decarboxylation of L-malic to L-lactic acid and carbon dioxide, by the action of lactic acid bacteria, such as *Oenococus oeni* (Cabrita *et al.*, 2008). The advantages of this process are still under controversy, since it can significantly improve or reduce the quality of wines. Malolactic fermentation causes a decrease in the acidity and has been more frequently used for wines from cold regions, exhibiting excessive acidity, than for those produced in warmer regions, normally presenting lower acidity (Jackson, 2000).

Much attention has been devoted to β-glucosidase of wine yeasts. In opposition, β-glucosidase of wine lactic acid bacteria has received little concern. Readily detectable activity of β-glucosidase in eleven commercial preparations of oenococci was found by Grimaldi *et al.* (2000). The hydrolysis of the sugar-bound anthocyanins liberates the sugar and the corresponding anthocyanidin. A slight (Vrhovsek *et al.*, 2002) and extended decrease (Keller *et al.*, 1999; Mazza *et al.*, 1999) in total anthocyanins was described after malolactic fermentation. Whether this decrease is a result of anthocyanin adsorption to lactic acid bacteria, as occurs in yeasts, was not confirmed. Mayen *et al.* (1994) found a decrease in individual anthocyanins during malolactic fermentation, which was accompanied by an increase in condensed pigments and colour intensity.

It has been suggested that the sugar moiety of glycosilated anthocyanins is used as an energy source by these bacteria (Vivas *et al.*, 1997). As referred above, anthocyanidin may be converted to brown or colourless compounds. So, glucosidase activity ultimately can result in a decolourizing effect. In general, these findings indicate that wine lactic acid bacteria have the potential to hydrolyse glycoconjugates and to affect wine colour.

A decrease in hydroxycinnamic acid derivatives, such as the tartaric esters of caffeic, *p*-coumaric and ferulic acids, and the rise of the corresponding free forms was observed (Cabrita *et al.* 2008; García-Falcón *et al.*, 2007; Hernández *et al.*, 2007b). However, the hydrolysis of those esters does not always account for total increase in hydroxycinnamic acids. Hydrolysis of cinnamoyl-glycoside anthocyanins by lactic acid enzymatic activity can also be a probable source of free acids (Cabrita *et al.* 2008).

The concentration of volatile phenols increased markedly during malolactic fermentation (Etiévant *et al.*, 1989), pointing that lactic acid bacteria might be involved. Whereas wine yeasts are, to a large extent, responsible for the decarboxylation of phenolic acids (Valentão *et al.*, 2008), wine lactic acid bacteria may also be able to do it. The catabolism of ferulic and *p*-coumaric acids by several wine lactobacilli and pediococci and the detection of the corresponding volatile phenols (4-ethylguaiacol and 4-ethylphenol) confirm this fact (Cavin *et al.*, 1993; *Couto et al.*, 2006).

During malolactic fermentation resveratrol levels were found to increase, accompanied by a decrease of piceid concentration. The β-glucosidase activity of lactic acid bacteria may explain the hydrolysis of piceid (Yunoki et al., 2004; Hernández *et al.*, 2007b).

Other studies on malolactic fermentation impact in the non-anthocyanic composition of red wine showed marked differences. Procyanidin dimers and a prodelphinidin dimer, not present in the initial wine, were found after malolactic fermentation (Hernández *et al.*, 2007b). Additionally, resveratrol, tyrosol, (+)-catechin, (-)-epicatechin, myricetin and quercetin increased after malolactic fermentation, for some lactic acid bacteria strains (Hernández *et al.*, 2007b). However, Gil-Muñez *et al.* (1999) found a decrease in (+)-catechin and (-)-epicatechin contents after this step.

The possible use of phenolic compounds with antimicrobial activity against lactic acid bacteria is nowadays under study, although they can act both as stimulators or inhibitors of bacterial growth in the concentrations found in wine (Cabrita *et al.*, 2008). This use can alter the profile of a wine, both qualitatively and quantitatively, depending on the composition of the phenolics additives. The use of wine phenolics as antimicrobial agents in winemaking must be conditioned by changes in both physicochemical and organoleptic properties, because inhibitory concentrations are much higher than those occurring naturally. Such concerns should also take into account the many antagonistic and synergistic effects between polyphenols and other wine constituents. Spiked wines, resulting from the addition of polyphenolic-rich extracts of wine or grapes, might be a solution for the widespread use of sulphur dioxide as preservative (García-Ruiz *et al.*, 2008) that may constitute a risk for asthmatics, by inducing bronchial constriction (Dahl *et al.*, 1986).

3.5. Enological Practices

The colour intensity of young red wines is known to be influenced by anthocyanins. Such intensity is highly dependant on the maceration conditions that occur during the winemaking process, such as fermentation temperature, must freezing, skin to juice ratio, maceration time and enzymes added (Jensen *et al.*, 2008).

Alcoholic fermentation of red wines is generally done on the skin or by thermovinification. The latter employs destemmed grapes that are heated to 60 or 87 °C, so that cell structure is disrupted and instant extraction of all cell constituents is initiated. This technique is usually applied in cool climate viticulture when grapes have low contents of anthocyanins, while fermentation on skin is applied worldwide and allows both aqueous and alcoholic extraction of phenolic compounds from several parts of the grape berry (Fischer *et al.*, 2000).

A factor of undisputed importance in relation to wine quality is skin contact with must. When the pomace contacts with the fermentating must, both flavonol glycosides and aglycones are gradually extracted and such process peaks at around 8 to 14 days, declining in the following 88 days (Makris *et al.*, 2006b). Kelebek *et al.* (2006) showed that maceration time has a considerable effect on the total phenolics present, namely anthocyanin glycosides, resulting in a maximum at the end of six days. A decrease is seen further on, probably due to fixation of compounds in yeast, degradation or condensation in the form of tannins. These timings apply with higher certainty to glycosides, whereas aglycones exhibited erratic behaviour, presumably because of glycoside hydrolysis (Kelebek et al., 2006).

Fermentation on skin can be combined with mash heating. This latter consists in heating the must up to 65 °C and then cooling it down until 30° for 24 hours, before the inoculation with yeasts. The combination of both techniques results in higher concentration of flavonoids and stilbenes, namely anthocyanins, flavan-3-ols, flavonols and resveratrol (Netzel et al., 2003).

The run-off treatment consists on the separation of a portion of the grape juice before fermentation. This methodology, tested by Bautista-Ortín et al. (2007a), allowed a higher skin-to-juice ratio. This study showed that monomeric anthocyanins exhibit a slight increase in early days of alcoholic fermentation, decreasing rapidly later on. Polymeric anthocyanins behave differently and were present in the highest amounts during the last days of fermentation.

Traditional punch down treatment yields lower anthocyanins and non-coloured phenolics extraction than modern fermentation equipment. Pump over treatment has been shown to extract seeds and stem constituents, such as gallic acid, catechin and epicatechin, better than mechanical punch down. This extraction is further enhanced in small berry size grape varieties, such as Pinot noir, which exhibit higher amounts of seed and stem mass per grape cluster (Fischer et al., 2000).

Flash release consists on heating the grapes quickly to over 95 °C using only biological vapour (released from grapes), at atmospheric pressure, and then applying a strong vacuum, which results in instant vaporization. Such method induces a degradation of cell walls and has been shown to produce an increase in over 50% of total phenolics in wines. Wines produced using this method exhibit higher amount of flavonols, catechins and proanthocyanidins than the control wines and similar contents of hydroxycinnamic acids. Increasing the temperature of heating or the length of the heating resulted in a favoured conversion of anthocyanins to orange or brown pigments. Flash release produces musts that are much richer in polyphenols than wines produced in the conventional way. However, their concentration decreases dramatically if pressing was achieved immediately after flash release. Pomace contact in flash release wines yields higher amounts of flavonols, catechins, anthocyanins and proanthocyanidins (Morel-Salmi et al., 2006).

The length of maceration of red wine grapes has been studied, revealing that longer maceration times depicted an increase of seeds' compounds, particularly catechins. The use of temperature has been shown to be important in the release of high weight phenolics from skin, such as proanthocyanidins. An increase of temperature from 25°C to 35°C in the last two days of the maceration enhanced anthocyanin contents (Vrhovsek et al., 2002). Wines produced without contact with stems presented the highest levels of anthocyanins, followed by those made by stem-contact and by carbonic maceration. Extended maceration seems to diminish the amount of free anthocyanins, either by adsorption by yeast, degradation or condensation with tannins.

Spranger et al. (2004) noted that, according to winemaking technology, namely stem contact maceration for 7 and 21 days, non-stem contact wine during 7 days and carbonic maceration at 35°C, marked differences in proanthocyanidins and catechins occour. The latter leads to the lowest amounts of both oligomeric and polymeric proanthocyanidins. Stem contact in maceration can extend the extraction of important flavan-3-ols, such as (+)-catechin, due to the contribution of stems to the wine overall phenolic composition. The most important explanation for this fact is that wines produced with stem contact have a higher level of alcohol, hence enhancing the diffusion rate of polyphenols from the grape to the must. Extended stem-contact maceration time to 21 days did not result in supplementary increase in procyanidins than those observed for 7 days. On the other hand, additional maceration time can result in more compounds from grape solids interacting with some procyanidins and thus, causing a decrease of these compounds in wine. Winemaking procedures were found to alter the structural composition of proanthocyanidins in wine. Carbonic maceration is mostly characterised by a decrease in the percentage of (-)-epicatechin gallate as terminal unit and a decrease of (+)-catechin and an increase of (-)-epicatechin as extension units (Spranger *et al.*, 2004).

Changes in the content of total polyphenols induced by the use of commercial pectolitic enzymes have been observed (Cabrita *et al.*, 2008). The application of pectolytic enzymes, a common practice in winemaking to increase phenolics content in wines, is responsible for the stability, taste and structure improvement of red wines, not only because more anthocyanins are released by degradation of cell walls, but also because tannins attached to the grape's skin are released as consequence of the enzymatic activity. Such technique is preferably employed for grapes with low content in anthocyanins, for which the ratio of extraction is more important. The use of pectolytic enzymes causes an increase in colour intensity. This results from raised polymeric anthocyanin content and from enhanced co-pigmentation due to enhanced extraction of non-coloured polyphenols (Kelebek *et al.*, 2007). Although anthocyanin extraction suffered an increase, no particular anthocyanin was preferably extracted, resulting in a similar profile. However, other studies have not found that the use of pectolytic enzymes lead to wines richer in anthocyanic compounds (Wightman *et al.*, 1997). These disparities concerning pectolytic enzyme addition and its role in the extraction of phenolic compounds from grape skin may be explained by the fact that different grape varieties display distinct amounts of pectin (Kelebek *et al.*, 2007).

The use of enological tannins may also contribute to wine colour stabilisation, improved wine structure, and elimination of reduction odours. However, the use of tannins, especially hydrolyzable tannins, must be undertaken with care, for such addition might result in loss of equilibrium in wines and consequent deterioration, due to a decrease in polymeric anthocyanins contents (Bautista-Ortín *et al.*, 2007a).

Red grapes co-winemaking effect on phenolic fraction is of high appeal for winemakers, since some varieties can be richer in certain anthocyanins, other polyphenols and other colours stabilisation co-factors. Therefore, some grape varieties may benefit from the presence of other different ones and such complementary effect may be achieved by co-maceration and co-fermentation. This method was restricted to grapes that ripen at the same period, but advances in modern refrigeration now allow co-maceration and co-fermentation of grapes that ripen at different times. Co-winemaking can give rise to co-pigmentation reactions during co-maceration, resulting in wine with different profiles of phenolic compounds (Lorenzo *et al.*, 2005). This technique is not always used since monovarietal wines are first produced and then mixed by *coupage* (blending of finer wines).

Manufacturers, in order to counter year-to-year variability in climate or grapes' characteristics, also blend ports from different years and grapes of different cultivars or geographical origin, exhibiting different phenolics content, so that quality and style consistency are not affected (Andrade *et al.,* 1998).

Some post-fermentation treatments, such as fining with agents, namely casein, bentonite and activated charcoal, were found to cause significant reduction in both flavonol glycosides and aglycones in Sherry wines (Makris *et al.,* 2006b).

3.6. Oxygenation

Wine colour is highly influenced by oxygen exposure. During the conservation of red wines, anthocyanins react with other phenolic compounds, mainly flavan-3-ols, being regarded as the cause for the colour change of wines during aging, from red-bluish in young wines towards orange-brown in matured wines (Revilla *et al.,* 1999).

Oak barrels show different porosity according to the species of oak used in the barrel manufacture. The amount of oxygen present in wines in early stages of maturation is a direct result of the porosity and the volume of the barrel, but the pores become progressively obstructed so that after several uses of a specific barrel the dissolved oxygen becomes very similar to those in wines stored in tanks. The favourable surface/volume ratio of smaller barrels may facilitate the polymerisation of phenolics, hence diminishing its contents in wines (Perez-Prieto *et al.,* 2003). Makris *et al.* (2006b) stated that the permeability of bottle cork can also contribute to the oxygen availability in bottled wines.

Oxygen exposure in wines has been employed for the sake of improving wine quality, by orienting the phenolic compounds reactions towards the oxidative ways, in search of more coloured and less astringent products. The pathway, thought to be favoured by the presence of oxygen, includes the formation of pyranoanthocyanins and ethyl-bridged adducts (Atanasova *et al.,* 2002) (Figure 4).

Wide diversity of pyranoanthocyanins can be obtained through this process, depending mostly on the nature and relative amounts of flavan-3-ols and anthocyanin molecules, but also on the availability of acetaldehyde. Acetaldehyde is a naturally occurring product of yeast metabolism during fermentation or of the oxidation of ethanol in the presence of phenolic compounds (Atanasova *et al.,* 2002).

Micro-oxygenation is used to mimic the oxygen input experienced by wines stored in wood barrels, for wines put to age in stainless steel and other containers (**Figure 10**). Micro-oxygenation is mainly linked to the condensation of anthocyanins with tannins. The presence of sulphur dioxide has the ability to delay this process.

Sulphur dioxide can reverse the oxidation of B ring catechol groups, remove peroxide radicals within the wine and interferes with the formation of carbocations at the 4 position of proanthocyanidins. The latter tampers with the formation of more complex polyphenols. Such effects have been found to be dose-related, once wines with high sulphur dioxide contents revealed retarded combination of anthocyanins with tannins while this formation was significantly faster in a low SO_2 environment (Tao *et al.,* 2007).

The influence of micro-oxygenation was measured by the increase of anthocyanin-ethyl-(epi)catechin, although the formation of pyranoanthocyanins was not affected (Atanasova *et al.,* 2002). Additionally, micro-oxygenation caused a decrease in quercetin, (+)-catechin and (-)-epicatechin, possibly due to its reactivity in an oxidant medium (Ferrarini *et al.,* 2001; Rice-Evans *et al.,* 1996).

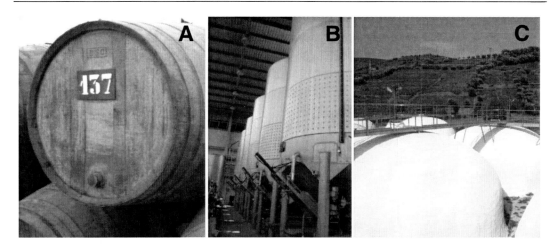

Figure 10. Containers for wine aging: wood barrels (A), steel reservoirs (B) and concrete tanks (C).

Once bottled, the formation of condensed pigments occurs in a gradual manner. These reactions yield polymeric compounds and can happen in the absence of oxygen. Due to the reduced availability of oxygen in bottles, the formation of co-pigments during this phase of the storage period is more influenced by temperature than by dissolved oxygen (García-Falcón et al., 2007). Moreover, the total concentration of phenolic acids exhibits a decrease, especially after the third month, largely due to the hydrolysis of *trans*-coutaric and *trans*-caftaric acids, in favour of the free form, or by acting as copigments with anthocyanins. When addressing flavan-3-ols, epicatechin exhibits a decrease over time while catechin increases. Glycosides of myricetin, kaempferol and quercetin decrease, possibly due to the hydrolysis of conjugated flavonols (García-Falcón et al., 2007).

3.7. Aging

Most wines are aged in wood barrels and this practice has been considered fundamental to the beneficial evolution of stored wines. Among other aspects, evaporation, extraction, oxidation and component reactions occur in wood barrels, but not in stainless steel or concrete containers (Figure 10), unless microoxygenation is employed. These factors have a large impact on wine characteristics and are favoured in small and new barrels (Perez-Prieto et al., 2003), once their extension is dependent on greater wood surface in contact with a unit of beverage. The surface/volume ratio of 220 L barrels may facilitate the polymerization of phenolics. Much of the literature focus on maturing wine in small oak barrels, although many of the world's wines are aged on mid to large barrels, such as 1000L ones.

Theextraction of different polyphenols from oak barrels into wine during aging produces changes in wine composition that are directly related to the potential extractable compounds present in wood and the duration of the contact. The chemical composition of oak wood is highly influenced by an array of factors. The species of oak, geographical origin and sylvocultural treatment of the tree account for major differences in wood chemical composition, along with the processing of wood in cooperage, method of seasoning and degree and technology of oak toasting during barrel manufacture (Alamo et al., 2000).

Due to high demand of quality wood and the need to preserve current supply areas, the use of other woods apart from the traditional French and American oak, such as the Spanish oak, has been tested. Several species grown in Spain (*Quercus robur*, *Q. petraea*, *Q. pyrenaica* and *Q. faginea*), France (*Q. robur* and *Q. petraea*) and America (*Q. alba*) have been studied (de Simón et al., 2003). The polyphenolic composition and its evolution throughout wine processing showed quantitative differences, especially between European and American species. A decrease in total anthocyanins was observed for all types of oak. American oak displayed values significantly lower than the rest of the species, reaching a minimum after 21 months. Since that total anthocyanins content was obtained based on the flavilium ion colour intensity and that the polymers of anthocyanins do not contribute to the colour of the wines, it appears that American oak favours these reactions. When addressing total polyphenols, total catechins and total proanthocyanidins, the initial decrease observed was dependent on the type of wood, but at the end of the aging period, the extension of that decrease was similar for all wood barrels. The differences between European and American species were explained by the ultra-structure of the wood of *Q. alba* (Chatonnet & Dubourdieu, 1998). This type of wood causes an increased difficulty for wine to penetrate into it, reduces evaporation of liquids and also diminishes the penetration of oxygen. That is, oxygen-promoted condensation processes are less favoured in American oak (Feuillat et al., 1994). In addition, Alamo et al. (2004) noticed that the degree of *O*-glycoside bonds cleavage of flavonols appears to be dependant on the type of wood used (*Q. alba*, *Q. robur* and *Q. sessilis*): *Q. alba* shows more cleavage than the other tested species. It has also been shown that wines aged in American oak (*Q. alba*) barrels for 24 months exhibited a lower total anthocyanins content, quercetin glycosides and aglycone and ellagic acid than that of French (*Q. rubor* and *Q. petraea*) and Spanish oak (*Q. rubor*, *Q. petraea*, *Q. pyrenaica* and *Q. faginea*) barrels (Hernández et al., 2007a).

Other studies regarding oak barrels' influence on phenolic compounds allowed to observe that the differences in concentration of total low-polymer polyphenols was statistically significant for barrel wood type and source cooperage, although the latter seems to exert greater influence (Alamo et al., 2000).

Levels of ellagic acid on toasted wood do not correlate with the contents found in wine, so its presence in the layer of toasted wood is not the only factor contributing to its availability in wine (de Simón et al., 2003).

Nagel & Wulf (1979) have described that during the aging of experimental wines the levels of anthocyanins drop between fermentation and 240 days. Moreover, anthocyanins exhibit a reduction of 97% in eight months, catechin, caftaric and *p*-coutaric acids are reduced by 57% in less than seven months. Flavan-3-ols also decrease with aging in oak barrels and the vast majority show clear changes in their concentrations at the end of several months (Hernández et al., 2007a). Additionally, Andrade et al., (1998) described how wine phenolics profile within the same variety differed from year to year during aging in wood barrels (**Figure 11**). These results indicate that the analysis of young wines is not enough to predict the characteristics of a wine by the time of consumption, for aging constitutes a major cause for wine phenolics alteration.

High-molecular-weight polymers, resultant from tannin polymerization, can be formed during the aging period, causing a decrease in total phenolics content. Additionally, the process of co-pigmentation with anthocyanins can account for diminished content in flavan-3-ols and flavonols (de Simón et al., 2003).

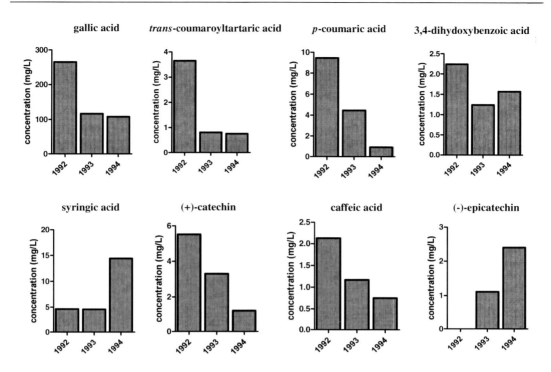

Figure 11. Concentration of phenolic compounds in experimental varietal wines in three distinct years (adapted from Andrade et al., 1998).

Perez-Prieto et al. (2003) observed such decrease of total phenols after six months of aging. However, contradictory studies either found a constant level for 12 months (Gómez-Cordovés & Gonzales, 1995), or a slight increase, due to the extraction of compounds form the wood (Jindra & Gallender, 1987), or an increase in (-) epicatechin due to procyanidin hydrolysis (Andrade et al., 1998).

Studies indicate that different concentrations of ethanol have a direct effect on the extraction of *cis* and *trans*-oak lactones from *Q. alba* and of phenolic aldehydes from Bulgarian *(Q. rubor)* oak chips, later oxidised to its respective phenolic acids (del Alamo Sanza et al., 2004). Moreover, the alcohol content seems to be more important than pH for the extraction of wood compounds. Cerdán et al. (2004) observed that Merlot wines exhibited a higher concentration of furanic aldehydes, oak lactones, phenolic aldehydes and phenolic alcohols than Cabernet wines, during aging in wooden barrels of *Q. alba,* due to the higher amount of alcohol in Merlot wines.

Oak chips are mainly used to accelerate the aging process (Sanza et al., 2004). Addition of chips is a valuable tool, tested in order to reduce costs while wine aging and quality is guaranteed. However, some authors noticed that the addition of chips may give a less satisfactory result. Therefore, the use of oak chips from various origins may influence or enhance a wine's sensorial and chemical profile, due to the extraction of gallic, ferulic, vanillic, syringic and ellagic acids, ellagitannins and tannins (Sartini et al., 2007).

The combination of this technique with lees or micro-oxygenation has also been examined. Wine colour intensity decreased with the use of wood chips, possibly due to the adsorption of anthocyanins. Additionally, the blue colour of wines is affected by polymerisation phenomena caused by ethyl bridges that generate red-violet compounds. The combined use of chips and micro-oxygenation has been proved to counterbalance the adsorption effect of the wood chips. Some compounds such as caftaric acid, quercetin and myricetin, more reactive towards oxygen, are protected from oxidation by yeast lees because they are able to use oxygen, removing it from the medium (Sartini *et al.*, 2007).

The most common method to simulate aging in wood barrels is the addition of oak wood extracts, mainly composed of gallic vanillic, syringic and ellagic acids, with or without treatment of the wood (del Alamo Sanza *et al.* 2004). This addition increases phenolic acids content in wines. These oak extracts lack aromatic aldehydes, which are present when wine/oak contact occurs. The lack of aromatic aldehydes is used in the control of some counterfeit aged-wines (Russo *et al.*, 2008).

3.8. Miscellaneous

Elderberries (*Sambucus nigra*) are rich sources of anthocyanins and, apart from the use for juices and jam as a food colorant source, are used illegally in wine manufacture, particularly port wines. Such adulteration was thought to accelerate wine fermentation and to produce red wine from white grapes. The detection of this adulteration was achieved by HPLC-UV, being found cyanidin-3-sambubioside-5-glucoside and cyanidin-3-sambubioside that are inexistent in wine anthocyanins composition. Additionally, elderberries can also produce cyanidin-3-glucoside, increasing the normally low content of this compound in wines (García-Viguera & Bridle, 1995). Contact time, temperature and alcoholic content enhance the extraction of elderberry anthocyanic pigments into wine. Despite the presence of gallic acid, 3,5-dihydroxybenzoic acid, rutin and quercetin in both elderberries and wines, the addition of these berries to wine resulted in very little differences on these compounds (García-Viguera & Bridle, 1995).

The synthesis of *trans*-resveratrol and other stilbenes is triggered by mould infections and physiological stresses. Thus, wines produced from grapes not affected by such aggressions exhibit lower amounts of this compounds (Revilla & Ryan, 2000). *Botrytis* infection of grape berries is widely regarded as a fungal infection with detrimental effects on the quality of wines produced. Grapes in contact with *Botrytis* exhibit enhanced flavonoids production as a result of their synthesis as phytoalexins in face of the fungal threat (Jeandet *et al.*, 1995). Despite this fact, heavily infected grapes exhibit a lower amount of resveratrol than would be expected, possibly because it undergoes degradation exerted by laccase-like stilbene oxidase (Pezet *et al.*, 1991). Even in the absence of symptoms of *Botrytis* infection, resveratrol levels are higher due to the comensal presence of *Botrytis* on fruits.

Gibberellins are an important class of natural growth regulators in plants. Its use for table grape production has been extensively studied and yield improvements in berry weight and juice quality. GA_3 reduces berry set, increases berry weight, increases petiole length, produces a less firm berry skin, enhances shoot growth and reduces the number of seeds. These GA_3-treated grapes are not yet used on wine production, but its interest is growing rapidly. Thinning in grape-wine production with gibberellic acid could decrease the risk of infections, such as by *Botrytis cinerea*, and bunch rot. It has been described that gibberellic acid leads to less compact grape clusters, which are less sensitive to fungal infection, with higher polyphenols contents, including anthocyanins (Teszlák *et al.*, 2005). The use of GA3 has been proven to diminish the number of botrytised berries, putatively leading to less oxidative destruction of polyphenols, namely anthocyanins, by tyrosinase and laccase, the main fungal polyphenol destruction enzymes. This effect is clearer when considering epicatechin, caftartic and gallic acids but different *Vitis* varieties exhibit distinct behaviour.

Recent years have seen an increase in ecological wines, produced from grapes without the use of chemical fertilizers, insecticides or other pest control substances. This approach seeks to replace industrial fertilizer with natural manure and pesticides by natural predators, both resulting in wines free from chemical residues. Moreover, grapes grown under ecological conditions are exposed to pests, so that its phenolic compounds might be produced to counteract this aggression. The resulting wines are said to be richer in polyphenols and constitute a great appeal for the consumers seeking safe products. Zafrilla *et al.* (2003) showed that conventional and ecological wines evolve very similarly. While conventional wines see a decrease of about 88% of anthocyanins during 7 months of storage in the dark, in ecological wines the decrease was 91% and no qualitative differences were observed between the two wines. In what concerns to hydroxycinnamic acids, no qualitative and quantitative differences were noticed. However, conventional red wine suffered a decrease on caffeic acid esters and an increase in free caffeic acid, but the total amount of hydroxycinnamic acids did not vary after storage.

Once a bottle of wine is open for consumption, polyphenols are influenced by the oxygen availability. The study performed by Tarola *et al.* (2007) showed that samples kept in a refrigerator, in contact with oxygen, exhibited a stabilization of (+)-catechin, (-)-epicatechin, gallic acid, *trans*-resveratrol, caffeic acid, chlorogenic acid, quercetin and rutin contents after three days, followed by a slight decrease. On the contrary, *cis*-resveratrol showed an increase, probably due to the isomerisation of the *trans* isomer. This stability is most likely caused by the antioxidant ability of the polyphenols in wine. Wines stored at 4°C and protected from light for up to a week did not differ significantly from those analyzed immediately after bottle opening.

4. CONCLUSION

The understanding of the changes in wine phenolics from grape to bottle is a valuable tool for manufactures and consumers, allowing to create specific wine products that not only retain or improve beneficial organoleptic properties of wines, but also may meet the demands of the market. Nevertheless, it has become clear that the consumption of moderate amounts of wine has undeniable health effects.

The herein presented chapter shows how the knowledge of red wine phenolics can be fundamental when addressing several aspects of wine technology. The factors affecting phenolic compounds and their combined influences can be modulated, enhanced or countered in order to produce wines that are richer in phenolic compounds and, hence, that might constitute an improved tool in health promotion. Further studies on these matters would be interesting to understand how the observed changes translate in modulated biological activities and whether additional beneficial effects might arise.

REFERENCES

Adrian, M., Jeandet, P., Bessis, R. & Joubert, J. M. (1996) Induction of Phytoalexin (Resveratrol) Synthesis in Grapevine Leaves Treated with Aluminum Chloride (AlCl$_3$). *Journal of Agricultural and Food Chemistry, 44,* 1979-1981.

Alamo, M., Bernal, J. L., & Gómez-Cordovés, C. (2000) Behaviour of monosaccharides, phenolic compounds, and colour of red wines aged in used oak barrels and in the bottle. *Journal of Agricultural and Food Chemistry, 48,* 4613-4618.

Amico, V., Napoli, E. M., Renda, A., Ruberto, G., Spatafora, C., & Tringali, C. (2004) Constituent of grape pomace from the Sicilian cultivar Nerello Mascalese. *Food Chemistry, 88,* 599-607.

Anderson, O. M. (2002) Anthocyanin occurrences and analysis *Proceedings of the international workshop on anthocyanins: Research and development of anthocyanins,* Adelaide, South Australia, April 17–19.

Andrade, P., Seabra, R., Ferreira, M., Ferreres, F., & Garcia-Viguera, C. (1998) Analysis of non-coloured phenolics in port wines by CZE. Influence of grape variety and ageing. *Zeitschrift fur Lebensmittel-Untersuchung Und-Forschung A, 206,* 161-164.

Andrade, P. B., Mendes, G., Falco, V., Valentão, P., & Seabra, R. M. (2001) Preliminary study of flavonols in port wine grape varieties. *Food Chemistry, 73,* 397-399.

Atanasova, V., Fulcrand, H., Cheynier, V., & Moutounet, M. (2002) Effect of oxygenation on polyphenol changes occurring in the course of wine-making. *Analytica Chimica Acta, 458,* 15-27.

Bakker, J., & Timberlake, C. F. (1985) The distribution and content of anthocyanins in young port wines as determined by high performance liquid chromatography. *Journal of the Science of Food and Agriculture, 36,* 1325-1333.

Barón, R., Mayén, M., Mérida, J., & Medina, M. (1997) Changes in Phenolic Compounds and Browning during Biological Aging of Sherry-Type Wine. *Journal of Agricultural and Food Chemistry, 45,* 1682 -1685.

Bautista-Ortín, A. B., Fernández-Fernandéz, J. I., López-Roca, J. M., & Gómez-Plaza, E. (2006) The effect of grape ripening stage on red wine color. *Journal International de la Vigne et du Vin, 40,* 14-24.

Bautista-Ortín, A. B., Fernández-Fernandéz, J. I., López-Roca, J. M., & Gómez-Plaza, E. (2007a) The effects of enological practices in anthocyanin, phenolic compounds and wine colour and their dependence on grape characteristics. *Journal of Food Composition and Analysis, 20,* 546-552.

Bautista-Ortín, A. B., Romero-Casales, I., Fernadéz-Fernández, J. I., López-Roca, J. M., & Gómez-Plaza, E. (2007b) Influence of the yeast strain on Monastrell wine colour. *Innovative Food Science and Emerging Technologies, 8,* 322-328.

Bridle, P., & García-Viguera, C. (1996) A simple technique for the detection of red wine adulteration with elderberry pigments. *Food Chemistry, 55,* 111-113.

Brouillard, R., & Delaporte, B. (1977) Chemistry of anthocyanin pigments: Kinetic and thermodynamic study of proton transfer, hydration, and tautometric reactions of malvidin-3-glucoside. *Journal of the American Chemical Society, 99,* 8461–8468.

Brouillard, R. (1982) *Chemical structure of anthocyanins. Anthocyanins as food colors.* New York, NY: Academic Press.

Bruneton, J. (1993). *Pharmacognosie: Phytochimie, plantes médicinales* (2nd edition), Paris, France: Lavoisier.

Budic-Leto, I., & Lovric, T. (2002) Identification of Phenolic Acids and Changes in their Content during Fermentation and Ageing of White Wines Posip and Rukatac. *Food Technology and Biotechnology, 40,* 221-225.

Cabornneau, M. A., Leger, C. L., Descomps, B., Michael, F., & Monnier, L. (1998) Improvement in the antioxidant status of plasm and low density lipoprotein in subjects receiving a red wine phenolics mixture. *Journal of the American Oil Chemists' Society, 75,* 235-240.

Cabrita, M. J., Torres, M., Palma, V., Alves, E., Patão, R., & Costa Freitas, A. M. (2008) Impact of malolactic fermentation on low molecular weight phenolic compounds. *Talanta, 74,* 1281-1286.

Caridi, A., Cufari, A., Lovino, R., Palumbo, R., & Tedesco, I. (2005) Influence of yeast on polyphenol composition of wine. *Food Technology and Biotechnology, 42,* 37-40.

Castillo-Muñoz, N., Gómez-Alonso, S., García-Romero, E., & Hermosín-Gutíerrez, I. (2007) Flavonol Profiles of *Vitis vinifera* Red Grapes and Their Single-Cultivar Wines. *Journal of Agricultural and Food Chemistry, 55,* 992-1002.

Cavin, J. F., Andioc, V., Etiévant, P. X., & Divies, C. (1993) Ability of wine lactic acid bacteria to metabolize phenol carboxylic acids. *American Journal of Enology and Viticulture, 44,* 76–80.

Cerdán, T. G., Goñi, D. T., & Azpilicueta, C. A. (2004) Accumulation of volatile compounds during ageing of two red wines with different composition. *Journal of Food Engineering, 63,* 349-356.

Chatonnet, P., & Dubourdieu, D. (1998) Comparative Study of the Characteristics of American White Oak (*Quercus alba*) and European Oak (*Quercus petraea* and *Q. robur*) for Production of Barrels Used in Barrel Aging of Wines. *American Journal of Enology and Viticulture, 49,* 79-85.

Cooke, D., Steward, W. P., Gescher, A. J., & Marczylo, T. (2005) Anthocyanins from fruits and vegetables – Does bright colour signal cancer chemopreventive activity? *European Journal of Cancer, 41,* 1931-1940.

Couto, J. A., Campos, F. M., Figueiredo, A. R., & Hogg, T. A. (2006) Ability of Lactic Acid Bacteria to Produce Volatile Phenols. *American Journal of Enology and Viticulture, 57,* 166-171.

da Costa, C. T., Horton, D., & Margolis, S. A. (2000) Analysis of anthocyanins in foods by liquid chromatography, liquid chromatography-mass spectrometry and capillary electrophoresis. *Journal of Chromatography A, 881,* 403-410.

Dahl, R., Henriksen, J. M., & Harving, H. (1986) Red wine asthma: A controlled study. *Journal of Allergy and Clinical Immunology, 78,* 1126-1129.

del Alamo Sanza, M., Dominguez, N., & Merino, S. G. (2004) Influence of different ageing systems and oak woods on aged wine color and anthocyanin composition. *European Food and Research Technology, 219,* 124-132.

de Simón, B. F., Hernández, T., Cadahía, E., Dueñas, M., & Estrella, I. (2003) Phenolic compounds in a Spanish red wine aged in barrels made of Spanish, French and American oak word. *European Food Research and Technology, 216,* 150-156.

de Simón, B. F., Hernández, T., Estrella, I., & Gómez-Cordovés, C. (1992) Variation in phenol content in grapes during ripening: low-molecular-weight phenols, *Zeitschrift fur Lebensmittel-Untersuchung Und-Forschung, 194,* 351-354.

Dopico-García, M. S., Fique, A., Guerra, L., Afonso, J. M., Pereira, O., Valentão, P., Andrade, P. B., & Seabra, R. M. (2008) Principal components of phenolics to characterize red *Vinho Verde* grapes: Anthocyanins or non-coloured compounds? *Talanta, 75,* 1190-1202.

Edlin, D. A. N., Narbad, A., Dickinson, J. R., & Lloyd, D. (1995) The biotransformation of simple phenolic compounds by *Brettanomyces anomalus. FEMS Microbiology Letters, 125,* 311-316.

Etiévant, P. X., Issanchou, S., Marie, S., Ducruet, V, & Flanzy, C. (1989) Sensory impact of volatile phenols on red wine aroma: influence of carbonic maceration and time of storage. *Sciences des Aliments, 9,* 19–33.

Fazal, F., Rahman, A., Greensill, J., Ainley, K., Hasi, S. M., & Parish, J. H. (1990) Strand scission in DNA by quercetin and Cu (II): Identification of free radical intermediates and biological consequences of scission. *Carcinogenesis, 11,* 2005-2008.

Ferrarini, R., Giraldi, F., De Conti, D., & Castellari, M. (2001) Esperienze di applicazione della microossigenazione come tecnica d'affinamento dei vini. *Industrie della bevande, 30,* 116-118, 122.

Feuillat, F., Perrin, R., & Keller, R. (1994). Experimental "stave interface" simulation: measurement of wood impregnation and surface evaporation dynamics. *Journal International des Sciences de la Vigne et du Vin, 28,* 227-246.

Fischer, U., Strasses, M., & Gutzler, K. (2000) Impact of fermentation technology on the phenolic and volatile composition of German red wines. *International Journal of Food Science and Technology, 35,* 81-94.

Gambelli, L., & Santaroni, G. P. (2004) Polyphenols content in some Italian red wines of different geographical origins. *Journal of Food Composition and Analysis, 17,* 613-618.

García-Falcón, M. S., Pérez-Lamela, C., Martínez-Carballo, E., & Simal-Gándara, J. (2007) Determination of phenolic compounds in wines: Influence of bottle storage of young red wines on their evolution. *Food Chemistry, 105,* 248-259.

García-Ruiz, A., Bartolomé, B., Martínez-Rodríguez, A. J., Pueyo, E., Martín-Álvarez, P. J., & Moreno-Arribas, M. V. (2008) Potencial of phenolic compounds for controlling lactic acid bacteria growth in wine. *Food Control, 19,* 835-841.

García-Viguera, C., & Bridle, P. (1995) Analysis of non-coloured phenolic compounds in red wines. A comparison of high-performance liquid chromatography and capillary zone electrophoresis. *Food Chemistry, 54,* 349-352.

Gil-Muñez, R., Gómez-Plaza, E., Martínez, A., & López-Roca, J. M. (1999) Evolution of Phenolic Compounds during Wine Fermentation and Post-fermentation: Influence of Grape Temperature. *Journal of Food Composition and Analysis, 12,* 259-272.

Gómez-Cordovés, C., & Gonzales, S. J. M. L. (1995) Interpretation of color variables during the aging of red wines: relationship with families of phenolic compounds. *Journal of Agricultural and Food Chemistry, 43,* 557-561.

Grimaldi, A., McLean, H., & Jiranek, V. (2000) Identification and partial characterization of glycosidic activities of commercial strains of the lactic acid bacterium, *Oenococcus oeni. American Journal of Enology and Viticulture, 51,* 362–369.

Guadalupe, Z., Palacios, A., & Ayestarán, B. (2007) Maceration Enzymes and Mannoproteins: A possible strategy to increase colloidal stability and colour extraction in red wines. *Journal of Agricultural and Food Chemistry, 55,* 4854-4862.

Harborne, J. B., (1964) Plant polyphenols – XI. The structure of acylated anthocyanins. *Phytochemistry, 3,* 151-160.

Haselgrove, L., Botting, D., van Heeswijck, R., Høj, P. B., Dry, P. R., Ford, C., & Illand, P. (2000) Canopy microclimate and berry composition: the effect of bunch exposure on the phenolic composition of *Vitis Vinifera* L. cv. Shiraz grape berries. *Australian Journal of Grape Wine Research, 6,* 141-149.

Hernández, T., Estrella, I., Carlavila, D., Martín-Álvarez, P. J., & Moreno-Arribas, M. V. (2006) Phenolic compounds in red wine subjected to industrial malolactic fermentation and ageing on lees. *Analytica Chimica Acta, 563,* 116-125.

Hernández, T., Estrella, I., Dueñas, M., de Simón, B. F., & Cadahía, E. (2007a) Influence of wood origin in the polyphenolic composition of a Spanish red wine aging in bottle, alter storage in barrels of Spanish, French and American oak Word. *European Food Research and Technology, 224,* 695-705.

Hernández, T., Estrella, I., Pérez-Gordo, M., Alegría, E. G., Tenorio, C., Ruiz-Larrrea, F., & Moreno-Arribas, M. V. (2007b) Contribution of malolactic fermentation by *Oenococcus Oeni* and *Lactobacillus Plantarum* to the changes in the nonanthocyanin polyphenolic composition of red wine. *Journal of Agricultural and Food Chemistry, 55,* 5260-5266.

Hipskind, J. D., Hanau, R., Leite, B., & Nicholson, R. L. (1990) Phytoalexin accumulation in sorghum: identification of an apigeninidin acyl ester. *Physiological and Molecular Plant Pathology, 36,* 381-396.

Hung, L.-M., Chen, J.-K., Huang, S.-S., Lee, R.-S., & Su, M.-J. (2000) Cardioprotective effect of resveratrol, a natural antioxidant derived from grapes. *Cardiovascular Research, 47,* 549-555.

Jackson, R. S. (2000). *Wine Science, Principles, practice and perception* (2nd edition). San Diego, California: Academic Press.

Jang, M., Cai, L., Udeani, G. O., Slowing, K. V., Thomas, C.F., Beecher, C. W. W., Fong, H. H. S., Farnsworth, N. R., Kinghorn, D., Mehta, R. G., Moon, R. C., & Pezzuto, J. M. (1997) Cancer Chemopreventive Activity of Resveratrol, a Natural Product Derived from Grapes. *Science, 275,* 218-220.

Jeandet, P., Bessis, R., Maume, B. F., Meunier, P., Peyron, D., & Trollat, P. (1995) Effect of enological practices on the resveratrol isomer content of wine. *Journal of Agricultural and Food Chemistry, 43,* 316-319

Jensen, J. S., Meniray, S., Egebo, M., & Meyer, A. S. (2008) Prediction of wine colour attributes from the phenolic profiles of red grapes (*Vitis vinifera*). *Journal of Agricultural and Food Chemistry, 56,* 1105-1115.

Jindra, J. A., & Gallender, J. F. (1987) Effect of American and French oak barrels on the phenolic composition and sensory quality of Sevyal blanc wine. *American Journal. of Enology and Viticulture, 38,* 133-138.

Kallithraka, S., Tsoutsouras, E., Tzourou, E., & Lanaridis, P. (2006) Principal phenolic compounds in Greek red wines. *Food Chemistry, 99,* 784-793.

Kanazawa, K., Yamashita, T., Ashida, H., & Danno, G. (1998) Antimutagenicity of flavones and flavonols to heterocyclic amines by specific and strong inhibition of the cytochrome P450 1A1 family. *Bioscience, Biotechnology and Biochemistry, 62,* 970-977.

Karagiannis, S., Economou, A., & Lanaridis, P. (2000) Phenolic and volatile composition of wines made from *Vitis vinifera* v. Muscat lefko grapes from the island of Samos. *Journal of Agricultural and Food Chemistry, 48,* 5369-5375.

Kelebek, H., Canbas, A., Selli, S., Saucier, C., Jourdes, M., & Glories, Y. (2006) Influence of different maceration times on the anthocyanin composition of wines made from *Vitis vinifera* L. cvs. Boğazkere and Öküzgözü. *Journal of Food Engineering, 77,* 1012-1017.

Kelebek, H., Canbas, A., Cabaroglu, T., & Selli, S. (2007) Improvement of anthocyanin content in the cv. Öküzgözü wines by using pectolytic enzymes. *Food Chemistry, 105,* 334-339.

Keli., U., Hertog, M. G. L., Feskens, E. J. M., & Kromhout, D. (1994) Dietary flavonoids, antioxidant vitamins and the incidence of stroke: the Zutphen study. *Archives of Internal Medicine, 154,* 637-642.

Keller, M., Pool, R. M., & Henick-Kling, T. (1999) Excessive nitrogen supply and shoot trimming can impair colour development in Pinot Noir grapes and wine. *Australian Journal of Grape and Wine Research, 5,* 45–55.

Langcake, P., & Pryce, R. J. (1976) The production of resveratrol by *Vitis vinifera* and other members of the Vitaceae as a response to infection or injury. *Physiology and Plant Pathology, 9,* 77-86.

Langcake, P., & Pryce, R. J. (1977) A new class of phytoalexins from grapevines. *Experientia, 33,* 151-152.

Lo, S.-C., Weiergang, I., Bonham, C., Hipskind, J., Wood, K., & Nicholson, R. L. (1996) Phytoalexin accumulation in sorghum: Identification of a methyl ether of luteolinidin. *Physiology and Molecular Plant Pathology, 49,* 21-31.

Lorenzo, C., Pardo, F., Zalacain, A., Alonso, G. L., & Salinas, M. R. (2005) Effect of red grapes co-winemaking in polyphenols and color of wines. *Journal of Agricultural and Food Chemistry, 53,* 7609-7616.

Macheix, J. J., Fleuriet, A., & Billot, J. (1990) Phenolic compounds in fruit processing. In: Macheix, J. J., Fleuriet, A., Billot, J., Eds., *Fruit phenolics* (1st edition, pp. 295–358). Boca Raton, FL: CRC Press.

Makris, D. P., Kallithraka, S., & Mamalos, A. (2006a) Differentiation of young red wines based on cultivar and geographical origin with application of chemometrics of principal polyphenolic constituents. *Talanta, 70,* 143-1152.

Makris, D. P., Kallithraka, S., & Kefalas, P. (2006b) Flavonols in grape, grape products and wines: Burden, profile and influential parameters. *Journal of Food Composition and Analysis, 19,* 396-404.

Martorell, N., Martí, M. P., Mestres, M., Busto, O., & Guasch, J. (2002) Determination of 4-ethylguaiacol and 4-ethylphenol in red wines using headspace-solid-phase microextraction-gas chromatography. *Journal of Chromatography A, 975,* 349–354.

Mateus, N., Oliveira, J., Santos-Buelga, C., Silva, A. M. S., & de Freitas, V. A. P. (2004) NMR structure characterization of a new vinylpyranoanthocyanin-catechin pigment. *Tetrahedron Letters, 45,* 3455-3457.

Mayen, M., Mérida, J. & Medina, M. (1994) Free anthocyanins and polymeric pigments during fermentation and post-fermentation standing of musts from Cabernet Sauvignon and Tempranillo grapes. *American Journal of Enology and Viticulture, 45,* 161–166.

Mazauric, J., & Salmon, J. (2005) Interaction between yeast lees and wine polyphenols during simulation of wine aging: I. Analysis of remnant polyphenolic compounds in the resulting wines. *Journal of Agricultural and Food Chemistry, 53,* 5647-5653.

Mazauric, J., & Salmon, J. (2006) Interaction between yeast lees and wine polyphenols during simulation of wine aging: II. Analysis of desorbed polyphenol compounds from yeast lees. *Journal of Agricultural and Food Chemistry, 54,* 3876-3881.

Mazza, G., Fukumoto, L., Delaquis P., Girard, B., & Ewert B. (1999) Anthocyanins, Phenolics, and Color of Cabernet Franc, Merlot, andPinot Noir Wines from British Columbia. *Journal of Agricultural and Food Chemistry, 47,* 4009-4017.

Mira, F. J. H., & Chozas, M. G. (1993) Compuestos fenólicos en vinos tintos. *Alimentación, equipos y tecnología, 8,* 37-42.

Monagas, M., Gómez-Cordovés, C., & Bartolomé, B. (2007) Evaluation of different *Saccharomyces cerevisiae* strains for red winemaking. Influence on the anthocyanin, pyranoanthocyanin and non-anthocyanin phenolic content and colour characteristics of wines. *Food Chemistry, 104,* 814-823.

Morel, L., Lescoat, G., Cillard, P., & Cillard, J. (1994) Role of flavonoids and iron chelation in antioxidant action. *Methods in Enzymology, 234,* 437-443.

Morel-Salmi, C., Souquet, J., Bes, M., & Cheynier, V. (2006) Effect of Flash Release treatment on phenolic extraction and wine composition. *Journal of Agricultural and Food Chemistry, 54,* 4270-4276.

Nagel, C. W., & Wulf, L. W. (1979) Changes in the anthocyanins, flavonoids and hydroxycinnamic acid esters during fermentation and aging of Merlot and Cabernet Sauvignon. *American Journal of Enology and Viticulture, 45,* 1-5.

Netzel, M., Strass, G., Bitsch, I., Christmann, M., & Bitsch, R. (2003) Effect of grape processing on selected antioxidant phenolics in red wine. *Journal of Food Engineering, 56,* 223-228.

Nip, W. K., & Burns, E. E. (1969) Pigment characterization in grain sorghum. I. Red varieties. *Cereal Chemistry, 46,* 490-495.

Noble, A. C. (1990). Bitterness and astringency in wine. In R. Rouseff, *Bitterness in Foods and Beverages* (1st edition, pp. 145-158). Amsterdam, Netherlands: Ed. Elsevier.

Ough, C. S., & Amerine, M. A. (1988) *Methods for analysis of musts and wines.* New York, NY: Wiley

Pérez-Margariño, S., & González-SanJosé, M. L. (2006) Polyphenols and colour variability of red wines made from grapes harvested at different ripeness grade. *Food Chemistry, 96,* 197-208.

Perez-Prieto, L. J., Hera-Orts, M. L., López-Roca, J. M., Fernández-Fernandéz, J. I., & Gómez-Plaza, E. (2003) Oak-matured wines: influence of the colour and sensory characteristics. *Journal of the Science of Food and Agriculture, 83,* 1445-1450.

Pezet, R., Pont, V., Hoang-Van, K. (1991) Evidence of oxidative detoxification of pterostilbene and resveratrol by a laccase-like stilbene oxigenase produced by *Botrytis cinerea*. *Physiological and Molecular Plant Pathology, 39,* 441-450.

Price, S. F., Breen, P. J., Valladao, M., & Watson, B. T. (1995) Cluster sun exposure and quercetin in Pinot Noir grapes and wine. *American Journal of Enology and Viticulture, 46,* 187-194.

Prior, R. L., & Wu, X. (2006) Anthocyanins: Structural characteristics that result in unique metabolic patterns and biological activities. *Free Radical Research, 40,* 1014-1028.

Quirós, A. R., López-Hernández, J., Ferraces-Casais, P., & Lage-Yusty, M. A. (2007) Analysis of non-anthocyanin phenolic compounds in wine samples using high performance liquid chromatography with ultraviolet and fluorescence detection. *Journal of Separation Science, 30,* 1262-1266.

Remy, S., Fulcrand, H., Labarbe, B., Cheynier, V., & Moutounet, M. (2000) First confirmation in red wine of products resulting from direct anthocyanin-tannin reaction. *Journal of the Science Food and Agriculture, 80,* 745-751.

Renaud, S., & de Lorgeril, M. (1992) Wine, alcohol, platelets and the French paradox for coronary heart disease. *The Lancet, 339,* 1523-1526.

Revilla, E., García-Beneytez, E., Cabello, F., Martín-Ortega, G., & Ryan, J. (2001) Value of high-performance liquid chromatographic analysis of anthocyanins in the differentiation of red grape cultivars and red wines made from them. *Journal of Chromatography A, 915,* 53-60.

Revilla, E., & Ryan, J.-M. (2000) Analysis of several phenolic compounds with antioxidant properties in grape extracts and wines by high-performance liquid chromatography – photodiode array detection without sample preparation. *Journal of Chromatography A, 881,* 461-469.

Revilla, I., Pérez-Margariño, S., González-SanJosé, M. L., & Beltrán, S. (1999) Identification of Anthocyanin derivatives in grape skin extracts and red wines by liquid chromatography with diode array and mass spectrometric detection. *Journal of Chromatography A, 847,* 83-90.

Ribéreau-Gayon, P. (1964) Les composés phénoliques du raisin et du vin. *Annales de Physiologie Vegetale, 6,* 119-147.

Rice-Evans, C. A., Miller, N. J., & Paganga, G. (1996) Structure-antioxidant activity relationships of flavonoids and phenolic acids. *Free Radical Biology and Medicine, 20,* 933-956.

Ritchey, J. G., & Waterhouse, A. L. (1999) A standard red wine: Monomeric phenolic analysis of commercial Cabernet Sauvignin wines. *American Journal of Enology and Viticulture, 50,* 91-100.

Ros Barcelo, A., Calderon, A. A., Zapata, J. M., & Munoz, R (1994) The histochemical localization of anthocyanins in seeded and seedless grapes (*Vitis vinifera*). *Scientia Horticulturae, 57,* 265-268.

Russo, P., Andreu-Navarro, A., Aguilar-Caballos, M., Fernández-Romero, J., & Gómez-Hens, A. (2008) Analytical Innovations in the detection of phenolics in wines. *Journal of Agricultural and Food Chemistry, 56,* 1858-1865.

Salas, E., Atanasova, V., Poncet-Legrand, C., Meudec, E., Mazauric, J. P., & Cheynier, V. (2004) Demonstration of the occurrence of flavanol–anthocyanin adducts in wine and in model solutions. *Analytica Chimica Acta, 513,* 325-332.

Sánchez-Torres, P., González-Candelas, L., & Ramón, D. (1998) Heterologous expression of a *Candida molischiana* anthocyanin-β-glucosidase in a wine yeast strain. *Journal of Agricultural and Food Chemistry, 46,* 354-360.

Sanza, M. A., Domínguez, I. N., Cárcel, L. M. C., & Gracia, L. N. (2004) Analysis for low molecular weight phenolic compounds in a red wine aged in oak chips. *Analytica Chimica Acta, 513,* 229-237.

Sartini, E., Arfelli, G., Fabiani, A., & Piva, A. (2007) Influence of chips, lees and micro-oxygenation during aging on the phenolic composition of a red Sangiovese wine. *Food Chemistry, 104,* 1599-1604.

Siemann, E. H., & Creasy L. L. (1992) Concentration of the Phytoalexin Resveratrol in Wine. *American Journal of Enology and Viticulture, 43,* 49-52.

Silva, L. R., Andrade, P. B., Valentão, P., Seabra, R. M., Trujillo, M. E., & Velázquez, E. (2005) Analysis of non-coloured phenolics in red wine: Effect of *Dekkera bruxellensis* yeast. *Food Chemistry, 89,* 185-189.

Somers, T. C., & Ziemelis, G. (1985) Spectral evaluation of total phenolic components in *Vitis vinifera*: Grapes and Wines. *Journal of the Science of Food and Agriculture, 36,* 1275-1284.

Spayd, S. E., Tarara, J. M., Mee, D. L., & Ferguson, J. C. (2002) Separation of sunlight and temperature effects on the composition of *Vitis vinifera* cv. Merlot berries. *American Journal of Enology and Viticulture, 53,* 171-182.

Spranger, M.I., Clímaco, M., Sun, B., Eiriz, N., Fortunato, C., Nunes, A., Leandro, M.C., Avelar, M.L., & Belchior, A.P. (2004) Differentiation of red winemaking technologies by phenolic and volatile composition. *Analytica Chimica Acta, 513,* 151-161.

Strack, D., & Wray, V. (1993). *The Flavonoids: Advances in Research Since 1986* (1st edition). London, United Kingdom: Chapman & Hall.

Subbaramaiah, K., Michaluart, P., Chung, W. J., & Dannenberg, A. J. (1998) Resveratrol inhibits the expression of cyclooxygenase-2 in human mammary and oral epithelial cells. *Pharmaceutical Biology, 36,* 35-43.

Tao, J., Dykes, S. I., & Kilmartin, P. A. (2007) Effect of SO_2 concentration on polyphenol development during red wine micro-oxygenation. *Journal of Agricultural and Food Chemistry, 55,* 6104-6109.

Tarola, A. M., Milano, F., & Giannetti, V. (2007) Simultaneous determination of phenolic compounds in red wines by HPLC-UV. *Analytical letters, 40,* 2433-2445.

Teszlák, P., Gaál, K., & Nikfardjam, M. S. P. (2005) Influence of grapevine flower treatment with gibberellic acid (GA_3) on polyphenol content of *Vitis vinifera* L. wine. *Analytica Chimica Acta, 543,* 275-281.

Tommaso, D. D., Calabrese, R., & Rotilio, D. (1998) Identification and Quantitation of Hydroxytyrosol in Italian Wines. *Journal of High Resolution Chromatography, 21,* 549-553.

Valentão, P., Seabra, R. M., Lopes, G., Silva, L. R., Martins, V., Trujillo, M. E., Velázquez, E., & Andrade, P. B. (2007) Influence of *Dekkera bruxellensis* on the contents of anthocyanins, organic acids and volatile phenols of Dão red wine. *Food Chemistry, 100,* 64-70.

Vidal, S., Francis, L., Noble, A., Kwiatkowski, M., Cheynier, V., & Waters, E. (2004) Taste and mouth-feel properties of different types of tannin-like polyphenolic compounds and anthocyanins in wine. *Analytica Chemical Acta, 513,* 57-65.

Vivas, N., Lonvaud-Funel, A., & Glories, Y, (1997) Effect of phenolic acids and anthocyanins on growth, viability and malolactic activity of a lactic acid bacterium. *Food Microbiology, 14,* 291-300.

Vrhovsek, U., Vanzo, A., & Nemani, J. (2002) Effect of red wine maceration techniques on oligomeric and polymeric pranthocyanidins in wine, cv. Blaufränkisch. *Vitis, 41,* 47-51.

Wang, H., Race, E. I., & Shrikhande, A. J. (2003) Anthocyanin Transformation in Cabernet Sauvignon Wine during Aging. *Journal of Agricultural and Food Chemistry, 51,* 7989 - 7994.

Waterhouse, A. (2002) Wine phenolics. *Annals of the New York Academy of Science, 957,* 21-36.

Wightman, J. D., Price, S. F., Watson, B. T., & Wrolstad, R. E. (1997) Some effect of processing enzymes on anthocyanins and phenolics in Pinot noir and Cabernet Sauvignon wines. *American Journal of Enology and Viticulture, 48,* 39-48.

Wu, X., & Prior, R. L. (2005) Identification and characterization of anthocyanins by HPLC-ESI-MS/MS in common foods in the United States: Vegetables, nuts and grains. *Journal of Agricultural and Food Chemistry, 53,* 3101–3113.

Yunoki, K., Yasui, Y., & Ohnishi, M. (2004) Changes in concentrations of resveratrol and its related compounds in red wine during alcoholic and malolactic fermentation. *Nippon Shokuhin Kagaku Kogaku Kaishi, 51,* 274-278.

Zafrilla, P., Morillas, J., Mulero, J., Cayuela, J. M., Martínez-Cachá, A., Pardo, F., & Nicolás, J. M. L. (2003) Changes during storage in convencional and ecological wine: Phenolic content and antioxidant activity. *Journal of Agricultural and Food Chemistry, 51,* 4694-4700.

In: Red Wine and Health
Editor: Paul O'Byrne

ISBN 978-1-60692-718-2
© 2009 Nova Science Publishers, Inc.

Chapter 4

ANTIOXIDANTS AND ANTIOXIDANT ACTIVITY OF RED AND WHITE WINES AFFECTED BY WINEMAKING AND OTHER EXTRINSIC AND INTRINSIC FACTORS

Lachman Jaromír and Šulc Miloslav

Department of Chemistry, Faculty of Agrobiology, Food and Natural Resources, Czech University of Life Sciences in Prague, Kamýcká 129, 165 21 Prague 6 – Suchdol, Czech Republic

ABSTRACT

The French have low coronary heart disease mortality with high fat consumption; this epidemiological anomaly known as the *"French Paradox"* is commonly attributed to the consumption of red wine. Phenolic compounds in wines, especially in red wines, possess strong antioxidant activity *in vitro*. Phenolic compounds obtained in red wine have the largest effect in decreasing atherosclerosis by both hypolipemic and antioxidant mechanisms. Phenolics (esp. catechins, resveratrol, phenolic acids and anthocyanins) show a positive effect on the human health and they may cause an increase of antioxidant activity of blood plasma. The long-term uptake of red wine has a positive impact on antioxidant activity [AA] of blood plasma in rats *in vivo* and increases AA by 15-20% compared to a control group. Major anthocyanins found in red wine are malvidin-3,5-O-diglucoside and 3-O-glucoside, cyanidin-3-O-galactoside, cyanidin-3-O-glucoside and 3,5-O-diglucoside, peonidin-3-O-glucoside, delphinidin-3-O-glucoside, and petunidin-3-O-glucoside. In this article the effect of total phenolics [TP], total anthocyanins [TA], individual anthocyanins, procyanidins and phenolics contained in red grapes, musts, grape seeds and skins and wines on the antioxidant activity [AA] is discussed. The significant impact of varieties, viticultural regions and locations, climate conditions and vintage has been shown. Likewise, the ways and individual stages of the vinification technology process (maceration in red wine production), and storage conditions affect color, TP, TA and AA and health aspects of produced wines. Likewise, resveratrol, another free radical scavenger mainly contained in the skins of grapes, inhibits the risk of cardiovascular diseases. Higher amounts of *trans*-resveratrol have been found in wines from cool and wet climate regions and lesser amounts are typical for warm and dry regions. During an attack with *Botrytis cinerea* the plant forms a resveratrol barrier surrounding the attacked site where the resveratrol concentration is low, but it is four times higher in the neighbor. Changes in the TP content and AA affected by grape variety, vineyard location and winemaking process in white and blue varieties from different vineyards of the Czech Republic were studied. Significant differences in TP among varieties were found. Analysis of variance showed statistically high differences among red and white wines and growing locations. Wines differed significantly in TP content and AA increased significantly during the winemaking process. Statistically significant differences in AA values were found among growing areas, wines and varieties. Significant positive correlations between TP and AA were determined. Total antioxidant status [TAS] of white and blue vine varieties (Czech Republic) revealed significant differences in AA between white and red wines. Moreover, differences were ascertained between individual varieties of red wine. The results obtained supported the assumption that variety plays a considerable role in TAS; the blue vine varieties showed a much higher TAS. Analysis of variance in AA showed statistically high significance between red and white wines. AA increased during the winemaking process, esp. in Zweigeltrebe, St. Laurent and Pinot Noir wines, suggesting thus higher AA of wines compared with grape musts at the beginning of the winemaking process. The highest increase was determined during fermentation and maturation stages of red wine.

ABBREVIATIONS

AA – antioxidant activity
EQA – ascorbic acid equivalent (mg/mL)
ABTS – 2,2'-azinobis(3-ethylbenzothiazolin)-6-sulfphonate
DPPH – 1,1'-diphenyl-2-picrylhydrazyl
HDL cholesterol – high-density lipoprotein cholesterol
LDL cholesterol – low-density lipoprotein cholesterol
RES – resveratrol
TA – total anthocyanins
TAS – total antioxidant status
TP – total phenolics

INTRODUCTION

It was recently determined that moderate red wine consumption improves endothelial function in normal volunteers and oxidative stress in patients with an acute coronary syndrome (Guarda et al., 2005). The "antioxidant power" of a food is an expression of its capability both to defend the human organism from the action of free radicals and to prevent degenerative disorders deriving from persistent oxidative stress (Di Majo et al., 2008).

Many epidemiological studies have shown a correlation between diets that are not well-balanced and coronary heart diseases, a few types of cancer and diabetes (Fernàndez-Pachòn et al., 2004; Landrault et al., 2001). Epidemiologists have observed that a diet rich in polyphenolic compounds may provide a positive effect due to their antioxidant properties (Frankel et al., 1995; Hertog et al., 1998). Red wine is particularly rich in polyphenol substances compared to white wine (Vinson et al., 2001). Polyphenols, measured as flavonoids in the diet, are inversely associated with coronary heart disease mortality and morbidity. Polyphenols are powerful *in vitro* antioxidants in preventing lower density lipoprotein oxidation, the cornerstone event in the oxidation theory of atherogenesis. Epidemiological studies suggest protective effects of moderate wine consumption against cardiovascular diseases. Some of these effects are attributed to wine antioxidant polyphenols, which have been shown to slow down LDL-cholesterol oxidation. Red wines raise plasma HDL-cholesterol, plasma triglyceride and total cholesterol concentrations (Goldberg et al., 1996a). Other mechanisms involving phenolics, such as inhibition of platelet aggregation, stimulation of nitric oxide and influence on prostaglandin synthesis, are also recognized as contributory in preventing cardiovascular diseases (Bartolomé et al., 2004). Wine is an important component in Mediterranean dietary tradition because it is very rich in antioxidant compounds. The polyphenolic contents of wine consist of two classes of components (flavonoids and non-flavonoids) and depend on the grape variety, vineyard location, cultivation system, climate, and soil type, vine cultivation practices, harvesting time, production process and ageing (Shahidi & Naczk, 1995). Grapes and wines contain large amounts of phenolic compounds, mostly flavonoids. At high concentrations of 1000–1800 mg/L, a large part of phenolics found in wines may act as antioxidants (Kanner et al., 1994). The polyphenolic molecules have a functional role in that they behave as antioxidants against the free radicals and show a physiological role as well; in fact, they increase the antioxidant capacity in the human body after red wine consumption (Serafini et al., 1998). The latter is due to the reduction-oxidation properties of the phenolic hydroxyl groups and the potential for delocalization of electrons within the individual ring. Functional ingredients of grape seeds, skins and musts include phenolics such as monomeric flavanols catechin and epicatechin, dimeric, trimeric and polymeric procyanidins, phenolic acids (gallic acid and ellagic acid) and anthocyanins (Yilmaz & Toledo, 2004). Polyphenolic antioxidants of grape are very effective in preventing cancer and cardiovascular diseases (Bianchini & Vainio, 2003). These phenolics were reported to exhibit antioxidant activity *in vivo* and *in vitro* in a number of studies (Karakaya et al., 2001; Borbalan et al., 2003; De Beer et al., 2003; Dugo et al., 2003) and are more effective than vitamin C and E (Matějková & Gut, 2000; Bartolomé & Nuñez, 2004). The highest values of antioxidant activity, inhibition of low-density lipoproteins and total polyphenols were determined in pomace, grapes and must (Yildirim et al., 2005). Grape skins proved to be rich sources of anthocyanins (Chicón et al., 2002), hydroxycinnamic acids, flavanols and flavonol glycosides, whereas flavanols are mainly present in seeds (Kammerer et al., 2004) and could exert antibacterial activities (Baydar et al., 2004). Katalinić et al. (2004) elucidated different reducing/antioxidant power of red and white wines in view of their different phenolic composition.

Another important compound contained in wine and grapes is resveratrol, which is a free radical scavenger and inhibits the risk of cardiovascular diseases (Filip et al., 2003; Frémont, 2000). Burkitt & Duncan (2000) have demonstrated that resveratrol behaves as a powerful antioxidant, both via classical, hydroxyl-radical scavenging and via a novel, glutathione-sparing mechanism. The French have low coronary heart disease mortality with high fat consumption; this epidemiological anomaly is known as the "French Paradox" and is commonly attributed to the consumption of red wine (Vinson et al., 2001). Red wine is a complex fluid containing grape, yeast, and wood-derived phenolic compounds, the majority of which have been recognized as potent antioxidants (Burns et al., 2001). Assessment of the antioxidant activity of a serving of 100 g fresh weight fruit, vegetables and beverages

(Paganga et al., 1999) confirmed very high antioxidant activity of red wine: 1 glass (150 mL) red wine = 12 glasses white wine = 2 cups of tea = 4 apples = 5 portions of onion = 5.5 portions of egg plant = 3.5 glasses of blackcurrant juice = 3.5 (500 mL) glasses of beer = 7 glasses of orange juice = 20 glasses of apple juice. Antioxidant capacity of wine on human LDL oxidation and antiplatelet properties are related to the content of polyphenols contained in wines (Hurtado et al., 1997), which improve aortic biomechanical properties (Mizutani et al., 1999). Wine may be protective against oxidative stress leading to hypertension, insulin resistance, and type 2 diabetes (T2D) (Banini et al., 2006). Daily intake of 150 mL of muscadine grape wine or dealcoholized muscadine grape wine with meals improved several metabolic responses among diabetics compared with diabetics given muscadine grape juice. Red wine has a beneficial effect on the modulation of endothelial progenitor cells, which play a significant role in regeneration of damaged blood vessels (Balestrieri et al., 2008). Probit analysis of Soleas et al. (2002) of the antitumorigenic activities of four major red wine polyphenols revealed that quercetin was the most ($ED_{50} < 1$ µmol) and gallic acid the least effective (ED_{50} 5–10 µmol). (+)-Catechin and *trans*-resveratrol were intermediate, with ED_{50} values of 5 and 6 µmol, respectively. However, *trans*-resveratrol is absorbed much more efficiently than (+)-catechin and quercetin in humans after oral consumption and it can be concluded that *trans*-resveratrol may be the most effective anticancer polyphenol present in red wine as consumed by healthy human subjects. Nevertheless, red wine phenolics can also interact with iron and protein in the lumen during digestion and, consequently, decrease the antioxidant capacity of phenolics, as Argyri et al. (2006) showed in their experiments under conditions of in vitro digestion. Likewise, Saura-Calixto & Díaz-Rubio (2007) take that a part of wine polyphenols (35–60% of total polyphenols in red wine and about 9% in white wine) are associated with dietary fibre, are not bioaccesible in the human small intestine, and reach the colon along with dietary fiber. Content of polyphenols, composition of phenolic complex and antioxidative or antiradical capacity of wines could be affected by many extrinsic and intrinsic factors, such as variety, wine growing area and climatic conditions, quality of wine, and, not least, technological procedures during wine-making (Faitová et al., 2004). Color evolution during vinification and ageing has been attributed to the progressive changes of phenolic compounds extracted from grapes (Vivar-Quintana et al., 2002). In recent years, many studies focused on the dynamics of polyphenol extraction during maceration processes of grape varieties (Budic-Leto et al., 2003, 2005). What is important is the evolution of grape polyphenol oxidase activity and phenolic content during wine maturation and vinification (Valero et al., 1989), changes and evolution of polyphenols in young red wines (Pellegrini et al., 2000), and changes of the hydrophilic and lipophilic antioxidant activity of white and red wines during the wine-making process (Alcolea et al., 2003). Some authors put more emphasis on the maceration process (Budic-Leto et al., 2005), others on grape maturation (Jordao et al., 2001), when quantitative changes in oligomeric phenolics occur. In addition, Echeverry et al. (2005) reported changes in antioxidant capacity of Tanat red wines during early maturation. The aging of sparkling wines manufactured from red and white grape varieties (Pozo-Bayon et al., 2003) and different copigmentation models by interaction of anthocyanins and catechins play an important role during the aging process of wine (Mirabel et al., 1999, Esparza et al., 2004, Monagas et al., 2005). Phenolic content and antioxidant activity could also be affected by storage conditions or a conventional or ecological way of wine production (Zafrilla et al., 2003).

GRAPE AND WINE ANTIOXIDANTS

Grapes contain a large number of different phenolic compounds in skins, pulp and seeds that are molecules (especially anthocyanins, catechins and procyanidins) partially extracted during wine-making (Revilla & Ryan, 2000). Catechin oligomers, procyanidin dimers and trimers, along with other monomeric wine phenolics were extracted and then purified from grapes and grape seeds (Teissedre & Landrault, 2000) and tested for their inhibition of LDL oxidation. Among the various phenolic antioxidants present in red wine, (+)-catechin, (-)-epicatechin, resveratrol, quercetin and its glucoside rutin are the most potent (Sakkiadi et al., 2001), since they have been found to protect human LDL against oxidation more efficiently than α-tocopherol on a molar basis (Frankel et al., 1993). Major anthocyanins found in red wines are 3-O-glucosides of malvidin, peonidin, petunidin, delphinidin, cyanidin, pelargonidin, malvidin-3,5-O-diglucoside, and cyanidin-3-O-galactoside (Fig. 1). Gao & Cahoon (1995) in the anthocyanin profile of *Vitis* hybrid cv. reliance detected by HPLC seven peaks, which were identified as delphinidin-3-O-glucoside (32%), cyanidin-3-O-glucoside (56%), peonidin-3-O-glucoside, cyanidin-3,5-O-diglucoside, petunidin-3-O-glucoside, malvidin-3-O-glucoside, and acylated cyanidin derivative. Krisa et al. (1999) identified in *Vitis vinifera* cell suspension cultures three major anthocyanin monoglucosides: cyanidin-3-O-β-glucoside, peonidin-3-O-β-glucoside and malvidin-3-O-β-glucoside. Mc Dougall et al. (2005) refer to over 20 identifiable anthocyanins contained in red wines of which the main components were 3-*O*-glucosides of malvidin, peonidin, petunidin, delphidin and cyanidin. Coumaroylated-glucoside derivatives of malvidin, petunidin, peonidin, and delphinidin were observed and acetylated glucosides of peonidin, petunidin and malvidin were identified (Jacob et al., 2008). Anthocyanins with modified aglycones similar to vitisin A derivatives of delphinidin, peonidin, petunidin and malvidin were also identified. Red wines contain carboxypyranomalvidine glucosides – vitisins: vitisin A – 5-carboxypyranomalvidin-3-O-β-D-glucoside (Fig. 2) (Asenstorfer & Jones, 2007), vitisin B – pyranomalvidin-3-O-β-D-glucoside. Proanthocyanidins are contained especially in grape seeds (Negro et al., 2003). Valentão et al. (2007) identified in Portugal red wines from Dão region as major anthocyanin malvidin-3-glucoside and from volatile phenols 4-ethylguaiacol. Silva et al. (2005) by analysis of non-anthocyanin phenolics in red wine found that phenolic acids predominated over flavonoids with major gallic acid and in lesser amounts present caffeic, *p*-coumaric, *trans*-caffeoyltartaric and *trans-p*-coumaroyltartaric acids. Yilmaz & Toledo (2006) found in grape seeds monomeric flavanols (catechin and epicatechin), dimeric, trimeric and polymeric procyanidins, and phenolic acids (gallic and ellagic acid). Gutiérrez et al. (2005) in the evaluation of young and briefly aged red wines made from single cultivar grapes grown in the warm climate region of La Mancha (Spain) determined the varietals' differentiation of these wines based on anthocyanin, flavonol and hydroxycinnamic profiles. Characteristic flavonols found were principally glycosides, the main ones being: myricetin 3-glucoside, quercetin 3-glucoside, and quercetin 3-glucuronide. Flavonoids, as well as abundant anthocyanins, especially malvidin-3-O-glucoside could contribute to copigmentation (Álvarez et al., 2006). Bravo et al. (2006) determined in Muscatel wines produced in Portugal resveratrol, piceid, gallic acid, protocatechuic acid, catechin, quercetin and quercetin glycosides.

These phenolics were reported to exhibit antioxidant activity *in vivo* and *in vitro* in a number of studies (Karakaya et al., 2001; Borbalan et al., 2003; De Beer et al., 2003; Dugo et al., 2003) and are more effective than vitamin C and E (Matějková & Gut, 2000; Bartolomé et al., 2004). The highest values of antioxidant activity, inhibition of low-density lipoproteins and total polyphenols were determined in pomace, grapes and must (Yildirim et al., 2005). Grape skins proved to be rich sources of anthocyanins (Chicón et al., 2002), hydroxycinnamic acids, flavanols and flavonol glycosides, whereas flavanols are mainly present in seeds (Kammerer et al., 2004) and could exert antibacterial activities (Baydar et al., 2004). Katalinić et al. (2004) elucidated different reducing/antioxidant power of red and white wines in view of their different phenolic composition.

Oxidation reactions involving phenolics might change the chemical and sensory profile of wines. While oxidation is a long-standing problem in winemaking, a definitive understanding of its chemical mechanisms is lacking, and such an understanding could allow us to better predict and control wine aging. The hypothesis of Waterhouse & Laurie (2006) suggests that catalytic iron converts wine's hydrogen peroxide into hydroxyl radical. This leads to a much stronger and less selective oxidant that could react with almost all wine components, in proportion to their concentration and with little selectivity for antioxidant properties. This reaction could produce many electrophilic oxidation products, mainly aldehydes and ketones that could further modify the chemical composition and sensory perception of wine.

Another important compound contained in wine and grapes is resveratrol (Fig. 3), which is a free radical scavenger and inhibits the risk of cardiovascular diseases (Filip et al., 2003; Frémont, 2000). Resveratrol is mainly contained in the skins of grapes (Matějková & Gut, 2000; Schmandke, 2002), while a low content of it was found in fresh musts (Kopec, 1994). High amounts of *trans*-resveratrol were found in wines from Bordeaux, Burgundy, Switzerland and Oregon and, on the contrary, lower amounts are typical of Mediterranean regions (Filip et al., 2003). During an attack of *Botrytis cinerea* the plant forms a resveratrol barrier (Šmidrkal et al., 2001). In recent time, Barger et al. (2008) reported that resveratrol in high doses (4.9 mg/kg/day), has been shown to extend lifespan in some studies in invertebrates and to prevent early mortality in mice fed a high-fat diet. Both, administration of resveratrol and calorie restricted diet in 14 and 30 months old mices caused a striking transcriptional overlap of calorie restricted diet and resveratrol in heart, skeletal muscle and brain. Both dietary interventions inhibit gene expression profiles associated with cardiac and skeletal muscle aging, and prevent age-related cardiac dysfunction. Dietary resveratrol also mimics the effects of calorie restricted diet in insulin mediated glucose uptake in muscle. Thus, both calorie restricted diet and resveratrol may retard some aspects of aging through alterations in chromatin structure and transcription.

In grape berries of some varieties piceid, a stilbene glucoside of resveratrol (Fig. 4) (Waterhouse & Lamuela-Raventos, 1994), was also detected, which is related to the biosynthesis of resveratrol and its levels in wine could affect the physiologically available amounts of resveratrol to consumers of wine. Together with resveratrol, its oligomers: dimer trans-ε-viniferin (Fig. 5) and trimer α-viniferin, also occur in wines (Price & Langcake, 1977, Rayne et al., 2008).

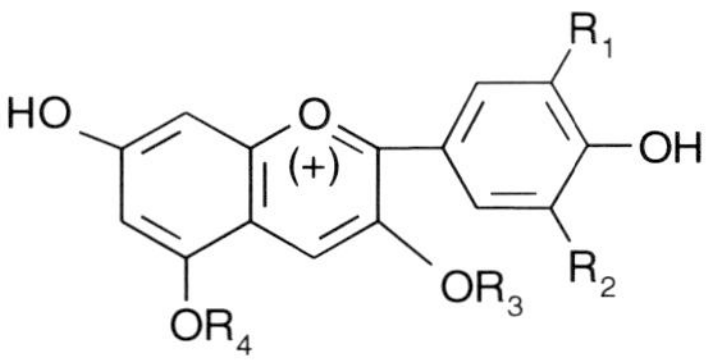

Figure 1. Major anthocyanins contained in red grapes and wine

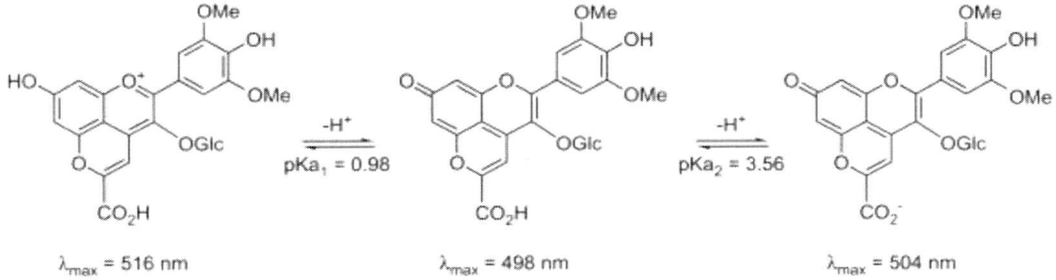

R₁=R₂=R₄=H, R₃=glu — pelargonidin-3-O-glucoside
R₁=OH, R₂=R₄=H, R₃=gal — cyanidin-3-O-galactoside
R₁=OH, R₂=R₄=H, R₃=glu — cyanidin-3-O-glucoside
R₁=OH, R₂=H, R₃=R₄=glu — cyanidin-3,5-O-diglucoside
R₁=R₂=OH, R₄=H, R₃=glu — delphinidin-3-O-glucoside
R₁=OCH₃, R₂=R₄=H, R₃=glu — peonidin-3-O-glucoside
R₁=OCH₃, R₂=OH, R₄=H, R₃=glu — petunidin-3-O-glucoside
R₁=R₂=OCH₃, R₄=H, R₃=glu — malvidin-3-O-glucoside
R₁=R₂=OCH₃, R₃=R₄=glu — malvidin-3,5-O-diglucoside

Figure 2. Structure of 5-carboxypyranomalvidin–3-O-β-D-glucoside (reprinted from Tetrahedron, 63 (22), Asenstorfer RE, Jones GP, Charge equilibria and pK values of 5-carboxypyranomalvidin-3-glucoside (vitisin A) by electrophoresis and absorption spectroscopy, 4788-4792, Copyright 1997, with permission from Elsevier)

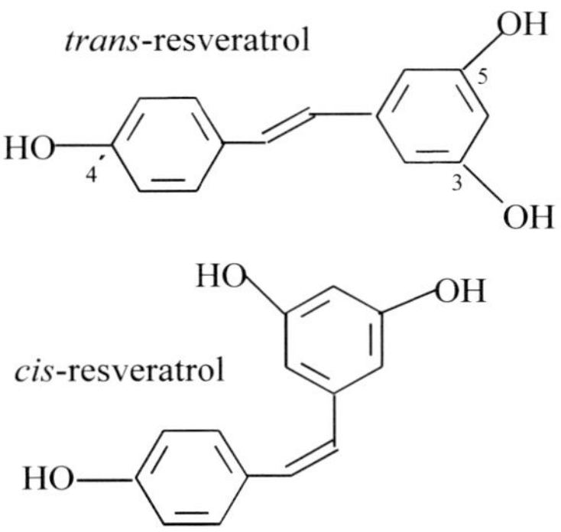

Figure 3. Structures of *trans*- and *cis*-resveratrol

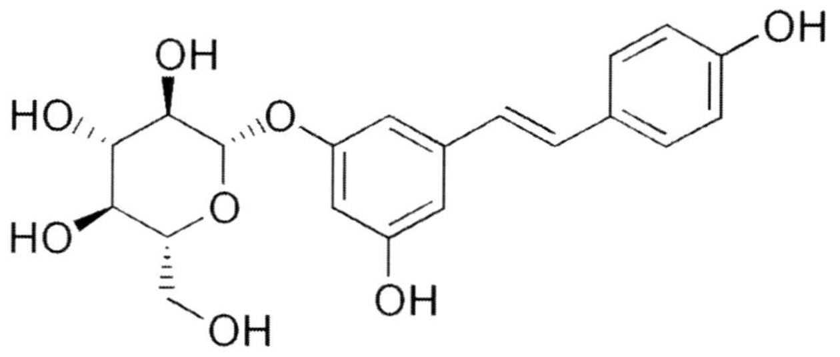

Figure 4. Structure of piceid – resveratrol 3-O-β-D-glucopyranoside

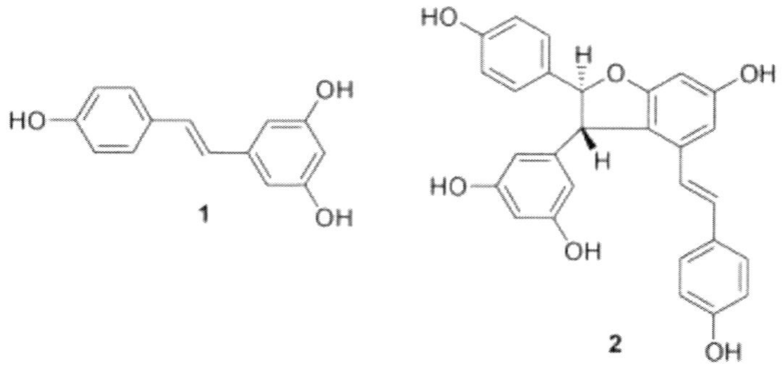

Figure 5. Structures of *trans*-resveratrol (1) and its dimer *trans*-ε-viniferin (2) in wine

La Torre et al. (2006) identified in Sicilian red wines twenty four phenolic compounds: gallic acid, protocatechuic acid, vanillic acid, syringic acid, caffeic acid, ferulic acid, *p*-coumaric acid, tyrosol, procyanidin B1, procyanidin B2, (+)-catechin, (-)-epicatechin, ethylgallate, rutin, isoquercitrin, isorhamnetin-3-O-glucoside, kaempferol-3-O-glucoside, myricetin, quercetin, kaempferol, isorhamnetin, rhamnetin, *trans*-resveratrol, *cis*-resveratrol, *trans*-piceid and *cis*-piceid.

USEFUL METHODS USED FOR THE DETERMINATION OF WINE ANTIOXIDANTS AND ANTIOXIDANT ACTIVITY

Preparation of Samples

From the grapes, juice was squeezed and from the solid remains, seeds and skins were separated. Immediately after pressing, juice was frozen and seeds and grapes lyophilized. Must was filtered through a course filter and frozen. Samples after lyophilization and stabilization in an exsiccator were ground in the laboratory mill and then extracted with 80% water ethanol in a Soxhlet apparatus for 20 hours. The weight of samples represented 6 – 10 g. Obtained extracts were placed in a 250 mL volumetric flask and adjusted with 80 % water ethanolic solution to the mark.

Determination of Total Polyphenol (TP) Content

For the determination of total polyphenols an adjusted method of Lachman et al. (1998) with Folin-Ciocalteau´s reagent was used. 1 mL of sample was pipetted into a 50 mL volumetric flask and diluted with distilled water. Then 2.5 mL of Folin-Ciocalteau's reagent was added and after agitation, 7.5 mL of 20% sodium carbonate solution was added. After 2 hours standing at laboratory temperature absorbance of samples was measured on the spectrophotometer Heλios γ (Spectronic Unicam, GB) at wavelength λ= 765 nm against a blank. Extract of seeds was diluted before measuring at a 1:50 ratio. Results were expressed as gallic acid (in mg/kg dry matter – DM and in the case of must mg/L fresh must, gallic acid Merck, Germany). Average results were obtained from three parallel determinations.

Determination of Resveratrol (RES) By HPLC

HPLC with isocratic elution on the chromatograph Waters^{TM} was used (pump Waters^{TM}, autosampler Waters^{TM} 717 plus, detector Waters^{TM} PDA 996 UV-VIS for the identification in UV and visible regions (Burns et al., 2000). A mixture of acetonitrile with water (75:25, V/V) as a mobile phase was used; its pH value was adjusted to 1.5 with trifluoracetic acid. Column ODS-Hypersil 250 x 4.6 mm, 5 µm was used, flow rate was 1 mL/ min. Detection was performed at wavelength λ = 307 nm. Before chromatographic analyses, samples were filtered through a Spartan 0.45 µm filter. As a standard *trans*-resveratrol of 99% purity (Sigma Aldrich®, USA) was used. Calibration range was 0.05-10 µg/mL, calibration linearity min. 0.05 – 10 µg/mL, detection limit 0.034 µg/mL and critical level of signal was 0.017 µg/mL.

DPPH Assay

DPPH decolorization was measured after the reaction of the sample with the free stable radical DPPH· according to Molyneux (2004). 2.5 mL of fresh methanolic solution DPPH$^{•}$ was transferred into plastic cuvettes 10 mm in length and absorbance at a wavelength of λ = 515 nm was measured. Absorbance at time t_0 ranged between 0.200 and 1.000 depending on the nature of the sample assayed. Then 5 µL of the sample was added and after stirring with a hand stirrer in cuvettes, the reaction mixture was left to stand for 5 minutes. The absorbance was again measured and the percentage of inactivation calculated from the decrease of absorbance according to the relation:

$$\% \text{ of inactivation} = 100-[(A_{t5}/A_{t0}) \times 100] \qquad (1)$$

The calibration curves of ascorbic acid (diluted in 13% ethanol V/V) were made for each DPPH absorbance at t_0.

ABTS Assay

The ABTS assay was performed according to the adjusted procedure of Pennycooke et al. (2005): 5 mM water stock solution of ABTS (25 mL) was prepared and 1 g of MnO_2 was added as an oxidizing agent (to produce activated $ABTS^{\bullet+}$ radical). The mixture was stirred and left for 20 min at room temperature. Afterwards the MnO_2 was removed by centrifugation and syringe-filter filtration (0.25 µm). The activated $ABTS^{\bullet+}$ stock solution was diluted in 5 mM phosphate buffer saline (pH 7.4) and adjusted to an absorbance ranging between 0.200 and 1.000, depending on the nature of the assayed sample. The absorbance in a plastic cuvette 10 mm in length at t_0 was recorded and an additional 10 µl of the sample was added, stirred and left to stand for 5 minutes. A decrease in absorption after 5 minutes was measured. The TAS was obtained as mentioned in formula (1) and standardized using the ABTS-ascorbic acid calibration curve for each starting (t_0) absorbance as mentioned above.

EFFECT OF RED WINE ON ANTIOXIDANT ACTIVITY OF BLOOD PLASMA OF *RATTUS NORVEGICUS* (WISTAR)

The French have a low level of coronary heart disease mortality in spite of high fat consumption; this epidemiological anomaly is known as the *"French Paradox"* and is commonly attributed to the consumption of red wine (Vinson et al., 2001). Moderate consumption of red wine has been associated with lowering the risk of developing coronary heart disease (Dell' Agli et al., 2004). Minussi et al. (2004) and De Beer et al. (2005) found a close relationship between total phenolic content and total antioxidant potential for wines, esp. red wines *in vitro*. Wine polyphenols could reinforce the endogenous antioxidant system and thereby diminish oxidative damage (Rodrigo et al., 2005). Cooke et al. (2005) found that anthocyanidins inhibited malignant cell survival. Studies in long-term models to understand the relationship between the bioavailability of polyphenols and their biological effects are still lacking. Šulc et al. (2006) assayed to prove the hypothesis that the AA of red wine from the Czech Republic (Blue Burgundy) is positively correlated with the AA of blood plasma in rats *in vivo*, after long-term wine consumption. From the results given in Table 1 and Fig. 6 it is evident that red wine increased antioxidant activity of blood plasma by approx. 6 – 12 % (with the exception of the first measuring). AA was highest at the beginning of the study and during the study gradually decreased. At P=0.05 statistically significant differences between the control and application groups were found. Both, red wine polyphenols and induction of plasma urate elevation could contribute to increase of plasma antioxidant capacity and thus involve two separate mechanisms in elevation of FRAP plasma values (Modun et al., 2008).

Table 1. Antioxidant activity (expressed as % of ABTS$^{\bullet+}$ solution decrease)

Group	Term of measurement*	Average	Minimum	Maximum	STD
Control	21	46.54	38.13	54.26	3.10
Experimental		38.62	23.40	43.87	3.10
Control	42	45.75	33.46	56.49	3.64
Experimental		54.29	45.05	59.70	2.94
Control	63	36.68	29.62	44.25	2.77
Experimental		42.32	36.36	47.86	1.92
Control	84	32.21	26.89	35.31	1.53
Experimental		38.61	35.27	41.91	1.40

* Days after start of experiment

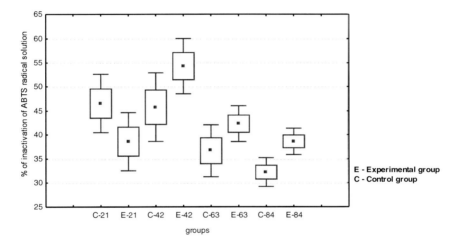

Figure 6. Box diagram of antioxidant activity of blood plasma (related to Table 1)

RELATIONSHIP BETWEEN ANTIOXIDANT ACTIVITY, POLYPHENOLIC ANTIOXIDANTS AND RESVERATROL IN GRAPE MUSTS, SKINS AND SEEDS

Šulc et al. (2005a) analyzed 25 samples of grape must, skins and seeds (Table 2). The average determined TP content was the highest in seeds (536.6 mg/g DM); lesser concentrations were found in must (273.1 mg/L) and skins (165.9 mg/g DM). Seeds contained 3.2 times more TP than grape skins. This is in agreement with the results of Yildirim et al. (2005), who found that concentrations of gallic acid, monomeric catechin, and epicatechin were lower in the winery by-product grape skins than in the seeds. Negro et al. (2003) also confirmed that grape seeds contained the highest quantities of proanthocyanidins. The condensed tannins are considered superior antioxidants as their potential oxidation may lead to oligomerisation via phenol coupling and enlargement of the number of reactive sites (Bors and Michel, 2002). However, Kammerer et al. (2004) evaluated grape skins as rich sources of anthocyanins, hydroxycinnamic acids, flavanols, and flavonol glycosides, whereas flavanols were major constituents present in the seeds. Especially dimeric, trimeric, oligomeric, or polymeric procyanidins account for most of the superior antioxidant capacity of grape seeds (Yilmaz and Toledo, 2004b). Contrary to TP the highest RES content was found in the grape skins and its levels were higher in comparison with the seeds apparently due to relation with the *Botrytis* infestation (Frémont, 2000). Free *trans*-resvetratrol in the musts was contained mainly below the detectable limit. In agreement with Nikfardjam et al. (2006a), our results show that *trans*-resveratrol content is mainly dependent on variety and vintage year.

Statistical analysis of variance of obtained results (Tables 3, 4) did not reveal any statistically significant differences between the vineyard regions and varieties in total polyphenol content in grape skins and seeds and between TP and AA in grape skins (Fig. 7). Regarding the vineyard regions only the highest TP content was measured in the samples from the Velké Žernoseky wine growing-area (858 mg/g DM grape seeds) and Karlštejn (426.4 mg/g DM grape seeds and 412.8 mg/L must). Peña-Neira et al. (2000) by multivariate analysis applied to the phenol compounds found both qualitative and quantitative differences in polyphenolic antioxidants of red and white Spanish wines of different geographical origin.

As expected, we can confirm significant varietal differences and differences between the blue and white grape varieties. All average TP contents were higher in the blue varieties (282.7 mg/g DM in grape skins, 546.3 mg/g DM in seeds and 326.7 mg/L in must) when compared with the white varieties (149.6 mg/g DM in skins, 531.2 mg/g DM in seeds and 242.9 mg/L in must). The blue grape varieties have 1.89 times higher TP content in grape skins and 1.35 times higher in must as compared with the white grape varieties, whereas the content in seeds was practically the same. These results are in full accordance with the results of Peña-Neira et al. (2000) and Cantos et al. (2002). The highest TP contents were found in the blue Zweigeltrebe from the Most vineyard area (Table 2). Higher TP contents were found in the blue grape varieties Alibernet and St. Laurent. On the contrary, lower TP contents were found out in the white grape varieties such as Rhine (White) Riesling, Müller-Thurgau, Kerner, Hibernal, and Green Sylvaner.

AA was measured in grape skins and seeds (Table 2). It follows from the results that AA expressed in ascorbic acid equivalents (EQA, mg/mL) was higher in grape skins of the white grape varieties (0.271 EQA) in comparison with the blue varieties (0.187 EQA), while in seeds the results were reciprocal (1.032 EQA in the blue varieties and 0.841 EQA in the white varieties, Fig. 8). Regarding these results, it could be concluded that anthocyanins contained mainly in blue varieties contribute to AA only to a lesser extent. Arnous et al. (2001) found that total flavanols contributed to hydroxyl free radical scavenging efficacy and to a lesser extent to antiradical and reducing ability, whereas there was a less significant relationship between the antioxidant properties and the total phenolics and only a weak relationship to total anthocyanin content. Kallithraka et al. (2005) also revealed a low and statistically insignificant correlation ($r^2=0.0724$, $p<0.05$) between antiradical activity and total anthocyanin content. Thus, AA will be dependent on special phenolics content, esp. in seeds (Fig. 8). The highest EQA values were found in Müller-Thurgau from the Karlštejn vineyard area (2.436 EQA in seeds, 0.440 EQA in grape skins), Blue Portugal (2.223 EQA in seeds from Kutná Hora and 1.799 EQA in seeds and 0.433 EQA in grape skins from Velké Žernoseky), White Chrupka (1.852 EQA in seeds and 0.482 EQA in grape skins from Kutná Hora) and St. Laurent (1.053 EQA in seeds from Roudnice nad Labem and 0.914 EQA from

Velké Žernoseky). Durak et al. (1999) found that red wine, white wine and grape juices were characterized by strong antioxidant activity in a similar way. Also Dávalos et al. (2005) confirm grape juice and wine vinegar as good dietary sources of antioxidants. The ORAC-FL values varied from 4.6 to 25.0 µmol of Trolox equivalents/mL for red grape juices, from 3.5 to 11.1 µmol of Trolox equivalents/mL for white grape juices, and from 4.5 to 11.5 µmol of Trolox equivalents/mL for wine vinegars. Differences in the antioxidant activities among grape juice, wine, and vinegar were attributed to their different phenol contents and compositions.

In Fig. 9 we compared AA of tannin >> gallic acid > ascorbic acid. This is in good accordance with the hypothesis of Bors and Michel (2002) that the condensed tannins are considered superior antioxidants as their eventual oxidation may lead to oligomerization via phenol coupling and enlargement of the number of reactive sites. In addition, gallic acid, monomeric catechin, and epicatechin – three major phenol constituents of grape seeds – contribute to antioxidant capacity in a greater deal (Yilmaz and Toledo, 2004b). Peroxyl radical scavenging activities of phenolics present in grape seeds or skins in decreasing order were resveratrol > catechin > epicatechin and gallocatechin > gallic acid and ellagic acid. Thus, functional ingredients of grape seeds – monomeric flavanols (catechin and epicatechin), dimeric, trimeric and polymeric procyanidins and condensed tannins, and phenol acids (gallic acid and ellagic acid) seem to be major contributors to antioxidant and antiradical activity (Yilmaz and Toledo, 2004b). In addition, resveratrol has stronger ability to inhibit lipid peroxidation as compared with other antioxidants: resveratrol > propyl gallate > tripolyphosphate > vanillin > phenol > butylated hydroxytoluene > α-tocopherol (Murcia and Martinez-Tome, 2001). De Beer et al. (2006) by analyzing of 139 Pinotage wines (2002 and 2003 vintages) suggest that synergy between phenol compounds does play a role in the wine TAC (16-23% synergic antioxidant activity).

Antioxidant and vasodilatation activity is correlated with the total phenol content and is especially associated with the content of gallic acid, resveratrol and catechin (Burns et al., 2000). Bartolomé et al. (2004), Dugo et al. (2003), and Karakaya et al. (2001) reported that total antioxidant activities of foods were well correlated with total phenols (r^2=0.95). Also Guendez et al. (2005) after the assessment of the *in vitro* antiradical activity employing the stable radical DPPH• showed that there is a significant correlation with total polyphenol content (r^2=0.6499, $P<0.01$), but the most effective was shown to be procyanidin in grape seed extracts (r^2 = 0.7934, $P<0.002$). Munoz-Espada et al. (2004) and Sanchez et al. (2003) found a relatively high correlation in red wine between oxygen radical absorbance capacity and malvidin glucosides (r^2=0.75, $P<0.10$), and proanthocyanidins (r^2=0.87, $P<0.05$) and white wines trimeric proanthocynidin fraction (r^2=0.86, $P<0.10$). In contrast to these studies Zafrilla et al. (2003) did not find a significant relationship between the total concentrations of phenol compounds in conventional and ecological red and white wines and the antioxidant activity ($p>0.05$). In red wines, no significant differences were observed in the antioxidant activity of ecological and conventional red wine ($p=0.28$), while in white wine significant differences were observed in the antioxidant activity between conventional and ecological wine ($p=0.006$).

Table 2. TP content in the grape skins, seeds and musts (in mg/g DM or mg/L in musts) and AA (in % of inactivation) or AA* (in EQA mg/mL) in the grape skins and seeds of analyzed varieties from five Czech vineyard areas

Variety	Grape skin TP	AA [%]	AA*	Seeds TP	AA [%]	AA*	Must TP [mg/L]
ROUDNICE NAD LABEM VINEYARD AREA							
Kerner[W]	38.6 ± 0.3	5.49 ± 0.15	0.213	475.0 ± 0.9	18.92 ± 0.12	0.642	590.0 ± 2.1
Müller-Thurgau[W]	43.4 ± 1.7	4.19 ± 0.32	0.171	538.7 ± 2.1	23.15 ± 1.03	0.777	212.1 ± 1.0
Rhine (White) Riesling[W]	86.3 ± 0.4	3.73 ± 0.18	0.156	515.3 ± 1.5	25.44 ± 0.28	0.851	187.1 ± 0.9
Green Sylvaner[W]	44.4 ± 0.5	7.16 ± 0.11	0.266	575.5 ± 2.3	22.97 ± 0.21	0.771	93.8 ± 1.3
Blue Portugal[B]	161.5 ± 1.3	2.59 ± 0.20	0.120	525.7 ± 2.2	21.51 ± 0.25	0.726	124.5 ± 1.2
St. Laurent[B]	488.5 ± 1.4	3.76 ± 0.31	0.157	666.6 ± 3.1	31.73 ± 0.12	1.053	140.3 ± 1.9
KARLŠTEJN VINEYARD AREA							
Hibernal[W]	42.4 ± 0.9	6.13 ± 0.32	0.233	553.1 ± 3.2	19.42 ± 1.02	0.658	193.1 ± 1.7
Bianca[W]	158.6 ± 1.5	6.49 ± 0.13	0.245	529.0 ± 3.5	17.88 ± 0.45	0.607	217.2 ± 1.5
Müller-Thurgau[W]	31.5 ± 1.7	12.57 ± 0.51	0.440	426.4 ± 2.4	74.91 ± 0.51	2.436	412.8 ± 2.5
KUTNÁ HORA VINEYARD AREA							
Müller-Thurgau[W]	49.1 ± 1.2	8.52 ± 0.20	0.310	385.1 ± 1.7	11.00 ± 0.21	0.390	326.8 ± 3.1
White – Chrupka[W]	162.5 ± 2.1	13.90 ± 1.02	0.482	426.9 ± 5.3	56.66 ± 0.78	1.852	591.5 ± 1.8
Traminer[W]	133.9 ± 2.3	3.39 ± 0.10	0.145	484.6 ± 2.8	16.05 ± 0.09	0.549	107.9 ± 0.9
Blue Portugal (Blauer Portugieser)[B]	206.0 ± 1.3	4.51 ± 0.20	0.181	420.8 ± 3.1	68.24 ± 0.33	2.223	346.3 ± 1.2
Blue Burgundy (Blauburgunder, Pinot Noir)[B]	72.0 ± 0.8	1.28 ± 0.17	0.078	558.3 ± 3.2	21.53 ± 0.25	0.727	147.5 ± 1.8

Table 2. Continued

Variety	Grape skin TP	AA [%]	AA*	Seeds TP	AA [%]	AA*	Must TP [mg/L]	AA*
MOST VINEYARD AREA								
Müller-Thurgau[W]	69.6 ± 0.9	8.87 ± 0.11	0.321	471.6 ± 1.5	14.99 ± 0.21	0.514	171.9 ± 0.8	
White Burgundy[W]	34.1 ± 0.5	4.04 ± 0.15	0.166	453.8 ± 3.2	21.65 ± 0.18	0.728	146.5 ± 0.7	
Red Traminer (Roter Traminer)[W]	389.1 ± 3.1	18.02 ± 0.78	0.614	440.9 ± 2.5	16.94 ± 0.22	0.577	128.1 ± 0.9	
Blue Franken (Lemberger, Blaufränkisch)[B]	318.6 ± 2.8	1.23 ± 0.03	0.076	513.3 ± 3.7	11.16 ± 0.15	0.391	299.6 ± 1.0	
Zweigeltrebe[B]	615.1 ± 3.8	4.19 ± 0.08	0.171	573.2 ± 3.7	28.14 ± 0.54	0.937	357.8 ± 2.1	
Alibernet[B]	400.9 ± 1.7	8.87 ± 0.10	0.321	737.9 ± 4.2	14.93 ± 0.23	0.514	874.3 ± 1.5	
VELKÉ ŽERNOSEKY VINEYARD AREA								
Müller-Thurgau[W]	53.4 ± 0.7	2.44 ± 0.07	0.115	858.0 ± 5.1	21.29 ± 0.32	0.718	164.1 ± 1.4	
White Burgundy[W]	234.1 ± 1.6	6.38 ± 0.13	0.241	502.6 ± 4.3	20.94 ± 0.27	0.706	142.3 ± 1.1	
Rhine (White) Riesling[W]	31.9 ± 0.9	5.56 ± 0.08	0.215	862.8 ± 5.0	20.08 ± 0.18	0.678	200.9 ± 2.0	
Blue Portugal (Blauer Portugieser)[B]	63.3 ± 0.8	12.36 ± 0.21	0.433	341.4 ± 2.7	55.03 ± 0.62	1.799	253.9 ± 1.9	
St. Laurent[B]	218.7 ± 1.7	3.50 ± 0.08	0.149	579.5 ± 3.4	27.41 ± 0.50	0.914	396.3 ± 1.8	
Average value of 25 samples	165.9 ± 1.44	6.37 ± 0.23	0.241	536.6 ± 3.1	27.21 ± 0.36	0.910	273.1 ± 1.5	

[W] white, [B] blue

Table 3. Analysis of variance of the content of total polyphenols

Grape part	Source of variability	P-values	Significance
Grape skins	vineyard area	0.056704	*
	variety	0.292673	-
Grape seeds	vineyard area	0.591718	-
	variety	0.757813	-

Table 4. Analysis of variance of antioxidant activity

Grape part	Source of variability	P-values	Significance
Grape skins	vineyard area	0.691572	-
	variety	0.828411	-
Grape seeds	vineyard area	0.433584	-
	variety	0.818846	-

* Significant differences ($P < 0.10$)

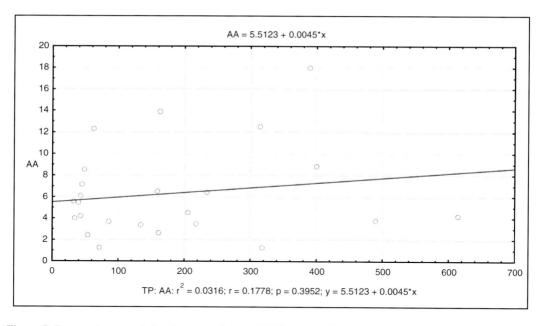

Figure 7. Regression correlation between AA and TP in grape skins

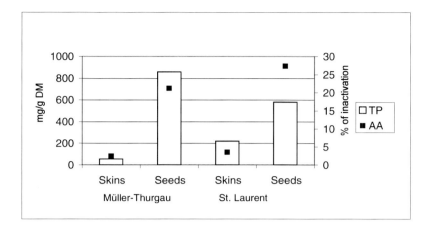

Figure 8. Relationship between TP and AA in V. Žernoseky vineyard area

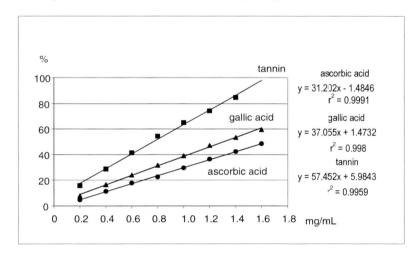

Figure 9. Antioxidant activity of standard grape constituents and ascorbic acid at different concentrations

FACTORS INFLUENCING LEVELS OF MAJOR ANTIOXIDANTS AND ANTIOXIDANT ACTIVITY IN GRAPES AND WINES

Effect of Grape/Vine Varieties and Cultivars

As Lachman et al. (2004) determined grape must contained relatively high content of total polyphenols (Table 5). White varieties contained lesser average amounts (213 mg/L) in comparison with blue varieties (306 mg/L). Average TP content varied from 173 mg/L to 254 mg/L in white varieties and 166 mg/L to 447 mg/L in blue varieties in the years 2001 and 2002. Average TP content in the year 2001 was 171 mg/L, in the year 2002 324 mg/L. Among analyzed blue grape varieties (Fig. 10), the highest amount was determined in cv. Royal (587 mg/L in the year 2002, average content 427 mg/L); lesser contents were found for

Blue Burgundy (av. 231 mg/L) and St. Laurent (236 mg/L). Significantly lesser contents were found in white varieties – the highest content is characteristic for Muscat Ottonel (av. 267 mg/L), the lowest one in Bacchus (116 mg/L) and Early Red Veltliner (160 mg/L).

The highest TP content was determined in the seeds (99.45 g/kg DM), higher in the year 2002 (107.4 g/kg DM) in comparison with the year 2001 (91.45 g/kg DM). Higher content was determined in blue varieties (110.8 g/kg DM) as compared with white varieties (93.44 g/kg DM). The highest content was found in the Blue Burgundy variety (120.5 g/kg DM), while lower amounts were found in Zweigeltrebe (101.2 g/kg DM) and St. Laurent (107.3 g/kg DM). Among white varieties the highest content was found in the seeds of cv. Aurelius (112.2 g/kg DM), the lowest one in cv. Kerner (72.92 g/kg DM). Average year content was higher in the year 2002 (15.6 g/kg DM) in comparison with the year 2001 (7.47 g/kg DM).

TP content in skins was in comparison with the seeds lesser, on av. 11.54 g/kg DM. Higher contents were found again in blue varieties (av. 18.13 g/kg DM) than in white varieties (av. 7.9 g/kg DM). Higher contents were found in the year 2002 (15.6 g/kg DM) than in the year 2001 (7.47 g/kg DM). The highest values were shown in cv. Zweigeltrebe (20.95 g/kg DM) and cv. Royal (19.2 g/kg DM). Among white varieties, the richest were Green Veltliner (10.49 g/kg DM) and Muscat Ottonel (10.44 g/kg DM). The lowest level was found in cv. Bacchus (4.14 g/kg DM in 2001) and Early Red Veltliner (5.52 g/kg DM).

Gonzáles-Nevez et al. (2004) evaluated in 2001 and 2002 the phenol potential of Tannat, Cabernet-Sauvignon and Merlot grapes and its correspondence with the color and composition of the respective wines. Tannat grapes presented anthocyanin and total polyphenols contents significantly higher in both years. Therefore, wines from this variety presented color intensity and phenol contents statistically higher than Cabernet-Sauvignon and Merlot. The correlations between the phenol contents of the grapes, skins, musts and wines were very significant. Color intensity and phenol contents of the wines were highly correlated with the total polyphenols of the grapes and with anthocyanins of the grapes, skins, musts and wines. Orak (2007) determined in sixteen red grape cultivars stronger correlation between antioxidant activity and total polyphenol content than antioxidant activity and total anthocyanins.

In grape musts, *trans*-resveratrol content was very low with the highest concentration in the blue varieties Royal and St. Laurent in the year 2002. Frémont (2000) found *trans*-resveratrol in red wines in concentrations that generally ranged between 0.1 and 15 mg/L. Romero-Pérez et al. (1996) have reported results of authors, who quantified the four monomeric forms of resveratrol in white wines of various origin. They found between 0.05 and 1.8 mg/L of total stilbenes. The mean values were aglycone, 0.13 (*trans*-) and 0.06 (*cis*-), piceid, 0.16 (*trans*-) and 0.12 (*cis*-). In rosé wines, the levels of resveratrol monomers were between levels in white and red wines. The maceration time with skin but also varietals' differences in the types of grapes used influence the resveratrol content of wine. Kolouchová-Hanzlíková et al. (2004) found the concentrations of *trans*-resveratrol in the Czech red wines from different vineyard regions ranging between 1.035 mg/L (St. Laurent, Mostecká vineyard region, 1998) to 6.253 mg/L (Pinot Noir, Roudnická vineyard, 1998), and *cis*-resveratrol between 0.683 mg/L (Blaufrankisch, Mutěnická vineyard, 1986) and 2.806 mg/L (Pinot Noir, Roudnická vineyard, 1998). In grape berries the contents of *trans*-resveratrol ranged more widely (0.201 – 5.841 mg/L); the highest contents were found in leaves (1.462 - 44.32 mg/L) and rachis (6.041 - 440.1 mg/L). Red wines featured higher *trans*-resveratrol content (av. 4.653 mg/L) compared to white wines (1.216 mg/L). Gürbüz et al. (2007) determined that wine samples from Turkey contained higher phenolics and *trans*-resveratrol levels than the corresponding musts. White wines and musts contained lower concentrations of phenolics than red wines and musts. Within the red wine and must cultivars, Boğazkere, Öküzgozü, and Cabernet contained the highest concentrations of flavan-3-ols and *trans*-resveratrol. Significantly higher amounts of total phenols, flavonoids and antioxidant activities in red wines compared to white wines were demonstrated elsewhere, e.g. in selected wines produced in the northeast of Thailand (Woraratphoka et al., 2007) or in white, rosé and red commercial *Terras Madeirenses* Portuguese wines from Madeira Island (Paixão et al., 2007).

From the statistical variance analysis, significant differences ($p<0.05$) were found between vintages for total polyphenols. Also between total polyphenol content in grape skins and seeds and between variety and the part of the plant significant differences were proved. Some varieties differed significantly from each other (Table 6). For the *trans*-resveratrol content vintages were significantly different – skins and seeds and vintage and the part of the plant. In *trans*-resveratrol content in the skins and the seeds, no statistical differences among varieties were found.

All analyzed varieties were cultivated at the Research Viticulture Station in Karlštejn under the same conditions of microclimate, soil and cultivation procedures. The blue varieties contained higher amounts of polyphenolic compounds in comparison with the white varieties due to enhanced biosynthesis of colorants and condensed tannins, which is in good correlation with the results of Cantos et al. (2002), Chicon et al. (2002), De Beer et al. (2003), Uhlig and Clingeleffer (1998). As determined by Makris et al. (2003), the total polyphenol concentration is principally correlated with the antioxidant potency and the antiradical activity. Also Borbalan et al. (2003) confirm a good correlation between the total polyphenol content and antioxidant power.

Obtained results also proved the effect of vintage. In the year 2001 lower TP levels were estimated in comparison with the year 2002. It could be correlated with an extraordinarily warm year in 2002 ($\Delta t = +1.7\ ^0C$) in comparison with the year 2001 ($\Delta t = +0.9\ ^0C$). Both years could be evaluated as humid. Zoecklein et al. (1998) illustrate the affect of microclimate manipulation on phenol-free grape glycosides. Higher TP levels in the year 2002 are in accordance with the results of Uhlig (1998) that total polyphenol concentrations in berry skin were higher in sun-exposed grapes. Also increased vine water deficit causes small increases in anthocyanins and decreases in flavonols (Kennedy et al., 2002).

The effect of an attack with *Botrytis cinerea* as a biotic stress factor (Montero et al., 2003) influenced apparently higher content in the year 2001. Lesser content in the skins in comparison with the seeds could be caused by its metabolization (Adrian et al. 1998) and the fact that only free *trans*-resveratrol was determined. Higher levels of *trans*-resveratrol were found in blue varieties as compared with white ones (Bianchini and Vainio, 2003), because resveratrol is more sensitive to oxidation in white musts (Castellari et al., 1998). Some statistically significant differences were found between some varieties, esp. Blue Burgundy x Bacchus, Royal, Kerner, Welschriesling and Kerner x Royal, St. Laurent, Zweigeltrebe and Royal x Welschriesling. Very low levels of *trans*-resveratrol in musts could be correlated with the activity of isoenzyme B_5, whose activity is the highest at pH 3.0 – 4.0 (Morales et al., 1997) and with the average pH values in our samples 3.18 (2001) and 3.33 (2002). Abril et al. (2005) evaluated concentrations of *trans*- and *cis*-resveratrol isomers of 98 commercial wines of the four designations of origin, from several vintages, and found concentration of *trans*-

resveratrol ranging from 0.32 to 4.44 mg/L in red wines and from 0.12 to 2.80 mg/L in rosé wines. The grape variety influenced resveratrol contents in wines from the different regions – the highest *trans/cis* ratios were found in Somontano (4.50) and Calatayud wines (2.90), both of the Tempranillo variety. However, a discriminant analysis applied to the concentrations did not show significant differences between young red wines or between rosé wines of the four designations of origin. Kallithraka et al. (2001) applied an improved method for resveratrol determination in 29 red Greek wines of appellation of origin; the concentrations found varied between 0.550 and 2.534 mg/L with the highest concentration for the grape variety Mandilaria.

Table 5. Content of total polyphenols in grape must, skins and seeds

WHITE VARIETIES	Grape must [g/L]		Grape skins [g/kg DM]			Grape seeds [g/kg DM]	
	2001	2002	2001	2002	Average	2001	2002
Aurelius	0.174	0.302	3.19	10.16	6.675	90.49	133.9
Bacchus	0.116	nd	4.14	nd	4.140	75.56	nd
Kerner	0.116	0.390	2.98	8.98	5.980	67.40	78.4
Muscat Ottonel	0.268	0.266	6.98	13.90	10.440	85.04	102.2
Welschriesling	0.344	0.132	6.40	11.90	9.150	76.99	78.9
Green Sylvaner	0.059	0.338	7.74	7.80	7.770	98.71	105.8
Green Veltliner	0.232	0.104	10.20	10.78	10.490	94.88	114.0
Early Red Veltliner	0.074	0.245	3.57	7.47	5.520	86.95	103.9
BLUE VARIETIES	Grape must [g/L]		Grape skins [g/kg DM]			Grape seeds [g/kg DM]	
	2001	2002	2001	2002	Average	2001	2002
Royal	0.267	0.587	14.30	24.09	19.20	98.8	129.6
Blue Burgundy	0.114	0.348	8.57	20.42	14.50	124.1	116.8
St. Laurent	0.086	0.385	10.52	25.25	17.89	107.9	106.7
Zweigeltrebe	0.196	0.468	11.02	30.87	20.95	90.6	111.8

nd – non determined in the year 2002 due to grape bunch atrophy

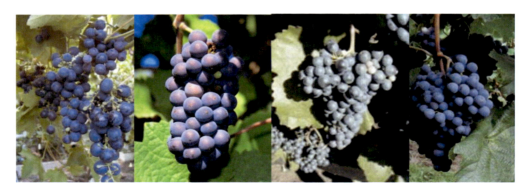

Figure 10. Blue grape varieties Royal, Blue Burgundy (Pinot Noir), St. Laurent and Zweigeltrebe

Table 6. T-test (for α=0.05) for varieties in total polyphenol content

VARIETY	Aurelius	Bacchus	Blue Burgundy	Kerner	Muscat Ottonel	Royal	Welschriesling	St. Laurent	Green Sylvaner	Early Red Veltliner	Green Veltliner	Zweigeltrebe
Aurelius	-	0.223177	0.939049	0.059593	0.964526	0.968896	0.230564	0.999977	0.999472	0.886194	1.000000	1.000000
Bacchus	0.223177	-	*0.023086	1.000000	0.807730	*0.029379	0.999986	0.097075	0.551503	0.905524	0.349346	0.147449
Blue Burgundy	0.939049	*0.023086	-	*0.002865	0.260512	1.000000	*0.013573	0.998703	0.543985	0.162766	0.800346	0.987315
Kerner	0.059593	1.000000	*0.002865	-	0.531049	*0.003858	0.999727	*0.018400	0.251814	0.701286	0.117864	*0.032821
Muscat Ottonel	0.964526	0.807730	0.260730	0.531049	-	0.323791	0.917146	0.745939	0.999987	1.000000	0.996644	0.880733
Royal	0.968896	*0.029379	1.000000	*0.003858	0.323791	-	*0.018563	0.999741	0.630770	0.207827	0.866668	0.995519
Welschriesling	0.230564	0.999986	*0.013753	0.999727	0.917146	*0.018563	-	0.082452	0.652498	0.977956	0.393430	0.138650
St. Laurent	0.999977	0.097075	0.998703	*0.018400	0.745939	0.999741	0.082452	-	0.958214	0.578276	0.997861	1.000000
Green Sylvaner	0.999472	0.551503	0.543985	0.251814	0.999987	0.630770	0.652498	0.958214	-	0.999283	0.999998	0.991978
Early Red Veltliner	0.886194	0.905524	0.162766	0.701286	1.000000	0.207827	0.977956	0.578276	0.999283	-	0.976114	0.744346
Green Veltliner	1.000000	0.349346	0.800346	0.117864	0.996644	0.866668	0.393430	0.997861	0.999998	0.976114	-	0.999920
Zweigeltrebe	1.000000	0.147449	0.987315	*0.032821	0.880733	0.995519	0.138650	1.000000	0.991978	0.744346	0.999920	-

* statistical significant level at $P<0.05$

Effect of Growing Locations (Altitude, Soil) and Climatic Conditions (Temperature, Sum of Precipitation, Vintage Years) on Major Grape and Wine Antioxidants and Antioxidant Activity

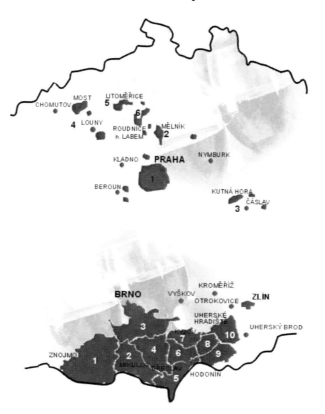

Figure 11. Wine growing sub-regions and locations in Bohemia and Moravia (Rejlová, 2007)

Faitová et al. (2004) using the spectrophotometric method determined in white Riesling from different vineyard subregions (Fig. 11, Table 7), kinds of wine (Table 8), vintages (Table 9) the content of total polyphenols (TP) and that of *trans*-resveratrol (RES) by the HPLC method. The TP content was presented as gallic acid equivalent per liter of wine, and the content of RES as *trans*-resveratrol per liter of wine (Table 7). TP values in the vineyard region of Bohemia ranged from 223.0 to 532.7 mg/L (average content 330.3 mg/L), and were higher than in the vineyard region of Moravia from 175.0 to 465.0 mg/L (average content 271.7 mg/L). RES values in the vineyard region of Bohemia ranged from < 0.033 to 0.421 mg/L (average content 0.117 mg/L), in the vineyard region of Moravia from < 0.033 to 0.875 mg/L (average content 0.123 mg/L). The highest average TP content (370.1 mg/L) and RES content (0.262 mg/L) were found in the sub-region Roudnická (the vineyard region of Bohemia). The harvest year of 1994 was evaluated as that providing the highest average levels of TP (386.5 mg/L) and RES (0.201 mg/L). The kind of wine with the highest average TP was the kind of "selected grapes" (327.2 mg/L), while the highest average RES content was found in the late harvest wine (0.141 mg/L). The differences in RES and TP contents affected by vintage years, vineyard sub-region or the kind of wine were not significant, and as the statistically significant correlation between TP and RES contents was not demonstrated

(5.73%). However, Dadáková et al. (2003) found increased concentrations of free and conjugated quercetin in Moravian red wines in 2000, which could be a consequence of a longer sunshine period in that year.

Table 7. Content of (TP) and (RES) in white Riesling related to the vineyard sub-regions (the first part of table is the vineyard region of Moravia and the second part of the table is the vineyard region of Bohemia)

Vineyard sub-regions	Frequency	Average (TP) content [mg/L]	Range of (TP) content [mg/L]	Average (RES) content [mg/L]	Range of (RES) content [mg/L]
Brněnská	1	-	265.0	-	0.045
Bzenecká	3	264.62	261.1 – 269.5	0.086	< 0.033 - 0.169
Kyjovská	1	-	243.4	-	0.004
Mikulovská	13	258.5	175.0 – 371.8	0.144	< 0.033 – 0.875
Mutěnická	9	238.7	171.7 – 288.3	0.132	< 0.033 – 0.447
Podluží	3	266.0	226.3 – 328.1	0.063	0.044 – 0.095
Strážnická	3	277.1	241.7 – 315.5	0.113	0.077 – 0.161
Uherskohradišťská	1	-	280.6	-	0.072
Velkopavlovická	6	298.9	212.1 - 465.0	0.145	0.038 – 0.185
Znojemská	12	263.1	171.7 – 358.0	0.149	< 0.033 – 0.466
Mělnická	7	305.1	223.0 – 443.8	0.092	< 0.033 – 0.145
Mostecká	1	-	353.5	-	-
Pražská	1	-	378.4	-	0.185
Roudnická	4	370.1	282.6 – 532.7	0.262	0.050 – 0.421
Žernosecká	6	321.3	245.0 – 392.0	0.051	< 0.033 – 0.070
Vineyard region of Bohemia	19	330.3	223.0 – 532.7	0.115	< 0.033 – 0.421
Vineyard region of Moravia	57	271.7	175.0 – 465.0	0.121	< 0.033 – 0.875

< 0.033 – below range of detection

Table 8. (TP) content and (RES) content in white Riesling related to the type of wine

Type of wine	Frequency	Range of (TP) content [mg/L]	Average (TP) content [mg/L]	Range of (RES) content [mg/L]	Average (RES) content [mg/L]
Quality wine	27	197.7 – 465.0	272.4	< 0.033 – 0.466	0.123
Late harvest	29	175.0 – 362.1	264.7	< 0.033 – 0.875	0.128
Archive	7	243.4 – 532.7	321.6	0.044 – 0.421	0.141
Cabinet wine	11	193.6 – 443.8	300.3	< 0.033 – 0.242	0.102
Selected grapes	2	282.6 – 371.8	327.2	0.050 – 0.090	0.070
Average	76	175.0 – 532.7	279.5	< 0.033 – 0.875	0.122

< 0.033 – below range of detection

Table 9. (TP) content and (RES) content in white Riesling related to vintage years

Vintage	Frequency	Range of (TP) content [mg/L]	Average (TP) content [mg/L]	Range of (RES) content [mg/L]	Average (RES) content [mg/L]
2002	7	171.7 – 394.5	267.1	< 0.033 – 0.144	0.076
2001	16	175.0 – 465.0	267.2	< 0.033 – 0.242	0.096
2000	23	171.7 – 443.8	293.7	< 0.033 – 0.875	0.135
1999	14	215.3 – 334.8	260.3	< 0.033 – 0.358	0.125
1998	6	188.8 – 370.2	281.3	0.057 – 0.218	0.156
1997	1	255.1	-	0.123	-
1996	1	201.2	-	0.075	-
1994	3	235.2 – 532.7	386.5	0.070 – 0.421	0.201
1990	1	243.4	-	0.162	-
1989	1	279.0	-	0.136	-
1985	1	349.0	-	0.057	-
Average	76	175.0 – 532.7	279.5	< 0.033 – 0.875	0.122

< 0.033 – below range of detection

Statistical analysis of variance of results of Šulc et al. (2005) (Table 3) revealed statistically significant differences among vineyard regions and varieties in total polyphenol content in grape skins at the level of statistic significance $p<0.05$. The variety Müller-Thurgau statistically differed regarding the vineyard area (Figs. 12, 13). Peña-Neira et al. (2000) by multivariate analysis applied to the phenol compounds found both qualitative and quantitative differences in polyphenolic antioxidants of red and white Spanish wines of different geographical origin. La Torre et al. (2006) identified and determined twenty-four phenol compounds in twenty-two different commercial Sicilian red wines using an HPLC with PDA detector coupled on-line with a MS system. The data on the levels of all the phenol compounds in the red Sicilian commercial wines showed that the wine samples from Merlot grapes generally had the highest phenol compounds content. In all our commercial wine samples, the predominant phenol constituents was gallic acid (mean value 86.23 mg/L in Merlot wines; 62.90 mg/L in Nero d´Avola wines and 74.53 mg/L in wines from allochthonous grapes) and procyanidin B1 (mean value 76.87 mg/L in Merlot wines; 43.17 mg/L in Nero d´Avola wines and 60.03 mg/L in wines from allochthonous grapes). Kallithraka et al. (2006) suggested some of the unexploited rare native Greek varieties (e.g. Karvouniaris, Thrapsa, Nerostafilo, Bakouri, Vertzami) contained appreciable amounts of non-colored phenols as well as anthocyanins as worthy of use for the production of quality wines. Furthermore, the antioxidant efficiency of red wines tested appears to be largely influenced by the proanthocyanidin level, with anthocyanins playing a minor role (Cimino et al., 2007). Similarly Goldberg et al. (1995) using a solid-phase extraction followed by direct-injection gas chromatography-mass spectrometry, measured the concentration of *trans*-resveratrol in a representative selection of wines from most of the prominent wine-producing countries and regions. High concentrations were measured in wines from Pinot Noir, irrespective of origin, but, on the other hand, Cabernet Sauvignon wines showed a wide range of concentrations, with relatively high values in those from cool-climate countries (Ontario, Bordeaux regions), whereas such wines from warmer climates (California, South America, and Australia) tended to have much lower concentrations. Kallithraka et al. (2001) determined that the red wines produced by grape varieties grown in the Greek islands (Rhodes, Crete and Paros) were richer in *trans*-resveratrol. In comparison with wines made from grapes grown in foreign countries, Greek wines had a much higher *trans*-resveratrol content than the Japanese wines (0.08–0.244 mg/L). It is noticeable however, that the concentration of the phytoalexin *trans*-resveratrol may vary considerably, since this substance is produced by grape berries as a response to fungal infection and UV irradiation. The results obtained by Sakkiadi et al. (2001) reflect previous reports on other southern European wines (Italian, Spanish and Portuguese) and support the conclusion that relatively low *trans*-resveratrol concentrations are present in Mediterranean wines. The results indicate that a novel clone of Xinomavro variety produced wine is the richest in phenol antioxidants among the traditional and new varieties cultivated in Greece. Californian wines made from Cabernet Sauvignon were also lower than the Greek wines in *trans*-resveratrol level 0.46–0.74 mg/L, 0.002 mg/L; 0.05 to 0.09 mg/L. However Californian wines made from blended varieties showed a higher *trans*-resveratrol content (2.74–5.77 mg/L). The richest California variety was Pinot Noir containing from 3.72 to 7.99 mg/L *trans*-resveratrol. Portuguese red wines had a similar *trans*-resveratrol content to the Greek wines (average values 1.0 mg/L for monovarietal and 1.5 mg/l for blended wines, whereas French (3 mg/L) and Spanish wines (5.13 mg/L from Pinot Noir grape varieties, 3.99 mg/L from Merlot and 2.43 mg/L from Grenache) were higher in *trans*-resveratrol level. However, Spanish wines made from Cabernet Sauvignon (1.42 mg/L) and Tempranillo (1.33 mg/L) grape varieties had similar *trans*-resveratrol content to the Greek wines. For Italian wines, it ranged between 0.5 and 10 mg/L depending on cultivar, area of cultivation, climate and winemaking technology. In another study, thirty-two Tuscan red wines were found to contain between 0.3 and 2.1 mg/L of *trans*-resveratrol. Wines from relatively warm and dry climatic conditions tended towards lesser resveratrol levels. Stervbo et al. (2007) found the highest *trans*-resveratrol levels in the wines made from Pinot Noir and St. Laurent; the average levels of *trans*-resveratrol in red wine varied greatly from one region to another, but no specific region was significantly different from all the others. Roggero (2000) found that intense UV irradiation leads to complete disappearance of *trans*- and *cis*-isomers of piceid and to a large decrease in resveratrol isomers content.

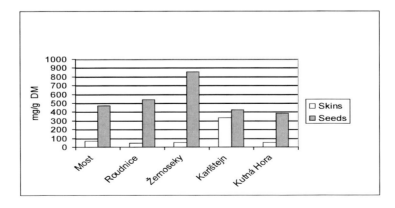

Figure 12. Total polyphenol (TP) content in skins and seeds of cv. Müller Thurgau from five vineyards

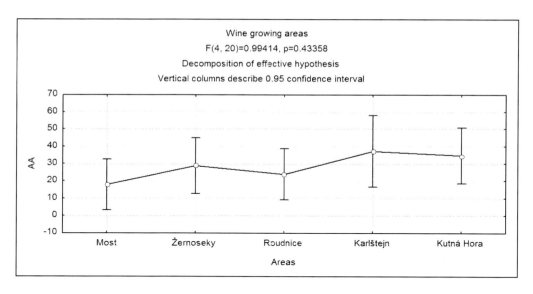

Figure 13. Analysis of variance of antioxidant activity in grape seeds of five vineyard areas

Comparison of Total Antioxidant Status of Bohemian Wines during the Winemaking Process and Effect of Technological Processing and Vinification

Phenol levels in wine and grape juice are affected by numerous processing conditions (crushing, pressing, sulphite addition, skin contact, oak aging). Lachman et al. (2007) measured TAS values during the winemaking process with the DPPH assay (Fig. 14) and the

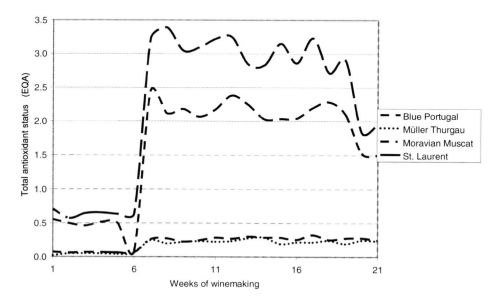

Figure 14. TAS of wines during the winemaking process analyzed by DPPH assay

ABTS assay (Fig. 15). Obtained results revealed significant differences between the white and red wines (Figs. 16 - 19). The TAS of the white wines was significantly lesser in comparison with the red wines. White wines showed a median value of approximately 0.227 EQA as compared to the red wines (2.212 EQA) and had ten times as much TAS when determined by DPPH assay. In the ABTS assay, the EQA values were higher (median 1.453 of white wines and 5.464 EQA of red wines); the TAS increase was 3.7 times higher in the red wines in comparison with the white wines. The difference between the white wines determined by both methods was nearly the same (14% by the DPPH assay, 12% by the ABTS assay). The TAS values determined by the ABTS and DPPH assays were strongly affected during the winemaking process. The highest values were determined in the St. Laurent wine (Figs. 14, 15) with a high increase by week 4 (15 EQA by ABTS assay) and between weeks 6 and 7 (3.4 EQA by DPPH). A similar tendency was found in the Blue Portugal wine with an increase during weeks 6 – 8 (5 EQA by the ABTS assay, 3.4 EQA by the DPPH assay). The St. Laurent wine has 40% higher TAS in comparison with the Blue Portugal wine when determined by the DPPH assay, and 45% higher when determined by the ABTS assay.

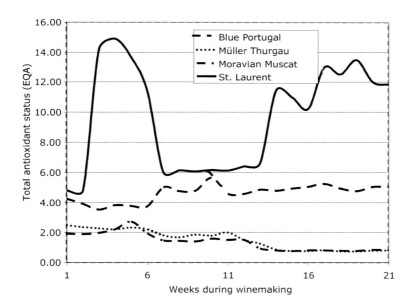

Figure 15. TAS of wines during winemaking process analyzed by ABTS assay

A significant difference was found between red and white wines and all analysed wines except Müller-Thurgau and Moravian Muscat (Table 10).

The TAS found by ABTS and DPPH assays in the white and red wines differed significantly (Figs. 16, 18), which is well in accordance with the recent data obtained by de Villiers et al. (2005) suggesting a high polyphenol content in red wines. Statistically significant differences were also found between individual red wines, contrary to white wines (Figs. 17, 19).

The winemaking process strongly affected the TAS (TAS has been determined by different methods – ABTS, DPPH and ORAC – Oxygen Radical Absorbance Capacity) and it is evidently in close relation to the content of polyphenolic antioxidant compounds, as Fernández-Pachón et al. (2006) in their study confirmed. This concerns especially gallic, protocatechuic, and caftaric acids and (-)-epigallocatechin gallate. In blue vine varieties, mostly the anthocyanin content is affected by different vinification methods (Gómez-Plaza et al., 2006). According to our previous results, the stage of maceration in particular affects the total polyphenol content in red wines. Differences in the anthocyanin and tannin extractability in grapes during the wine-making process seem to be one of the main factors affecting anthocyanin and polyphenol content and thus the TAS of wines indicate similar results reported by Ortega-Regules et al. (2006) and Netzel et al. (2003). Our results are in good accordance with the results obtained by Villaño et al. (2006) determined by ORAC, DPPH and ABTS and confirm the impact of oenological practices on the TAS of wines. The maceration and fermentation methods used for red wines have a positive effect on the antioxidant potential. Grapes for the production of red wines were in our study cold macerated for 14 days using a standard technology procedure. The significant difference between the blue vine varieties Blue Portugal and St. Laurent also confirms behavioural differences during vinification, depending on the grape variety. As Rivero-Pérez et al. (2008a) showed, free anthocyanins fraction is main responsible for of the total antioxidant capacity and scavenger activity of red wines. Among anthocyanins, glycosylated and methoxylated anthocyanidins (e.g. malvidin 3-O-glucoside) are the type of anthocyanins with higher participation on antioxidant activity of red wines.

Another very important factor influencing the TAS results (determined by ABTS and DPPH assays) in the study was the addition of SO_2, which acts both as a reducing agent and provides antibacterial effects. The sharp TAS increase recorded between weeks 6 and 7 (see Figs. 14, 15) we ascribe mainly to the addition of SO_2. Fifty percent of the determined values in red wines ranged from 4.5 to 10.5 EQA and 0.5 – 2 EQA in white wines (determined with the ABTS assay) and from 0.6 to 2.7 EQA in the red wines determined by the DPPH assay. From this comparison, it is evident that the ABTS assay gives higher values than the DPPH assay. From the linear correlation and regression analysis of the ABTS and DPPH assays of all wines, a medium correlation between ABTS and DPPH values has been found (r^2=0.7156 and r=0.8459, y=1.6597+1.3889x). In red wines the results were similar (Fig. 20), and in white wines, only a very weak correlation could be found (r^2=0.5512, r=0.7424, y=2.3731-4.7292x, Fig. 21). The absolute results obtained by both methods are in good interpretation agreement with the same conclusions (Table 10). However, the lack of strong correlation between these two assays is likely attributable to the fact that every individual phenol compound contained in wine causes a different response to the specific radical used in the assay. These different phenol compounds contained in different concentrations depend on the selected technological procedure and duration of its individual phases (especially the period of fermentation, period of remaining in the barrel, and storage temperature). A similar lack of correlation between the TAS measured by the Trolox equivalent antioxidant assay (TEAC) and other assays (ABTS, FRAP – Ferric Reducing Ability of Plasma) was reported recently by Wang et al. (2004). Thus, according to these results, more different methods should be used in parallel for the estimation of the TAS of biological materials (Prior & Cao, 1999). $ABTS^{•+}$ and $DPPH^{•}$ radicals have a different stereochemical structure and another method of genesis and thus they lend, after the reaction with the antioxidants, a qualitatively different response to the inactivation of their radical.

According to used winemaking technologies total antioxidant capacity determined by a chemiluminiscence assay also suffered a decrease; the highest decrease (30-50 %) was found after the clarification procedure, which may be due to the fining agents used and to oxygen contact (Girotti et al., 2006). Monagas et al. (2007) investigated the possible industrial use of three previously selected *Saccharomyces cerevisiae* strains (1EV, 2EV and 7EV) in musts derived from Tempranillo and Cabernet Sauvignon. With the exception of hydroxycinnamic acids and derivatives, no particular influence of the yeast strain was observed on the remaining non-anthocyanin phenol compounds (i.e. hydroxybenzoic acids and flavanols). Pyranoanthocyanins and metabolites resulting from the alcoholic fermentation such as tyrosol and tryptophol, seemed to be more influenced by the must composition and pH, and thus, by the grape variety, than by the yeast strain. Combined treatment with bentonite, egg albumin and Polyclar AT both, in wines and musts decreases the amounts of catechins, flavonols, anthocyanins and leucoanthocyanidins (Gorinstein et al., 1993); polyphenols (32 – 17%) and anthocyanogens (64 – 48%) were removed by this technological process.

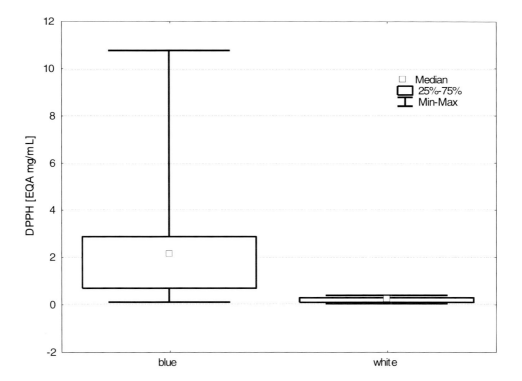

Figure 16. Comparison of TAS of red wines (blue varieties) and white wines (white varieties) determined by DPPH assay

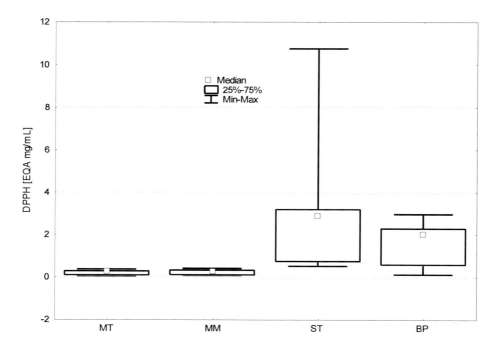

Figure 17. Comparison of TAS of varietal wines (MT – Müller Thurgau, MM – Moravian Muscat, ST – St. Laurent, BP – Blue Portugal) determined by DPPH assay

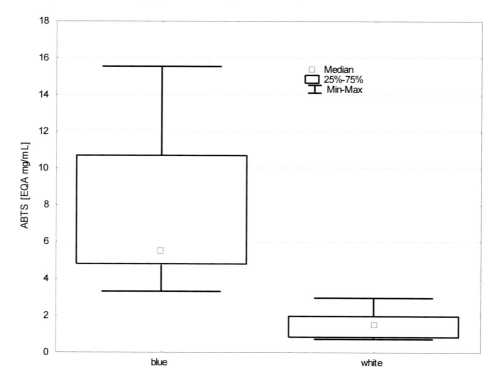

Figure 18. Comparison of TAS of red wines (blue varieties) and white wines (white varieties) determined by DPPH assay

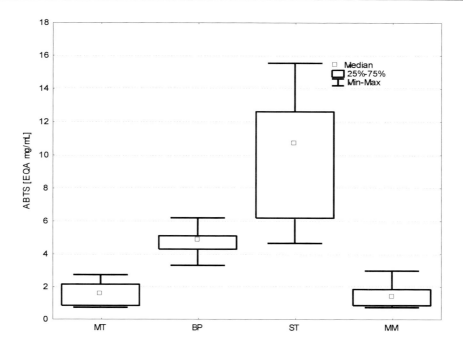

Figure 19. Comparison of TAS of varietal wines (MT – Müller Thurgau, MM – Moravian Muscat, ST – St. Laurent, BP – Blue Portugal) determined by DPPH assay

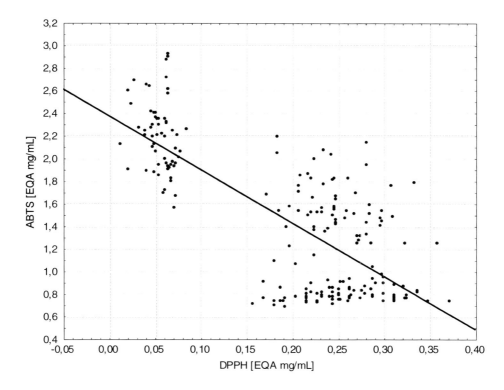

Figure 20. Correlation and regression between values provided with ABTS/DPPH assays in red wines

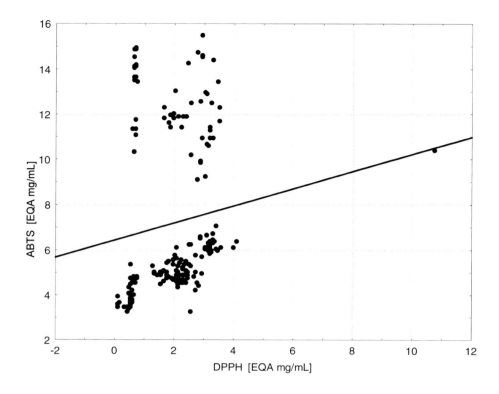

Figure 21. Correlation and regression between values provided with ABTS/DPPH assays in white wines

According to technologically different winemaking procedures of white and red wines (in white wine vinification mashing is lacking) Lachman et al. (2006) found that at the end of the winemaking process red wines contained on av. 1.426 g/L TP, whereas white wines only 0.162 g/L (Figs. 22 -25). Thus, red wines contained on average two times more TP in comparison with grape must at the beginning of winemaking, whereas TP content decreased to 86 % of origin content in grape musts. The highest TP contents were found in Pinot Noir (1.935 g/L), Zweigeltrebe (1.522 g/L) and Blue Portugal (1.318 g/L). Analysis of variance (Scheffé test) at level of significance P<0.05 showed statistically high significance between red and white wines in TP content (P=0.000), Zweigeltrebe and all other varieties (P=0.000 – 0.013), St. Laurent and Blue Portugal from all other varieties except Pinot Noir. Differences among white varieties were not significant. Variance analysis among wine growing areas confirmed highly significant differences (P=0.000 – 0.041). Higher values were found in the Mělník area (Zweigeltrebe 1.258 g/L) as compared with the Kutná Hora area (Zweigeltrebe 0.387 g/L). These results confirm the suggestions of Burns et al. (2001) that the extraction of the phenolics was influenced by vinification procedure, grape quality, and grape variety. We can confirm the high influence of winemaking techniques on the polyphenolic composition as Budic-Leto et al. (2003, 2005) referred to in specific Croatian wines. White and red wines differed significantly in TP content course during the vinification process. In all measured cases from the preparation of must and its fermentation in October a moderate increase could be seen followed by almost constant content during further fermentation and maturation

(November – December 2004, January – February 2005), followed finally by a moderate decrease in March – April 2005 during and after bottling. TP content changes in white wines during their vinification were insignificant. On the contrary, the procedures of winemaking of red wines are characterized by dramatic changes in their TP content. Maceration and mashing in October was characterized by a moderate or medium TP increase, while during fermentation in November – December an intense increase of TP occurred followed by constant content or its moderate decrease during the January – March 2005 period (maturation of wine) and then decrease in April (bottling and aging). As a result, an increase of TP and AA esp. in red wines during vinification was found (Figs. 14, 15, 22-25). As Pellegrini et al. (2000) suggested aging is the main factor influencing the antioxidant activity and TP contents of wines. During maturation, quantitative changes of catechins and oligomeric procyanidins were recorded (Jordao et al., 2001). Relative constant total polyphenol content during maturation of wine is in accordance with results of Echeverry et al. (2005), suggesting the relevance of qualitative changes of phenolics. It could be concluded that red and white wines differ not only in final contents of phenolics, but also in their extreme increase in red wines during fermentation. Different evolution patterns during aging depending on the grape variety were also confirmed by Monagas et al. (2005). Decrease is caused mainly by flavanols condensation reactions. Villaño et al. (2006) evaluated the impact of enological practices included maceration for red wines, pressing degree for white wines and clarification in both types of wines on antioxidant activity of wines. Maceration time had a positive effect on antioxidant potential of red wines depending on the variety and a pressure increase caused higher antioxidant activity of white wines. Clarification treatments did not significantly affect the phenol composition or the antioxidant activity of wines. Castillo-Sánchez et al. (2006) found that red wines prepared from a single batch of Vinhão grapes treated with fining agents (polyvinylpyrrolidine, gelatin, egg albumin, and casein) as well as by carbonic maceration tended to have somewhat lower anthocyanin levels, but after two years storage the color density differences were negligible.

Table 10. Comprehensive statistical evaluation of DPPH and ABTS assays

		DPPH assay			ABTS assay	
	N	Median	Minimum	Maximum	Median	Minimum	Maximum
All varieties	420	0.329	0.012	10.727	3.095	0.693	15.494
Blue varieties	210	2.113	0.082	10.727	5.464	3.263	15.494
White varieties	210	0.227	0.013	0.372	1.453	0.693	2.927
Blue Portugal	105	2.005	0.082	2.925	4.785	3.263	6.157
Müller-Thurgau	105	0.215	0.013	0.333	1.554	0.693	2.684
Moravian Muscat	105	0.247	0.040	0.372	1.380	0.704	2.927
St. Laurent	105	2.844	0.479	10.727	10.663	4.607	15.494

Analysis of variance (Scheffé test) at level of significance P<0.05 showed statistically high significance differences of AA between red and white wines (P = 0.000). AA increased during the wine-making process, esp. in Zweigeltrebe, St. Laurent and Pinot Noir wines (Figs. 23, 25), suggesting thus better AA of wines compared with grape juices at the beginning of the wine-making process (Alcolea et al., 2003). The highest increase was determined during fermentation and maturation of wine. Multiple correlation coefficients between TP and AA revealed significant correlations in the Kutná Hora (r = 0.4701) and Mělník (r = 0.7379) vineyard regions.

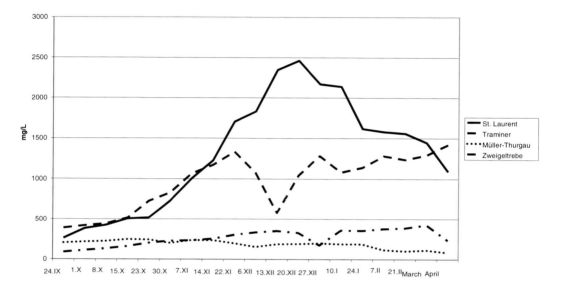

Figure 22. Content of total polyphenols [mg/L] during winemaking in wines from the Kutná Hora vineyard area

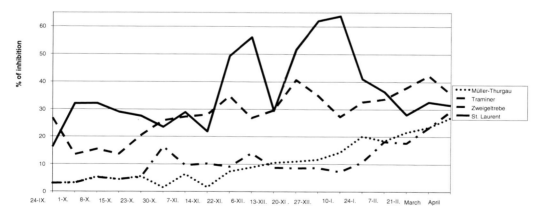

Figure 23. Changes of antioxidant activity [%] of wines during winemaking from the Kutná Hora vineyard area

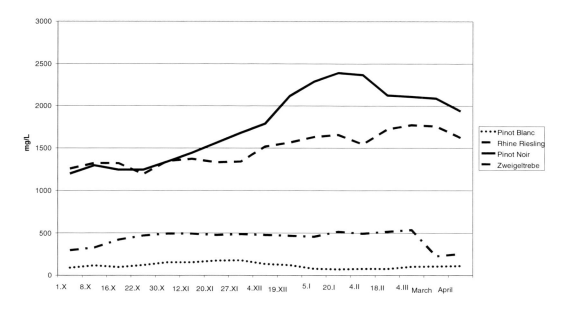

Figure 24. Content of total polyphenols [mg/L] during winemaking in wines from the Mělník vineyard area

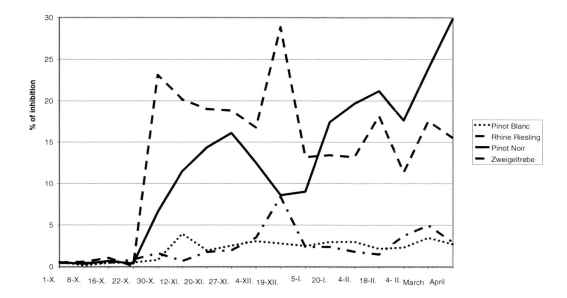

Figure 25. Changes of antioxidant activity [%] during wine-making in wines from the Mělník vineyard area

Sun et al. (2006) analyzed stilbene levels in grape skins of three *Vitis vinifera* varieties (Castelão, Syrah and Tinta Roriz) and in their corresponding wines made by traditional winemaking technologies. Skins are the major source of these compounds in wine. The evolution of these compounds during the elaboration of wines (from the end of alcoholic fermentation until the second racking, i.e., just before bottling) showed that in general, *trans-*

resveratrol concentration decreases gradually, *trans*-piceid stays constant, while *cis*-resveratrol increases slightly. The important finding of this work is that there was a significant correlation between the concentration of total piceid in grape skins and that in the respective wine.

USE OF ANTIOXIDANTS FROM WINEMAKING WASTES

Spigno & Faveri (2007) assessed the feasibility of extracting antioxidant compounds from winemaking wastes (grape stalks and marc) by solvent extraction. Together with the type of raw material they also investigated the influence of some process parameters on final antioxidants yields and extract purity: a treatment, type of solvent (ethanol or a mixture of ethylacetate:water = 9:1), temperature (28 or 60 degrees C) and length of maceration (5 or 24 h). Solvent and temperature were statistically influent ($p < 0.05$), and the yields were higher with ethanol (but with lower purities) and at 60 degrees C. The results of Bonilla et al. (1999) revealed a higher extraction of phenol compounds from red grape marc for use as food lipid antioxidants by the ethyl acetate acting on crushed marc, so the cost of this last operation can be largely compensated. Antioxidant activity of the phenols of the extract was close to that of BHT, mostly because of its catechin content. Rayne et al. (2008) investigated grape cane waste as a potential source of high-value phytochemicals with medicinal and anti-phytopathogenic applications. Extraction yields of *trans*-resveratrol and *trans*-viniferin from *Vitis vinifera* cv. Pinot Noir grape cane were 3.45±0.04 and 1.30±0.07 mg/g DM, respectively. The study suggested that these compounds can be quantitatively extracted from grape cane residue using low-cost, environmentally benign, and non-toxic aqueous alcoholic solvent systems such as ethanol:water mixtures. Lafka et al. (2007) confirmed that ethanol extract of winery waste exhibited the highest antioxidant activity compared to the other solvent extracts, to synthetic food antioxidants BHT, ascorbyl palmitate and to the natural food antioxidant, vitamin E. HPLC analysis of the extracts showed that gallic acid, catechin and epicatechin were the major phenol compounds in winery waste. Hydroxytyrosol, tyrosol, cyanidin glycosides and various phenol acids such as caffeic, syringic, vanillic, *p*-coumaric and *o*-coumaric acids were also identified. Bozan et al. (2008) recommend seeds of red grape varieties as dietary supplement due to high amount of total phenolic content and antioxidant activity. While (+)-catechin (4.71–23.8 mg/g seed) was found as main flavanol, galloylated catechin monomer and dimeric procyanidin amounts varied between 2.89–17.2 and 0.97–2.97 mg/g seed, respectively. Other two by-products of the winemaking process, namely stem and pomace, of Manto Negro red grape variety native to Mallorca have been characterized recently by Llobera & Cañellas (2007). These products present considerably high contents in dietary fibre with associated polyphenols and excellent antioxidant properties, particularly in the case of the stem, which confer on them a wide range of applications as food ingredients. The pomace has high protein (12.2%), oil (13.5%) values, and the stem large amounts of extractable polyphenols (11.6%). Hwang et al. (2008) added red grape wine lees to ice cream, improved thus its rheological properties, and increased radical scavenging activity.

EFFECT OF STORAGE CONDITIONS AND WINE AGE

Faitová et al. (2004b) investigated in twelve bottles of Traminer (vintage 2000, late harvest, wine growing area Žernoseky), total content of polyphenols and resveratrol to determine the variability of the content of measured substances in various bottles of the same batch and from the same manufacturer. Although the bottles were of the same batch with exactly the same conditions for bottling and bottle storage, the content of TP and R slightly oscillated. The differences in the content of measured substances could be likely explained by storage and transport conditions (bottles placed in the upper part of a storage area are more exposed to light and temperature changes than bottles stored in lower layers (Goldberg et al., 1996b). The packaging material can also influence the content of the measured substances. The outer conditions (light and heat exposure) can also cause the degradation of one group of polyphenols – anthocyanins (Bakowska et al., 2003, Garcia–Beneytez et al., 2002, Morais et al., 2002). It is possible to conclude that the light exposure causes significant changes for anthocyanins, which can cause the differences in the content of total polyphenols. As Monagas et al. (2006a) determined in young red wines during 26 months of ageing in bottle, total anthocyanins markedly decreased. They suggested the occurrence of condensation reactions during ageing in bottle, due to the disappearance of monomeric anthocyanins, an increase of catechins and procyanidins and a decrease of low-polymerized polyphenols. Monagas et al. (2006b) investigated the relationships between the color parameters (colorimetric indexes and CIELAB variables) and the phenol components (anthocyanins, pyranoanthocyanins, hydroxybenzoic and hydroxycinnamic acids, flavanols and flavonols) of young red wines from *Vitis vinifera* L. cv. Tempranillo, Graciano and Cabernet Sauvignon (vintage 2000, Navarra, Spain), during 26 months of wine aging in bottles (a period embracing their commercial life), through the application of different statistical analysis (principal component, correlation and polynomial regression). It was found that for each variety the color parameters were correlated with the anthocyanins during aging in bottles. Finally, by the application of polynomial regression analysis, both anthocyanins (simple glucosides and acetyl-glucosides) and pyranoanthocyanins (anthocyanin-pyruvic acid adducts) were selected as the variables that best described the different color parameters during aging in bottles. The level of monomeric phenolics and low molecular-weight phenol oligomers decreases with age, while the level of high molecular-weight phenolics increases (Roginsky et al., 2006). Versari et al. (2008) reported that the total color of wines was an aggregate number of three components: copigmentation (8–30%), total free anthocyanins (24–35%), and polymeric pigment (35–63%). The level of copigmentation can be almost completely described by the levels of monomeric pigments ($r^2 = 0.9464$) and not by the tannin content as has often been suggested (copigmentation vs tannin: $r^2 = 0.4827$). A progressive decline in both antioxidant capacity and total anthocyanin content of a grape skin ingredient (43 and 40% decrease, respectively) was observed over a 60 day storage period (45 degrees C and 75% relative humidity), demonstrating its weak stability under these conditions (Monagas et al., 2006b). The pyranoanthocyanins of cyanidin, petunidin, malvidin and pelargonidin showed a high capacity to scavenge superoxide anion radicals but did not scavenge hydroxyl radicals. Current data indicate that formation of anthocyanin adducts with pyruvic acid, which may occur during wine ageing or fruit juice processing, decreases the hydroxyl and superoxide anion scavenging and thus could decrease the antioxidant potential of these compounds (Garcia-Alonso et al., 2005). Cliff et al. (2007) found that younger wines had higher concentrations of copigmented, monomeric and total anthocyanins than did older wines. In addition, the harvesting date of grapes (directly correlated with the degree of maturity of the grapes) influences the chromatic characteristics of the wines. In general, higher intensities of blue or violet tones were detected in wines made from the grapes collected on the second harvesting date, in which the ratios anthocyanins/proanthocyanidins and anthocyanins/(proanthocyanidins + catechins) were the lowest. These ratios are proposed as probable indicators of the aptitude for wine ageing (Pérez-Magariño and González-San José, 2006). The assay methods of Rivero-Pérez et al. (2008b) on red wines aged in barrels and botttles showed different behaviours for the same wines, thus the young wines presented higher indices for ABTS, DPPH and DMPD (a mechanism that predominates in this assay method, is sharply reduced when it coincides with the formation of more complex and stable compounds, such as newly formed pigments (vitisins, pyro-anthocyanins, aryl-anthocyanins), whereas those that were aged showed higher indices for ABAP-LP [2,2'- diazobis-(2-aminodinopropane)-dihydrochloride] and ORAC. Also the reductive capacity of the wines evaluated in FRAP assays showed higher indices in wines aged for 12 months in the barrel (probably due to the greater transfer of ellagitannins from the wood to the wine).

INCREASING OF *TRANS*-RESVERATROL AND PHENOLICS IN WINES

Todaro et al. (2008) used *trans*-resveratrol content in Sicilian wines using β-glucosidase (EC 3.2.1.21) from different sources to increase the *trans*-resveratrol in some Sicilian wines by hydrolyzing resveratrol glucoside piceid. Belhadj et al. (2008) determined that the methyl jasmonate/sucrose treatment was effective in stimulating phenylalanine ammonia lyase, chalcone synthase, stilbene synthase, UDP glucose:flavonoid-O-glucosyltransferase, proteinase inhibitor and chitinase gene expression, and triggered accumulation of both piceids and anthocyanins in cells, and *trans*-resveratrol and piceids in the extracellular medium. Hence, methyl jasmonate treatment might be an efficient natural strategy to both protect grapevine berries in the vineyard and increase *trans*-resveratrol content in grapes and wines. Analogically Nikfardjam et al. (2006b) investigated *trans*-resveratrol content in quality Hungarian and German wines from botrytized grapes and determined these values as very high, which is particularly true for the Tokay wines. Another approach is use of an organic way of cultivation (Dani et al., 2007). Organic grape juices showed statistically different ($p < 0.05$) higher values of total polyphenols and resveratrol as compared conventional grape juices. Purple juices presented higher total polyphenol content and *in vitro* antioxidant activity as compared to white juices, and this activity was positively correlated ($r = 0.680$; $p < 0.01$) with total polyphenol content. Fuhrman et al. (2001) have been looking for a way of making white wine with higher polyphenol levels. Whole, crushed grapes were stored for different lengths of time before removing the skins, and they tried adding various concentrations of ethanol to see if that aided polyphenol extraction. Leaving the skins with the juice for two to 18 hours gave a gradual increase in the white wine's polyphenol content, though it was still 10 times less than red. Adding alcohol gave 60% higher polyphenol levels, in a dessert wine with a final alcohol content of 18% and high sugar content. Its antioxidant capacity was directly proportional to its polyphenol content. Despite the overall levels of polyphenols being over four-fold less than in the red wine, its antioxidant effect was similar to that of the red, suggesting that only the more potent polyphenols were extracted from the grape skins. It was concluded that processing white wine by imposing a short period of grape skin contact in the presence of alcohol leads to extraction of grape skin polyphenols and produces polyphenol-rich white wine with antioxidant characteristics similar to those of red wine. Another approach is to enhance procyanidin oligomers in Tannat red wine. Tannat is considered one of the most concentrated varieties of *Vitis vinifera* concerning total polyphenol content and it name comes from this characteristic, as a tannic grape. In young wines, procyanidins are found mainly in dimeric and trimeric form and in aged wines the relative degree of polymerization increases to 8-10 (Brouillard et al., 1997). There is an interest in developing grape varieties with high anthocyanin levels with antioxidative and antiproliferative properties through traditional breeding of selected high-polyphenol grape lines (Jacob et al., 2008). As Pardo et al. (1999) determined, the enzyme preparations (endoenzyme contact pelliculatire, biopectinase, Ultrazym 100Q and Rapidase excolor) during the maceration carried out during vinification produced an increase in the quantity of polyphenols extracted from the solid parts (the highest values were obtained in color density, anthocyanins and index of total polyphenols). Talcott et al. (2005) evaluated changes in maximum absorbance, total soluble phenolics, isoflavonoids, and anthocyanins in muscadine juice and wine following the addition of isoflavonoid extracts from red clover with maximum color enhancement found at an anthocyanin to cofactor ratio of 1:8. Thus, red clover isoflavonoids proved to be novel and effective color enhancing compounds when used in low concentrations in young muscadine wines.

CONCLUSION

Grape berries, grape juices, grape wines, especially blue grape cultivars, and red wines produced from them by fermentation of grapes by natural yeasts present in the fruit have many health benefits due to contained amounts of effective constituents. They have strong antioxidant impact, heart health effect; decrease harmful LDL-cholesterol, have a stroke sparing effect on the nerves that could be damaged by strokes, have a longevity effect when used in diet, and increase the elasticity of the arteries. The efficient constituents are phenol antioxidants, among them catechins, phenol acids, flavonoids, stilbene phytoalexins in white wines and in addition anthocyanins and monomeric and oligomeric proanthocyanidins. Their total content, total antioxidant capacity and the content of individual major antioxidants typical for grapes and wines – anthocyanins (malvidin-3,5-O-diglucoside and 3-*O*-glucosides of malvidin, peonidin, petunidin, delphidin and cyanidin, coumaroylated-glucoside derivatives), oligomeric and polymeric procyanidins, monomeric flavanols (catechin and epicatechin), phenol acids (gallic acid, ellagic acid, protocatechuic acid, caffeic acid, *p*-coumaric acid, and *trans*-caffeoyltartaric and *trans*-*p*-coumaroyltartaric acids), flavonoids (myricetin 3-glucoside, quercetin 3-glucoside, and quercetin 3-glucuronide), and stilbene phytoalexins (*trans*- and *cis*-resveratrol and their glucosides – piceids, their dimer trans-ε-viniferin and trimer α-viniferin) and carboxypyranomalvidine glucosides (vitisins: vitisin A – 5-carboxypyranomalvidin-3-O-β-D-glucoside, vitisin B – pyranomalvidin-3-O-β-D-glucoside) – are affected by many factors, which have been intensively studied in recent times. The main impacts on the content of these constituents are made by variety and cultivar, vineyard regions, climatic conditions, year of cultivation (vintage), way of cultivation, date of harvest, wine-making procedures (especially differences between white and red wines related to the first stage of fermentation – maceration, while the skins are still in contact with the liquid), wine storage conditions and wine aging. Antioxidant activity is related to the content of total phenolics, but very efficient among them are monomeric flavanols (catechin and epicatechin), dimeric, trimeric and polymeric procyanidins and condensed tannins, and phenol acids (gallic acid and ellagic acid) and other antioxidants like resveratrol. Statistically significant differences between white and red wines have been found; red wines contain higher amounts of antioxidants and show higher antioxidant activity. Other major factors seem to be variety/cultivar and the individual stages of the winemaking process – vinification. The phase of maceration of grape skins increases largely antioxidant content and activity. Vineyard regions and subregions with cooler and more humid climatic conditions have a tendency towards higher *trans*-resveratrol content, because of considerable infestation with *Botrytis cinerea*. Regarding the beneficial health effect of wine antioxidants, the possibilities of increasing their contents in wines are provided, e.g. with botrytized wines, methyl jasmonate treatment or using enzymatic hydrolysis to increase resveratrol content. Also highly appreciated are wine wastes or grape skins and seeds, as a rich source for obtaining of contained active principles and selection of optimal conditions of the extraction and extractive solvents. On the basis of the evaluation of grape berries, skins and seeds and produced white and red wines originating in the vineyard regions of the Czech Republic (Bohemia, Moravia) and subregions the impact of these factors on antioxidant content and total antioxidant status is described and evaluated in detail and compared with the most recent knowledge in connection with obtaining highly quality wines and grape products, as well as valuable beneficial phytochemicals and preparations from wine-making by-products, esp. grape skins and seeds.

In conclusion, the present findings support our knowledge from experimental and epidemiological studies, suggesting that the supply of antioxidant phenols through a moderate daily consumption of red wines may provide additional protection against in vivo oxidation and other damages of cellular bioconstituents. Thus, vine-breeders and wine producers can try to produce grape products and wines with the highest content of phenolic antioxidants and antioxidant activity, as well as with the optimal organoleptic properties.

ACKNOWLEDGEMENT

This study was supported by the Research Project of the Ministry of Education, Youth and Sports of the Czech Republic, MSM 6046070901.

REFERENCES

Abril, M.; Negueruela, A.I.; Pérez, C.; Juan, T. & Estopañán, G. (2005). Preliminary study of resveratrol content in Aragón red and rosé wines. *Food Chemistry*, 92, 729-736.

Adrian, M.; Rajaei, H.; Jeandet, P.; Veneau, J. & Bessis, R. (1998). Resveratrol oxidation in *Botrytis cinerea* conidia. *Phytopathology*, 88, 472-476.

Alcolea, J.F.; Cano, A.; Acosta, M. & Arnao, M.B. (2003). Determination of the hydrophilic and lipophilic antioxidant activity of white- and red wines during the wine-making process. *Italian Journal of Food Science*, 15, 207-214.

Álvarez, I.; Aleixandre, J.L.; García, M.J. & Lizama, V. (2006). Impact of prefermentative maceration on the phenolic and volatile compounds in Monastrell red wines. *Analytica Chimica Acta*, 563, 109-115.

Argyri, K.; Komaitis, M. & Kapsokefalou, M. (2006). Iron decreases the antioxidant capacity of red wine under conditions of in vitro digestion. *Food Chemistry*, 96, 281-289.

Arnous, A.; Makris, D.P. & Kefalas, P. (2001). Effect of principal polyphenolic components in relation to antioxidant characteristics of aged red wines. *Journal of Agricultural and Food Chemistry*, 49, 5736-5742.

Asenstorfer, R.E. & Jones, G.P. (2007). Charge equilibria and pK values of 5-carboxypyranomalvidin-3-glucoside (vitisin A) by electrophoresis and absorption spectroscopy. *Tetrahedron*, 63, 4788-4792.

Bakowska, A.; Kucharska, A.Z. & Oszmianski, J. (2003). The effects of heating, UV-irradiation, and storage on stability of the anthocyanin – polyphenol copigment complex. *Food Chemistry*, 81, 349-355.

Balestrieri, M.L.; Fiorito, C.; Crimi, E.; Felice, F.; Schiano, C.; Milone, L.; Casamassimi, A.; Giovane, A.; Grimaldi, V.; Del Giudice, V.; Minucci, P.B.; Mancini, F.P.; Servillo, L.; D´Armiento, F.P.; Farzati, B. & Napoli, C. (2008). Effect of red wine antioxidants and minor polyphenolic constituents on endothelial progenitor cells after physical training in mice. *International Journal of Cardiology*, 126, 295-297.

Banini, A.E.; Boyd, L.C.; Allen, J.C.; Hengameh, G.A. & Derrick, L.S. (2006). Muscadine grape products intake, diet and blood constituents of non-diabetics and type 2 diabetic subjects. *Nutrition*, 22, 1137-1145.

Barger, J.L.; Kayo, T.; Vann, J.M.; Arias, E.B.; Wang, J.; Hacker, T.A.; Wang, Y.; Raederstorff, D.; Morrow, J.D.; Leeuwenburgh, C.; Allison, D.B.; Saupe, K.W.; Cartee, G.D.; Weindruch, D. & Prolla, T.A. (2008). A low dose of dietary resveratrol partially mimics caloric restriction and retards aging parameters in mice. *PloS ONE*, 3, (6), e2264, 1-10, doi: 10.1371/journal.pone0002264.

Bartolomé, B.; Nuñez, V.; Monagas, M. & Gómez-Cordovés, C. (2004). In vitro antioxidant activity of red grape skins. *European Food Research and Technology*, 218, 173–177.

Baydar, N.G.; Ozkan, G. & Sagdic, O. (2004). The phenolic contents and antibacterial activities of grape (*Vitis vinifera* L.) extracts. *Food Control*, 15, 335-339.

Belhadj, A.; Telef, N.; Saigne, C.; Cluzet, S.; Barrieu, F.; Hamdi, S. & Mérillon, J.M. (2008). Effect of methyl jasmonate in combination with carbohydrates on gene expression of PR proteins, stilbene and anthocyanin accumulation in grapevine cell cultures. *Plant Physiology and Biochemistry*, 46, 493-499.

Bianchini, F. & Vainio, H. (2003). Wine and resveratrol: mechanismus of cancer prevention? *European Journal of Cancer Prevention*, 12, 417-425.

Bonilla, F.; Mayen, M.; Merida, J. & Medina, M. (1999). Extraction of phenolic compounds from red grape marc for use as food lipid antioxidants. *Food Chemistry*, 66, 209-215.

Borbalán, A.M.A.; Zorro, L.; Guillén, D.A. & Barroso, C.G. (2003). Study of the polyphenol content of red and white grape varieties by liquid chromatography – mass spectrometry and its relationship to antioxidant power. *Journal of Chromatography* A, 1012, 31–38.

Bors, W. & Michel, C. (2002). Chemistry of the antioxidant effect of polyphenols. Alcohol & Wine in Health and Disease Annals of N.Y. *Academy of Sciences*, 957, 57-69.

Bozan, B.; Tosun, G. & Özcan, D. (2008). Study of polyphenol content in the seeds of red grape (*Vitis vinifera* L.) varieties cultivated in Turkey and their antiradical activity. *Food Chemistry*, 109, 426-430.

Bravo, M.N.; Silva, S.; Coelho, A,V.; Boas, L.V. & Bronze, M.R. (2006). Analysis of phenolic compounds in Muscatel wines produced in Portugal. *Analytica Chimica Acta*, 563, 84-92.

Brouillard, R.; George, F. & Fougerousse, A. (1997). Polyphenols produced during red wine ageing. *Biofactors*, 6, 403-410.

Budic-Leto, I.; Lovric, T. & Vrhovsek, U. (2003). Influence of different maceration techniques and ageing on proanthocyanidins and anthocyanins of red wine cv. Babic (*Vitis vinifera* L.). *Food Technology and Biotechnology*, 41, 299-303.

Budic-Leto, I.; Lovric, T.; Pezo, I. & Kljusuric, J.G. (2005). Study of dynamics of polyphenol extraction during traditional and advanced maceration processes of the Babic grape variety. *Food Technology and Biotechnology*, 43, 47-53.

Burkitt, M.J. & Duncan, J. (2000). Effects of *trans*-resveratrol on copper-dependent hydroxyl-radical formation and DNA-damage: evidence for hydroxyl-radical scavenging and a novel, glutathione-sparing mechanism of action. *Archives of Biochemistry and Biophysics*, 381, 253-263.

Burns, J.; Gardner, P.T.; O´Neil, J.; Crawford, S.; Morecroft, I.; Mc Phail, D.B.; Lister, C.; Matthews, D.; Mac Lean, M.E.J.; Duthie, G.G. & Crozier, A. (2000). Relationship among antioxidant activity, vasodilatation capacity, and phenolic content of red wines. *Journal of Agricultural and Food Chemistry*, 48, 220-230.

Burns, J.; Gardner, P.T.; Metthews, D.; Duthie, G.G.; Lean, M.E.J & Crozier, A. (2001). Extraction of phenolics and changes in antioxidant activity of red wines during vinification. *Journal of Agricultural and Food Chemistry*, 49, 5797-5808.

Cantos, E.; Espin, J.C. & Tomas-Barberan, F.A. (2002). Varietal differences among the polyphenol profiles of seven table grape cultivars studied by LC/DAD/MS/MS. *Journal of Agricultural and Food Chemistry*, 50, 5691-5696.

Castellari, M.; Spinabelli, U.; Riponi, C. & Amati, A. (1998). Influence of some technological practices on the quantity of resveratrol in wine. *Zeitschrift für Lebensmittel Untersuchung-Forschung A*, 206, 151-155.

Castillo-Sánchez, J.J.; Mejuto, J.C.; Garrido, J. & García-Falcón, S. (2006). Influence of wine-making protocol and fining agents on the evolution of the anthocyanin content, colour and general organoleptic quality of Vinhão wines. *Food Chemistry*, 97, 130-136.

Chicón, R.M.; Sanchez-Palomo, E. & Cabezudo, M.D. (2002). The colour and polyphenol composition of red wine varieties in Castilla – La Mancha (Spain). *Afinidad*, 59, 435–443.

Cimino, F.; Sulfaro, V.; Trombetta, D.; Saija, A. & Tomaino, A. (2007). Radical-scavenging capacity of several Italian red wines. *Food Chemistry*, 103, 75-81.

Cliff, M.A.; King, M.C. & Schlosser, J. (2007). Anthocyanin, phenolic composition, colour measurement and sensory analysis of BC commercial red wines. *Food Research International*, 40, 92-100.

Cooke, D.; Steward, W.P.; Gescher, A.J. & Marczylo, T. (2005). Anthocyans from fruits and vegetables – Does bright colour signal cancer chemopreventive activity? *European Journal of Cancer*, 41, 1931-1940.

Dadáková, E.; Vrchotová, N.; Tříska, J. & Kyseláková, M. (2003). Determination of free and conjugated quercetin in Moravian red wines. *Chemické listy*, 97, 558-561.

Dani, C.; Oliboni, L.S.; Vanderlinde, R.; Bonatto, D.; Salvador, M. & Henriques, J.A.P. (2007). Phenolic content and antioxidant activities of white and purple juices manufactured with organically- or conventionally-produced grapes. *Food and Chemical Toxicology*, 45, 2574-2580.

Dávalos, A.; Bartolomé, B. & Gómez-Cordovés, C. (2005). Antioxidant properties of grape juices and vinegars. *Food Chemistry*, 93, 325-330.

De Beer, D.; Joubert, E.; Gelderblom, W.C.A. & Manley, M. (2003). Antioxidant activity of South African red and white cultivar wines: Free radical scavenging. *Journal of Agricultural and Food Chemistry*, 51, 902–909.

De Beer, D.; Joubert, E.; Gelderblom, W.C.A. & Manley, M. (2005). Antioxidant activity of South African red and white cultivar wines and selected phenolic compounds: In vitro inhibition of microsomal lipid peroxidation. *Food Chemistry*, 90, 569-577.

De Beer, D; Joubert, E.; Marais, J. & Manley, M. (2006). Unravelling the total antioxidant capacity of pinotage wines: Contribution of phenolic compounds. *Journal of Agricultural and Food Chemistry*, 54, 2897-2905.

Dell' Agli, M.; Busciala, A. & Bosisio, E. (2004). Vascular effects of wine polyphenols. *Cardiovascular Research*, 63, 593-602.

De Villiers, A.; Majek, P.; Lynen, F.; Crouch, A.; Lauer, H. & Sandra, P. (2005). Classification of South African red and white wines according to grape variety based on the non-coloured phenolic content. *European Food Research and Technology*, 221, 520-528.

Di Majo, D.; Guardia, M.L.; Giammanco, S.; Neve, L.L. & Giammanco, M. (2008). The antioxidant capacity of red wine in relationship with its polyphenolic constituents, *Food Chemistry*, 111, 45-49.

Durak, I.; Avci, A.; Kacmaz, M.; Buyukkocak, S.,; Cimen, M.Y.B.; Elgun, S. & Ozturk, H.S. (1999). Comparison of antioxidant potentials of red wine, white wine, grape juice and alcohol. *Current Medical Research and Opinion*, 15, 316-320.

Dugo, G.; Salvo, F.; Dugo, P.; La Torre, G.L. & Mondello, L. (2003). Antioxidants in Sicilian wines: Analytic and compositive aspects. *Drugs under Experimental and Clinical Research*, 29, 189–202.

Echeverry, C.; Ferreira, M.; Reyes-Parada, M.; Abin-Carriquiry, J.A.; Blasina, F.; Gonzales-Neves, G. & Dajas, F. (2005). Changes in antioxidant capacity of Tannat red wines during early maturation. *Journal of Food Engineering*, 69, 147-154.

Esparza, I.,; Salinas, I.; Caballero, I.; Santamaría, C.; Calvo, I.; García-Mina, J.M. & Fernández, J.M. (2004). Evolution of metal and polyphenol content over a 1-year period vinification: sample fractionation and correlation between metals and anthocyanins. *Analytica Chimica Acta*, 524, 215-224.

Faitová, K.; Hejtmánková, A.; Lachman, J.; Pivec, V. & Dudjak, J. (2004). The contents of total polyphenolic compounds and trans-reveratrol in white Riesling originated in the Czech Republic. *Czech Journal of Food Sciences*, 22, 215-221.

Faitová, K.; Hejtmánková, A.; Lachman, J.; Dudjak, J.; Pivec, V. & Šulc, M. (2004b). Variability of the content of total polyphenols and resveratrol in Traminer bottles of the same batch. *Scientia Agriculturae Bohemica*, 35, 64-68.

Fernàndez-Pachòn, M. S., Villano, D., Garcia-Parrilla, M. C., & Troncoso, A. M. (2004). Antioxidant activity of wines and relation with their polyphenolic composition. *Analytica Chimica Acta*, 513, 113-118.

Fernández-Pachón, M.S., Villaño, D., Troncoso, A.M., & García-Parrilla, M.C. (2006). Determination of the phenolic composition of sherry and table white wines by liquid chromatography and their relation with antioxidant activity. *Analytica Chimica Acta*, 563, 101-108.

Filip, V.; Plocková, M.; Šmidrkal, J.; Špičková, Z.; Melzoch, K. & Schmidt, S. (2003). Resveratrol and its antioxidant and antimicrobial effectiveness. *Food Chemistry*, 83, 585–593.

Frankel, E.N.; Kanner, J.; German, J.B.; Parks, E. & Kinsella, J.E. (1993). Inhibition of oxidation of human low-density-lipoprotein by phenolic substance in red wine. *Lancet*, 341, 454-457.

Frankel, E.N.; Waterhouse, A.L. & Teissedre, P.L. (1995). Principal phenolic phytochemicals in selected California wines and their antioxidant activity in inhibiting oxidation of human low-density lipoproteins. *Journal of Agricultural and Food Chemistry*, 43, 890-894.

Frémont, L. (2000). Minireview. Biological effects of resveratrol. *Life Sciences*, 66, 663–673.

Fuhrman, B.; Volkova, N.; Suraski, A. & Aviram, M. (2001). White wine with red wine-like properties: increased extraction of grape skin polyphenols improves the antioxidant capacity of the derived white wine. *Journal of Food and Agricultural Chemistry*, 49, 3164-3168.

Gao, Y. & Cahoon, G.A. (1995). High performance liquid chromatographic analysis of anthocyanins in the red seedless table grape Reliance. *American Journal of Enology and Viticulture*, 46, 339-345.

Garcia-Alonso, M.; Rimbach, G; Sasai, M.; Nakashara, M.; Matsugo, S.; Uchida, Y.; Rivas-Gonzalo, J.C. & de Pascual, T.S. (2005). Electron spin resonance spectroscopy studies on the free radical scavenging activity of wine anthocyanins and pyranoanthocyanins. *Molecular Nutrition & Food Research*, 49, 1112-1119.

Garcia–Beneytez, E.; Revilla, E. & Cabello, F. (2002). Anthocyanin pattern of several red grape cultivars and wines made from them. *European Research Technology*, 251, 32-37.

Girotti, S.; Fini, F.; Bolelli, L.; Savini, L.; Sartini, E. & Arfelli, G. (2006). Chemiluminescent determination of total antioxidant capacity during wine-making. *Luminiscence*, 21, 233-238.

Goldberg, D.M.; Garovic-Kocic, V.; Diamandis, E.P. & Pace-Asciak, C.R. (1996a). Wine: does the colour count? *Clinica Chimica Acta*, 246: 183-193.

Goldberg, D. M.; Tsang, E.; Kuramanchiri, A.; Diamandis, E.P.; Soleas, G. & Ng, E. (1996b). Method to assay the concentrations of phenolic constituents of biological interest in wines. *Analytical Chemistry*, 68, 1688-1694.

Goldberg, D.; Yan, J.; Ng, E.; Diamandis, E.P.; Karumanchiri, A.; Soleas, G. & Waterhouse, A.L. (1995). A global survey of trans-resveratrol concentrations in commercial wines. *American Journal of Enology and Viticulture*, 46, 159-165.

Gómez-Plaza, E., Miñano, A., & López-Roca, J.M. (2006). Comparison of chromatic properties, stability and antioxidant capacity of anthocyanin-based aqueous extracts from grape pomace obtained from different vinification methods. *Food Chemistry*, 97, 87-94.

Gonzáles-Neves, G.; Charamelo, D.; Balado, J.; Barreiro, L.; Bochicchio, R.; Gatto, G.; Gil, G.; Tessore, A.; Carbonneau, A. & Moutounet, M. (2004). Phenolic potential of Tannat, Cabernet-Sauvignon and Merlot grapes and their correspondence with wine composition. *Analytica Chimica Acta*, 513, 191-196.

Gorinstein, S.; Weisz, M.; Zemser, M.; Tilis, K.; Stiller, A.; Flam, I. & Gat, Y. (1993). Spectroscopic analysis of polyphenols in white wines. *Journal of Fermentation and Bioengineering*, 75, 115-120.

Guarda, E.; Godoy, I.; Foncea, R.; Perez, D.D.; Romeo, C.; Venegas, R. & Leighton, F. (2005). Red wine reduces oxidative stress in patients with acute coronary syndrome. *International Journal of Cardiology*, 104, 35-38.

Guendez, R.; Kallithraka, S.; Makris, D.P. & Kefalas, P. (2005). Determination of low molecular weight polyphenolic constituents in grape (*Vitis vinifera* sp.) seed extracts: Correlation with antiradical activity. *Food Chemistry*, 89, 1-9.

Gutiérrez, I.H.; Lorenzo, E.S.P. & Espinosa, A.V. (2005). Phenolic composition and magnitude of copigmentation in young and shortly aged red wines made from the cultivars, Cabernet Sauvignon, and Syrah. *Food Chemistry*, 92, 269-283.

Gürbüz, O.; Göçmen, D.; Dağdelen, F.; Gürsoy, M.; Aydin, S.; Şahin, I.; Büyükuysal, L. & Usta, M. (2007). Determination of flavan-3-ols and trans-resveratrol in grapes and wine using HPLC with fluorescence detection. *Food Chemistry*, 100, 518-525.

Hertog, M.G.L. (1998). Flavonols in wine and tea and prevention of coronary heart disease. In: Vercauteren, J.; Chèze, C. & Triaud, J. (eds.), Polyphenols 96, July 15–18, 1996, Bordeaux. Paris, *INRA*, 117–131.

Hurtado, I.; Caldu, P.; Gonzalo, A.; Ramon, J.M.; Minguez, S. & Fiol, C. (1997). Antioxidative capacity of wine on human LDL oxidation in vitro: Effect of skin contact in wine-making of white wine. *Journal of Agricultural and Food Chemistry*, 45, 1283-1289.

Hwang, J.Y.; Shyu, Y.S. & Hsu, C.K. (2009). Grape wine lees improves the rheological and adds antioxidant properties to ice cream. *LWT – Food Science and Technology*, 42, 312-318.

Jacob, J.K.; Hakimuddin F.; Paliyath, G. & Fisher, H. (2008). Antioxidant and antiproliferative activity of polyphenols in novel high-polyphenol grape lines. *Food Research International*, 41, 419-428.

Jordao, A.M.; Ricardo-Da-Silva, J.M. & Laureano, O. (2001). Evolution of catechins and oligomeric procyanidins during grape maturation of Castelao Frances and Touriga Francesa. *American Journal of Enology and Viticulture*, 52, 230-234.

Kallithraka, S.; Arvanytoiannis, I.; El-Zajouli, A. & Kefalas, P. (2001). The application of an improved method for trans-resveratrol to determine the origin of Greek red wines. *Food Chemistry*, 75, 355-363.

Kallithraka, S.; Mohdaly, A.A.; Makris, D.P. & Kefalas, P. (2005). Determination of major anthocyanin pigments in Hellenic native grape varieties (*Vitis vinifera* sp.). Association with antiradical activity. *Journal of Food Composition and Analysis*, 18, 375-386.

Kallithraka, S.; Tsoutsouras, E., Tzourou, E. & Lanaridis, P. (2006). Principal phenolic compounds in Greek red wines. *Food Chemistry*, 99, 784-793.

Kammerer, D.; Claus, A.; Carle, R. & Schieber, A. ((2004). Polyphenol screening of pomace from red and white grape varieties (*Vitis vinifera* L.) by HPLC-DAD-MS/MS. *Journal of Agricultural and Food Chemistry*, 52, 4360-4367.

Kanner, J.; Frankel, E.; Granit, R.; German, B. & Koinsella, J.E. (1994). Natural antioxidants in grapes and wines. *Journal of Agricultural and Food Chemistry*, 42, 64-69.

Karakaya, S.; El, S.N. & Tas, A.A. (2001). Antioxidant activity of some foods containing phenolic compounds. *International Journal of Food Sciences and Nutrition*, 52, 501–508.

Katalinić, V.; Milos, M.; Modun, D.; Musić, I. & Boban, M. (2004). Antioxidant effectiveness of selected wines in comparison with (+)-catechin. *Food Chemistry*, 86: 593–600.

Kennedy, J.A.; Matthews, M.A. & Waterhouse, A.L. (2002). Effect of maturity and vine water status on grape skin and wine flavonoids. *American Journal of Enology and Viticulture*, 53, 268-274.

Kolouchová-Hanzlíková, I.; Melzoch, K.; Filip, V. & Šmidrkal, J. (2004). Rapid method for resveratrol determination by HPLC with electrochemical and UV detections in wines. *Food Chemistry*, 87, 151-158.

Kopec, K. (1994). Resveratrol – a chemoprotective constituent of grapes. Zahradnictví – *Horticultural Science* (Prague), 26, 135–138.

Krisa, S.; Téguo, P.W.; Decendit, A.; Deffieux, G.; Vercauteren, J. & Mérillon, J.M. (1999). Production of ^{13}C-labelled anthocyanins by *Vitis vinifera* cell suspension cultures. *Phytochemistry*, 51, 651-656.

Lachman, J.; Hosnedl, V.; Pivec, V. & Orsák, M. (1998). Polyphenolics in Cereals and Their Positive and Negative Role in Human and Animal Nutrition. *International Conference Human Health and Preventive Nutrition. Mendel University of Agriculture and Forestry in Brno*, 7. – 11.07.1998 Brno, Czech Republic. *Proceedings*, 118-125.

Lachman, J.; Šulc, M.; Hejtmánková, A.; Pivec, V.; Orsák, M. (2004). Content of polyphenolic antioxidants and *trans*-resveratrol in grapes of different varieties of grapevine (*Vitis vinifera* L.). *Horticulture Sciences* (Prague), 31, 63-69.

Lachman, J. & Šulc, M. (2006). Phenolics and antioxidant activity of wines during the wine-making process. Control Applications in Post – *Harvest and Processing Technology* (CAPPT 2006). *4th IFAC/CIGR Workshop*. Section Measurement and Modelling of Crop or Product Responses for Quality Enhancement during Storage or Processing. *Leibniz-Institut für Agrartechnik Potsdam-Bornim*, 26. – 29.03.2006 Potsdam. *Abstracts*, 33-34.

Lachman, J.; Šulc, M. & Schilla, M. (2007). Comparison of the total antioxidant status of Bohemian wines during the wine-making process. *Food Chemistry*, 103, 802-807.

Lafka, T.I.; Sinanoglou, V. & Lazos, E.S. (2007). On the extraction and antioxidant activity of phenolic compounds from winery wastes. *Food Chemistry*, 104, 1206-1214.

Landrault, N.; Poucheret, P.; Ravel, P.; Gasc, F.; Cros, G. & Teissedre, P. (2001). Antioxidant capacities and phenolics levels of French wines from different varieties and vintages. *Journal of Agricultural Food Chemistry*, 49, 3341-3348.

La Torre, G.L.; Saitta, M.; Vilasi, F.; Pellicanò, T. & Dugo, G. (2006). Direct determination of phenolic compounds in Sicilian wines by liquid chromatography with PDA and MS detection. *Food Chemistry*, 94, 640-650.

Llobera, A. & Cañellas, J. (2007). Dietary fibre content and antioxidant activity of Manto Negro red grape (*Vitis vinifera*): pomace and stem. *Food Chemistry*, 101, 659-666.

Makris, D.P.; Psarra, E.; Kallithraka, S. & Kefalas, P. (2003). The effect of polyphenolic composition as related to antioxidant capacity in white wines. *Food Research International*, 36, 805-814.

Matějková, Š. & Gut, I. (2000). Polyphenols in nutrition as protective compounds. *Remedia*, 10, 272–281.

Mc Dougall, G.J.; Fyffe, S.; Dobson, P. & Stewart, D. (2005). Anthocyanins from red wine – their stability under simulated gastrointestinal digestion. *Phytochemistry*, 66, 2540-2548.

Minussi, R.C.; Rossi, M.; Bologna, L.; Cordi, L.; Rotilio, D.; Pastore, G.M. & Durán, N. (2003). Phenolic compounds and total antioxidant potential of commercial wines. *Food Chemistry*, 82, 409-416.

Mirabel, M.; Saucier, C.; Guerra, C. & Glories, Y. (1999). Copigmentation in model wine solutions: Occurrence and relation to wine aging. *American Journal of Enology and Viticulture*, 50, 211-218.

Mizutani, K.; Ikeda, K.; Kawai, Y. & Yamori, Y. (1999). Extract of wine phenolics improves aortic biomechanical properties in stroke-prone spontaneously hypertensive rats (SHRSP). *Journal of Nutritional Science and Vitaminology*, 45, 95-106.

Modun, D.; Musić, I.; Vuković, J.; Brizić, I.; Katalinić, V.; Obad, A.; Palada, I.; Dujić, Z. & Boban, M. (2008). The increase in human plasma antioxidant capacity after red wine consumption is due to both plasma urate and wine polyphenols. *Atherosclerosis*, 197, 250-256.

Molyneux, P. (2004). The use of the stable free radical diphenylpicrylhydrazyl (DPPH) for estimating antioxidant activity. Songklanakarin *Journal of Science and Technology*, 26, 211-219.

Monagas, M.; Bartolomé, B. & Gómez-Cordovés, C. (2005). Evolution of polyphenols in red wines from *Vitis vinifera* L. during aging in the bottle – II. Non-anthocyanin phenolic compounds. *European Food Research and Technology*, 220, 331-340.

Monagas, M.; Gómez-Cordovés, C. & Bartolomé, B. (2006a). Evolution of the phenolic content of red wines from *Vitis vinifera* L. during ageing in bottle. *Food Chemistry*, 95, 405-412.

Monagas, M.; Hernández-Ledesma, B.; Gómez-Cordovés, C. & Bartolomé, B. (2006b). Commercial dietary ingredients from Vitis vinifera L. leaves and grape skins: Antioxidant and chemical characterization. *Journal of Agricultural and Food Chemistry*, 54, 319-327.

Monagas, M; Gómez-Cordovés, C. & Bartolomé, B. (2007). Evaluation of different *Saccharomyces cerevisiae* strains for red wine-making. Influence on the anthocyanin, pyranoanthocyanin and non-anthocyanin phenolic content and colour characteristics of wines. *Food Chemistry*, 104, 814-823.

Montero, C.; Cristescu; S.M.; Jimenéz, J.B.; Orea, J.M.; Hekkert; S.T.L.; Harren, F.J.M. & Urena A.G. (2003). *trans*-Resveratrol and grape disease resistance. A dynamical study by high-resolution laser-based techniques. *Plant Physiology*, 131, 129-138.

Morales, M.; Alcántara, J. & Barceló, A.R., (1997). Oxidation of *trans*-resveratrol by a hypodermal peroxidase isoenzyme from Gamay rouge grape (*Vttis vinifera*) berries. *American Journal of Enology and Viticulture*, 48, 33-39.

Morais, H.; Ramos, C.; Forgacs, E.; Cserhati, T.; Matos, N.; Almeida, V. & Oliveira, J. (2002). Stability of anthocyanins extracted from grape skins. *Chromatographia*, 56, Supplement, 173-175.

Muňoz-Espada, A.C.; Wood, K.V.; Bordelon, B. & Watkins, B.A (2004). Anthocyanin quantification and radical scavenging capacity of Concord, Norton, and Marechal Foch grapes and wines. *Journal of Agricultural and Food Chemistry*, 52, 6779-6786.

Murcia, M.A. & Martinez-Tome, M. (2001). Antioxidant activity of resveratrol compared with common food additives. *Journal of Food Protection*, 64, 379-384.

Negro, C.; Tommasi, L. & Miceli, A. (2003). Phenolic compounds and antioxidant activity from red grape marc extracts. *Bioresource Technology*, 87, 41-44.

Netzel, A.; Strass, G.; Bitsch, I.; Konitz, R.; Christmann, M. & Bitsch, R. (2003). Effect of grape processing on selected antioxidant phenolics in red wine. *Journal of Food Engineering*, 56, 223-228.

Nikfardjam, M.S.P.; László, M.; Avar, P.; Figler, M. & Ohmacht, R. (2006a). Polyphenols, anthocyanins, and trans-resveratrol in red wines from the Hungarian Villa´ny region. *Food Chemistry*, 98, 453-462.

Nikfardjam, M.S.P.; László, G. & Dietrich, H. (2006b). Resveratrol-derivatives and antioxidative capacity in wines made from botrytized grapes. *Food Chemistry*, 96, 74-79.

Orak, H.H. (2007). Total antioxidant activities, phenolics, anthocyanins, polyphenoloxidase activities of selected red grape cultivars and their correlations. *Scientia Horticulturae*, 111, 235-241.

Ortega-Regules, A.; Romero-Cascales, I.; Ros-García, J.M.; López-Roca, J.M. & Gómez-Plaza, E. (2006). A first approach towards the relationship between grape skin cell-wall composition and anthocyanin extractability. *Analytica Chimica Acta*, 563, 26-32.

Paganga, G.; Miller, N. & Rice-Evans, C.A. (1999). The polyphenolic content of fruit and vegetables and their antioxidant activities. What does a serving constitute? *Free Radical Research*, 30, 153-162.

Paixão, N.; Perestrelo, R.; Marques, J.C. & Câmara, J.S. (2007). Relationship between antioxidant capacity and total phenolic content of red, rosé and white wines. *Food Chemistry*, 105, 204-214.

Pardo, F.; Salinas, M.R.; Alonso, G.L.; Navarro, G. & Huerta, M.D. (1999). Effect of diverse enzyme preparations on the extraction and evolution of phenolic compounds in red wines. *Food Chemistry*, 67, 135-142.

Pellegrini, N.; Simonetti, P.; Gardana, C.; Brenna, O.; Brighenti, F. & Pietta, P. (2000). Polyphenol content and total antioxidant activity of Vini novelli (young red wines). *Journal of Agricultural and Food Chemistry*, 48, 732-735.

Peña-Neira, A.; Hernández, T.; García-Valejjo, C. & Suarez, J.A. (2000). A survey of phenolic compounds in Spanish wines of different geographical origin. *European Food Research and Technology*, 210, 445-448.

Pennycooke, J.C.; Cox, S. & Stushnoff, J.C. (2005). Relationship of cold acclimation, total phenolic content and antioxidant capacity with chilling tolerance in petunia (*Petunia* x *hybrida*). *Environmental and Experimental Botany*, 53, 225-232.

Pérez-Magariño, S. & González-San José, M.L. (2006). Polyphenols and colour variability of red wines made from grapes harvested at different ripeness grade. *Food Chemistry*, 96, 197-208.

Pozo-Bayon, M.A.; Hernandez, M.T.; Martin-Alvarez, P.J. & Polo, M.C. (2003). Study of low molecular weight phenolic compounds during the aging of sparkling wines manufactured with red and white grape varieties. *Journal of Agricultural and Food Chemistry*, 51, 2089-2095.

Price, R.J. & Langcake, P. (1977). Viniferin: An antifungal resveratrol trimer from grapevines. *Phytochemistry*, 16, 1452-1454.

Prior, R.L., & Cao, G. (1999). In vivo antioxidant capacity: comparison of different analytical methods. *Free Radical Biology and Medicine*, 27, 1173-1181.

Rayne, S.; Karacabey, E. & Mazza, G. (2008). Grape cane waste as a source of *trans*-resveratrol and *trans*-viniferin: High-value phytochemicals with medicinal and anti-phytopathogenic applications. *Industrial Crops and Products*, 27, 335-340.

Rejlová, P. (2007). Vineyard regions. University of Hradec Králové, *Faculty of Informatics and Management*, http://lide.uhk.cz/fim/student/fsrejlp1/oblasti.html

Revilla, E. & Ryan, J.M. (2000). Analysis of several phenolic compounds with potential antioxidant properties in grape extracts and wines by high-performance liquid chromatography – photodiode array detection without sample preparation. *Journal of Chromatography* A, 881, 461-469.

Rivero-Pérez, M.D.; Muñiz, P. & González-Sanjosé, M.L. (2008a). Contribution of anthocyanin fraction to the antioxidant properties of wine. *Food and Chemical Toxicology*, 46, 2815-2822.

Rivero-Pérez, M.D.; González-Sanjosé, M.L.; Ortega-Herás, M. & Muñiz, P. (2008b). Antioxidant potential of single-variety red wines aged in the barrel and in the bottle. *Food Chemistry*, 111, 957-964.

Rodrigo, R.; Castillo, R.; Carrasco, R.; Huerta, P. & Moreno, M. (2005). Diminution of tissue lipid peroxidation in rats is related to the in vitro antioxidant capacity of wine. *Life Sciences*, 76, 889-900.

Roggero, J.P. (2000). Study of the ultraviolet irradiation of resveratrol and wine. *Journal of Food Composition and Analysis*, 13, 93-97.

Roginsky, V.; de Beer, D.; Habertson, J.F.; Kilmartin, P.A.; Barsukoval, T. & Adams, T.O. (2006). The antioxidant activity of Californian red wines does not correlate with wine age. *Journal of the Science of Food and Agriculture*, 86, 834-840.

Romero-Pérez, A.I.; Lamuela-Raventos, R.M.; Waterhouse, A.L. & de la Torre-Boronat, M.C. (1996). Levels of *cis*- and *trans*-resveratrol and their glucosides in white and rosé *Vitis vinifera* wines from Spain. *Journal of Agricultural and Food Chemistry*, 44, 2124-2128.

Sakkiadi, A.V.; Haroutounian, S.A. & Stavrakakis, M.N. (2001). Direct HPLC assay of five biologically interesting phenolic antioxidants in varietal Greek red wines. *Lebensmittel-Wissenschaft & Technologie*, 34, 410-413.

Sanchez-Moreno, C.; Cao, G.H.; Ou, B.X. & Prior, R.L. (2003). Anthocyanin and proanthocyanidin content in selected white and red wines. Oxygen radical absorbance capacity comparison with nontraditional wines obtained from highbush blueberry. *Journal of Agricultural and Food Chemistry*, 51, 4889-4896.

Saura-Calixto, F. & Díaz-Rubio, M.E. (2007). Polyphenols associated with dietary fibre in wine. A wine polyphenols gap? *Food Research International*, 40, 613-619.

Schmandke, H. (2002). Resveratrol and piceid in grapes and soybeans and products made from them. *Ernährungs-Umschau*, 49, 349–352.

Serafini, M., Maiani, M. & Ferro-Luzzi A. (1998). Alcohol-free red wine enhances plasma antioxidant capacity in humans. *Journal of Nutrition*, 128, 1003-1007.

Shahidi, F. & Naczk, M. (1995). Wine in food phenolics: sources, chemistry, effects, applications, *Pennsylvania: Technomic Publishing Co.*, 136-148.

Silva, L.R.; Andrade, P.B.; Valentão, P.; Seabra, R.M.; Trujillo, M.E. & Velázguez, E. (2005). Analysis of non-coloured phenolics in red wine: Effect of *Dekkera bruxellensis* yeast. *Food Chemistry*, 89, 185-189.

Soleas, G.J.; Grass, L.; Josephy, P.D.; Goldberg, D.M. & Diamandis, E.P. (2002). A comparison of the anticarcinogenic properties of four red wine polyphenols. *Clinical Biochemistry*, 35, 119-124.

Spigno, G. & Faveri D.M. (2007). Antioxidants from grape stalks and marc: Influence of extraction procedure on yield, purity and antioxidant power of the extracts. *Journal of Food Engineering*, 78, 793-801.

Stervbo, U.; Vang, O. & Bonnesen, Ch. (2007). A review of the content of the putative chemoprevetive phytoalexin resveratrol in red wine. *Food Chemistry*, 101, 449-457.

Sun, B.; Ribes, A.M.; Leandro, M.C.; Belchior, A.P. & Spranger, M.I. (2006). Stilbenes: Quantitative extraction from grape skins, contribution of grape solids to wine and variation during wine maturation. *Analytica Chimica Acta*, 563, 382-390.

Šmidrkal, J.; Filip, V.; Melzoch, K.; Hanzlíková, I.; Buckiová, D. & Kriša, B. (2001). Resveratrol. *Chemické Listy*, 95, 602–609.

Šulc, M.; Lachman, J.; Hejtmánková, A. & Orsák, M. (2005a). Relationship between antiradical activity, polyphenolic antioxidants and free *trans*-resveratrol in grapes (*Vitis vinifera* L.). *Horticulture Sciences (Prague)*, 32, 154-162.

Šulc, M.; Pivec, V.; Lachman, J. & Orsák, M. (2005b). Antiradical activity and polyphenolic antioxidants in grapes (*Vitis vinifera* l.) in the Czech vineyard area. *ChemZi, 1*, 283-284.

Šulc, M.; Lachman, J. & Masopustová, R. (2006). Effect of red wine from the Mělník vineyard region on antioxidant activity of blood plasma of *Rattus norvegicus* (Wistar). Biotechnology 2006, Section Animal Biotechnology. 15. – 16.02.2006, *South Bohemian University, České Budějovice. Proceedings*, 409-411.

Talcott, S.T.; Peele, J.E. & Brenes, C.H. (2005). Red clover isoflavonoids as anthocyanin color enhancing agents in muscadine wine and juice. *Food Research International*, 38, 1205-1212.

Teissedre, P.L. & Landrault, N. (2000). Wine phenolics: contribution to dietary intake and bioavailability. *Food Research International*, 33, 461-467.

Todaro, A.; Palmeri, R.; Barbagallo, R.N.; Pifferi, P.G. & Spagna, G. (2008). Increase of *trans*-resveratrol in typical Sicilian wine using β-Glucosidase from various sources. *Food Chemistry*, 107, 1570-1575.

Uhlig, B.A. (1998). Effects of solar radiation on grape (*Vitis vinifera* L.) composition and dried fruit colour. *Journal of Horticulture Science & Biotechnology*, 73, 111-123.

Uhlig, B.A. & Clingeleffer, P.R., (1998). Ripening characteristics of the fruit from *Vitis vinifera* L. drying cultivars sultana and Merbein seedless under furrow irrigation. *American Journal of Enology and Viticulture*, 49, 375-382.

Valentão, P.; Seabra, R.M.; Lopes, G.; Silva, L.R.; Martins, V.; Trujillo, M.E.; Velázquez, E. & Andrade, P.B. (2007). Influence of *Dekkera bruxellensis* on the contents of anthocyanins, organic acids and volatile phenols of Dão red wine. *Food Chemistry*, 100, 64-70.

Valero, E.; Sanchezferrer, A.; Varon, R. & Garciacarmona, F. (1989). Evolution of grape polyphenol oxidase activity and phenolic content during maturation and vinification. *Vitis*, 28, 85-95.

Versari, A.; Boulton, R.B. & Parpinello, G.P. (2008). A comparison of analytical methods for measuring the color components of red wines. *Food Chemistry*, 106, 397-402.

Villaño, D.; Fernández-Pachón, M.S.; Troncoso, A.M. & García-Parrilla, M.C. (2006). Influence of enological practices on the antioxidant activity of wines. *Food Chemistry*, 95, 394-404.

Vinson, J.A.; Teufel, K. & Wu, N. (2001). Red wine, dealcoholized red wine, and especially grape juice, inhibit atherosclerosis in a hamster model. *Atherosclerosis*, 156, 67-72.

Vivar-Quintana, A.M.; Santos-Buelga, C. & Rivas-Gonzalo, J.C. (2002). Anthocyanin-derived pigments and colour of red wines. *Analytica Chimica Acta*, 458, 147-155.

Wang, C.C.; Chu, C.Y.; Chu, K.O.; Choy, K.W.; Khaw, K.S.,; Rogers, M.S. & Pang, C.P. (2004). Trolox-equivalent antioxidant capacity assay versus oxygen radical absorbance capacity assay in plasma. *Clinical Chemistry*, 50, 952-954.

Waterhouse, A.L. & Lamuela-Raventos, R.M. (1994). The occurrence of piceid, a stilbene glucoside, in grape berries. *Phytochemistry*, 37, 571-573.

Waterhouse, A.L. & Laurie, V.F. (2006). Oxidation of wine phenolics: A critical evaluation and hypotheses. *American Journal of Enology and Viticulture*, 57, 306-313.

Woraratphoka, J.; Intarapichet, K.O. & Indrapichate, K. (2007). Phenolic compounds and antioxidative properties of selected wines from the northeast of Thailand. *Food Chemistry*, 104, 1485-1490.

Yildirim, H.K.; Akcay, Y.D.; Guvenc, U.; Altindisli, A. & Sozmen, E.Y. (2005). Antioxidant activities of organic grape, pomace, juice, must, wine and their correlation with phenolic content. *International Journal of Food Science and Technology*, 40, 133–142.

Yilmaz, Y. & Toledo, R.T. (2004a). Health aspects of functional grape seed constituents. *Trends in Food Science & Technology*, 15, 422-433.

Yilmaz, Y. & Toledo, R.T. (2004b). Major flavonoids in grape seeds and skins: Antioxidant capacity of catechin, epicatechin, and gallic acid. *Journal of Agricultural and Food Chemistry*, 52, 255-260.

Zafrilla, P.; Morillas, J.; Mulero, J.; Cayuela, J.M.; Martinez-Cacha, A.; Pardo, F. & Nicolas, J.M.L. (2003). Changes during storage in conventional and ecological wine: Phenolic content and antioxidant activity. *Journal of Agricultural and Food Chemistry*, 51, 4694-4700.

Zoecklein, B.W.; Wolf, T.K.; Duncan, S.E.; Marcy, J.E. & Jasinki, Y. (1998). Effect of fruit zone removal on total glycoconjugates and conjugate fraction concentration of Riesling and Chardonnay (*Vitis vinifera* L.) grapes. *American Journal of Enology and Viticulture*, 49, 259-265.

In: Red Wine and Health
Editor: Paul O'Byrne

ISBN 978-1-60692-718-2
© 2009 Nova Science Publishers, Inc.

Chapter 5

METHODS FOR THE DETERMINATION OF NATURAL ANTIOXIDANTS IN RED WINES

L.M. Ravelo-Pérez, A.V. Herrera-Herrera, J. Hernández-Borges and M.A. Rodríguez-Delgado[1]

Department of Analytical Chemistry, Nutrition and Food Science, University of La Laguna, Avda. Astrofísico Fco. Sánchez s/nº, 38071 La Laguna, Tenerife, Canary Islands, Spain.

ABSTRACT

Wine can be considered one of the most consumed drinks in the world, subjected to strict regulations concerning its quality in regards to truth-to-label and absence of additives. Among the different types of wines available, red wine is particularly important especially for its high antioxidant content. In this sense, research interest in this field has been intensified in the light of recent evidence regarding their important role in human health, particularly, several preventive effects on cancer, coronary heart diseases, neurological degeneration, inflammatory disorders, etc. Analytical methods for the analysis of antioxidants in red wines include mainly high-performance liquid chromatography (HPLC) and, with less applications, gas chromatography (GC). However, in recent years, the popularity of capillary electrophoresis (CE) has also increased the amount of works dealing with this subject. Therefore, the aim of this chapter is to describe the applications of the different analytical methods that have been developed so far for the analysis of natural antioxidants in red wine.

ABBREVIATIONS

BGE	Background electrolyte
BSTFA	bis(trimethylsilyl)trifluoroacetamide
CE	Capillary electrophoresis

CL	Chemiluminiscence
CMC	Critical micelle concentration
CZE	Capillary zone electrophoresis
DAD	Diode array detection
EC	Electrochemical detector
EOF	Electroosmotic flow
ESI	Electrospray ionization
FL	Fluorimetric detector
GC	Gas chromatography
HPLC	High-performance liquid chromatography
ITP	Isotacophoresis
LLE	Liquid-liquid extraction
LOD	Limit of detection
LOQ	Limit of quantification
LTFS	Low-temperature fluorescence spectroscopy
MEKC	Micellar electrokinetic chromatography
MEOH	Methanol
MS	Mass spectrometry
MSPD	Matrix solid-phase dispersion
ODS	Octadecylsilica
OS	Octylsilica
PA	Polyacrylate
PDA	Photodiode array detection
QqQ	Triple quadrupole
RPLC	Reversed-phase-liquid-chromatography
SDS	Sodium dodecyl sulphate
SIM	Single ion monitoring
SPE	Solid-phase extraction
SPME	Solid-phase microextraction
UPLC	Ultra performance liquid chromatography
UV	Ultraviolet

1. INTRODUCTION

Wine is a beverage of international trade widely consumed around the world. It has been part of human culture for more than 6000 years playing, in most cases, an important role in ceremonial life (i.e. ancient Greece, Rome and Egypt) [1]. From a chemical point of view, wine is a complex mixture of several hundred compounds at different concentrations levels being water, ethanol, glycerol, organic acids, sugars and salts the major ones while, for example, aliphatic and aromatic alcohols, amino acids and phenolic compounds are present at much lower concentrations. Chemical analysis of this complex mixture is becoming more and more important for quality control purposes for winemaking industries and consumers.

---

1 Corresponding author: Dr. Miguel Ángel Rodríguez-Delgado, Tel: +34 922 318046; Fax: +34 922 318003; email: mrguez@ull.es

Particularly, differentiation according to vine variety, geographical origin, winemaking process and year of production is of great importance.

In the late years, the medical community has cited beneficial health effects of wine based on the presence of other components different from alcohol. Much of the new data supports the basic premise that moderate consumption of wine and other alcoholic beverages is associated with a healthier and longer life than that of abstainers. As an example, red wine consumption has been proposed as an explanation for the lower death rate from coronary heart disease in France referred to as *"The French Paradox"* (despite high fat intake, mortality from coronary heart disease is lower in some regions of France than in the other developed countries due to regular wine consumption) [1]. Most of the benefits of wine consumption appear to be derived from the consumption of low quantities of alcohol, however other, less precisely defined, appear to be derived from other components: antioxidants (which can be found in higher amounts in red wines).

Generally speaking (not only in the wine field), the term *antioxidant* involves different types of compounds such as phenols (simple phenols, phenolic acids, flavonoids, coumarins, isocoumarins, xanthones, etc.), vitamins like vitamin C (ascorbic acid), B_2 (riboflavin) or E (tocopherol), carotenoids, etc. many of which are present in popular beverages in the world including tea, coffee, cocoa, fruits/vegetables juices, beer and wine. Their study has become an intense focus of research interest because of their recognised role in the prevention or management of several diseases and disorders (cerebral, cardiovascular, rheumatoid diseases, etc.) [2-4].

The antioxidant properties of red wines have been correlated especially with their content in anthocyanins [5], flavanols [6], and tannic acid [7]. However, it is highly believed that red wines' antioxidant properties are more linked with the total polyphenol concentration rather than individual polyphenols [8]. In fact, owing to the alcohol content, polyphenol compounds can be easily absorbed through the alimentary tract [9].

As a result, the determination of red wines antioxidant compounds is especially important in fields like nutrition but also in others like medicine or health [10-12]. This increasing interest has developed the need of the development of analytical procedures able to handle the complexity of the wine matrix.

Recent advances in separation science have helped to identify and quantify many different compounds in wines, including antioxidants. In this sense, the analytical technique most commonly used for the analysis of this type of compounds is high-performance liquid chromatography (HPLC), normally in reversed-phase, although other techniques like gas chromatography (GC) and capillary electrophoresis (CE) have also provided good results. The aim of this chapter is to provide an updated overview of the different analytical methods that exist nowadays for the determination of antioxidants in red wines, the different sample pretreatment available, detection systems most frequently used as well as some of their content in samples of different origin.

2. ANTIOXIDANTS PRESENT IN RED WINE

In general, antioxidants can be classified according to their action mechanism into primary, secondary and synergistic antioxidants. The first of them, terminate the oxidation chain reaction by the donation of either electrons or a hydrogen atom to free radicals. Secondary antioxidants prevent oxidation by the decomposition of the lipid peroxides into stable end products, while synergistic antioxidants are oxygen scavengers and chelators. Another classification can also be developed taking into account the chemical family they belong to.

Flavonoid Polyphenols

Flavonoids are a group of more than 4000 polyphenolic compounds that occur naturally in foods of plant origin. They are consumed in considerable amounts (it is estimated that the human intake of all flavonoids is a few hundreds of milligrams per day [13]) and are also heat stable. Their concentration in the wine depends highly on the grape variety, vineyard location, cultivation system, climate, soil type, vine cultivation practices, harvesting time, production process and ageing. The flavonoid class includes anthocyanidins, flavones, flavonols, flavanoids (leucoanthocyanidins), aurones, biflavonoids, chalcones, dichydrochalcones, flavanones, dihydroflavonols, flavans and isoflavonoids. There are also polymeric compounds called tannins. In all cases, further subdivision in other classes can also take place depending on the type and quantity of substituents. Although flavonoids are responsible for the color of fruits and vegetables, colorless flavonoids are also present in nature.

The flavonol class is mainly represented by quercetin, myricetin, kaempferol and isorhamnetin (see Figure 1). They constitute the most biologically important phenolics present in wine. Their antioxidative effect has been of interest for considerable time, although the specific mode of oxidation is not fully clear. The content of flavonols in wine highly depends on their extraction from the skins and thus on the extraction time and temperature. Also, significant changes in the amounts of flavonols during wine vinification processes have been found [14]. In red wines, flavonol compounds have been found up to total concentrations of approx. 200 mg/L [14]. *McDonald et al.* [15] developed a comparative study of free and conjugated myricetin and quercetin in 65 red wine samples. The analytical survey of the 65 samples of different origin showed that quercetin, myricetin and their glycosides were at concentrations between 4.6 and 41.6 mg/L. In many of the samples no aglycones were detected, which was attributed to their relative instability. An interesting comparison of flavonol contents of wines, grapes and grapes products of different variety and origin can be found in the work of *Makris et al.* [14].

The flavanol group which is also known as catechins, includes compounds such as catechin and epicatechin (which are optically active) and their gallates (see Figure 2). Like flavonoids, catechins are generally bound to sugars in order to increase their solubility. Red wine as well as green, black and oolong teas, fruits like plum, apples, peach, strawberry and cherry, and beans and grains like broad bean, lentil and cocoa are rich in catechins. They are released from both grape skins and seeds during the winemaking which, as well as the ageing, they undergo structural transformations (oxidation and condensation reactions) having a high influence on the astringency and color of the wine [16]. Their concentration in red wines is higher than all the other flavonoid compounds [17].

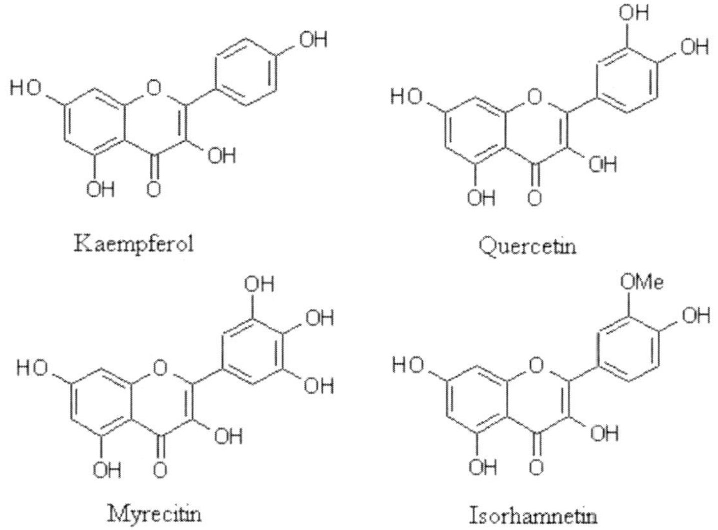

Figure 1. Chemical structures of the four common flavonol aglycones encountered in red wines.

Tannins are polymeric structures of a few to over 100 flavonoid units of high molecular weight [18]. In the so called condensed tannins, the monomeric forms are responsible for most of the red color of young wines, and they contribute to the development of more stable red polymeric pigments during wine aging. They are composed of monomer units of dihydroxylated catechins (i.e. (+)-catechin and (-)-epicatechin) forming procyanidins polymers, and/or trihydroxylated gallocatechins (i.e. (+)-gallocatechin and (-)-epigallocatechin) forming prodelphinidin polymers. Monomer units are linked by C_4–C_6 or C_4–C_8 bonds and are sometimes esterified by gallic acid on C_3, especially (-)-epicatechin (epicatechin 3-gallate) [19]. Condensed tannins are found in grape skins (procyanidins and prodelphinidins) and seeds (procyanidins only) and are extracted during winemaking.

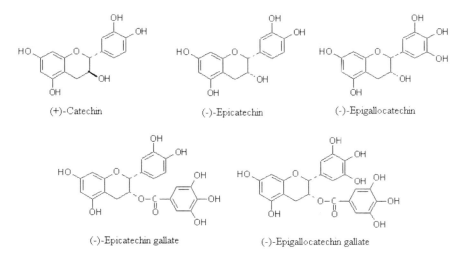

Figure 2. Chemical structures of the major catechins.

Resveratrol

Resveratrol (3,4,5-*N*-trihydroxystilbene), known for its ability to protect plants from bacteria and fungi, is a phytoalexin present also in grapes and wines that belong to the stilbene class. It exists in both *trans* and *cis* isomers (see Figure 3) and also in the glycoside form known as piceid. Both resveratrol and piceid can be found in wines at concentrations of the glycoside usually higher that the aglycone. The concentrations of each isomer in different grape cultivars and the respective wines are very variable, depending also on geographical origin, wine-making processes and fungal presence [20]. In fact, *trans*-resveratrol (the most stable) isomerizes to *cis*-resveratrol when exposed to UV light [21] causing changes in the respective concentrations of grapes, must and wine. It is one of the most studied antioxidants because it is believed to be the main responsible for red wine benefits on human health. Resveratrol in all its forms is found at much higher concentrations in red wines than in white or rose wines. At present, analysis of red wine originating from diverse countries show some variations in ranges of resveratrol concentrations (around 10 mg/L) while piceid can be found at higher concentrations, frequently three times higher [22, 23]. Various factors during the wine making process also affects the levels of resveratrol in the final red wines; increased temperature, higher levels of SO_2 and/or decreased pH results in higher resveratrol levels [24].

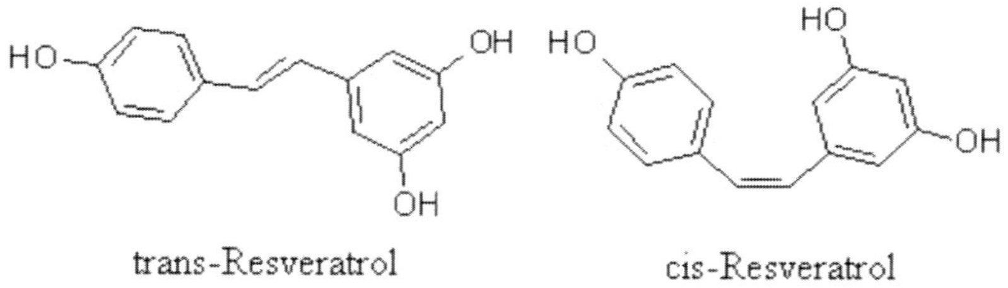

Figure 3. Chemical structure of resveratrol (3,4,5-*N*-trihydroxystilbene).

Non-Flavonoid Polyphenols

Non-flavonoid polyphenols are also abundant constituents of wine. They are simple phenols with a variety of different functional groups present (see Figure 4), like benzaldehydes (i.e. syringealdehyde, vanillin...), benzoic-based phenols (i.e. gallic acid, protocatechuic acid, vanillic acid...), cinnamic acids (i.e. ferullic acid, *p*-coumaric acid, caffeic acid, etc.) and cinnamaldehydes (i.e. sinapaldehyde, coniferaldehyde, etc.). These smaller phenolic acids are responsible for the wine bitterness while those volatile ones contribute to apart from the bitterness to the pungency and smokiness.

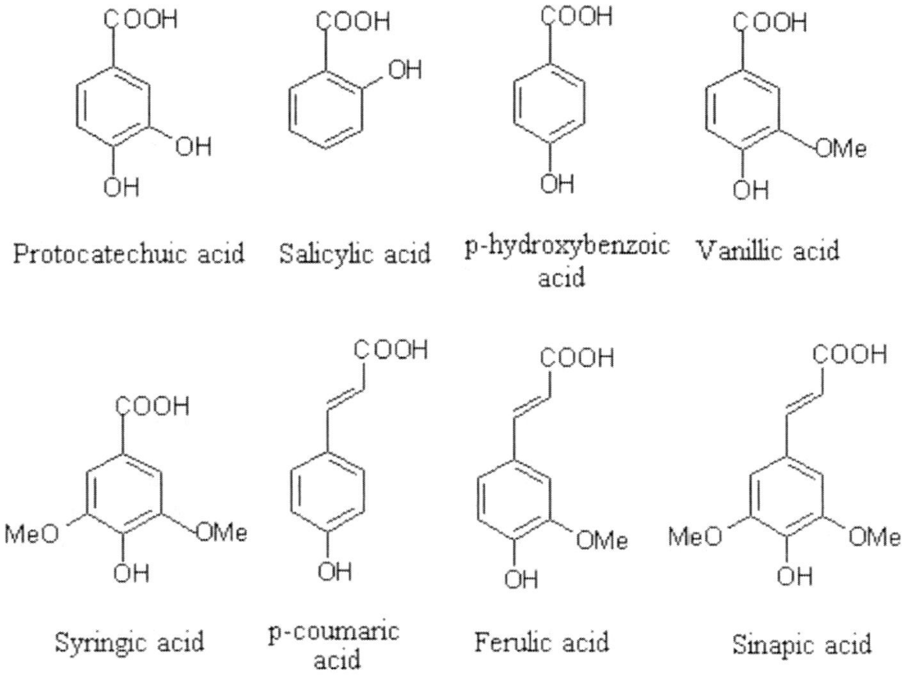

Figure 4. Chemical structures of common non-flavonoid polyphenols found in red wines.

3. ANALYSIS OF ANTIOXIDANTS IN RED WINES BY HPLC

Up to the present, HPLC technology has been the most widely used analytical approach to assay antioxidants compounds either individually or in combination, especially for the analysis of red wines (by reversed-phase-liquid-chromatography, (RPLC)). Most stationary phases are based on silica that has been chemically modified with octadecyl (C_{18} or ODS) or octyl (C_8 or OS) chains. Table 1 shows some examples of the application of HPLC for the analysis of antioxidants in red wines. In most of the applications either ultraviolet (UV) or diode array detector (DAD) have been used.

Total phenols and polyphenols are usually quantified by employing Folin-Ciocalteu's reagent. This procedure is also employed in the wine industry, where gallic acid is usually selected as a standard. On the other hand, total antioxidant activity values are measured from induction times in free radical mediated processes and/or from the bleaching of stable free radicals [25]. However, these methods can not specifically show the individual concentration of each compound. For this purpose, HPLC methods are highly used. This is also the case of the work developed by *Zhang et al.* [26]. In this work, a selective and sensitive method was developed for the determination of 20 phenolic compounds (*m*-aminophenol, tyrosine, phloroglucinol, gallic acid, pyrogallol, 3,5-dihydroxybenzoic acid, resorcinol, 2,5-dihydroxybenzoic acid, *p*-hydroxybenzoic acid, 2,4-dihydroxybenzoic acid, 2,3-dihydroxybenzoic acid, *m*-hydroxybenzoic acid, phenol, puerarin, salicylic acid, *trans*-resveratrol, quercetin, 1-naphthol, kaempferol and isorhamnetin) in Chinese red wine by HPLC with DAD and chemiluminiscence detection, which is not a frequent detection system used in this field. In this case, wine samples were filtered and directly introduced in the HPLC system. Chemiluminiscence detection was based on a Cerium (IV)-rhodamine 6G system. The reaction between cerium (IV) and rhodamine 6G in a strong sulfuric acid medium undertakes weak chemiluminiscence (CL), which can be greatly enhanced by different phenolic compounds [27]. The chromatographic profile of phenolic compounds in red wine by CL detection showed that there is no interference of the sample matrix. Six of the 20 phenolic compounds were identified and quantified in the wine (gallic acid, *p*-hydroxybenzoic acid, 2,4-dihydroxybenzoic acid, salicylic acid, *trans*-resveratrol and kaempferol). The use of a DAD could only allow the quantification of one of these six phenolic compounds (the LOD of the DAD was higher). Another example is the work of *García-Falcón et al.* [28] who developed various HPLC-DAD methods for the determination of 38 phenolic compounds in Spanish red wines. One method was developed for the analysis of anthocyanins, another for the simultaneous analysis of phenolic acids, catechins and flavonols, and another one for the analysis of procyanidins. Among the phenolic compounds, gallic acid, protocatechuic acid, *p*-hydroxybenzoic acid, *trans*-caftaric acid, *cis*-coutaric acid, *trans*-coutaric acid, vanillic acid, (+)-catechin, trans-caffeic acid, syringic acid, (-)-epicatechin, *trans p*-coumaric acid, procyanidin B3, procyanidin B1, trimer, procyanidin B4 and procyanidin B2 could be found. Concerning sample preparation, anthocyanins and hydroxycinnamic acids were determined by direct injection of the samples (after filtration) while hydroxybenzoic acids, catechins, procyanidins and flavonols required a more complex analytical pretreatment involving liquid-liquid extraction (LLE) with ethyl ether followed by solid phase extraction (SPE) on C_{18} stationary phases. The determination of hydroxybenzoic acids, catechins, procyanidins and flavonols entailed their fractionation into phenolic acids, catechins and flavonols (fraction 1) on the one hand and procyanidins (fraction 2) on the other. Fraction 1 was the result of the LLE with diethyl ether while fraction 2 was the result of the SPE of the residual wine previously extracted with diethyl ether (see Figure 5). Because of the overlap between some catechins and procyanidins with interferences from the sample matrix (as well as low recovery values for gallic and protocatechuic acids), the SPE procedure was not enough and thus the LLE procedure was introduced. In this case, mean recovery values were in the range 51-100% for all phenolic acids also for gallic and protocatechuic acids (the ones with the lowest molecular weight).

Concerning the analysis of resveratrol, HPLC is presently the method of choice for its quantification in wines based upon the number of reported applications [26, 29-33]. In a very beginning, only *trans*-resveratrol was analyzed, but later on, methods were developed for the quantification of both isomers. Very recently *Mercolini et al.* [32] developed a new HPLC method for the determination of resveratrol isomers together with melatonin in red and white Italian wines using fluorescence detection (all these analytes have native fluorescence). Separation of the isomers together with melatonin was obtained by using a RP column (C_8) and a mobile phase composed of 79% aqueous phosphate buffer at pH 3.0 and 21% acetonitrile. Fluorescence intensity was monitored at λ_{em} = 386 nm while exciting at λ_{exc}= 298 nm, mirtazapine was used as the internal standard. In this case the samples were previously extracted by SPE using BondElut C_{18} cartridges. As it has been previously reported (and also expected), the concentration of resveratrol was found to be higher in the red wine than in white wine and *trans*-resveratrol was also found at higher concentrations than *cis*-resveratrol in both wines.

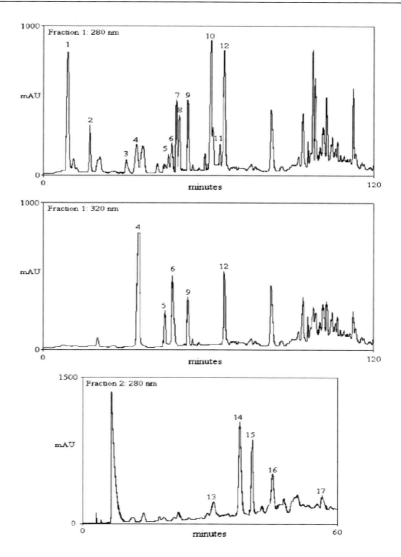

Figure 5. Chromatograms of the fraction 1 (phenolic acids and catechins at 280 and 320 nm) and fraction 2 (procyanidins at 280 nm) of Mencia red wine. Peaks identification: (1) gallic acid, (2) protocatechuic acid, (3) p-hydroxybenzoic acid, (4) trans-caftaric acid, (5) cis-coutaric acid, (6) trans-coutaric acid, (7) vanillic acid, (8) (+)-catechin, (9) trans-caffeic acid, (10) syringic acid, (11) (-)-epicatechin, (12) trans p-coumaric acid, (13) procyanidin B3, (14) procyanidin B1, (15) trimer, (16) procyanidin B4 and (17) procyanidin B2. Reprinted from [28] with permission from Elsevier.

Ultra-high performance liquid chromatography (UPLC) as a recent implementation of HPLC has also been applied to the analysis of antioxidants in wines [34, 35] despite the fact that, up to now, few applications of UPLC in food analysis have been published (more works will sure come out in a relatively short period of time). When compared to HPLC, it is clear that UPLC, which is manufactured for the use of columns with sub-2 μm particles, provides a higher peak capacity, greater resolution, increased sensitivity and higher speed of analysis. *Spáčil et al.* [34] compared an HPLC and UPLC method for the determination of 34 phenolic substances in red wines and tea among which gallic acid, protocatechuic acid, vanillic acid, caffeic acid, syringic acid, *p*-coumaric acid, ferulic acid, sinapic acid and *o*-coumaric acid could be found. For this purpose, similar conditions and analytical columns with analogous particle size were used. The HPLC mobile phase consisted of 0.1% formic acid–methanol, from 85:15 to 50:50 (v/v) pumped at 1.0 mL/min; while the UPLC mobile phase also consisted of 0.1% formic acid–methanol, from 88.5:11.5 to 30:70 (v/v) pumpted at 0.45 mL/min. In this case, the UPLC method performed 4.6 times faster than the HPLC approach. While the HPLC method indicated problems with the resolution of chlorogenic, vanillic and caffeic acid (partial peak overlap) this poor resolution was not observed by UPLC (see Figure 6). A similar comparison was carried out for the separation of coumarins and flavonoids but only the method developed for phenolic acids was used for the their identification in red wines.

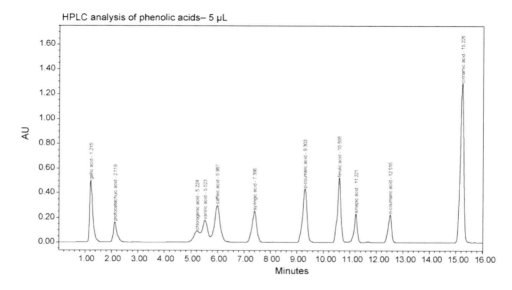

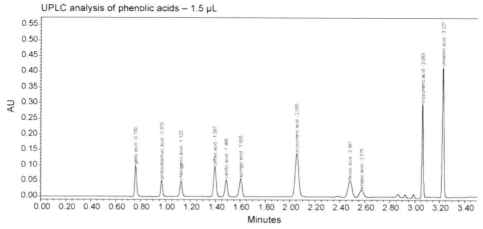

Figure 6. Separation of 11 phenolic acids by HPLC and UPLC. Mobile phase composition: HPLC, 0.1% formic acid–methanol, from 85:15 to 50:50 (v/v), 1.0 mL/min; UPLC, 0.1% formic acid–methanol, from 88.5:11.5 to 30:70 (v/v), 0.45 mL/min. Reprinted from [34] with permission from Elsevier.

4. ANALYSIS OF ANTIOXIDANTS IN RED WINES BY GC

GC has also been used for the analysis of antioxidants in red wines; however, the fact that a suitable derivatization reaction is required in order to increase the volatility and thermal stability of these polar compounds and thus the sensitivity of the determination, has only originated few applications in this field. Table 2 shows some of these works.

Contrary to what frequently happens in HPLC methods, with GC determination a more complex sample pretreatment in required. In this sense, SPE is the most applied technique. As an example, *Soleas et al.* [46] developed a method for the analysis of 15 polyphenols (the phenolic acids gentisic, vanillic, ferulic, *m*-coumaric, *p*-coumaric, caffeic, and gallic acid; the trihydroxystilbenes *cis*- and *trans*-resveratrol and *cis*- and *trans*-polydatin; and the flavonoids catechin, epicatechin, quercetin, and morin) in red and white wines. An assay involving SPE (on C_8) followed by derivatization with 1:1 bis(trimethylsilyl)trifluoroacetamide (BSTFA) and GC-MS was used to quantify the polyphenols. Overlapping values between red and white wines were observed for gentisic, ferulic, *p*-coumaric, and caffeic acid, while the concentrations of the other polyphenols were 5-20-fold higher in red wines, apart from *m*-coumaric acid and morin, which could not be detected in any of these wines. Another example of the application of SPE for the analysis of antioxidants in red wine by GC is the work of *Minuti and Pellegrino* [47], who employed matrix solid-phase dispersion (on silica gel) for the analysis of 23 phenolic compounds (homovanillic acid, catechin, gallic acid, homogentisic acid, 3,4-dihydroxyphenylacetic acid, vanillic acid, syringic acid, tyrosol, caffeic acid, (−)-epicatechin, fisetin, sinapinic acid, vanillin, *p*-hydroxybenzoic acid, ferulic acid, coumaric acid, quercetin, veratric acid, kaempferol, *trans*-cinnamic acid, *trans*-resveratrol and flavonone) from red wine samples prior their determination by GC-MS. LODs were between 2 and 8 µg/L. In another work of the same group, *Minuti et al.* [48] also determined 22 phenolic compounds (vanillin, *trans*-cinnamic acid, tyrosol, veratric acid, vanillic acid, homovanillic acid, 3,4-dihydroxyphenylacetic acid, homogentisic acid, syringic acid, *p*-coumaric acid, gallic acid, flavonone, ferulic acid, caffeic acid, sinapinic acid, *trans*-resveratrol, (−)-epicatechin, catechin, fisetin, quercetin and myricetin) in red wines by GC-MS. In this case, three extraction and derivatization procedures were compared: LLE with ethyl acetate; SPE on C_{18}; and LLE with ethyl acetate and salt addition. In all cases, derivatization with BSTFA/pyridine was assayed. The third extraction procedure (LLE with ethyl acetate and salt addition and derivatization with BSTFA) was selected as the optimal extraction method. The recoveries for all the compounds were in a range of 73-107%, which were generally better than those found with the other two methods. The whole method was applied to four different red wine samples, finding that gallic acid, tyrosol, caffeic acid and catechin were the most abundant components in all these samples analyzed. Moreover, LODs achieved were in the range of 1-8 µg/L for all the analytes, except for quercetin (30 µg/L) and myricetin (360 µg/L).

Resveratrol has also been analyzed several times by GC [10, 49-54]. In most of these methods a derivatization with bis(trimethylsilyl)trifluoroacetamide is developed in order to increase the sensitivity and selectivity of the determination (resveratrol is a polar compound that tends to absorb onto the GC column). Although the GC separation allows the determination of both *cis*- and *trans*- isomers, the fact that a suitable derivatization and extraction procedure has to be developed, increases the analysis time. One example is the

Table 1. Some examples of HPLC methods for the determination of antioxidants in red wines.

Analytes	Column	Amount found	Detection	Comments	Reference
Gallic acid, protocatechuic acid, vanillic acid, caffeic acid, syringic acid, p-coumaric acid, ferulic acid, sinapic acid, o-coumaric acid	HPLC: Zorbax SB C$_{18}$ (50mm×4.6mm, 1.8µm) UPLC: bridged ethylene hybrid (BEH) C$_{18}$ (100mm×2.1mm, 1.7µm)	-	UV (280nm)	Samples were filtrated and directly injected. UPLC gradient method brought a substantial saving in time (a factor of 2–8)	[34]
Gallic acid, procyanidin B1, *trans*-caffeoyltartaric acid, (+)-catechin, *trans*-coumaroyltartaric acid, procyanidin B2, (-)-epicatechin, delphinidin-3-*O*-glucoside, cyanidin-3-*O*-glucoside, petunidin-3-*O*-glucoside, peonidin-3-*O*-glucoside, malvidin-3-*O*-glucoside, rutin, quercetin-3-*O*-glucuronoside, malvidin-3-*O*-glucoside-acetate, *trans*-resveratrol, malvidin-3-*O*-glucoside-(*p*-coumarate)	Nova-Pak C$_{18}$ (250 mm×3.9 mm, 5µm)	-	DAD (250-600 nm)	-	[29]
Hydroxybenzoic acids: gallic, protocatechuic, *p*-hydroxybenzoic, vanillic, syringic. Hydroxycinnamic acids: *cis*-caftaric, *trans*-caftaric, *cis*-coutaric, *trans*-coutaric, *trans*-caffeic, *trans*-*p*-coumaric, *trans*-ferulic, catechins: (+)-catechin, (-)-epicatechin. Procyanidins: trimer, procyanidin B1, procyanidin b4, procyanidin b2. Flavonols: glycosylated flavonol, myricetin, kaempferol, quercetin. Anthocyanins: delfinidin 3-glucoside, cyanidin, petunidin 3-glucoside, peonidin 3-glucoside, malvidin 3-glucoside, peonidin 3-(6-acetyl glucoside), malvidin 3-(6-acetyl glucoside), malvidin 3-(6-coumaryl glucoside), polymeric anthocyanin	Anthocyanins: Symmetry C$_{18}$ (150 x 4.6 mm i.d., 5 µm). Phenolic acids, catechins, procyanidins and flavonols: ODS Hypersyl (250 x 4.6 mm i.d., 5 µm)	Hydroxybenzoic acids: 28-38 mg/L Hydroxycinnamic acids: 55-164 mg/L Catechins: 25-50 mg/L Procyanidins: 31-68 mg/L Flavonols: 3-17 mg/L Anthocyanins: 10-205 mg/L	DAD (280, 320, 360, 520 nm)	LLE (ethyl ether) and SPE (Sep-Pak Plus C$_{18}$) for hydroxybenzoic acids, catechins, procyanidins and flavonols. LOQs: 0.2-1 mg/L	[28]
Anthocyanins: Delphinidin-3-*O*-glucoside, cyanidin-3-*O*-glucoside, petunidin-3-*O*-glucoside, peonidin-3-*O*-glucoside, malvidin-3-*O*-glucoside, delphinidin-3-glucosylacetate, petunidin-3-glucosylacetate, malvidin-3-glucosylacetate, delphinidin-3-glucosylcoumarate, petunidin-3-glucosylcoumarate, and malvidin-3-glucosylcoumarate. Phenolic acids: gallic acid, *cis*-caftaric acid, *trans*-caftaric acid. Flavonols: rutin, acid, *cis*-coutaric acid, *trans*-coutaric acid, caffeic acid and *p*-coumaric, myricetin-3-glucoside, kaempferol, myricetin, quercetin, isorhamnetin-3-glucoside. Flavanols: catechin, epicatechin and epigallocatechin.	Kromasil 100-C$_{18}$ (200mm×46mm i.d., 5 µm)	Total proanthocyanidin: 238-2411mg/L	DAD (280, 310, 365, 515 nm)	Fractionation of wine phenolics by gel permeation chromatography (GPC). LOD 0.01mg/L.	[36]

Table 1. (Continued)

Analytes	Column	Amount found	Detection	Comments	Reference
Myricetin, luteolin, quercetin, kaempferol, isorhamnetin and galanin.	LiChrospher 100RP-18e (250 x 4.0 mm i.d., 5 μm)	Quercetin: 0.17–4.87 mg/L, myricetin: 1.57–4.45 mg/L, luteolin: 0.18–0.96 mg/L, kaempferol: 0.06–0.20 mg/L, isorhamnetin: 0.03–0.54 mg/L and galangin: 0.01–0.04 mg/L	UV (360 nm)	Sample filtration (organic solvents elimination). LOD: 0.010 –0.036 mg/L	[37]
Catechin, epicatechin and *trans*-resveratrol.	C_{18} Hypersil H5 ODS column (250 x 4.6 mm i.d.)	Catechin: 5.823-14.357 mg/L, Epicatechin: 0.873-3.232 mg/L, Resveratrol: 0.176-4.403 mg/L	FL ($\lambda_{Exc}/\lambda_{Em}$ 280/315 nm for catechin and epicatechin, 324/370 nm for *trans*-resveratrol).	Sample centrifugation and directly injection	[30]
Gallic acid, protocatechuic acid, tyrosol, vanillic acid, syringic acid, caffeic acid, ferulic acid, *p*-coumaric acid, procyanidin B1, procyanidin B2, (+)-catechin, (-)-epicatechin, ethylgallate, rutin, isoquercitrin, isorhamnetin-3-o-glucoside, kaempferol-3-o-glucoside, myricetin, quercetin, kaempferol, isorhamnetin, rhamnetin, *trans*-resveratrol, *cis*-resveratrol, *trans*-piceid, *cis*-piceid	C_{18} Discovery (150 mm x 2.1 mm i.d, 5 μm)	Gallic acid: 28.34-107.83 mg/L Protocatechuic acid: 0.85-4.05 mg/L Tyrosol: 3.11-75.66 mg/L Vanillic acid: 4.60-11.19 mg/L Syringic acid: 3.62-9.90 mg/L Caffeic acid: 2.25-24.42 mg/L Ferulic acid: 0.04-1.96 mg/L *p*-Coumaric acid: 0.18-2.78 mg/L Procyanidin B1: 8.06-127.5 mg/L Procyanidin B2: 4.66-80.98 mg/L (+)-Catechin: 5.45-99.00 mg/L (-)-Epicatechin: 23.23-136.01 mg/L Ethylgallate: 5.45-31.83 mg/L Rutin: 1.86-29.75 mg/L Isoquercitrin: 9.06-58.44 mg/L Isorhamnetin-3-O-glucoside: 0.61-21.89 mg/L Kaempferol-3-O-glucoside: 0.87-44.86 mg/L. Myricetin: 1.91-30.92 mg/L Quercetin: 3.19-16.70 mg/L Kaempferol: 0.13-0.57 mg/L Isorhamnetin: 0.10-0.90 mg/L Rhamnetin: 0.08-0.22 mg/L *trans*-Resveratrol: 0.10-2.44 mg/L *cis*-Resveratrol: 0.04-1.81 mg/L *trans*-Piceid: 0.25-3.74 mg/L *cis*-Piceid: 0.05-1.97mg/L	PDA (258-370 nm)-MS	Sample filtration and direct injection. LODs:0.001-0.160 mg/L	[31]

Table 1. (Continued)

Analytes	Column	Amount found	Detection	Comments	Reference
Trans- and *cis-*resveratrol,	RP column C$_8$ (150 mm x4.6 mm id, 5 μm)	*Trans-*resveratrol: 210 ng/mL; *cis-*resveratrol: 50 ng/mL	FL ($\lambda_{Exc}/\lambda_{Em}$ 298/386 nm)	SPE (BondElut C$_{18}$). LOD: 1 ng/mL for *trans-*resveratrol and 0.3 ng/mL for *cis-*resveratrol.	[32]
Pyranomalvidin 3-glucoside-dimer B3, pyranomalvidin 3-glucoside-(+)-catechin, pyranomalvidin 3-glucoside-(-)-epicatechin, pyranomalvidin 3-(coumaroyl) glucoside-dimer B1, pyranomalvidin 3-(coumaroyl) glucoside-(+)-catechin, pyranomalvidin 3-(coumaroyl) glucoside-(-)-epicatechin	DAD: RP C$_{18}$ (250mm×4.6mm i.d.); MS: AQUA RP C$_{18}$ (150mm×4.6 mm, 5μm)	Pyranomalvidin 3-glucoside-dimer B3: 7.86-10.59 mg/L, Pyranomalvidin 3-glucoside-(+)-catechin: 0.75-2.51 mg/L, Pyranomalvidin 3-glucoside-(-)-epicatechin: 1.91-6.30 mg/L Pyranomalvidin 3-(coumaroyl) glucoside-dimer B1: 3.33-6.62 mg/L, Pyranomalvidin 3-(coumaroyl) glucoside-(+)-catechin: 0.54-0.82 mg/L, Pyranomalvidin 3-(coumaroyl) glucoside-(-)-epicatechin: 1.65-2.39 mg/L.	DAD (510 nm), Electrospray ionization-mass spectrometry (ESI-MS)	Isolation with TSK Toyopearl gel HW-40 (S)	[38]
Polyphenols: gallic acid, tyrosol, caftaric acid, catechin, grp, procyanidin B2, caffeic acid, epicatechin, *p*-coumaric acid, fertaric acid, rutin, ferulic acid, quercetin, *trans-*resveratrol, anthocyanins: delphinidin-3-glucoside, petunidin-3-glucoside, peonidin-3-glucoside, malvidin-3-glucoside	Polyphenols and anthicyanins: ChromSep LiChrospher RP-18 end-capped (250x4.6 mm i.d, 5 μm); *trans-*resveratrol: C$_{18}$ (250x4.6 mm i.d, 6 μm)	Polyphenols: Gallic acid: 29.7-79.2 mg/L Tyrosol: 46.7-117 mg/L Caftaric acid: 42.1-87.0 mg/L Catechin: 62.1-103 mg/L GRP: 0.0-4.7 mg/L Procyanidin B2: 3.0-83.2 mg/L Caffeic acid: 5.9-37.4 mg/L Epicatechin: 64.6-126 mg/L *p*-coumaric acid: 0.0-10.5 mg/L Fertaric acid: 0.0-11.5 mg/L Rutin: 6.8-20.2 mg/L Ferulic acid: 0.0-2.6 mg/L Quercetin: 2.4-13.4 mg/L *trans-*Resveratrol: 0.8-3.9 mg/L Anthocyanins: Delphinidin-3-glucoside: 24.3-152 mg/L Petunidin-3-glucoside: 14.0-220 mg/L Peonidin-3-glucoside: 11.4-128 mg/L Malvidin-3-glucoside: 129-1810 mg/L	PDA (280, 306, 520 nm)	-	[33]

Table 1. (Continued)

Analytes	Column	Amount found	Detection	Comments	Reference
Epicatechin-peonidin-3-O-glucoside, epicatechin-malvidin-3-O-glucoside, delphinidin-3-O-glucoside, diepicatechin-malvidin-3-O-glucoside, cyanidin-3-O-glucoside, epicatechin-malvidin-3-O-glucoside, diepicatechin–malvidin-3-O-glucoside, petunidin-3-O-glucoside, peonidin-3-O-glucoside, malvidin-3-O-glucoside, malvidin-3-O-glucoside pyruvate, malvidin-3-O-glucoside acetaldehyde, malvidin-3-O-glucoside-8-ethyl-epicatechin, malvidin-3-O-glucoside-8-ethyl-epicatechin, malvidin-3-O-glucoside-4-vinyl-diepicatechin, malvidin-3-O-glucoside-8-ethyl-epicatechin, malvidin-3-O-glucoside-4-vinyl-diepicatechin, malvidin-3-O-glucoside-8-ethyl-epicatechin, epicatechin-malvidin-3-O-coumarylglucoside, malvidin-3-O-coumarylglucoside pyruvate, peonidin-3-O-acetyl-glucoside, malvidin-3-O-acetyl-glucoside, delphinidin-3-O-coumarylglucoside, malvidin-3-O-acetyl-glucoside-4-vinyl-epicatechin, malvidin-3-caffeoylglucoside, cyanidin-3-O-coumarylglucoside, petunidin-3-O-coumarylglucoside, malvidin-3-O-coumarylglucoside, malvidin-3-O-coumarylglucoside-4-vinyl-diepicatechin, malvidin-3-O-coumarylglucoside-4-vinylepicatechin, peonidin-3-O-coumarylglucoside-8-ethyl-epicatechin, malvidin-3-O-coumarylglucoside-8-ethyl-epicatechin, peonidin-3-O-coumarylglucoside, malvidin-3-O-coumarylglucoside, malvidin-3-O-glucoside-4-vinylcatechol, malvidin-3-O-coumarylglucoside-4-vinylepicatechin, malvidin-3-O-coumarylglucoside-4-vinyl-epicatechin, malvidin-3-O-coumarylglucoside-4-vinyl-epicatechin, malvidin-3-O-glucoside-4-vinylphenol, malvidin-3-O-glucoside-4-vinylguaiacol, malvidin-3-O-coumarylglucoside-8-ethyl-epicatechin.	Luna C$_{18}$ column (150 x 2.0 mm i.d., 5 µm)	-	UV (520 nm)-ESI-MS	-	[39]
Gallic acid, p-hydroxybenzoic acid, 2,4-dihydroxybenzoic acid, salicylic acid, trans-resveratrol, kaempferol	Zorbax Eclipse XDB-C$_8$, (150mm×4.6mm i.d., 5µm)	Gallic acid: 5314.2 ng/mL p-Hydroxybenzoic acid: 2871.5 ng/mL 2,4-Dihydroxybenzoic acid: 938.6 ng/mL Salicylic acid: 463.7 ng/mL trans-Resveratrol: 244.3 ng/mL Kaempferol: 43.9 ng/mL	DAD (254, 270, 290, 306, 365 nm). Chemiluminescence detection	LOD: 2.9-814.2 ng/mL	[26]

Table 1. (Continued)

Analytes	Column	Amount found	Detection	Comments	Reference
Gallic acid, caffeic acid, catechin, epicatechin, procyanidin, myricetin 3-glucoside, quercetin 3-glucoside, quercetin 3-glucuronide, rutin, myricetin, quercetin, kaempferol, isorhamnetin, delphinidin-3-glucoside, cyaniding-3-glucoside, petunidin, peonidin glucosides, malvidin-3-glucoside, four unidentified acylated anthocyanins	-	Average flavonols: 5.16 mg/L	DAD and electrochemical detector (EC)	Flavanols were determined by the reaction with *p*-(dimethylamino)-cynnamaldehyde	[40]
cis- and *trans*-resveratrol, *cis*- and *trans*-resveratrol glucoside (astringin), *cis*- and *trans*-piceatannol and *cis*- and *trans*-piceatannol glucoside (piceid)	C$_{18}$ column (250mmx2.1mm i.d.) packed in laboratory, with Kromasil particle size 5 µm	*cis*-resveratrol: 0.48-3.10 mg/L *trans*-resveratrol: 0.63-2.24 mg/L *cis*-astringin (only detected in three varieties of wine): 0.51-1.59 mg/L **trans-astringin (only detected in two varieties of wine): 0.51-1.83 mg/L** *trans*-piceatannol: 0.54-1.80 mg/L *trans*-picied: 0.47-9.31 mg/L *cis*-piceid (only detected in two varieties of wine): 3.81-38.47 mg/L	MS (QqQ)	SPE (Sep-Pak C$_{18}$). LOD: 48.0 ng/mL for *cis*- and *trans*-resveratrol and for *cis*- and *trans*-resveratrol glucoside, and 50.0 ng/mL for *cis*- and *trans*-piceatannol.	[41]
***trans*-resveratrol, *cis*-resveratrol, *trans*-piceid and *cis*-piceid**	A Synergi Hydro-RP 80 (150 x 2 mm i.d., 4µm)	*trans*-resveratrol: 1.06-6.48 mg/L *cis*-resveratrol: 1.92-5.15 mg/L *trans*-picied: 1.07-2.65 mg/L *cis*-piceid: 1.22-12.9 mg/L	DAD-ESI-MS/MS	Sample filtration and direct injection	[42]
***trans*-resveratrol**	Nova-Pak C$_{18}$ (150x3.9 mm i.d., 4 µm)	0.18-5.66 mg/L (DAD), 0.25-5.46 mg/L (FL)	DAD(280 nm) and FL(λexc=360 nm / λem=374 nm)	SPE (Sep-Pak Plus C$_{18}$ cartridges). LOD: 0.02 mg/L (DAD), 0.003mg/L (fluorescence)	[43]

Table 1. (Continued)

Analytes	Column	Amount found	Detection	Comments	Reference
Gallic acid, protocatechuic acid, protocatechuicaldehyde, (+)-catechin, vanillic acid, caffeic acid, syringic acid, (-)-epicatechin, syringaldehyde, p-coumaric acid, ferulic acid, *trans*-resveratrol, myricetin, quercitrin, quercetin, kaempferol	Nova-Pak C$_{18}$ (150x3.9-mm i.d., 4μm).	Gallic acid: 15.13-43.09 mg/L (DAD) Protocatechuic acid: nd-1.10 mg/L (DAD) Protocatechuicaldehyde: 0.60-1.17 mg/L (DAD) (+)-Catechin: 102.22-132.04 mg/L (DAD), 10.60-31.69 mg/L (FL) Vanillic acid: 0.80-1.58 mg/L (DAD), 1.22-2.11mg/L (FL) Caffeic acid: 2.12-4.42 mg/L (DAD) Syringic acid: 1.04-2.73 mg/L (DAD), 1.64-2.64 mg/L (FL) (-)-Epicatechin: 7.04-19.77 mg/L (FL) Syringaldehyde: 7.11-44.51 mg/L (DAD) p-Coumaric acid: 0.11-0.30 mg/L (DAD) Ferulic acid: 0.55-0.78 mg/L (DAD) *trans*-Resveratrol: 1.36-2.70 mg/L (DAD) Myricetin: nd-0.56 mg/L (DAD) Quercitrin: nd-3.52 mg/L (DAD) Quercetin: 2.88-21.06 mg/L (DAD) Kaempferol: 0.57-2.37 mg/L (DAD)	DAD (280 nm) and FL (λexc=278 nm and λem=360 nm over 17.5 min and λexc=330 nm and λem=374 nm for 16.5 min.). LOD: 0.03-0.54 mg/L (DAD), 0.03-0.093 mg/L(FL)	LLE (diethyl ether)	[44]
Gallic acid, protocatechuic acid, protocatechuicaldehyde, (+)-catechin, vanillic acid, caffeic acid, syringic acid, (-)-epicatechin, syringaldehyde, p-coumaric acid, ferulic acid, *trans*-resveratrol, myricetin, quercitrin, quercetin, kaempferol	Nova-Pak C$_{18}$ (150x3.9-mm i.d., 4μm).	Gallic acid: 5.16-4.69 mg/L Protocatechuic acid: 0.40-5.96 mg/L Protocatechuicaldehyde: 0.05-0.94 mg/L (+)-Catechin: 30.53-85.30 mg/L Vanillic acid: 0.74-3.84 mg/L Caffeic acid: 3.04-6.24 mg/L Syringic acid: 1.05-5.41 mg/L (-)-Epicatechin: 7.64-28.25 mg/L Syringaldehyde: 3.33-23.52 mg/L p-Coumaric acid: 0.54-19.59 mg/L Ferulic acid: 0.15-1.12 mg/L *trans*-Resveratrol: 0.48-5.45 mg/L Myricetin: 0.20-2.17 mg/L Quercitrin: nd-3.87 mg/L Quercetin: 0-38.55 mg/L and Kaempferol: nd-6.49 mg/L	DAD (280 nm)	SPE (Sep-Pak Plus C$_{18}$ cartridge) and LLE (diethyl ether) were compared to establish the best conditions for extraction. LLE shows the best results. LOD: in the range 0.02 mg/L for *trans*-resveratrol to 1.51 mg/L for quercitrin.	[45]

work of *Luan et al.* [53] in which a solid phase microextraction (SPME) procedure was developed prior to the derivatization and GC/MS determination. The silylation of *trans*-resveratrol was carried out onto a polyacrylate (PA) fiber coating. A linear response of *trans*-resveratrol over a concentration range of 10 ng/L-1 mg/L with a correlation coefficient of 0.9997 and LOD of 5 ng/L were obtained. The analytical recoveries in wine ranged from 84 to 106% with precision below 10% RSD. Another on-fiber derivatization was also carried out by *Shao et al.* [54] also using a PA fiber. However, in this case, the SPME method incorporated a modification to the procedure to remove moisture and permit the use of water sensitive derivatizing reagents and also, GCxGC-MS allowing the separation of resveratrol from potential interferences that cause peak overlap in single column GC analysis of complex red wine samples.

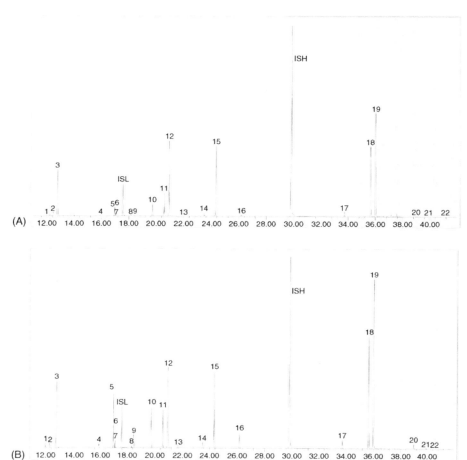

Figure 7. GC chromatogram: (A) silylated standard compounds present in a calibration standard solution; (B) silylated compounds present in the extract of a red wine. Peak identification: (1) vanillin; (2) *trans*-cinnamic acid; (3) tyrosol; (4) veratric acid; (5) hydroxytyrosol; (6) vanillic acid; (7) homovanillic acid; (8) 3,4-dihydroxyphenylacetic acid; (9) homogentisic acid; (10) syringic acid; (11) *p*-coumaric acid; (12) gallic acid; (13) flavonone; (14) ferullic acid; (15) caffeic acid; (16) sinapinic acid; (17) *trans*-resveratrol; (18) (-)-epicatechin; (19) catechin; (20) fisetin; (21) quercetin; (22) myricetin; (ISL) phenanthrene; (ISH) 2,3-benzophenanthrene. Reprinted from [48] with permission from Elsevier.

Table 2. Some examples of GC methods for the determination of antioxidants in red wines.

Analytes	Column	Amount found	Detection	Comments	Reference
Homovanillic acid, catechin, gallic acid, homogentisic acid, 3,4-dihydroxyphenylacetic acid, vanillic acid, syringic acid, tyrosol, caffeic acid, (−)-epicatechin, fisetin, sinapinic acid, vanillin, p-hydroxybenzoic acid, ferulic acid, coumaric acid, quercetin, veratric acid, kaempferol, trans-cinnamic acid, trans-resveratrol, flavonone	DB-5MS	Total: 68–326 mg/L	MS (SIM)	MSPD (silica gel); LOD: 2-8 µg/L	[47]
Vanillin, trans-cinnamic acid, tyrosol, veratric acid, vanillic acid, homovanillic acid, 3,4-dihydroxyphenylacetic acid, homogentisic acid, syringic acid, p-coumaric acid, gallic acid, flavonone, ferulic acid, caffeic acid, sinapinic acid, trans-resveratrol, (−)-epicatechin, catechin, fisetin, quercetin, myricetin	DB-5MS	Total: 135-182 mg/L	MS (SIM)	LLE (ethyl acetate); LOD: 1-360 µg/L	[48]
Cis-resveratrol, trans-resveratrol	DB-17HT	Total: 1.78-7.13 mg/L	MS (SIM)	SPE (C_{18}); LOD: 10 µg/L	[50]
Cis-resveratrol, trans-resveratrol, monohydroxystilbene, dihydroxystilbene, tetrahydroxystilbene	DB-5	Total: 0.1-71.5 mg/L	MS (SIM)	SPE (C_{18})	[52]
Trans-resveratrol	HP-5MS	0.10-0.95 mg/L	GCxGC-MS	SPME (PA)	[54]
Gentisic acid, vanillic acid, ferulic acid, m-coumaric acid, p-coumaric acid, caffeic acid, gallic acid, cis-resveratrol, trans-resveratrol, cis-polydatin, trans-polydatin, catechin, epicatechin, quercetin, morin	DB-5HT	Gentisic acid: 0.44-0.46 mg/L; Vanillic acid: 2.3-3.7 mg/L; Ferulic acid: <1.0; 2.86 mg/L; m- and p-coumaric acid: 2.61-4.5 mg/L; Caffeic acid: 3.15-12.95 mg/L; Gallic acid: >20; 13.08 mg/L; cis-resveratrol: 0.27-0.88 mg/L; trans-resveratrol: 0.71-2.50 mg/L; cis-polydatin: 0.02-0.68 mg/L; trans-polydatin: 0.02-0.98 mg/L; Catechin and epicatechin: 1.2-213 mg/L; Quercetin: 0.50-5.26 mg/L	MS (SIM)	SPE (C_8)	[46]

5. ANALYSIS OF ANTIOXIDANTS IN RED WINES BY CAPILLARY ELECTROMIGRATION METHODS

CE is increasingly becoming a versatile analytical tool for the routine determination of a wide variety of analytes due to its high efficiency, high resolution power, low analysis time and low consumption of sample and reagents, as it has been shown in different review articles [55, 56]. The term "capillary electromigration methods" refers to a group of separation techniques of CE with different operation characteristics and separation principles, but with a common operative line. They include capillary zone electrophoresis (CZE) and micellar electrokinetic chromatography (MEKC) modes [57] which are the ones mostly used, also for the analysis of antioxidants in red wines. Table 3 shows some examples of the application of capillary electromigration methods for the analysis of antioxidants in these samples.

CZE is probably the simplest CE mode of all. It is based on the separation of charged analytes in a conductive liquid placed in a capillary under the influence of a high voltage electric field. The separation is based on the difference in the charge to mass ratio of the analytes. Since most of wine antioxidants can be ionized in aqueous solution (depending on the pH value), CZE is a suitable technique for their separation as it can be seen in the different works shown in Table 3 [58-63] although when dealing with anionic compounds, coelectroosmotic CZE is more appropriate in order to decrease the analysis time (surfactants are introduced into the background electrolyte (BGE) at a concentration lower than the critical micelle concentration (CMC) to reverse the electroosmotic flow (EOF)). *Minussi et al.* [62] developed a CZE-DAD method for the determination of (+)-catechin, (-)-epicatechin, tyrosol, *cis-* and *trans*-resveratrol, hydroxytyrosol, sinapic acid, epicatechin gallate, syringic acid, *o*-coumaric acid, *p*-coumaric acid, vanillic acid, gentisic acid, *p*-hydroxybenzoic acid, salicylic acid, caffeic acid, gallic acid and protocatechuic acid in red wine using a BGE composed of 25 mM phosphate and 10 mM borate pH 8.8. Extraction of the analytes was developed following a LLE approach with diethyl ether. CZE showed that, in the red wines analyzed, gallic acid was the highest of the phenolic acids and (+)-catechin and (-)-epicatechin were the next most abundant phenolics. Also, these compounds were found to be strictly correlated with the total antioxidant potential of wines. Another example of the application of CZE is the work of *Woraratphoka et al.* [59] developed for the separation of *trans*-resveratrol, (+)-catechin, (-)-epicatechin, rutin, syringic acid, *p*-coumaric acid, caffeic acid, gallic acid, protocatechuic acid, cinnamic acid, *p*-hydroxybenzoic acid, quercetin, gentisic acid and salicylic acid using a BGE of 25 mM phosphate, 10 mM borate, pH 8.5. Figure 8 shows the electropherogram of the separation of these 14 compounds. Eleven red wine samples were extracted with diethyl ether and injected in the CE system after evaporation and reconstitution with methanol.

Contrary to CZE, MEKC is able to provide the separation of either charged or non changed analytes. In this separation mode an ionic surfactant solution is used as running buffer at a higher concentration that the CMC. The most commonly used is sodium dodecyl sulphate (SDS). As a result, the separation principle is based on their differential partitioning between the aqueous and micellar phases according to their polarity. When these antioxidants are analyzed by MEKC suitable control of the pH and surfactant concentration should be achieved [64-68]. One example is the work developed by *Rodríguez-Delgado et al.* [65] in which a group of five antioxidants (quercetin, rutin, myricetin, quercetrin and kaempferol) were analyzed by MEKC-DAD after the LLE of red wine samples from the Canary Islands with diethyl ether. Separation was achieved by a BGE composed of 150 mM boric acid (pH 8.5), 50 mM SDS and 5% v/v methanol. Analyte concentration in the samples were in the range nd-52.40 mg/L (quercetrin was found at a concentration of 52.4 mg/L in one of the analyzed sample which also had a high concentration of quercetin, 11.70 mg/L, rutin, 20.10 mg/L and myricetin, 5.42 mg/L). Another application of MEKC is the work by *Sun et al.* [67] developed for the separation of catechin, naringenin, quercetin, apigenin, kaempferol, myricetin. In this case the BGE was 40 mM borate, 40 mM SDS, pH 9.0, 20% 1-propanol with 16 min of analysis time. The method was also applied to the determination of these compounds in ten red wine samples after extraction with diethyl ether.

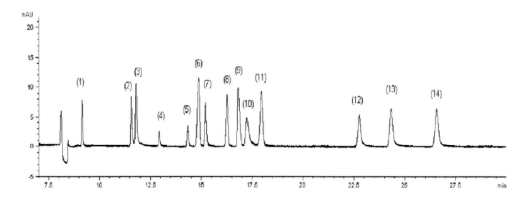

Figure 8. Electropherogram of the separation of twelve antioxidants by CZE. Peak identification: (1) *trans*-resveratrol, (2) (-)-epicatechin, (3) (+)-catechin, (4) rutin, (5) syringic acid, (6) cinnamic acid, (7) *p*-coumaric acid, (8) gentisic acid, (9) *p*-hydroxybenzoic acid, (10) quercetin, (11) salicylic acid, (12) caffeic acid, (13) gallic acid and (14) protocatechuic acid. BGE: 25 mM phosphate, 10 mM borate, pH 8.5. Separation voltage: 15 kV. Temperature: 25°C. Sample injected for 7 s. Reprinted from [59] with permission from Elsevier.

One of the main drawbacks in CE its low sensitivity compared to GC or HPLC. This low sensitivity is associated to both the small path-length of the capillary and the small volumes injected, usually a few nanoliters. In order to improve the poor limits of detection (LODs) of CE several alternatives have been proposed. Among them, special mention deserve the development of on-line preconcentration strategies as, for instance, sample stacking [69-71], sweeping [72] and on-line SPE [73-75]. *Hsieh and Lin* [64] applied the sweeping technique for the on-line preconcentration of *trans*-resveratrol previously extracted from red wine by LLE using ethyl acetate as extracting solvent. MEKC was used as separation mode with low-temperature fluorescence spectroscopy (LTFS) as detection system. Up to approx. 1500 fold increase in sensitivity was obtained with respect to non-stacking conditions which represents a LOD of 5 µg/L (much lower than LODs frequently achieved in CE, which are in the low mg/L level). Despite this on-line preconcentration attempt, the fact that antioxidants in red wine are generally at high concentrations (enough for CE) and the inherent characteristics of the technique (cheap capillaries that can be easily replaced) has provided the development of the direct injection of the sample [61] or only a dilution [60, 63, 66] prior to their CE determination in a relative high number of occasions (depending on the analyte) without a previous sample pretreatment/preconcentration step.

Table 3. Some examples of CE methods for the determination of antioxidants in red wines.

Analytes	CE mode	Background electrolyte	Amount found	Detection	Comments	Reference
Quercetin, rutin, myricetin, quercetin, kaempferol	MEKC	150 mM boric acid (pH 8.5), 50 mM SDS, 5% v/v MeOH	nd-52.40 mg/L	DAD (280 nm)	LLE (diethyl ether). LOD: 0.10-0.40 mg/L	[65]
Cis- and trans-resveratrol, quercetin, (+)- catechin, gallic acid	MEKC	50 mM sodium deoxycholate, 10 mM Na$_2$HPO$_4$, 6 mM disodium tetraborate (pH 9.3)	-	UV (220 nm)	Dilution and direct injection of the samples.	[66]
tyrosol, (±)-epicatechin, (+)-catechin, syringic acid, p-coumaric acid, caffeic acid, gallic acid, 3,4-dihydroxybenzoic acid, cis- and trans-coumaroyl tartaric	CZE	100 mM sodium borate (pH 9.5)	Total content: 147.97-319.10 mg/L	UV (280 nm)	Effect of ageing studied	[58]
Resveratrol, (+)-catechin, (-)-epicatechin, rutin, syringic acid, p-coumaric acid, caffeic acid, gallic acid, protocatechuic acid, cinnamic acid, p-hydroxybenzoic acid, quercetin, gentisic acid and salicylic acid	CZE	25 mM phosphate, 10 mM borate, pH 8.5	Nd- 25.90 mg/L	DAD (206, 217 nm)	LLE (diethyl ether)	[59]
Caffeic acid, ferulic acid, gallic acid, p-coumaric acid, protocatechuic acid, syringic acid vanillic acid, apigenin, epicatechin, kaempferol, catechin, quercetin, quercitrin and rutin	ITP-CZE	ITP: leading electrolyte 10 mM HCl pH 7.2 with Tris, the terminating electrolyte 50mM boric acid pH 8.2. CZE: 25mM β-hydroxy-4-morpholinopropanesulfonic acid (MOPSO), 50Mm Tris, 15mM boric acid and 5 mM β-cyclodextrin of pH 8.5	Nd-22.04 mg/L	EC (conductimetric for ITP) and UV (254 nm)	LOD: 30 µg/L for phenolic acids, quercitrin and rutin, 100 µg/L for quercetin, kaempferol and epicatechin, and 250 µg/L for catechin. Dilution of the sample.	[60]
Catechin, naringenin, quercetin, apigenin, kaempferol, myricetin	MEKC	40 mM borate, 40 mM SDS, pH 9.0, 20% 1-propanol	Nd-190.7 mg/L	UV (214 nm)	LLE (diethyl ether); LODs: $1.48 \cdot 10^{-2} - 2.31 \cdot 10^{-2}$ mg/L	[67]
Quercitin, rutin, quercetin, myricetin, flavona, D-catechin, epicatechin, protocatechuic acid, ferulic acid, caffeic acid, chlorogenic acid	CZE	30 mM NaH$_2$PO$_4$ and 30 mM Na$_2$HPO$_4$ (pH 8.85).	-	UV (220 nm)	Direct injection of the samples. Use of marker index tenchnique.	[61]

Table 3. (Continued)

Analytes	CE mode	Background electrolyte	Amount found	Detection	Comments	Reference
(+)-catechin, (-)-epicatechin, tyrosol, *cis*- and *trans*-resveratrol, hydroxytyrosol, sinapic acid, epicatechin gallate, syringic acid, *o*-coumaric acid, *p*-coumaric acid, vanillic acid, gentisic acid, *p*-hydroxybenzoic acid, salicylic acid, caffeic acid, gallic acid, protocatechuic acid	CZE	Phosphate 25 mM, borate 10 mM pH 8.8.	Nd-58.3 mg/L	DAD (206, 217 and 312 nm)	LLE (diethyl ether)	[62]
Trans-resveratrol	MEKC	75 mM SDS, 5 mM Na$_2$HPO$_4$, 5 mM boric acid, and 15% acetonitrile, pH 8.18.	1.3 mg/L	UV (306 nm)	SPE (C$_{18}$)	[68]
Trans-resveratrol	MEKC	150 mM SDS, 30 mM H$_3$PO$_4$ in a mixed methanol-water solution (25:75 v/v), pH 2.5	-	LTFS (low-temperature fluorescence spectroscopy) (λ_{exc} 313 nm, λ_{em} 400)	Sweeping (LOD: 5 µg/L, ~1500 fold sensitivity improvement). LLE (ethyl acetate).	[64]
Trans-resveratrol, (+)-catechin, (-)-epicatechin	CZE	100 mM borate buffer (pH 9.2)	2.12-45.8 mg/L	EC (amperometric)	LODs: 2·10^{-7} to 5·10^{-7} g/mL. Sample neutralization and dilution with BGE	[63]

6. CONCLUSIONS

Antioxidants are ubiquitously present in foods including vegetables, fruit, tea and especially in wine in which their content is higher in red wine samples. In this last case, due to their structure (which includes OH groups) they are responsible for oxidation processes and other chemical reactions playing an important role in the whole winemaking technology from grape to wine. They have a strong involvement in the organoleptic characteristics of wine, affecting color, astringency and bitterness. Besides, the antioxidant composition of wine can be strongly affected, not only qualitatively but also quantitatively, by grape varieties, cultivation methods, maturity, the ageing process as well as enological techniques.

Numerous studies have been performed to gather scientific evidence of red wine beneficial health as well as data regarding the exact mechanism of action and possible toxicological aspects of these products. Most of these studies have been carried out *in vitro* and still, a lot of information is unknown.

Based on the overview/revision of more than 150 papers it can be concluded that analytical methods used for the quantification of antioxidants in red wine samples are important for various reasons. On the one hand, they can provide objective and specific information on their content in wine samples, allowing its classification attending to their origin, grape variety, etc... which can be of especial importance in "origin denominations" productions. Furthermore, the information provided by these methods can help to identify the real antioxidant effect/mechanisms of these compounds. On the other hand, since they have a strong influence on wine organoleptic characteristics, their analysis can clearly indicate specific alterations of the wine.

These analytical methods are mainly based on the use of HPLC with either UV and MS detection. In this case, the relative recent introduction of UPLC has expanded the application and importance of the technique and it will surely expand its application in this field with low analysis times and high peak efficiencies and sensitivity. Even though, GC and CE applications have also found their space in this field although the number of works using GC is very low.

In most cases, samples pretreatments for the analysis of antioxidants in red wines are not very complicated nor time consuming, despite the complexity of the sample, especially when CE is used. In many cases, suitable dilution or LLE is enough, although SPE has also been applied in relatively high number of occasions.

REFERENCES

[1] Fehér, J; Lengyel, G; Lugasi, A. The cultural history of wine-theoretical background to wine therapy. *Central Europ. J. Medic.*, 2007, 2, 379-391.

[2] Ren, W; Qiao, Z; Wang, H; Zhu, L; Zhang, L. Flavonoids: Promising anticancer agents. *Medic. Res. Rev.,* 2003, 4, 519-534.

[3] Delmas, D; Jannin, B; Latruffe, N. Resveratrol: Preventing properties against vascular alterations and ageing. *Molec. Nutr. Food Res.,* 2005, 49, 377-395.

[4] Le Corre, L; Chalabi, N; Delort, L; Bignon, YJ; Bernard-Gallo, DJ. Resveratrol and breast cancer chemoprevention: *Molecular mechanisms Molec. Nutr. Food Res.*, 2005, 49, 462-471.

[5] Pellegrini, N; Simonetti, P; Gardana, C; Brenna, O; Brighenti, F; Pietta, P. Polyphenol content and total antioxidant activity of Vini Novelli (youngred wines). *J. Agric. Food Chem.*, 2000, 48, 732-735.

[6] Simonetti, P; Pietta, P; Testolin, G. Polyphenol content and total antioxidant potential of selected Italian wines. *J. Agric. Food Chem.*, 1997, 45, 1152-1155.

[7] Larrauri, JA; Sánchez-Moreno, C; Rupérez, P; Saura-Calixto, F. Free radical scavenging capacity in the aging of selected red Spanish wines. *J. Agric. Food Chem.*, 1999, 47, 1603-1606.

[8] Burns, J; Gardner, PT; O'Neil, J; Crawford, S; Morecroft, I; McPhail, DB; Lister, C; Matthews, D; MacLean, MR; Lean, ME; Duthie, GG; Crozier, A. Relationship among antioxidant activity, vasodilation capacity, and phenolic content of red wines. *J. Agric. Food Chem.*, 2000, 48, 220-230.

[9] Hagymasi, K; Blazovics, A; Feher, J; Lugasi, A; Kristo, ST; Kery, A. The in vitro effect of dandelions antioxidants on microsomal lipid peroxidation. *Phytother Res.*, 2000, 14, 43-44.

[10] Siemann, EH; Creasy, LL. Concentration of the phytoalexin resveratrol in wine. *Am. J. Enol. Vitic.*, 1992, 43, 49-52.

[11] Jang, M; Cai, L; Udeani, GO; Slowing, KV; Thomas, CF; Beecher, ChWW; Fong, HHS; Farnsworth, NR; Kimghorn, AD; Mehta, RG; Moon, RC; Pezzuto, JM. Cancer chemopreventive activity of resveratrol, a natural product derived from grapes. *Science*, 1997, 275, 218-220.

[12] Saito, M; Hosoyama, H; Ariga, T; Kataoka, S; Yamajo, N. Antiulcer activity of grape seed extract and procyanidins. *J. Agric. Food Chem.*, 1998, 46, 1460-1464.

[13] Hollman PC; Katan, MB. Dietary flavonoids: Intake, health effects and bioavailability. *Food Chem. Toxicol.*, 1999, 37, 937-942.

[14] Makris, DP; Kallithraka, S; Kefalas, P. Flavonols in grapes, grape products and wines: Burden, profile and influential parameters. *J. Food Compos. Anal.*, 2006, 19, 396-404.

[15] McDonald, MS; Hughes, M; Burns, J; Lean, MEJ; Matthews, D; Crozier, A. Survey of the free and conjugated myricetin and quercetin content of red wines of different geographical origins. *J. Agric. Food Chem.*, 1998, 46, 368-375.

[16] Cheynier, V. In: Martens, S; Treutter, D; Forkmann, G, editors. *Polyphenols*. Freising-Weihenstephan, 2000, 1-14, Germany.

[17] Goldberg DM; Karumanchiri A; Tsang E; Soleas GL. Catechin and epicatechin concentrations of red wines: regional and cultivar-related differences. *Am. J. Enol. Vit.*, 1998, 49, 23-34.

[18] Santos-Buelga C; Scalbert A. Proanthocyanidins and tannin-like compounds-nature, occurrence, dietary intake and effects on nutrition and health. *J. Sci. Food Agric.*, 2000, 80, 1094-1117.

[19] Cheynier, V; Moutounet, M; Sarni-Manchado, P. Les composés phénoliques. In: Flanzy, C, editor. Enologie: fondements scientifiques et technologiques. Lavoisier TEC & DOC, 1998, 123-162, Paris.

[20] Giaccio, M; Del Signore, A; Di Giacomo, F; Sanna, G; Manca, G. Effect of some yeasts on resveratrol content during alcoholic fermentation. *J. Commodity Sci.*, 2004, 43, 191-209.
[21] Kolouchova, I; Zamostny, P; Belohlav, Z; Melzoch, K; Siristova, L. Red wine as resveratrol protective system. *Czech. J. Food Sci.*, 2004, 22, 166-168.
[22] Stervbo, U; Vang, O; Bonnesen, C. A review of the content of the putative chemopreventive phytoalexin resveratrol in red wine. *Food Chem.*, 2007, 101, 449-457.
[23] Wenzel, E; Somoza, V. Metabolism and bioavailability of trans-resveratrol. *Molec. Nutr. & Food Res.*, 2005, 49, 472-481.
[24] Gambuti, A; Strollo, D; Ugliano, M; Lecce, L; Moio, L. *trans*-Resveratrol, quercetin, (+)-catechin, and (-)-epicatechin content in south Italian monovarietal wines: relationship with maceration time and marc pressing during winemaking. *J. Agric. Food Chem.*, 2004, 52, 5747-5751.
[25] Campodonico, P; Barbieri, E; Pizarro, M; Sotomayor, CP; Lissi, EA. A comparison between total phenol content of wines and their TRAP values measured by the bleaching of ABTS radical cations. *Boletin de la Sociedad Chilena de Química*, 1998, 43, 281-285.
[26] Zhang, Q; Cui, H; Myint, A; Lian, M; Liu, L. Sensitive determination of phenolic compounds using high-performance liquid chromatography with cerium(IV)-rhodamine 6G-phenolic compound chemiluminescence detection. *J. Chromatogr. A*, 2005, 1095, 94-101.
[27] Cu, H; Zhang, Q; Myint, A; Ge, X; Liu, L. Chemiluminescence of cerium (IV)–rhodamine 6G–phenolic compound system. *J. Photochem. Photobiol. A. Chem.*, 2006, 181, 238-245.
[28] García-Falcón, MS; Pérez-Lamela, C; Martínez-Carballo, E; Simal-Gándara, J. Determination of phenolic compounds in wines: Influence of bottle storage of young red wines on their evolution. *Food Chem.*, 2007, 105, 248-259.
[29] Revilla, E; Ryan, JM. Analysis of several phenolic compounds with potential antioxidant properties in grape extracts and wines by high-performance liquid chromatography–photodiode array detection without sample preparation. *J. Chromatogr. A*, 2000, 881, 461-469.
[30] Gürbüz, O; Göçmen, D; Dağdelen, F; Gürsoy, M; Aydin, S; Şahin, I; Büyükuysal, L; Usta, M. Determination of flavan-3-ols and trans-resveratrol in grapes and wine using HPLC with fluorescence detection. *Food Chem.*, 2007, 100, 518-525.
[31] La Torre, GL; Saitta, M; Vilasi, F; Pellicanò, T; Dugo, G. Direct determination of phenolic compounds in Sicilian wines by liquid chromatography with PDA and MS detection. *Food Chem.*, 2006, 94, 640-650.
[32] Mercolini, L; Saracino, MA; Bugamelli, F; Ferranti, A; Malaguti, M; Hrelia, S; Raggi, MA. HPLC-F analysis of melatonin and resveratrol isomers in wine using an SPE procedure. *J. Sep. Sci.*, 2008, 31, 1007-1014.
[33] Nikfardjam, MSP; Márk, L; Avar, P; Figler, M; Ohmacht, R. Polyphenols, anthocyanins, and trans-resveratrol in red wines from the Hungarian Villány region. *Food Chem.*, 2006, 98, 453-462.
[34] Spáčil, Z; Nováková, L; Solich, P. Analysis of phenolic compounds by high performance liquid chromatography and ultra performance liquid chromatography. *Talanta*, 2008, 76, 189-199.

[35] Gruz, J; Novák, O; Strnad, M. Rapid analysis of phenolic acids in beverages by UPLC–MS/MS. *Food Chem.*, 2008, 111, 789-794.

[36] Guadalupe, Z; Soldevilla, A; Sáenz-Navajas, MP; Ayestarán, B. Analysis of polymeric phenolics in red wines using different techniques combined with gel permeation chromatography fractionation. *J. Chromatogr. A*, 2006, 1112, 112-120.

[37] Fang, F; Li, JM; Pan, QH; Huang, WD. Determination of red wine flavonoids by HPLC and effect of aging. *Food Chem.*, 2007, 101, 428-433.

[38] He, J; Santos-Buelga, C; Mateus, N; de Freitas, V. Isolation and quantification of oligomeric pyranoanthocyanin-flavanol pigments from red wines by combination of column chromatographic techniques. *J. Chromatogr. A*, 2006, 1134, 215-225.

[39] Pati, S; Losito, I; Gambacorta, G; La Notte, E; Palmisano, F; Zambonin, PG. Simultaneous separation and identification of oligomeric procyanidins and anthocyanin-derived pigments in raw red wine by HPLC-UV-ESI-MS. *J. Mass Spectrom.*, 2006, 41, 861-871.

[40] Brenna, OV; Pagliarini, E. Multivariate Analysis of Antioxidant Power and Polyphenolic Composition in Red Wines. *J. Agric. Food Chem.*, 2001, 49, 4841-4844.

[41] Buiarelli, F; Coccioli, F; Jasionowska, R; Merolle, M; Terracciano, A. Analysis of some stilbenes in Italian wines by liquid chromatography/tandem mass spectrometry. *Rapid Commun. Mass Spectrom.*, 2007, 21, 2955-2964.

[42] Lee, J; Rennaker, C. Antioxidant capacity and stilbene contents of wines produced in the Snake River Valley of Idaho. *Food Chem.*, 2007, 105, 195-203.

[43] Rodríguez-Delgado, MA; González, J; Pérez-Trujillo, JP; García-Montelongo, FJ. *Trans*-resveratrol in wines from the Canary Islands (Spain). Analysis by high performance liquid chromatography. *Food Chem.*, 2002, 76, 371-375.

[44] Rodríguez-Delgado, MA; Malovaná, S; Pérez, JP; Borges, T; García-Montelongo, FJ, Separation of phenolic compounds by high-performance liquid chromatography with absorbance and fluorimetric detection. *J. Chromatogr. A*, 2001, 912, 249-257.

[45] Malovaná, S; García-Montelongo, FJ; Pérez, JP; Rodríguez-Delgado, MA. Optimisation of sample preparation for the determination of trans-resveratrol and other polyphenolic compounds in wines by high performance liquid chromatography. *Anal. Chim. Acta*, 2001, 428, 245-253.

[46] Soleas, GJ; Dam, J; Carey, M; Goldberg, DM. Toward the fingerprinting of wines: Cultivar-related patterns of polyphenolic constituents in Ontario wines. *J. Agric. Food Chem.*, 1997, 45, 3871-3880.

[47] Minuti, L; Pellegrino, RM. Determination of phenolic compounds in wines by novel matrix solid-phase dispersion extraction and gas chromatography/mass spectrometry. *J. Chromatogr. A*, 2008, 1185, 23-30.

[48] Minuti, L; Pellegrino, RM; Tesei, I. Simple extraction method and gas chromatography–mass spectrometry in the selective ion monitoring mode for the determination of phenols in wine. *J. Chromatogr. A*, 2006, 1114, 263-268.

[49] Goldberg, DM; Yan, J; Ng, E; Diamandis, EP; Karumanchiri, A; Soleas, G; Waterhouse, AL. Direct-injection gas-chromatographic mass-spectrometric assay for *trans*-resveratrol. *Anal. Chem.*, 1994, 66, 3959-3963.

[50] Goldberg, DM; Karumanchiri, A; Ng, E; Yan, J; Diamandis, EP; Soleas, GJ. Direct gas-chromatographic mass-spectrometric method to assay *cis*-resveratrol in wines-

preliminary survey of its concentration in commercial wines. *J. Agric. Food Chem.*, 1995, 43, 1245-1250.

[51] Soleas, GJ; Goldberg, DM; Diamandis, EP; Karumanchiri, A; Yan, J; Ng, E. A derivatized gas-chromatographic mass-spectrometric method for the analysis of both isomers of resveratrol in juice and wine. *Am. J. Enol. Vitic.*, 1995, 46, 346-352.

[52] Lamikanra, O; Grime, CC; Rodin, JB; Inyang, ID. Hydroxylated Stilbenes in Selected American Wines. *J. Agric. Food Chem.*, 1996, 44, 1111-1115.

[53] Luan, T; Li, G; Zhang, Z. Gas-phase postderivatization following solid-phase microextraction for rapid determination of *trans*-resveratrol in wine by gas chromatography-mass spectrometry. *Anal. Chim. Acta*, 2000, 424, 19-25.

[54] Shao Y; Marriott P; Hugel, H. Solid-phase microextraction-on-fibre derivatization with comprehensive two dimensional gas chromatography analysis of *trans*-resveratrol in wine. *Chromatographia*, 2003, 57, S349-S353.

[55] Hernández-Borges, J; Frías-García, S; Cifuentes, A; Rodríguez-Delgado, MA. Pesticide analysis by capillary electrophoresis. *J. Sep. Sci.*, 2004, 27, 947-963.

[56] Herrero, M; Ibáñez, E; Cifuentes, A. Analysis of natural antioxidants by capillary electromigration methods. *J. Sep. Sci.*, 2005, 28, 883-897.

[57] Khaledi, MG (Ed). High Performance Capillary Electrophoresis, Theory, techniques and applications, Vol. 146 in Chemical Analysis: A series of monographs on Analytical Chemistry and its Applications. Series Editor J.D. Winefordner. John Wiley & Sons, 1998, New York.

[58] Gil, MI; García-Viguera, C; Bridle, P; Tomás-Barberán, FA. Analysis of non-coloured phenolics in port wines by capillary zone electrophoresis. *Z. Lebensm. Unters. Forsch.*, 1995, 200, 278-281.

[59] [59] Woraratphoka, J; Intarapichet, K; Indrapichate, K. Phenolic compounds and antioxidative properties of selected wines from the northeast of Thailand. *Food Chem.*, 2007, 104, 1485-1490.

[60] Hamoudová, R; Urbánek, M; Pospíšilová, M; Polášek, M. Assay of phenolic compounds in red wine by on-line combination of capillary isotachophoresis with capillary zone electrophoresis. *J. Chromatogr. A*, 2004, 1032, 281-287.

[61] Kulomaa A; Siren, H; Riekkola, M. Identification of antioxidative compounds in plant beverages by capillary electrophoresis with the marker index technique. *J. Chromatogr. A,* 781, 1997, 523-532.

[62] Minussi, RC; Rossi, M; Bologna, L; Cordi, L; Rotilio, D; Pastore, GM; Durán, N. Phenolic compounds and total antioxidant potential of commercial wines. *Food Chem.*, 2003, 82, 409-416.

[63] Peng, YY; Chu, QC; Liu, FH; Ye, JN. Determination of phenolic constituents of biological interest in red wine by capillary electrophoresis with electrochemical detection. *J. Agric. Food Chem.*, 2004, 52, 153-156.

[64] Hsieh, MC; Lin, CH. On-line identification of *trans*-resveratrol in red wine using a sweeping technique combined with capillary electrophoresis/77 K fluorescence spectroscopy. *Electrophoresis*, 2004, 25, 677-682.

[65] Rodríguez-Delgado, MA; Pérez, J; Sánchez, MJ; García-Montelongo, FJ. Optimization of the separation of flavonoids by micellar electrokinetic capillary chromatography: Effect of organic solvents. *Chromatographia*, 2000, 52, 289-294.

[66] Prasongsidh, BC; Skurray, CR. Capillary electrophoresis analysis of *trans-* and *cis-*resveratrol, quercetin, catechin and gallic acid in wine. *Food Chem.,* 1998, 62, 355-358.

[67] Sun, Y; Fang, N; Chen, DDY; Donkor, KK. Determination of potentially anti-carcinogenic flavonoids in wines by micellar electrokinetic chromatography. *Food Chem.,* 2008, 106, 415-420.

[68] Fan, EG; Zhang, K; Yao, CY; Yan, C; Bai, YH; Jiang, S. Determination of *trans-*resveratrol in China Great Wall "Fazenda" red wine by use of micellar electrokinetic chromatography. *Chromatographia,* 2005, 62, 289-294.

[69] Quirino, JP; Terabe, S. Sample stacking of cationic and anionic analytes in capillary electrophoresis. *J. Chromatogr. A,* 2000, 902, 119-135.

[70] Shihabi, ZK. Stacking in capillary zone electrophoresis. *J. Chromatogr. A,* 2000, 902, 107-117.

[71] Kim, JB; Terabe, S. On-line sample preconcentration techniques in micellar electrokinetic chromatography. *J. Pharm. Biomed. Anal.,* 2003, 30, 1625-1643.

[72] Quirino, JP; Kim, JB; Terabe, S. Sweeping: concentration mechanism and applications to high-sensitivity analysis in capillary electrophoresis. *J. Chromatogr. A,* 2002, 965, 357-373.

[73] Guzmán, NA. Improved solid-phase microextraction device for use in on-line immunoaffinity capillary electrophoresis. *Electrophoresis,* 2003, 24, 3718-3727.

[74] [74] Petersson, M; Wahlund, KG; Nilsson, S. Miniaturised on-line solid-phase extraction for enhancement of concentration sensitivity in capillary electrophoresis. *J. Chromatogr. A,* 1999, 841, 249-261.

[75] Yang, Q; Tomlinson, AJ; Naylor, S. Membrane preconcentration CE. *Anal. Chem.,* 1999, 71, 183A-189A.

In: Red Wine and Health
Editor: Paul O'Byrne

ISBN 978-1-60692-718-2
© 2009 Nova Science Publishers, Inc.

Chapter 6

BIOGENIC AMINES IN WINES: A REVIEW

Fernanda Galgano, Marisa Caruso and Fabio Favati
Dept. of Biology, DBAF, University of Basilicata
Viale dell'Ateneo Lucano, 10, 85100 – Potenza - Italy

ABSTRACT

Biogenic amines are basic nitrogen compounds that can have toxicological effects on human health when present in foods and beverages at significant levels. These compounds are produced in small amounts in all living organisms and play an important role in cell growth and development, as well as in protecting stressed cells. Their presence at dangerous levels is principally attributed to microbial decarboxylation of the corresponding amino acids, and hence the occurrence of biogenic amines can be related to both food safety and food spoilage, becoming a useful index for the assessment of food quality and of the related manufacturing practices.

Nowadays an increasing attention is given to the presence in wine of biogenic amines, whose level and the possible synergic effect with ethanol may represent a significant risk for some consumers. The major toxicological implications are related to aromatic amines, such as histamine, tyramine, and 2-phenylethylamine; nevertheless, for these amines it is quite difficult to establish the exact threshold of toxicity, which depends on the efficiency of the detoxification mechanisms of different individuals. However, some countries have set limits for histamine in wine ranging from 2 to 10 mg/L, while for tyramine levels exceeding 10 mg/L in beverages should be considered unsafe. Several other amines may be found in wine, among them polyamines, that can enhance the adverse effect of aromatic amines, or cause negative consequences on wine aroma. Moreover, spermine and spermidine, that have secondary group, are involved in nitrosamine formation, compounds with a known cancerous action. Volatile amines, such as methylamine and ethylamine, come from amination of non-nitrogen compounds, such as aldehydes and ketones, and they have not a toxic action, but can exert a negative effect on wine aroma.

Biogenic amines usually found in wine are cadaverine, histamine, 2-phenylethylamine, putrescine and tyramine; agmatine and ethanolamine can be abundant, but they are generally little investigated. Low biogenic amine amounts, as normal constituents of the raw materials, can be released in must from grape and pulp during the winemaking process, and the biogenic amine concentration may increase as consequence of alcoholic fermentation, yeast autolysis, malolactic fermentation and wine aging, usually being red wines richer in amines than white wines.

In this work an overview of the presence of biogenic amines in wine is given, with a focus on the main factors affecting their presence and concentration in this alcoholic beverage.

1. INTRODUCTION

Biogenic amines [BA] are organic nitrogenous compounds of low molecular weight with biological activity that can be found in several living organisms (animals, plants and micro-organisms), where they may be formed or metabolized. BA play an important role in cell growth division and differentiation processes, but they are also of the utmost importance because, when present in foodstuffs at high concentration levels can cause direct or indirect toxicity; for this reason, some countries have set specific limits for their presence in various kinds of edible products [1-3]. In foods and beverages BA are mainly produced from amino acids through substrate-specific decarboxylase activity of microorganisms, which can be those responsible for fermentation processes and/or those related to food contamination or spoilage. Therefore, the qualitative and quantitative presence of BA has been suggested and recommended as an index of both food quality and poor manufacturing practices [4-7].

BA can be divided into three groups [8, 9]:

1) aromatic and the heterocyclic amines, such as histamine (HIM), tyramine (TYR), 2-phenylethylamine (PHE) and tryptamine (TRYPT), to which are associated pronounced toxicological risks for human health;
2) aliphatic mono, di- and polyamines, such as ethanolamine (ETHA), putrescine (PUT), cadaverine (CAD), agmatine (AGM), spermidine (SPD) and spermine (SPM), traditionally related to deficient sanitary conditions of foodstuffs, that enhance microbial activity;
3) aliphatic volatile amines, such as ethylamine (ETHY), methylamine (MET), isoamylamine (ISO), to which are not associated toxicological problems for human health; however, they can play a role in determining the sensory characteristics of foodstuffs.

Many microorganisms are capable to decarboxylate amino acids; it can be generally assumed that three important conditions have to be satisfied in order to producing BA, and precisely the presence of precursor moieties (i.e. amino acids), the presence of microorganisms able to decarboxylate amino acids and environmental conditions enabling microbial growth and enzymatic activity [10]. While the decarboxylase activity is not strictly associated with a specific microbial species, being usually strain dependent, the enzymes are generally induced at acidic pH and therefore they play a fundamental role in maintaining pH homeostasis or prolonging the microbial growth period by detoxification of the extracellular medium [11, 12]. Usually all foodstuffs containing proteins or free amino acids can contain BA, even if their qualitative and quantitative presence is strongly related to the food characteristics and to the microorganisms involved in BA production.

In the literature can be found several reviews dealing with the presence of BA in foods [4, 5, 13-15], as well as their biological activities [1, 10, 16]. In addition, analytical methods for the determination of these compounds have been reviewed [17], with also specific attention to wine [18].

In wine BA occur as odorless salts, but at the pH prevailing in the mouth amines are partly liberated and their flavor becomes apparent, affecting the sensory characteristics of the wine [18-20]. Furthermore, in alcoholic beverages it is important to consider the synergistic effect between amines and ethanol, because alcohol and acetaldehyde have been found to increase the sensitivity to BA [21, 22]. Determination of BA is not simple, because of their structure and because they are usually present at low levels in a complex matrix, such as wine. Among the different analytical techniques, high performance liquid chromatography (HPLC) is generally the most extensively utilized due to its high resolution, sensitivity, great versatility, and simple treatment [3].

The presence of BA in wine has been reported to range from a few to about 50 mg/L, and the type and concentration of these moieties depends on several factors, such as winemaking processes, time and storage conditions, raw material quality, and microbial contamination during winery operations. Moreover, some amines are normal constituents of grapes, and their level may vary with grape variety and degree of ripening, as well as with soil type and composition. Therefore, the geographical characterization based on the BA content has been also proposed as a criterion to discriminate several types of wines from different countries or regions [23-28].

In this work an overview of the presence of biogenic amines in wine is given, with a focus on the main factors affecting their presence and concentration in this alcoholic beverage.

2. BIOGENIC AMINES IN WINE

2.1. Origin

The presence of BA in wines has been studied extensively for 30 years and particularly over the last 10 years, as a consequence of the increasing attention to consumer protection. The study of BA in wines is of interest for two reasons: the toxicological risk associated with the BA content, and the evaluation of hygienic-sanitary conditions occurring during the winemaking process.

Biogenic amines are found in wines in variable quantities and their origin is different; in particular, non volatile amines, such as PUT, CAD, SPM, SPD, AGM, TYR, TRYPT, HIM and PHE, which is a volatile amine, are of microbial origin. In particular CAD, HIM, PHE, TYR and TRYPT derive from decarboxylation of the corresponding precursor amino acids (lysine, histidine, phenylalanine, tyrosine, and tryptophane respectively), while PUT can derive either from decarboxylation of ornithine or from AGM. Little is known about the significance of this latter polyamine in food and beverages, but besides being a precursor of PUT, SPM and SPD, it has also been related to food spoilage [29]. The pathway formation of PUT through AGM or via ornithine has been described in several wine lactic acid bacteria

(LAB), which can develop during malolactic fermentation (MLF) [30, 31]. Which of the two pathways prevails in any given situation has not yet been determined.

However, Bauza et al. [29] have shown a positive correlation between the concentration of AGM in must and the concentration of PUT in the finished wine after MLF, then supporting the hypothesis that the principal biosynthetic pathway for PUT is via arginine-AGM rather than via ornithine. In the study this theory found further support in fact that the arginine level, from which AGM derives, resulted to be higher in the must than in the finished wine. Whit regard to SPM and SPD, it is known that their synthesis is not the result of a simple amino acid decarboxylation, but it depends on a complex biosynthetic pathway [1].

Another biogenic amine found in wine is ETHA, and its exact metabolic origin has not yet been definitely assessed. ETHA was initially considered the precursor of 1,2-ethanediol, which is a normal product of yeast metabolism, being some yeasts able to form 1,2-ethanediol from ETHA [32]. In fact ETHA can be oxidized by an amino oxidase to glycol aldehyde that is then reduced by alcohol dehydrogenase to the diol. More recently, Choi et al. [33] have reported that ETHA is a precursor of phosphatidylcholine, the most abundant phospholipid in the membranes of eukaryotic cells, and because of regulation phenomena in the metabolism of phospholipids, it is probably released outside in the medium, and this fact could explain the increase of this amine during alcoholic fermentation.

With regard to the volatile amines, such as ETHY, MET and ISO, they can conceivably come from the amination of non-nitrogen compounds, such as aldehydes and ketones [29].

In order to control the BA level in wine, it would be necessary to identify the source of these compounds. However, despite the many studies carried out throughout the years, actually the research has not yet definitely clarify this point, and at present three different origins may be assumed for the BA found in wine: they are already present in the must, they are formed by the yeasts during the alcoholic fermentation, and/or they are formed in wine by the action of bacteria involved in the MLF. However, BA can be formed also during aging of wine, and there are reports indicating the possibility that BA are formed in wine by the action of contaminant microorganisms or by those not directly implicated in the fermentation process. Therefore, BA have been associated with a lack of hygiene during the winemaking process and have been suggested as an index of quality or of poor sanitary conditions of grapes [11] or poor manufacturing practices [6, 7, 28, 34-36]. Anyway, the formation of BA in fermented foods is related to the presence of certain microorganisms with decarboxylase activity, as well as to conditions allowing microbial growth [3].

Generally, MLF is considered a crucial factor for BA production, even if it has been reported that BA can also be produced by yeasts during alcoholic fermentation [36-40]. The connection between MLF and biogenic amine formation is a matter of controversy; some authors have found that during aging there is a greater increase in amines than during MLF, supporting the opinion that MLF has not a direct effect on the BA content of wines [11, 26, 41-45]. Conversely, several authors have presented evidence that in winemaking, BA are mainly formed during MLF [27, 28, 30, 36, 46-50]. In particular, Romero et al. [50] have reported that TYR, HIM and PUT, BA related to MLF and present in higher amounts in red wines than in white ones, could be used as chemical descriptors to discriminate wines on the basis of the vinification technology. Furthermore, the presence and the amount of TYR in wine could be utilized for assessing the extent of any irregular process in wine.

MLF appears to be the main source of TYR and PUT for the red wines, as opposed to white wines, where the source relies on the levels initially present in the musts [26]. During

MLF Landete et al. [27] have reported an increase in HIM, TYR and PHE, while PUT, CAD, and TRYPT concentrations were not affected, and this is also in accord with lactic acid bacteria being responsible of HIM, TYR and PHE levels in wine. Conversely, Bauza et al. [29] have observed an increase of PUT levels during fermentation from must to alcoholic fermentation to MLF, in agreement with Soufleros et al. [28]. The increased concentrations of PUT from must to wine may be explained taking into account that during winemaking this molecule can be formed either from yeast decarboxylation of ornithine, or from amino acids such as arginine via AGM. Nevertheless, there is a correlation between the production of these ammines and the presence of lactic acid bacteria during winemaking and aging [27, 49, 52, 53].

In general the data available in the literature are quite controversial, and contrary to the results of Soufleros et al. [28], who found a significant correlation between the levels of TYR and HIM during the fermentation processes, Herbert et al. [26] have reported that during either alcoholic or malolactic fermentative processes there were no significant changes in the levels of HIM, while PUT and TYR increased in red wines immediately after MLF. On the other side, Del Prete et al. [54] reported that during MLF, TYR disappeared, while the concentration of PUT was almost unchanged, while AGM level increased during MLF.

2.2. Microorganisms Producers of BA Isolated from Wine

A different role has been attributed to microorganisms performing the two different fermentation processes: alcoholic fermentation and MLF.

2.2.1. Alcoholic Fermentation

The contribution of yeasts performing alcoholic fermentation to BA production in wine is not clear [28, 34, 55, 56]. Experimental research has established that there is no relationship between alcoholic fermentation and BA, such as HIM, TYR, and CAD [28, 51]; however, despite the general opinion which ascribes the formation of BA to the activity of lactic acid bacteria involved in MLF, some authors have attributed mainly [36, 37, 39] or partially [38, 40] to yeasts the BA production.

Differently from what has been done for other microorganisms, only a few studies have been carried out concerning the qualitative evaluation of the aminobiogenic activity of yeasts on a synthetic medium [54, 57, 58]. Generally this activity has been evaluated quantitatively after alcoholic fermentation in grape must, and in particular Caruso et al. [38] have assessed the BA production of 50 yeast strains inoculated in grape must. These microorganisms belonged to five genera/species and were isolated from grapes or during grape must fermentation. Even if no strain resulted a high BA producer, the principal yeast species, *Saccharomyces cerevisiae,* resulted capable to produce ETHA and AGM and this latter amine was also produced from strains of all the species considered. *S. cerevisiae* and *Candida stellata* strains resulted to be the only producers of ETHA, as already observed by Arena and Manca de Nadra [31], while the highest concentration of total BA was produced by *Brettanomyces bruxellensis* strains, which produced also significant amounts of PHE and AGM, confirming the general spoilage aptitude of *B. bruxellensis* species in wine [59, 60].

Torrea Goñi and Ancín-Azpiculeta [40, 61] after inoculation of grape must with different *S. cerevisiae* strains, have reported some differences in BA concentration in wines. In particular, in both rosé and white wines, PUT resulted the most representative nonvolatile amine, but in all the wines tested its concentration never reached levels sufficiently high to cause toxic effects or to have a negative impact on the sensory characteristics of the beverage. In addition, Torrea Goñi, and Ancín-Azpiculeta [40] have also observed the production of volatile amines, such as ISO and ETHY, by yeasts.

Landete et al. [58] have tested for BA production 36 yeast strains of wine origin and belonging to different species, inoculating them in a synthetic medium and in grape must supplemented with amino acids. The results pointed out that no strain was able to produce the BA investigated (HIM, TYR, PHE, PUT, CAD, TRYPT).

Recently, Del Prete et al. [54], after alcoholic fermentation of grape musts inoculated with *S. cerevisiae* pure cultures, have reported that of the various BA originally present in musts, namely ETHA, ETHY and PUT, only ETHA increased during fermentation, while ETHY and PUT decreased, being the reduction of the latter much more significant. Conversely, low quantities of AGM and TYR, initially not present in musts, could be found at the end of the alcoholic fermentation and the AGM level raised also during MLF. The authors attributed the presence in wine of AGM and TYR after alcoholic and MLF not to any possible decarboxylation activity, but to the hydrolysis of AGM and TYR-hydroxycinnamic acid complexes, coming from the grapes, due to the action of yeasts and lactic acid bacteria.

Even if, to date, yeasts seem to be poor producers of BA, their role in BA accumulation in wine must be considered, because of their interaction with bacterial strains involved in fermentation processes, being the overall wine quality closely related to the diversity and composition of the microbial species and/or strains that develop during the whole fermentation process [62-64]. The growth of each wine yeast species is characterized by a specific metabolic activity, which may contribute to the aroma and flavor characteristics of wine, but that can also supply precursors for undesired amine biosynthesis by malolactic or contaminant bacteria [65, 66]. Moreover, low amounts of BA produced from yeasts added to those produced from bacteria, can contribute to reach the toxicological threshold or to have a negative impact on the organoleptic characteristics of wine. On the other hand, it is of importance to evaluate the potentiality of yeasts to reduce BA in wine, as recently reported for PUT and ETHY [54].

2.2.2. Malolactic Fermentation

MLF is a secondary fermentation, generally occurring after alcoholic fermentation, which is widely appreciated for its improvement of the flavor characteristics of wine, and is usually carried out principally by the species *Oenococcus oeni* [52, 67] or, more occasionally, by other lactic acid bacteria species belonging to the genera *Lactobacillus, Leuconostoc* and *Pediococcus*, which may develop during the winemaking process [8, 31, 68-70]. Generally the homofermentative lactobacilli, that are the major type of LAB present in grapes, disappear quickly after the beginning of the alcoholic fermentation in favor of *Leuc. mesenteroides*, which, at the end of the fermentation, is replaced by *O. oeni* [71]. *O. oeni*, due to its acid tolerance, is the most important species involved in converting into lactic acid the malic acid, present in grape juice and characterized by a strong acidic taste, and is also one of the species more industrially utilized in formulation of malolactic starters, in order to perform MLF in controlled conditions [48, 71].

HIM has been often detected in wines, but in rather low concentrations compared to that of other fermented foods, such as cheese [72]; however, wine contains alcohol and other moieties that may enhance the toxicity of HIM. For a long time, enologists have considered *Pediococcus* strains as the sole responsible for HIM production in wine [73], and this genus has always been found in the wine microflora during MLF, but usually at low concentration. Delfini [74], comparing the ability of several strains of *Leuconostoc* spp., *Lactobacillus* spp. and *Pediococcus* spp. to produce HIM, observed that only *P. damnosus* [*P. cerevisiae*] had the capability to produce significant amounts of HIM, while *Leuconostoc oenos* (*O. oeni*) strains were poor producers of this BA. In 1990, Choudhury et al. [75] showed that a strain of *O. oeni* was able to produce TYR in a laboratory medium, and later, in 1995, a strain of *O. oeni* able to produce HIM, via histidine decarboxylase (HDC), was isolated from wine [76]. However, in 2003 Moreno Arribas et al. [12] testing about 80 strains of lactic acid bacteria for production of TYR, HIM and PUT reported that no potential to form BA was observed in the *O. oeni* strains studied.

Leitão et al. [11] tested a total of 220 isolates of *O. oeni* for decarboxylase and proteolytic activity in wine: only six isolates showed both activities and only after a period of adaptation in a growth medium containing wine. These results suggest that the ability of *O. oeni* to use wine peptides and to produce BA is not a constant characteristic of this species, but it is strain dependent; furthermore, the enzymatic system expression appears to be closely dependent on nutritional and energetic composition of the medium. The authors concluded that wine is a medium which limits the formation of BA, so the synthesis of significant amounts of these compounds does not normally occur under common and careful winemaking conditions. According to previous works, they attributed the presence of low concentrations of BA in wine to undesirable bacteria like *Pediococcus* spp., originating from the grapes and/or wineries, and to the viticultural and enological practices adopted. Conversely, other authors have shown that *O. oeni* strains, together with *Lactobacillus hilgardii*, are the more important producers of BA in wine [8, 30, 48, 49, 58].

The role of *O. oeni* in HIM formation is unclear and controversial. Different studies suggest that HDC^+ strains of this species are frequent or rare in wine, and they are considered either weak or strong HIM producers [12, 27, 67]. The discordance among the different reports can be partially attributed to the different growth conditions and analytical procedures used to test bacterial strains. Fortunately, from the last decade it is possible to detect the presence of undesirable histamine-producing strains by rapid, sensitive and specific PCR test or DNA probe based on the gene encoding HDC [30, 67, 77]. Procedures for the detection of tyrosine decarboxylase and ornithine decarboxylase gene in LAB have also been developed [58, 78]. Moreover, recently in *O. oeni* and in *L. hilgardii* the gene coding for HDC was detected on an unstable plasmid, which could explain the erratic phylogenetic distribution of HDC^+ strains [77, 79]. This plasmid are probably unstable and rapidly lost during bacterial cultures, then HDC^+ strains could be easily converted in HDC^- strains during subcultures of the bacteria in laboratory. This could explain some surprising experimental results, such as the low abundance of HDC^+ strains in laboratory collections in contrast to the high frequency of these strains in environmental samples [12, 48, 80]. However, it can be stated that as regards *Pediococcus*, although the percentage of HIM producers is low, some strains can produce the highest concentration of HIM, whereas *O. oeni* producing HIM (HDC^+) are very frequent in wine, but they produce low amounts of HIM. The production of HIM by *O. oeni* is enhanced in the poorest growth conditions, such as low concentrations of sugar and malic acid, suggesting that histidine decarboxylation can be used as an additional mechanism for energy production in microbial cells deprived of other substrates [8]. HDC specifically decarboxylates only histidine, its optimum pH of activity is 4.8 and, unlike most amino acid decarboxylases, is pyridoxal-5'-phosphate (PLP) independent; furthermore the HDC activity of *O. oeni* increases in presence of ethanol concentrations up to 10%. Generally HIM accumulation increases if maceration, or storage with yeast lees, is prolonged, since more substrate (histidine) is available from yeast autolysis [8, 30]. After MLF, wine is sulfited in order to eliminate yeasts and bacteria and prevent any changes in composition due to microorganisms. On the other hand, in order to meet consumer demand, the wines produced nowadays are less acidic than in the past; grape maturity is prolonged as far as possible to increase the extractability of phenolic compounds and the concentration of aroma precursors, hence, total acidity is lower and pH higher [8]. Due to high pH, SO_2 results to be less active and particularly in red wines because of its combination with polyphenols. Then, viable but not-cultivable forms of LAB that retain some biological activities in order to survive, such as amino-acids decarboxylation, may be considered [8, 81]. Coton et al. [30] evaluated the HDC activity during the storage in wine at 20°C of a strain of *O. oeni*. After about two months, no viable cells can be detected, but HDC activity persist, having after four months 39% of the initial activity. Recently, some authors evaluated also the capability of acid lactic bacteria, and particularly of *O. oeni*, to produce PUT [53, 67], even if PUT production is generally attributed to some strains of *L. hilgardii* and *Lactobacillus buchneri* [12, 82].

PUT accumulation in wine is dependent on the presence of both PUT producer strains and ornithine, its precursor amino acid. Usually in wine ornithine can be found at low concentrations, but its amount may increase, like that of other amino acids, because of technological and biological factors, such as extended contact with lees and microbiological proteolysis [53]. Strains of *O. oeni* possess also ornithine, tyrosine and lysine decarboxylases, that have been shown to be PLP-dependent [8, 30, 52].

Guerrini et al. [53] have evaluated the biogenic amine-producing capability of several *O. oeni* strains originally isolated from different Italian wines. Under optimal growth conditions, more than 60% of the strains were able to produce HIM, at concentration ranging from 1.0 to 33 mg/l, and about 16% showed the additional capability to form PUT and CAD, to different extents and variable relative proportions. The amine-producing behavior of the strains was confirmed under stress culture conditions, while performing MLF. No strains were able to produce significant amounts of TYR, SPM, SPD or PHE under optimal growth conditions, while a few strains produced low amounts of SPD during MLF.

Mangani et al. [67] have reported that *O. oeni* strains in wine can produce PUT, not only from ornithine, but also from arginine, one of the major amino acid found in wine. In this case PUT could either derive from the metabolic activity of strains having a complete enzyme system allowing to convert arginine to PUT, or from a metabiotic association between strains characterized by different and complementary enzyme systems. Practically in the latter case PUT would be obtained by the combined activity of strains capable of metabolizing arginine to ornithine, but unable to produce PUT, and strains capable of producing PUT from ornithine but unable to degrade arginine. The PUT production pathway has been shown to take place when the MLF is completed, while the conversion of ornithine to PUT by a single culture of the decarboxylating strain may take place at the same time with the degradation of malic acid [8]. Due to the limited quantities of ornithine found in wines, the presence of low amounts of PUT should be expected, because ornithine decarboxylation is rapid and concurrent with MLF, besides being widespread among *O. oeni* strains. Conversely, using malolactic starters which are ornithine-decarboxylase-negative and/or unable to use arginine, the risk of an undesirable PUT increase could be not completely removed, because of the possible presence in wine of indigenous strains able to degrade arginine to ornithine. Consequently, in order to reduce PUT production in wine it would be necessary to remove malolactic bacteria or inhibit their activity immediately after MLF [67].

In the literature there are only a few reports dealing with the role of *Leuconostoc* strains in the formation of BA in wine. Moreno Arribas et al. [12] have reported that *Leuconostoc mesenteroides* strains possess a high potential for producing TYR, but also other *Leuconostoc* strains, together with *Lactobacillus brevis* strains, can be responsible for TYR production in wine [49, 83]. Strains of *L. buchneri* from wine were reported as PUT producers from ornithine decarboxylation [12].

Among the various microorganisms found in wine, strains of *L. brevis* and *L. hilgardii* have been reported to be TYR producers [58, 84] and those producing the highest amounts of this biogenic amine resulted also to be producer of PHE, as observed for other TYR producers microorganisms in foods [85-88]. Among the *Lactobacillus* species involved in MLF, *L. hilgardii* has been shown to be one of microorganisms higher BA producer [31]. Besides the decarboxylation of tyrosine, it was able to produce amines from arginine and ornithine precursors, producing HIM, AGM and PUT in high concentrations. PUT is formed by the decarboxylation of either ornithine or arginine via AGM, which is then converted into PUT either directly (by AGM deaminase enzyme) or indirectly via carbamyl PUT [31, 89]. The presence of phenols, natural compounds of red wines, can affect BA production by wine lactic acid bacteria. Alberto et al. [90] studied the influence of phenolic compounds on the growth survival and PUT formation from AGM of *L. hilgardii* X1B, a bacterium from wine able to produce important levels of PUT. PUT formation from AGM diminished in the presence of protocatechuic, vanillic and caffeic acids, and the flavonoids catechin and rutin; the phenolic compounds, besides already known properties to human health, seem to be a natural way of diminishing PUT formation, because the phenolics them selves could protect the cells against oxidative stress. The fact that PUT formation could be inhibited by phenolic compounds in wines is desirable from a hygienical-sanitary point of view. A negative correlation between phenolic compounds and PUT in wines seems to exist. In fact, wines with lower content in PUT, resulted characterized by a higher content in total poliphenols and higher content in AGM and vice versa [24]. Mazzoli et al. [91] have been reported that there is reciprocal interference between histidine decarboxylation and arginine deamination in a *L. hilgardii* strain: when arginine and histidine are present simultaneously in the culture medium, there is some delay in both HIM and ornithine accumulation. No influence of histidine on the kinetics of malate metabolization and vice versa was detected, while despite the poor survival rate in 11% ethanol, a slight but progressive HIM accumulation was observed.

Recently, *Lactobacillus zeae* has been identified as one of the predominant species in sherry-type wines during the biological aging and seemed to be one of the main PUT production [92].

2.3. Toxicological Aspects

BA exhibit interactions with normal metabolism in sensitive humans, mainly for their vasoactive and psychoactive properties that justify their research in foods [93]. Among BA, the most toxic for human health are the aromatic amines HIM and TYR and important physiological effects are also shown by TRYPT and PHE. When ingested in high concentrations, BA may induce headache, respiratory distress, hearth palpitation, hypo- or hypertension, enteric histaminosis, several allergic disorders, anaphylactic shock and, sometimes, death [5, 12, 15, 83, 94]. BA are physiologically inactivated in the intestinal tract by amine oxidases (monoamine oxidase and diamine oxidase), which catalyze their oxidative deamination with the production of an aldehyde, hydrogen peroxide and ammonia; moreover, HIM can be metabolized by the enzyme HIM-methyl transferase [10, 47, 95, 96]. Together with some antidepressive drugs, ethanol and acetaldehyde are known to be the most active inhibitors of amine oxidases and for this reason the presence of BA in alcoholic beverages can have toxic effects even if they are present in small amounts [8].

The polyamines PUT, AGM, CAD, SPM and SPD, have been identified as potentiators that may enhance the toxicity of HIM, TYR and PHE in humans, interfering with the enzymes that metabolize the above mentioned amines [97, 98]. However, in low concentrations the aliphatic polyamines, particularly PUT, SPM and SPD, can naturally occur in living organisms, as endogenous products of the normal metabolism, being essential for cell growth and have been correlated with many anabolic processes including synthesis of DNA, RNA and proteins [99-101].

BA with secondary amine groups, such as SPM and SPD, can react with nitrous acid and its salts to form nitrosamines, compounds with cancerous action [6, 18]; moreover, it has been demonstrated that polyamines, such as SPM, SPD, PUT and CAD, inhibit the oxidation of polyunsatured fatty acids, α-tocopherol and carotenoid pigments, because of their ability to scavenge superoxide radicals and hydroxyl radicals. The efficiency of the polyamine-scavenging activity appears to be linked to the amination degree, suggesting the involvement of amino groups [102].

Volatile amines do not have a toxic action on the human organism, even if three volatile amines, such as dimethylamine, pyrrolidine and diethylamine, can react with nitrites and produce nitrosamines [5]. On the other hand, volatile amine can have an influence on the sensorial characteristics of wine, even if in the literature no report can be found about an exact definition and quantification of such activity [18, 40]. Only for beer, Palamand et al. [103] have observed that concentrations of 50 µg/L of dimethylamine or 2000 µg/L of ETHY can negatively affect the aroma of this beverage. Besides volatile amines, also PUT has been reported to cause a significant negative change of wine sensorial quality at concentrations of 15-20 and 20-30 mg/L in white and red wines, respectively [31].

Arginine is the most abundant amino acid in grape berries [104], and through decarboxylation by means of the microbial enzymatic activities, AGM can originate from arginine. Other enzymes can then convert AGM in other BA, such ad PUT, SPD and SPM [47]; moreover, through deamination, arginine can be converted in NH_3, ornithine, carbamyl phosphate and ATP [31, 47, 105]. These metabolites have a negative effect on health: ammonia is toxic, ornithine can be decarboxylate to the polyamines PUT, SPM and SPD which, such as AGM, can potentiate the effect of HIM, while carbamyl phosphate can combine with ethanol, in wine, originating ethyl carbamate, a carcinogenic molecule [106]. The abundance of arginine in grape can justify the fact that PUT and AGM are generally the BA present in the highest concentration in wines [29, 40, 54, 107].

Another amine that, even if rarely investigated, can be found in significant amounts in wine is ETHA [54, 107]. Negative effects on humans have not been reported for ETHA; on the contrary, this moiety may be involved in several metabolic pathways, particularly in the synthesis of membrane components [108, 109].

The published studies concerning the toxicological effects of BA in humans are contradictory. Some authors considered that the presence of BA in wine could be an important food safety problem, due to some described implication of these compounds in cases of food intolerance and intoxication [110, 111]. Conversely, other authors have reported that no correlation could be found between the occurrence of symptoms and BA levels in wine, underlining that the amounts of HIM have no clinical or biological effects in healthy subjects, while the toxicological effects are a function of the efficiency of the system responsible for degradation of the HIM absorbed by the alimentary tract [112, 113].

Actually is it quite difficult to precisely and unambiguously define the toxic dose for amines in wine, due to the different human sensitivity to these compounds, and also taking into account the simultaneous ingestion of other moieties, that could interact with BA metabolism and eventually enhance their activity.

Although the toxicological threshold for PHE is not well defined, Soufleros et al. [28] have indicated as 3 mg/L the limit beyond which the wine might provoke negative physiological effects in humans. Also the toxic doses of HIM and TYR are difficult to be established, as the toxicity of these amines depends on the efficiency of enzymes, such as monoamine and diamine oxidase, which metabolize the BA and whose activity can vary in different individuals [10]. Soufleros et al. [28] have suggested that wines with concentrations of HIM between 8 and 20 mg/L may have toxic effects if consumed in large quantities, while in the case of TYR, wines with concentrations ranging from 25 to 40 mg/L should be consumed with precaution.

The regulatory limits for BA in wines have not yet been established by OIV (Organization International de la Vigne et du Vin); however, several European countries have set specific limits for HIM, even if often the values span over a too wide range (10 mg/L in Switzerland, 3,5 mg/L in Netherlands, 2 mg/L in Germany, 5 mg/L in Finland, 8 mg/L in France and 6 mg/L in Belgium) [18].

2.4. BA Content in Grape and Wines

The type and concentration of BA in wines can be significantly different, depending of several factors, even if some amines are normal constituents of grapes, with amounts varying with grape cultivar and degree of maturation [6]. Among the BA found in grapes, PUT and SPD are usually abundant, whereas ETHA, AGM, CAD, SPM, HIM, TYR and PHE have been found in smaller amounts [2, 6, 36, 114-118]. In addition, the grapes are also considered to be the main source of volatile amines and ammonia in wines [119]. Agnolucci et al. [46] have reported that MET, ETHY, PHE and CAD are present in grapes and can increase or be degraded during wine-making, while Del Prete et al. [54] studying 7 different cultivars of grapes, have found in all the samples investigated only ETHA, ETHY and PUT.

The presence of BA in must and wines is well documented in the literature, even if the processes that generate these amines, as well as the factors that influence their quantitative and qualitative presence, are in some cases not yet clearly understood and, sometimes, agreement is lacking between the published results. Different research has been carried out to investigate the BA content in wines from different producing areas, including, among others, wines produced in Argentina [120], China [121], France [28, 94, 122], Greece [45, 123, 124], Hungary [25, 125], Italy [24, 107, 126], Portugal [2, 9, 127], Spain [36, 39, 50, 78, 128-130], South Africa [131], Turkey [3] and United States [6]. In all these different works, red wines, whose winemaking process normally involves MLF, have been clearly shown to have a higher biogenic amine content than white wines, in which MLF does not take place or occurs to a lesser degree (Tables 1 and 2). In addition, it is possible to discriminate red and white wines on the basis of the biogenic amine type and content; in particular, Csomós et al. [132] have reported that a PCA analysis is able to characterize white wines principally according to TIR and SPM content, and red wines on the basis of PUT, HIM, AGM and CAD. Galgano et al. [24] have shown that red wines are definitely discriminated from white ones on the basis of HIM, TIR and SPD, being these BA lower in white wines. Moreover, Héberger et al. [25] have reported that BA could be useful for differentiating wines according to the wine-making technology and, although to a lesser extent, also to the geographical origin, grape variety, and year of vintage.

Usually the most investigated amines in wines have been HIM, TYR, PHE, PUT and CAD [2, 3, 6, 9, 18, 24, 28, 32, 37, 39, 45, 50, 94, 107, 120, 121, 123, 124, 126,128, 129, 131,133]. AGM and ETHA can be abundant in wines, but they have been little investigated [3, 6, 9, 24, 32, 37, 94, 107, 124, 126, 128].

From the data reported in Tables 1 and 2, ETHA results the most abundant amine both in red and white wines, being present in some Italian red wines at concentrations higher than 20 mg/L [24]. Buteau et al. [37] have indicated that ETHA is the only amine formed in substantial concentrations during alcoholic fermentation, as also reported more recently by Del Prete et al. [54], confirming the fact that yeasts are involved in ETHA production [38]. In addition, in a study of Pfeiffer et al. [32] ETHA concentration in German grape must has been reported as ranging from 3 to 8 mg/L, while during the alcoholic fermentation ETHA content increased, reaching values up to 17 mg/L.

Generally PUT and AGM can significantly contribute to the total amine content in alcoholic beverages [6, 47, 134], while the presence of the other amines seems to be dependent on the wine considered, thus on the winemaking process [6, 37, 47, 94, 135]. For AGM the concentration has been reported to vary from not detected to 21.6 mg/L in red wines and from not detected to 6.45 mg/L in white wines, while PUT has been reported to be present in red wines at concentrations ranging from 0.60 to 20.91 mg/L and from not detected to 9.07 mg/L in white wines (Tables 1 and 2).

CAD has been found in all wines at mean concentrations generally not higher than 2 mg/L, with the exception of some Italian [24], Chinese [121] and Turkish wines [3]. The presence of polyamines, such as SPD and SPM, has been little investigated, being the concentration of these BA usually quite limited and rarely exceeding 1 mg/L. In any case, SPD content found in wines is higher than that of SPM, due to the fact that plant-derived products usually contain more SPD than SPM, while animal-derived products contain more SPM than SPD [1]. TYR levels exceeding 10 mg/L in beverages should be considered unsafe for patients taking monoamine oxidase inhibitors [28], but in all the wines of Tables 1 and 2 this limit has never been exceeded. HIM has been found in all red and white wines considered, but at concentrations lower than the maximum limit generally considered to be safe for consumers in alcoholic beverages (10 mg/l) [18]. PHE level in wine over 3 mg/L has been indicated as potentially toxic [28] and only in a few red wines, namely from China, Italy, Portugal and Turkey this value has been reported as being higher, with a maximum level of 8.6 mg/L in the Turkish ones. Finally, as far as the volatile aliphatic monoamines are concerned, in the wine studied MET concentration has always been found to be lower than 1 mg/L, with the exception of some Greek red wines, whose MET content has been assessed as ranging from 0.59 to 1.50 mg/L.

3. FACTORS INFLUENCING BIOGENIC AMINE PRODUCTION IN WINES

A great variability characterizes the BA content of wines produced in different geographical areas, but also products with the same origin can differ in the content of these moieties. In fact, the capacity to produce amines is principally related to the bacterial strain and not to the species; moreover, the type and degree of ripeness of the grapes, level of amino acids in must, the climate and soil of the viticulture area, as well as the vinification techniques, may have an effect on the BA content in wine [6, 21, 30, 31, 110, 117, 118, 127, 136].

3.1. Raw Material and Viticulture Practices

Several authors have reported that precursor amino acids and amino nitrogen are fundamental factors, among others, which contribute to the final level of BA in wines, as well the presence of microorganisms able to decarboxylate the amino acids [26-28]. The concentration of these moieties in grape can be affected by fertilization treatments [137], while the amounts found in wine are also a function of the by winemaking procedures, such as time of maceration with skins, addition of nutrients, and racking protocols [47, 36, 138]. A high concentration of amino acids in the medium can produce more BA during wine aging, since amino acid decarboxylation constitutes part of the microorganism defense mechanisms against the acid environment [8]. Moreover, Martín Álvarez et al. [111] working on wines whose only difference was the production year (2001 and 2002), have reported that 2001 wines had significantly higher values of amines than those produced in 2002, and this fact could be justified by a higher significant concentration of most of the precursor amino acids in 2001 wines with respect to 2002 wines. Conversely, other authors have found no relationship between the formation of BA and the content of amino acids during alcoholic fermentation in wine [61, 139]. In addition, Nouadje et al. [122] have reported a limited correlation between amines and amino acids precursors during ripening in French red wines; this could be explained by the fact that the rate of degradation of wine proteins into amino acids was faster than the rate of degradation of amino acids into amines.

Table 1. Principal biogenic amine content found in different red wines from several countries

Country	AGM	CAD	ETHA	HIM	MET	PHE	PUT	SPM	SPD	TRYPT	TYR	N[a]	Reference
Argentina	-	nd-0.39	-	nd-5.22	-	nd-1.71	0.61-14.21	-	0-0.60	n.d.-3.49	0-5.38	38	120
China	-	nd- 13.0	-	nd-9.64	-	nd-4.58	0.3-13.06	nd-0.75	n.d.-3.82	n.d.	n.d.-6.94	38	121
France	-	0.28	-	7.47	0.32	0.71	18.86	-	-	-	7.84	92	28
France	21.6	0.2	-	3.7	-	1.9	10.8	0.1	0.6	-	3.7	54	94
Greece	-	0.52	-	0.31	0.10	0.59	1.17	0.12	0.27	-	0.43	45	45
Greece	-	0.04-0.53	-	0.28-2.63	0.59-1.50	-	0.90-3.15	-	-	-	0.52-1.58	5	123
Greece	nd- 0.63	nd-0.21	nd -0.71	0.98-1.65	nd-0.59	-	nd-2.70	-	-	nd-1.32	nd-0.46	15	124
Italy	8.95	2.88	25.77	3.20	0.50	4.23	6.24	0.50	0.65	8.63	2.83	73	24
Italy	9.92	2.46	10.97	1.07	nd	0.53	2.04	nd	nd	1.26	0.58	5	107
Italy	-	0.13	15.9	4.76	0.04	2.34	11.7	1.32	6.7	-	8.16	3	126
Oregon-USA	0.42	0.49	-	5.45	-	0.08	20.91	0.34	1.01	0.12	1.27	59	6
Not reported	-	0.22	-	1.9	0.19	1.34	4.84	-	0.16	0.08	1.87	32	133
Portugal	-	0.19	-	-	-	0.853	6.90	0.03	0.341	-	1.44	6	2
Portugal	-	0.64	15.56	1.21	0.68	4.87	3.61	-	-	-	0.81	6	9
South Africa	-	-	-	4.8	-	-	-	-	-	-	0.5	117	131
Spain	-	0.54	-	4.67	<0.4	0.59	7.80	-	-	-	3.39	5	39
Spain	-	1.45	-	2.75	-	-	9.59	0.16	-	-	2.91	6	50
Spain	-	0.17	-	3.62	0.32	0.10	7.06	-	-	-	1.40	61	78
Spain	nd-3.2	0.2	-	3.9	-	0.5	27.9	-	0.3	0.3	3.3	27	128
Spain	0.50	0.65	-	2.74	-	0.04	8.16	-	2.67	0.06	1.09	18	129
Turkey	0.5-15	0.11-4	-	0.03-2.8	-	0.10-8.6	0.94-15.6	0.05-3.4	0.015-1	0.4-8.80	0.04-3.5	30	3

[a] number of samples examined
n.d. not detected
When one figure is reported, the value represents the mean BA content in wine; otherwise, the data represent the minimum and maximum BA value reported by the authors.

Table 2. Principal biogenic amine content found in different white wines from several countries

Country	AGM	CAD	ETHA	HIM	MET	PHE	PUT	SPM	SPD	TRYPT	TYR	N[a]	Reference
France	-	0.14	-	1.09	0.30	1.57	4.53	-	-	-	1.14	20	28
France	10.3	0.1	-	0.1	-	0.9	1.9	0.1	0.3	-	2.2	15	94
Greece	-	0.81	-	0.41	0.13	0.50	0.98	0.27	0.17	-	0.42	47	45
Greece	-	0.12-0.21	-	0.25-0.99	0.51-0.90	-	0.53-2.54	-	-	-	n.d.-1.29	5	123
Greece	nd	nd-0.13	nd-0.22	0.34-1.13	nd-0.49	-	nd-9.07	-	-	nd-0.51	nd-1.16	17	124
Italy	6.45	2.57	15.30	0.95	0.25	0.87	2.19	0.12	0.56	1.92	0.58	39	24
Italy	2.46	nd	2.22	n.d.	nd	n.d.	2.15	nd.	nd	nd	nd	5	107
Italy	-	0.07	6.01	1.66	-	1.09	1.99	0.96	6.08	-	0.86	3	126
Not reported	-	0.06	-	1.10	0.14	2.26	1.20	-	0.04	<0.1	0.98	43	133
Portugal	-	0.07	-	-	-	0.38	2.08	-	0.075	-	0.057	6	2
Portugal	-	0.63	11.32	1.20	0.96	0.75	2.14	-	-	-	0.54	6	9
Spain	nd	0.1	-	0.2	-	0.3	4.0	-	0.3	0.4	0.2	10	128
Spain	-	0.66	-	1.17	-	-	4.31	-	-	-	0.48	6	50
Spain	0.70	0.23	-	0.30	-	0.04	6.16	-	0.93	0.10	0.91	14	129
Spain	-	< 0.2	-	0.30	0.80	0.79	1.96	-	-	-	<0.4	5	39
South Africa	-	-	-	0.1	-	-	-	-	-	-	0.1	62	131

[a] number of samples examined

n.d. not detected

When one figure is reported, the value represents the mean BA content in wine; otherwise, the data represent the minimum and maximum BA value reported by the authors.

Types and levels of amines in wines are influenced by several factors, such as degree of maturation of grape, soil type [6], viticulture practices [115] and content of nitrogen compounds in grape juice [30, 118]. Nitrogen fertilization can influence the amine content in wine, and the supply of 100 kg N/ha/year has been shown to cause a two fold increase of these compounds in wine [140]. Also soil nutrient deficiencies may affect the occurrence of BA in wine; for example, a potassium deficit in the soil may induce the formation and accumulation of PUT in grape, that then can be found in wine [115].

Several factors, such as nutrient starvation, osmotic shocks or presence of pollutant in the environment, can have a deep impact on the metabolism of di- and polyamines [141]. However, in a study carried out to evaluate whether the degree of irrigation may affect the endogenous amine content in grape, as well its evolution during the wine making process, the authors concluded that water-stress does not seem to be a factor influencing the BA level in wines [128].

Also the presence of *Botritis cinerea* in grapes appears to influence both quantity and quality of amines in grapes and wines [117], and bad grape hygienic conditions have been associated with the presence of higher amine levels, especially isopenthylamine and PHE [142]. Moreover, the anti-fungi treatments could have a positive influence on biogenic amine formation, as reported by Marques et al. [143], who found lower levels of BA, especially ISO, PHE and TYR, in wines obtained from grapes treated with fungicides.

Bauza et al. [29] have investigated the evolution of polyamines (AGM, PUT, SPD and SPM) during both the growth stages of the grapeberry and the winemaking, finding significant differences in the amine levels during the various ripening stages. These amines were present only in small quantities at grape maturity, and in particular PUT concentration decreased throughout the whole ripening period. However arginine, a precursor of PUT, increased in the berries, therefore, due to the low levels of polyamines at grape maturity, the amount of PUT found in the wine at the end of the winemaking process could be reasonably ascribed only to the microbial activity.

Also grape variety seems to be a relevant factor influencing the quantitative and qualitative content of BA in wines. In fact it has been possible to differentiate various wine varieties on the basis of their BA content. In particular Landete et al. [27] were able to discriminate wines made with three Spanish grape varieties (Bobal, Garnacha and Tempranillo) on the basis of the HIM, TYR and PUT content, while Hernández-Orte et al. [43] have shown that, with respect to wines obtained from grapes of the Cabernet Sauvignon variety, during aging higher levels of amines were produced in wines obtained from the Tempranillo variety. Also Marques et al. [143] found differences in wines obtained from the 6 different Portuguese grape varieties, whereas Herbert et al. [26] have reported that the varieties with the highest final concentration of BA were also the richer in assimilable amino acid level.

Further evidence of the importance of grape variety on the BA content in wine has been shown by several other authors. Soufleros et al. [45] have reported that PUT, CAD and SPD levels were significantly different in wines made from several grape varieties. Glória et al. [6] have found differences in HIM, PUT and TYM concentrations between Pinot noir and Cabernet Sauvignon wines originating from the same region; Hajós et al. [117] have reported significant differences in some amine levels in grapes and wines of 3 grape varieties of the Tokaj region in Hungary. Del Prete et al. [54] found a significant difference between the content of individual BA and the cultivars, with AGM being the only exception; taking into account that the cultivars were grown in the same pedoclimatic conditions and with the same training system, the observed differences could be attributed solely to genetic variety characteristics. Total BA level has been shown to vary significantly also in Brazilian wines obtained from different cultivars, being higher for Cabernet Sauvignon wines (4.33 to 7.60 mg/L) in comparison with Cabernet Franc (2.07 to 4.27 mg/L) and Merlot (4.27 to 4.93 mg/L) wines [144]. Finally, significant differences in BA content have also been found in Cabernet Sauvignon and Pinot grigio grape varieties cultivated in the Trentino region in Italy, with high levels of PUT and HIM in Cabernet Sauvignon and high levels of ETHY in Pinot grigio [114].

The observed differences among grape cultivars are probably due to the amino acids composition and the respective amounts in grape varieties, as well to the natural bacteria microflora present in grapes [143].

Organic viticulture has aroused great interest among ecologically aware consumers and is regulated by Council Regulation (EEC) No 2092/91. A study has been conducted in order to determine the effect of organic viticulture on the BA levels in wines from different organic and non-organic grapes of *Vitis vinifera* varieties [145], resulting the PUT and ETHY content greater in organic wines than in non-organic ones. This differences could be explained considering some of the different processing steps (spontaneous fermentation/pure culture, pressing process, quantities of SO_2, fining process) involved in organic and non-organic wine production.

3.2. Winemaking Procedures

MLF has usually a greater importance in red wines than in white ones, and this fermentation process plays a key role in the generation of BA. During MLF the main BA generated by decarboxylation of the corresponding amino acids are PUT, HIM and TYR, but also the pH of wine should be taken into account, because at relatively high pH values biogenic amines are always produced in large amounts; therefore, red wines, generally less acidic, present higher levels of these moieties than white wines [8, 24, 50, 82].

Several enological treatments can influence the BA content in wine, being in general HIM, TYR and PUT the amines mainly affected by the highest number of enological factors [111]. During alcoholic fermentation, the length of maceration is one the main factors influencing the extraction of the compounds present in the grape skin, such as the amino acids, precursors of the BA. However, while some authors have reported that long maceration times could favor a greater production of BA [21, 111], others have not found any correlation between skin contact time and BA concentration in wine [136].

Also the use of starter yeasts during fermentation can affect the BA level in wine. Torrea Goñi and Ancín-Azpilicueta [40] have reported that wines obtained from musts inoculated with different strains of *S. cerevisiae* had a higher content of non volatile amines and PHE; this could be probably ascribed to the fact that during fermentation a higher consumption of the precursor amino acids occurred in the inoculated samples.

In addition, the use of malolactic starters can contribute to minimize BA production when MLF is conducted by indigenous malolactic bacteria, high BA producers [43, 143, 144]. In particular, HIM, TYR and CAD content has been shown to be significantly lower in inoculated wines, although the mechanisms through which the malolactic starters prevent BA accumulation in susceptible wines is still not well known [111]. Results in vitro have demonstrated that some commercial malolactic bacteria do not produce HIM, TYR and PUT [12], and, in addition, Marques et al. [143] have reported higher concentrations of TYR, PUT and HIM in control wines than in wines inoculated with malolactic starters.

Commercial pectolytic enzymes can be used in winemaking process to increase juice yields, facilitate pressing and filtering, and to provide greater clarity to must and wine. However, these enzymes may also produce concomitant effects, such as an important proteolytic activity, which can lead to hydrolysis of proteins and peptides and the release of amino acids. One only study has been carried out about the influence of pectolytic enzymes on BA accumulation, reporting that the addition of pectolytic enzymes did not favor the accumulation of any biogenic amine [111].

3.3. Aging and Storage

Aging is one of the most important steps in wine making, affecting to a large extent the quality of the final product. The process can be carried out in bottles or in barrels and in this case the wine can be aged as it is or after filtration. In the latter case producers can avoid the racking step, thus saving on costs. However, the role of filtration in wine making is debated, because of its possible influence on the aroma and color of wine, due to the removal of yeasts, colloids, bacteria, which when present can alter the organoleptic characteristics of wine. One of the most utilized filtering aids is represented by diatomaceous earth, that can be characterized by a relatively large negative surface charge when used for wine filtration, due to the relatively low pH values of the product. This negative charge can cause a partial adsorption on the surface of some nitrogenous compounds, such as cationic amino acids and proteins, therefore influencing the final content of BA in wine. At this regard, recently Alcaide–Hidalgo et al. [146] have reported that wines with the lowest mean values of HIM were those racked and clarified before aging, while in contrast Jiménez-Moreno and Ancín Azpilicueta [147] in a specific study on the influence of turbidity on the accumulation of BA during aging, did not observe any influence of wine turbidity on the accumulation of BA.

Also the evolution of amines during wine storage in both bottles and barrels has been studied, but the results of the research are controversial. Some authors have reported a different evolution of BA during aging in oak barrels [148, 149]; in particular, PUT and CAD increased during aging and not underwent degradation, in agreement with the data of González Marco and Ancín Azpilicueta [149]. HIM and TYR were produced at the beginning of the aging process, although they were not accumulated in wine, probably due to their degradation, according to the data reported by Alcaide-Hidalgo et al. [146], Jiménez Moreno and Ancín Azpilicueta, [147] and Vidal-Carou [150], and in disagreement with Gerbaux and Monamy [151], who observed an increase of HIM and TYR during aging of wine in bottles. Bauza et al. [47] and Hernández-Orte et al. [43] have reported an increase in PUT and HIM during aging in oak barrels, while González Marco and Ancín Azpilicueta [149], and Landete et al. [27] have observed, in bottled wines, only an increase of HIM during the first 45 days and during the first 6 months of aging, respectively. Moreover, Jimenéz Moreno and Ancín Azpilicueta [147] have reported an increase of PHE and SPD during the aging period of wine.

With regard to the evolution of non-volatile amines, some authors have reported that during aging of wine in barrels the concentration of these moieties did not change, while a decrease of dimethylamine and isobuthylamine was observed [146, 149]. These latter amines could have been consumed by residual bacteria present in the wine for the production of carbon skeletons or amino groups. The increase in the concentrations of ETHY and pyrrolidine in wines aged in oak barrels could be due to yeast autolysis and/or to a reductive amination of the corresponding aldehyde or to the transamination of the aldehyde from an amino acid [35].

It has been shown that also wine acidity may influence the BA level, and it is noteworthy that less acid wines gave rise to higher HIM contents [124]. At higher pH values BA produced by *O. oeni* in a model system were in considerable amount, whereas high ethanol concentrations reduced their accumulation [52]. It has been reported that wines with higher pH generally have higher amine concentrations and this relationship between pH and amines may be explained by the fact that at higher pH a greater number of bacteria can develop, thus increasing the probability of having strains able to form amines [130].

Traditionally, during aging only some wines were left in contact with their lees, while nowadays, wine aging on lees is more recurrent in all viticultural areas. Wine less contact seems to be positive concerning the removal of most undesirable compounds from wine, but harmful in the case of BA, being the role of lees critical for their release of amino acids, besides representing a reservoir of microorganisms [152, 153].

Several studies have reported a higher concentration of BA in wines matured on lees than those elaborated in the traditional way and kept in bottle [21, 111, 143, 146, 148, 149]. In particular, González Marco and Ancín Azpilicueta [149] and Martín-Álvarez et al. [111] have reported that PUT is the biogenic amine most affected by the presence of lees, in agreement with the data of Bauza et al. [21] and Alcaide-Hidalgo [146], who also found a higher production of PUT in wines inoculated with bacteria by lees addition, while the level of this amine remained stable in those aged without lees. The increased PUT content in wines aged in the presence of lees was explained by Marcobal et al. [78] on the basis of an ornithine decarboxylase gene in the PUT-producer *O. oeni* BIFI-83 strain, which was isolated from lees from a wine with high concentration of PUT. Conversely, Jimenez-Moreno et al. [148] did not observe a decrease of PUT during aging of wines in presence or not of lees. Moreover, Marques et al. [143] have found higher levels only of TYR and CAD in wines stored on lees with respect to wines stored without, while PUT remained stable in both assays. This appreciable difference in the BA content between the wine stored in bottle and the same wine aged on lees could be due to the fact that during lees contact the wine composition changes, as a consequence of the hydrolysis of various biomolecules within the yeast cell. In fact due to the proteolytic processes taking place, proteins are hydrolyzed to amino acids and peptides, and these peptides are later degraded further to amino acids and amines.

In addition, also stirring during aging can increase the final BA content in wine aged on lees [146]; in particular, González Marco and Ancín Azpilicueta [149] have observed a higher concentration of TYR and HIM in wines aged on lees and weekly stirred than in wines obtained without stirring.

Storage temperature has an influence on the quality of wine, since the reactions which take place in bottled product intensify with an increase in temperature. Although wine should never be kept at a temperature above 20 °C, climatic or transport conditions may cause an increase of the wine temperature up to 30 °C, and several authors have reported how BA content in foodstuffs may depend also on temperature, increasing with time and storage temperature [4, 154, 155]. Little work has been done on the relationship between accumulation of BA in wine and temperature, during both the fermentation and the storage steps. In particular, while Vidal-Carou et al. [150] have reported that wine storage under conditions of spoilage at various temperatures did not affect the HIM and TYR levels in the final product, González Marco and Ancín Azpilicueta [156] have reported a slight influence of the temperature on the BA evolution in wine. In particular, in wines stored at different temperatures (4, 20 and 35°C) for a period up to 105 days, the recorded SPM level decreased up to undetectable values, while PUT, TYR and CAD concentrations did not show appreciable variations throughout the whole period. With regard to HIM, the amount of this amine was not significantly different ($p<0.05$) after 45 or 75 days, whereas when extending the storage period up to 105 days, the HIM content significantly increased in the wines kept at room temperature in comparison with those stored at the more extreme conditions of 4 and 35 °C, therefore suggesting that wine storage at room temperature favors the HDC activity.

3.4. Influence of Vintage and Provenance

Biogenic amines are generally considered markers more useful for discriminating wines according to the provenance [24, 26] or the winemaking technology [24, 25, 27] rather than to the production year or the grape variety. However, several studies have reported differences in the BA levels depending on the vintage [45, 54, 111, 118, 143]. In particular, Sass-Kriss et al. [118] have reported that the qualitative and quantitative content of biologically active amines in wine was mostly influenced by the vintage and the winemaking technology, and to a lesser extent by the grape variety. Marques et al. (143) and Del Prete et al. (54) have suggested that the observed levels of BA in wines produced in different years could be ascribed to the diversity of the wine microorganisms naturally and differently selected each year, probably because of the climatic conditions and the consequent viticulture/oenological practices.

Conversely, other authors have reported that the production year did not differentiate wines from different regions on the basis of BA [6, 24, 26, 82, 150].

Also the viticulture region may affect the amount of amines, since wines of some regions have been shown to contain higher amounts of amines than wines from other regions or countries [24-28, 125, 127, 143]. In particular, important differences in PUT and HIM concentrations were observed among three different Spanish wine-producing regions, while no differences were observed for TYR and PHE among all wines. Some authors have reported that PUT content seems to be more influenced by the geographical origin and grape variety than by the type of winemaking, and the different PUT levels in musts could be to some extent explained taking into account the soil chemical composition, with special regard to the potassium level [24, 27]. In addition, also other authors have reported differences in the BA level among wines produced in the same region, and they found these differences to be correlated with the type of grape and the type of wine-making process [6, 21, 136].

4. CONCLUSION

The study of BA in wines is of interest from a toxicological point of view, related to the ingestion of elevate amounts of these moieties in this alcoholic beverage; in addition BA have been associated with a lack of hygiene during the winemaking process and therefore they have been suggested as an index of quality or of poor sanitary conditions of grapes or of poor manufacturing practices.

Biogenic amines are mainly produced from microbial decarboxylation of the corresponding amino acids. In wines it has been reported that these moieties increase especially after MLF, red wines usually being richer in amines than white wines. Generally the most investigated amines in wines are HIM, TYR, PHE, PUT and CAD. AGM and ETHA resulted to be abundant in wines, but they have been little investigated. Even though the toxicological role of BA in wine is still not well-known, it is desirable to avoid the formation and accumulation of these moieties in wine; therefore, the sources and critical control points for amine formation during winemaking should be determined, in order to limit their presence and accumulation of BA in wine. Moreover, the variability in the amount of BA produced among the strains of the same species underlines the importance to utilize yeasts and lactic acid bacteria as starters in winemaking process and selected also for being low-producers of BA.

REFERENCES

[1] Bardócz, S. (1995). Polyamines in foods and their consequences for food quality and human health. *Trends in Food Science and Technology*, 6, 341-346.

[2] Fernandes, J.O. and Ferreira, M.A. (2000). Combined ion-pair extraction and gas chromatography-mass spectrometry for the simultaneous determination of diamines, polyamines and aromatic amines in Port wines and grape juice. *Journal of Chromatography A*, 886, 183-195.

[3] Anli, R.E., Vural, N., Yilmaz, S. and Vural, Y.H. (2004). The determination of biogenic amines in Turkish red wines. *Journal of Food Composition and Analysis* 17, 53-62.

[4] Halász, A., Baráth, A., Simon-Sarkadi, L. and Holzapfel, W. (1994). Biogenic amines and their production by micro-organisms in food. *Trends in Food Science and Technology*, 5, 42-48.

[5] Silla Santos, M.H. (1996). Biogenic amines: their importance in foods. *International Journal of Food Microbiology*, 29, 213-231.

[6] Glória, M.B., Watson, T., Sarkadi, L.S. and Daeschel, M.A. (1998). A survey of biogenic amines in Oregon Pinot noir and Cabernet Sauvignon wines. *American Journal of Enology and Viticulture*, 49, 279-282.

[7] Moret, S. and Conte, L.S. (1996). High-performance liquid chromatographic evaluation of biogenic amines in foods. An analysis of different methods of sample preparation in relation to food characteristics. *Journal of Chromatography A*, 729, 363-369.

[8] Lonvaud-Funel, A. (2001). Biogenic amines in wines: role of lactic acid bacteria. *FEMS Microbiology Letters*, 199, 9-13.

[9] Mafra, I., Herbert, P., Santos, L., Barros, P. and Alves, A. (1999). Evaluation of biogenic amines in some Portuguese quality wines by HPLC fluorescence detection of OPA derivatives. *American Journal of Enology and Viticulture*, 50, 128–132.

[10] Ten Brink, B., Damink, C., Joosten, H.M.L.J. and Huis in t' Veld, J.H.J. (1990). Occurrence and formation of biologically active amines in foods. *International Journal of Food Microbiology*, 11, 73-84.

[11] Leitão, M.C., Teixeira, H.C., Barreto Crespo, M.T. and San Romão, M.V. (2000). Biogenic amines occurrence in wines. Amino acid decarboxylase and proteolytic activities expression by *Oenococcus oeni*. *Journal of Agricultural and Food Chemistry*, 48, 2780-2784.

[12] Moreno-Arribas, M.V., Polo, M.C., Jorganes, F. and Muñoz, R. (2003). Screening of biogenic amine production by lactic acid bacteria isolated from grape must and wine. *International Journal of Food Microbiology*, 84, 117-123.

[13] Karovicova, J. and Kohajdovà, Z. (2004). Biogenic amine in food. *Chemical Papers*, 59, 70-79.

[14] Rice, S., Eitenmiller, R.R. and Koehler, P.E. (1976). Biologically active amine in food. A review. *Journal of Milk and Food Technology*, 39, 353-358.

[15] Shalaby, A.R. (1996). Significance of biogenic amines to food safety and human health. *Food Research International*, 29, 675-690.

[16] Kalač, P. and Krausová, P. (2005). A review of dietary polyamines: formation, implications for growth and health and occurrence in foods. *Food Chemistry*, 90, 219-230.

[17] Önal, A. (2007). A review: current analytical methods for the determination of biogenic amines in foods. *Food Chemistry*, 103, 1475-1486.

[18] Lehtonen, P. (1996). Determination of amines and amino acids in wine-a review. *American Journal of Enology and Viticulture*, 47, 127-133.

[19] Achilli, G. and Cellerino G.P. (1994). Determination of amines in wines by high-performance liquid chromatography with electrochemical coulometric detection after precolumn derivatization. *Journal of Chromatography A*, 661, 201-205.

[20] Tomera, J.F. (1999). Current knowledge of the health benefits and disadvantages of wine composition. *Trends in Food Science and Technology*, 10, 129-138.

[21] Bauza, T., Blaise, A., Mestres, J.P., Teissedre, P.L., Daumas, F. and Cabanis, J.C. (1995). Évolution des teneurs en amines biogènes des moûts et des vins au cours de la vinification. *Science des Aliments*, 15, 367-380.

[22] Busto, O., Miracle, M., Guasch, J. and Borrul, F. (1997). Determination of biogenic amines in wines by high-perfomance liquid chromatography with on column fluorescence derivatization. *Journal of Chromatography A*, 757, 311-318.

[23] Arvanitoyannis, I.S., Katsota, M.N., Psarra, E.P., Soufleros, E.H. and Kallitharaka, S. (1999). Application of quality control methods for assessing wine authenticity: use of multivariate analysis (chemometrics). *Trends in Food Science and Technology*, 10, 321-336.

[24] Galgano, F., Favati, F., De Giorgio, A., Caruso, M. and Lacertosa, G. (2004). Health and consumption of wine: study of polyphenols and biogenic amines in wines of South Italy. In "*Ricerche e innovazioni per l'industria alimentare*", Vol VI. A cura di S. Porretta, Chiriotti Editori Pinerolo (TO), pp. 1021-1028.

[25] Héberger, K., Csomós, E. and Simon-Sarkadi, L. (2003). Principal component and linear discriminant analyses of free amino acids and biogenic amines in Hungarian wines. *Journal of Agricultural and Food Chemistry*, 51, 8055-8060.

[26] Herbert, P., Cabrita, M.J., Ratoa, N., Laureano, O. and Alves, A. (2005). Free amino acids and biogenic amines in wines and musts from the Alentejo region. Evolution of amines during alcoholic fermentation and relationship with variety, sub-region and vintage. *Journal of Food Engineering,* 66, 315–322.

[27] Landete, J.M., Ferrer, S., Polo, L. and Pardo, I. (2005). Biogenic amines in wines from three Spanish regions. *Journal of Agricultural and Food Chemistry*, 53, 1119-1124.

[28] Soufleros, E., Barrios, M.L. and Bertrand, A. (1998). Correlation between the content of biogenic amines and other wine compounds. *American Journal of Enology and Viticulture,* 49, 266-278.

[29] Bauza, T., Kelly, M.T. and Blaise, A. (2007). Study of polyamines and their precursor amino acids in Grenache noir and syrah grapes and wine of the Rhone Valley. *Food Chemistry*, 105, 405-413.

[30] Coton, E., Torlois, S., Bertrand, A. and Lonvaud-Funel, A. (1999). Amines biogènes et bactéries lactiques du vin. *Bulletin O.I.V.*, 72, 23-35.

[31] Arena, M. E. and Manca De Nadra, M.C. (2001). Biogenic amines production by *Lactobacillus. Journal of Applied Microbiology*, 90, 158-162.

[32] Pfeiffer, P. and Radler, F. (1992). Determination of ethanolamine in wine by HPLC after derivatization with 9-fluorenylmethoxycarbonilchloride. *American Journal of Enology and Viticulture,* 43, 315-317.

[33] Choi, J.Y., Martin, W.E., Murphy, R.C. and Voelker, D.R. (2004). Phosphatidylcholine and N-methylated phospholipids are nonessential in *Saccharomyces cerevisiae. Journal of Microbiology and Biotechnology*, 18, 159-163.

[34] Baucom, T.L., Tabacchi, M.H., Cottrell, T.H.E. and Richmond, B.S. (1986). Biogenic amines content of New York state wines. *Journal of Food Science*, 51, 1376-1377.

[35] Buteau, C., Duitschaever C.L. and Ashton, G.C. (1984). High-performance liquid chromatographic detection and quantitation of amines in must and wine. *Journal of Chromatography,* 284, 201-210

[36] Vidal-Carou, M.C., Ambatlle-Espunyes, A., Ulla-Ulla, M.C. and Mariné-Font, A. (1990). Histamine and tyramine in Spanish wines: their formation during the winemaking process. *American Journal of Enology and Viticulture*, 41, 160-167.

[37] Buteau, C., Duitschaever C.L. and Ashton, G.C. (1984). A study of biogenesis of amines in a Villard noir wine. *American Journal of Enology and Viticulture*, 35, 228-236.

[38] Caruso, M., Fiore, C., Contursi, M., Salzano, G., Paparella, A. and Romano, P. (2002). Formation of biogenic amines as criteria for the selection of wine yeast. *World Journal of Microbiology and Biot*echnology, 18, 159-163.

[39] Iñiguez Crespo, M.B. and Vázquez Lasa M.(1994). Determination of biogenic amines and other amines in wine by an optimized HPLC method with polarity gradient elution. *American Journal of Enology and Viticulture*, 45, 460-463

[40] Torrea Goñi, D. and Ancín-Azpilicueta, C. (2002). Content of biogenic amines in a Chardonnay wine obtained through spontaneous and inoculated fermentations. *Journal of Agricultural and Food Chemistry,* 50, 4895-4899.

[41] Cavazza, A., Cerutti, G. and Gozzi, G. (1995). Ceppo di lievito e biogenesi di ammine nella fermentazione del mosto d'uva. *Vignevini*, 23, 8–12.

[42] Cerutti, G., Margheri, G. and Bongini, F. (1987). Sulla correlazione tra fermentazione malolattica ed ammine biogene vasoattive. *Vignevini*, 14, 39–42.

[43] Hernández-Orte, P., Lapeña, A.C., Peña-Gallego, A., Astrain, J., Baron, C., Pardo, I., Ferrer, S., Cacho, J. and Ferreira, V. (2008). Biogenic amine determination in wine fermented in oak barrels: factors affecting formation. *Food Research International*, 41, 697-706.

[44] Lafon-Lafourcade, S. (1995). L'histamine des vins. *Connaissance de la Vigne et du Vin*, 2, 103-115.

[45] Soufleros, E.H., Bouloumpasi, E., Zotou, A. and Loukou, Z. (2007). Determination of biogenic amines in Greek wines by HPLC and ultraviolet detection after dansylation and examination of factors affecting their presence and concentration. *Food Chemistry*, 101, 704-716.

[46] Agnolucci, M., Scarano, S., Sassano, C., Toffanin, A. and Nuti M.P. (2007). Influence of different winemaking technologies on the malolactic bacteria and the occurrence of biogenic amine in Chianti wines. *Proceeding of "1st International Symposium on Environment Identities and Mediterranean Areas"*, Corte-Ajaccio, France, 10-13 July pp. 625-628.

[47] Bauza, T., Blaise, A., Mestres, J.P., Teissedre, P.L., Cabanis, J.C., Kanny, G. and Moneret-Vautrin, A. (1995). Les amines biogènes du vin. Métabolisme et toxicité. *Bulletin de l'OIV*, 68, 42–67.

[48] Lonvaud-Funel, A. and Joyeux, A. (1994). Histamine production by wine lactic-acid bacteria-isolation of a histamine-producing strain of *Leuconostoc eonos*. *Journal of Applied Bacteriology*, 77, 401-407.

[49] Moreno-Arribas, M.V., Torlois S., Joyeux A., Bertrand, A. and Lonvaud Funel, A.(2000). Isolation, properties and behaviour of tyramine-producing lactic acid bacteria from wine. *Journal of Applied Microbiology*, 88, 584-593.

[50] Romero, R., Sánchez-Viñas, M., Gázquez, D. and Gracia Bagur, M. (2002). Characterization of selected Spanish table wine samples according to their biogenic amine content from liquid chromatographic determination. *Journal of Agricultural and Food Chemistry*, 50, 4713-4717.

[51] Marcobal, A., Martín-Álvarez, P.J., Polo, M.C., Muñoz, R. and Moreno-Arribas, M.V. (2006). Formation of biogenic amines throughout the industrial manufacture of red wine. *Journal of Food Protection*, 69, 397-404.

[52] Gardini, F., Zaccarelli A., Belletti, N., Faustini, F., Cavazza, A., Martuscelli, M., Mastrocola D. and Suzzi, G. (2005). Factors influencing biogenic amine production by a strain of *Oenococcus oeni* in a model system. *Food Control*, 16, 609-616.

[53] Guerrini, S., Mangani, S., Granchi, L. and Vincenzini, M. (2002). Biogenic amine production by *Oenococcus oeni*. *Current Microbiology*, 44, 374-378.

[54] Del Prete, V., Costantini, A., Cecchini, F., Morassut, M. and Garcia-Moruno, E. (2009). Occurrence of biogenic amines in wine: role of grapes. *Food Chemistry*, 112, 474-481.

[55] Pogorzelski, E. (1992). Studies of the formation of histamine in must and wines from edelberry fruit. *Journal of the Science of Food and Agriculture*, 60, 239-244.

[56] Izquierdo-Pulido, M., Font-Fábregas, J. and Vidal-Carou, C. (1995). Influence of *Saccharomyces cerevisiae* var. *uvarum* on histamine and tyramine formation during beer fermentation. *Food Chemistry*, 54, 51-54.

[57] Caruso, M., Romano, P. and Zirpoli, E. (2004). Detection of decarboxylase-positive *Saccharomyces cerevisiae* wine strains by a screening on plate medium. *Proceeding of "11th International Congress on Yeasts"*, Rio De Janeiro, Brasil, 15-20 August, p. 158.

[58] Landete, J.M., Ferrer, S., Polo, L. and Pardo, I. (2007). Biogenic amines production by lactic acid bacteria and yeast isolated from wine. *Food Control*, 18, 1559-1574.

[59] Sponholz, W.R. (1993). Wine spoilage by microorganisms. In: Wine microbiology and biotechnology. Fleet, G.H. (Ed). Chur, Switzerland: Harwood Academy Press, pp. 289-326.

[60] Heresztyn, T. (1986). Metabolisim of volatile phenolic compounds from hydroxycinnamic acids by *Brettanomyces* yeast. *Archives of Microbilogy*, 146, 96-98.

[61] Torrea Goñi, D. and Ancín-Azpilicueta, C. (2001). Influence of yeast strain on biogenic amines content in wines: relationship with the uitilization of amino acids during fermentation. *American Journal of Enology and Viticulture*, 52, 185-190.

[62] Fleet, G.H. (1993). Yeast interactions and wine flavour. *International Journal of Food Microbiology*, 86, 11-22.

[63] Romano, P., Caruso, M., Capece, A., Lipani, G., Paraggio, M. and Fiore, C. (2003). Metabolic diversity of *Saccharomyces cerevisiae* strains from spontaneously fermented grape must. *World Journal of Microbiology and Biotechnology*, 19, 311-315.

[64] Romano, P., Fiore, C., Paraggio, M., Caruso, M. and Capece, A. (2003). Function of yeast species and strains in wine flavour. *International Journal of Food Microbiology*, 86, 169-180.

[65] Lambrechts, M.G. and Pretorius, I.S. (2000). Yeast and its importance to wine aroma: a review. *South African Journal of Enology and Viticulture*, 21, 97-129.

[66] Brandolini, V., Salzano, G., Maietti, A., Caruso, M., Tedeschi, P., Mazzotta, D. and Romano, P. (2002). Automated multiple development for determination of glycerol produced by wine yeasts. *World Journal of Microbiology and Biotechnology*, 18, 481-485.

[67] Mangani, S., Guerrini, S., Granchi, L. and Vincenzini, M. (2005). Putrescine accumulation in wine: role of *Oenococcus oeni*. *Current Microbiology*, 51, 6-10.

[68] Davis, C.R., Wibowo, D., Eschenbruch R. and Lee, R. (1985). Practical implications of malolactic fermentation: a review. *American Journal of Enology and Viticulture*, 36, 290-301.

[69] Henick-Kling, T. (1993). *Malolactic fermentation*. In: Fleet, G.H. (ed). Wine microbiology and biotechnology. Chur, Switzerland, Harwood Academy Press, pp. 289-326.

[70] Kunkee, R.E. (1991). Some roles of malic acid in the malolactic fermentation in wine making. *FEMS Microbiological Reviews*, 88, 55-72.

[71] Lonvaud-Funel, A. (1999). Lactic acid bacteria in the quality improvement and depreciation of wine. *Antonie van Leeuwenhoek*, 76, 317-331.

[72] Stratton, J.E., Hutkins, R.W. and Taylor, S.L. (1991). Biogenic amines in cheese and other fermented foods: a review. *Journal of Food Protection*, 54, 460-470.

[73] Aerni, J. (1985). Origine de l'histamine dans les vins. Connaissances actuelles. *Bulletin de l'Office International du Vin*, 1016-1019.

[74] Delfini, C. (1989). Ability of wine malolactic bacteria to produce histamine. *Sciences des Aliments*, 9, 413-416.

[75] Choudhury, N., Hansen, W., Engesser, D., Hammes, W.P. and Holzapfel, W.H. (1990). Formation of histamine and tyramine by lactic acid bacteria in decarboxylase assay medium. *Letters in Applied Microbiology*, 11, 278-281.

[76] Straub, B.W., Kicherer, M., Schilcher, S.M. and Hammes, W.P. (1995). The formation of biogenic amines by fermentation organisms. *Zeitschrift für Lebensmittel Untersuchung und-Forschung*, 201, 79-82.

[77] Lucas, P.M., Claisse, O. and Lonvaud-Funel, A. (2008). High frequency of histamine-producing bacteria in the enological environment and instability of the histidine decarboxylase production phenotype. *Applied and Environmental Microbiology*, 74(3), 811-817.

[78] Marcobal, A., Polo, de las Rivas, B., Moreno-Arribas, M.V. and Muñoz, R. (2004). Biogenic amine content of red Spanish wines: comparison of a direct ELISA and an HPLC method for the determination of histamine in wines. *Food Research International*, 38, 387-394.

[79] Lucas, P.M., Wolken, W.A., Claisse, O., Lolkema, J.S. and Lonvaud-Funel, A. (2005). Histamine-producing pathway encoded on an unstable plasmid in *Lactobacillus hilgardii* 0006. *Applied and Environmental Microbiology*, 71, 1417-1424.

[80] Coton, E., Rollan, G., Bertrand, A. and Lonvaud-Funel, A. (1998). Histamine-producing lactic acid bacteria in wines: early detection, frequency, and distribution. *American Journal of Enology and Viticulture,* 49, 199-204.

[81] Rollan, G.C., Coton, E., and Lonvaud-Funel, A. (1995). Histidine decarboxylase activity of *Leuconostoc oenos* 9204. *Food Microbiology*, 12, 455-461.

[82] Marcobal, A., Polo, M.C., Martín-Álvarez, P.J. and Moreno-Arribas, M.V. (2005). Identification of the ornithine decarboxylase gene in the putrescine-producer *Oenococcus oeni* BIFI-83. *FEMS Microbiology Letters*, 239, 213-220.

[83] Moreno Arribas, V., and Lonvaud-Funel, A. (1999). Tyrosine decarboxylase activity of *Lactobacillus brevis* IOEB 9809 isolated from wine and *L. brevis* ATCC 367. *FEMS Microbiology Letters*, 180, 55-60.

[84] Le Jeune, C., Lonvaud-Funel, A., Ten BrinK, B., Hofstra, H. and Van Der Vossen, J.M.B.M. (1995). Development of a detection system for histamine decarboxylating lactic acid bacteria based on DNA probes, PCR and activity test. *Journal of Applied Bacteriology*, 78, 316-326.

[85] Galgano, F., Suzzi, G., Favati, F., Caruso M., Martuscelli, M., Gardini, F. and Salzano. G. (2001). Biogenic amines during ripening in "Semicotto Caprino" cheese: role of enterococci. *International Journal of Food Science and Technology,* 36, 153-160.

[86] Gardini, F., Martuscelli, M., Caruso, M., Galgano, F., Crudele, M.A., Favati, F., Guerzoni, M.A. and Suzzi, G. (2001). Effects of pH, temperature and NaCl concentration on the growth kinetics, proteolytic activity and biogenic amines production of *Enterococcus faecalis*. *International Journal of Food Microbiology*, 64, 105-117.

[87] Gonzales del Llano, D., Cuesta, P. and Rodríguez, A. (1998). Biogenic amine production by wild lactococcal and leuconostoc strains. *Letters in Applied Microbiology*, 26, 270-274.

[88] Montel, M.C., Masson, F. and Talon, R. (1999). Comparison of biogenic amine content in traditional and industrial French dry sausages. *Sciences des Aliments*, 19, 247-254.

[89] Landete, J.M., Arena, M.E., Pardo, I., Manca de Nadra, M.C. and Ferrer, S. (2008) Comparative survey of putrescine production from agmatine deamination in different bacteria. *Food Microbiology*, 25, 882-887.

[90] Alberto, M.R., Arena, M.E. and Manca De Nadra, M. (2007). Putrescine production from agmatine by *Lactobacillus hilgardii*: Effect of phenolic compounds. *Food Control*, 18, 898–903.

[91] Mazzoli, R., lamberti, C., Coisson, J.D., Purrotti, M., Arlorio, M., Giuffrida, M.G., Giunta, C. and Pessione, E. (2008). Influence of ethanol, malate and arginine on histamine production of *Lactobacillus hilgardii* isolated from an Italian red wine. *Amino Acids* DOI: 10.1007/s00726-008-0035-8.

[92] Moreno-Arribas, M. V. and Polo, M.C. (2008). Occurrence of lactic acid bacteria and biogenic amine in biologically aged wines. *Food Microbiology*, 25, 875-881.

[93] Alberto, M.R., Arena, M.E. and Manca De Nadra, M.C. (2002). A comparative survey of two analytical methods for identification and quantification of biogenic amines. *Food Control,* 13, 125-129.

[94] Bauza, T., Blaise, A., Daumas, F. and Cabanis, J.C. (1995). Determination of biogenic amines and their precursor amino acids in wines of the Vallée du Rhône by high-performance liquid chromatography with precolumn derivatisation and fluorimetric detection. *Journal of Chromatography A*, 707, 373-379.

[95] Cooper, R.A. (1997). On the amine oxidases of *Klebsiella aerogenes* strain W70. *FEMS Microbioloy Letters*, 146, 85-89.

[96] Chou, C.H. and Bejdanes, L.F. (1981). Effect of diamines, polyamines and tuna fish extracts on the binding of histamine to mucin in vitro. *Journal of Food Science,* 47, 79.

[97] Taylor, S.L. (1986). Histamine food poisoning: Toxicology and clinical aspects. *Critical Review in Toxicology,* 17, 91-128.

[98] Bauza, T. and Teissedre, P.L. (1995). Les amines biogénes du vin. Métabolism et toxicité. *Bulletin de l'Office International du Vin*, 68, 42-67.

[99] Seiler, N. (1992). *The role of polyamines in cell biology*. In: Chemistry of the Living Cell; Bittar, E.E., Ed.: JAI Press: Greenwich, CT.

[100] Bardócz, S., Grant, G., Brown, D.S., Ralph, A. and Pusztai, A. (1993). Polyamines in food-implications for growth and health. J*ournal of Nutritional Biochemistry*, 4, 66-71.

[101] Smith, TK., Mogridge, J.L. and Graça Sousadias, M. (1996). Growth-promoting potenzial and toxicity of spermidine, a polyamine and biogenic amine found in foods and feedstuffs. *Journal of Agriculture and Food Chemistry*, 44, 518-521.

[102] Lovaas, E. (1991). Antioxidative effects of polyamines. *Journal of the American Oil Chemists' Society*, 68, 353- 358.

[103] Palamand, S.R., Hardwick, W.A. and Marki, K.S. (1969). Volatile amines in beer and their influence on beer flavour. *Proceedings of the American Society of Brewing Chemists*, 54-58.

[104] Henschke, P.A. and Jiranek, V. (1993). *Yeast-metabolism of nitrogen compounds*. In: Fleet, G.H. (ed). Wine microbiology and biotechnology. Chur, Switzerland: Harwood Academy Press, pp. 289-326.

[105] Liu, S., Pritchard, G.G., Hardman, M.J. and Pilone, G.J. (1995). Occurrence of arginine deiminase pathway in arginine catabolism by wine lactic acid bacteria. *Applied and Environmental Microbiology*, 61(1), 310-316.

[106] Terrade, N. and Mira de Orduna, R. (2006). Impact of winemaking practices on arginine and citrulline metabolism during and after malolactic fermentation. *Journal of Applied Microbiology*, 101, 406-411.

[107] Galgano, F., Caruso, M., Favati, F. and Romano, P. (2003). HPLC determination of agmatine and other amines in wine. *International Journal of Vine and Wine Sciences*, 37, 237-242.

[108] Darvey, I.G. (1998). Is free ethanolamine required as a catalist for the *de novo* biosynthesis of phosphatidylethanolamine and ethanolamine in mammals? *Biochemical Education*, 26, 24-26.

[109] Maeba, R., Sawada, Y., Shimasaki, H., Takahashi, I. and Ueta, N. (2002). Ethanolamine plasmalogens protect cholesterol-rich liposomal membranes from oxidation caused by free radicals. *Chemistry and Physics of Lipids*, 120, 145-151.

[110] Ferreira, I.M.P.L.V.O. and Pinho, O. (2006). Biogenic amines in Portuguese traditional foods and wine. *Journal of Food Protection*, 69, 2293-2303.

[111] Martín-Álvarez, P.J., Marcobal, A., Polo, C. and Moreno-Arribas, M.V. (2006). Influence of technological practices on biogenic amine contents in red wines. *European Food Research and Technology*, 220, 420-424.

[112] Jansen, S.C., van Dusseldorp, M., Bottema, K.C. and Dubois A.E. (2003). Intolerance to dietary biogenic amines. A review. *Annals of Allergy, Asthma, and Immunology*, 91, 233-240.

[113] Kanny, G., Gerbaux, V., Olszewski, A., Frémont S., Empereue F., Nabet F., Cabanis, J.C. and Moneret-Vautrin D.A. (2001). No correlation between wine intolerance and histamine content of wine. *Journal of Allergy and Clinical Immunology*, 107, 375-378.

[114] Bertoldi, D., Larcher, R. and Nicolini, G. (2004). Content of some free amines in grapes from Trentino. *Industrie delle bevande*, 33, 437-441.

[115] Brodequis, M., Dumery, B. and Bouard, J. (1989). Mise en évidence de polyamines putrescine, cadavérine, nor- spermidine et spermine dans les feuilles et les grapes de *V. vinifera. Connaissance de La Vigne et du Vin*, 23, 1-6.

[116] Feuillat, M. (1998). Les acides amines du mout de raisin et du vin. In: *Enologie-Fondements scientifiques et technologiques*, Collection Sciences and Techniques Agroalimentaires, Technique and Documentation, Paris, pp.94-121.

[117] Hajós, G., Sass-Kiss, A., Szerdahelyi, E. and Bardócz, S. (2000). Changes in biogenic amines content in Tokai grapes, wines, and aszu-wines. *Journal of Food Science* 65, 1142-1144.

[118] Sass-Kiss, A., Szerdahelyi, E. and Hajós, G. (2000). Study of biologically active amines in grapes and wines by HPLC. *Chromatographia Supplement*, 51, 316-320.

[119] Ough, C.S. Daudt, C.E. and Crowell, E.A. (1981). Identification of new volatile amines in grapes and wines. *Journal of Agricultural and Food Chemistry*, 29, 938-941.

[120] Díaz, E.G., Santamaría, C., Gozzi, M. and Ferrari Costa, A. (2006). Biogenic amines in Argentine wines. *Toxicology Letters*, 164 S 1-S324.

[121] Zhijun, L., Yongning, W., Gong, Z., Yunfeng, Z. and Changhu, X. (2007). A survey of biogenic amines in chinese red wines. *Food Chemistry*, 105, 1530-1535.

[122] Nouadje, G., Siméon, N., Dedieu, F., Nertz, M., Puig, P. and Coudere, F. (1997). Determination of twenty eight biogenic amines and amino acids during wine aging by micellar electrokinetic chromatography and laser-induced fluorescence detection. *Journal of Chromatography A, 765*, 337-343.

[123] Loukou, Z. and Zotou, A. (2003). Determination of biogenic amines as dansyl derivates in alcoholic beverages by high- performance liquid chromatography with fluorimetric detection and characterization of the dansylated amines by liquid chromatography-atmospheric pressure chemical ionization mass spectrometry. *Journal of Chromatography* A, 996, 103-113.

[124] Proestos, C., Loukatos, P. and Komaitis, M. (2008). Determination of biogenic amines in wines by HPLC with precolumn dansylation and fluorimetric detection. *Food Chemistry*, 106, 1218-1224.

[125] Csomós, E., Héberger, K. and Simon-Sarkadi, L. (2002). Principal Component Analysis of biogenic amines and polyphenols in Hungarian wines. *Journal of Agricultural and Food Chemistry*, 50, 3768-3774.

[126] Hernández-Borges, J., D'Orazio, G., Aturki, Z. and Fanali, S. (2007). Nano-liquid chromatography analysis of dansylated biogenic amines in wines. *Journal of Chromatography A, 1147*, 192–199.

[127] Leitão, M.C., Marques, A.P. and San Romão, M.V. (2005). A survey of biogenic amines in commercial Portuguese wines. *Food Control*, 16, 199-204.

[128] Bover-Cid, S., Izquierdo-Pulido, M, Mariné-Font, A. and Vidal-Carou, M.C. (2006). Biogenic mono-, di- and polyamine contents in Spanish wines and influence of a limited irrigation. *Food Chemistry*, 96, 43-47.

[129] Gòmez-Alonso, S., Hermosin-Gutierrez, I. and Garsia-Romero, E. (2007). Simultaneous HPLC analysis of biogenic amines, amino acids, and ammonium ion as aminoenone derivatives in wine and beer samples. *Journal of Agricultural and Food Chemistry*, 55, 608-613.

[130] Vázquez-Lasa, M.B., Iñiguez-Crespo M., González-Larraina, M.A. and González-Guerrero, A. (1998). Biogenic amine in Rioja wines. *American Journal of Enology and Viticulture*, 49, 229-234.

[131] Cilliers, M.I. and Van Wyk, C.J. (1985). Histamine and tyramine content in South African wines. *South African Journal of Enology and Viticulture*, 6, 35-40.

[132] Csomós, E. and Simon-Sarkadi, L. (2002). Determination of biologically active compounds in Hungarian wines. *Periodica Polytechnica Series Chemical Engineering*, 46, 73-81.

[133] Ibe, A., Saito, K., Nakazato, M., Kikuchi Y., Fujinuma K., and Nishima, T. (1991). Quantitative determination of amines in wine by liquid chromatography. *Journal of the Association of Official Analytical Chemists*, 74, 695-698.

[134] Izquierdo-Pulido, M., Jover, T.H. and Vidal-Carou, C. (1996). Biogenic amines in European beers. *Food Chemistry*, 44, 3159-3163.

[135] Vecchio, A., Finoli, C., Cerutti G. and Moller, F. (1989). Ammine biogene in vini italiani. *Vignevini*, 16, 57-59.

[136] Soleas, G.J., Carey, M., and Goldberg, D.M. (1999). Method development and cultivar-related differences of nine biogenic amines in Ontario wines. *Food Chemistry*, 64, 49-58.

[137] Spayd, S.E., Wample, E.L., Evans, R.G., Seymour, B.J. and Nagel, C.W. (1994). Nitrogen fertilization of white Riesling grapes in Washington must and wine composition. *American Journal of Enology and Viticulture*, 45, 34-42.

[138] Vidal-Carou, M. C., Codony-Salcedo, R. and Mariné-Font A. (1990). Histamine and tyramine in Spanish wines: relationships with total sulfur dioxide level, volatile acidity and malolactic fermentation intensity. *Food Chemistry*, 35, 217–227.

[139] Pramateftaki, P.V., Metafa, M., Kallithraka, S. and. Lanaridis, P. (2006). Evolution of malolactic bacteria and biogenic amines during spontaneous malolactic fermentation in a Greek winery. *Letters in Applied Microbiology*, 43, 155-160.

[140] Bertrand, A., Ingargiola, M.C. and Delas, J. (1991). Incidence de la fumure azotée de la vigne et du greffage sur la composition des vins de merlot en particulier sur présence de carbamate d'ethyle et des amines biogènes. *Revue Francaise d'Oenologie*, 31, 7-13.

[141] Bouchereau, A., Aziz, A., Larher, F. and Martin-Tangui, J. (1999). Polyamines and environmental challenges: recent development. *Plant Science*, 140, 103-125.

[142] Eder, R., Brandes, W. and Paar, E. (2002). Einfluss von Traubenfäulnis und Schönungsmitteln auf Gehalte biogener Amine in Mästen Und Weinen. *Mitteilungen Klosterneuburg, Rebe und Wein, Obstbau und Fruchteverwertung*, 52, 204-217.

[143] Marques, A. P., Leitão, M.C. and San Romão, M.V. (2008). Biogenic amines in wines. Influence oenological factors. *Food Chemistry*, 107, 853-860.

[144] Souza, S.C., Theodoro, K.H., Souza É.R., Da Motta, S. and Abreu Glória, M.B. (2005). Bioactive amines in Brazilian wines: types, levels and correlations with physico-chemical parameters. *Brazilian Archives of Biology and Technology*, 48, 53-62.

[145] Kalkan Yildirim, H., Üren, A.L. and Yücel, U. (2007). Evaluation of biogenic amines in organic and non-organic wines by HPLC OPA derivatization. *Food Technology and Biotechnology*, 45, 62-68.

[146] Alcaide-Hidalgo, J.M., Moreno-Arribas, M.V., Martín-Alvarez, P.J. and Polo, M.C. (2007). Influence of malolactic fermentation, postfermentative treatments and aging with lees on nitrogen compounds of red wines. *Food Chemistry*, 103, 572-581.

[147] Jiménez Moreno, N. and Ancín Azpilicueta, C. (2004). Influence of wine turbidity on the accumulation of biogenic amines during aging. *Journal of the Science of Food and Agriculture*, 84, 1571-1576.

[148] Jiménez Moreno, N., Torrea Goñi, D. and Ancìn Azpilicueta, C. (2003). Changes in amine concentrations during aging of red wine in oak barrels. *Journal of Agricultural and Food Chemistry*, 51, 5732-5737.

[149] González-Marco, A. and Ancín-Azpilicueta, C. (2006). Influence of lees contact on evolution of amines in Chardonnay wine. *Journal of Food Science*, 71, 544-548

[150] Vidal-Carou, M.C., Codony-Salcedo, R. and Mariné-Font, A. (1991). Changes in the concentration of histamine and tyramine during wine spoilage at various temperature. *American Journal of Enology and Viticulture*, 42, 145-149.

[151] Gerbaux, V. and Monamy, C. (2000). Biogenic amines in Burgundy wines. Contents and origin in wines. *Revue Francaise d'Oenologie*, 183, 25-28.

[152] Pérez-Serradilla, J.A. and Luque de Castro, M.D. (2008). Role of lees in wine production: a review. *Food Chemistry,* 111, 447-456.

[153] Martínez-Rodríguez, A. and Polo, M.C (2000). Characterization of the nitrogen compounds released during yeast autolysis in a model wine system. *Journal of Agricultural and Food Chemistry*, 48, 1081-1085.

[154] Nadon, C.A., Ismond, M.A. and Holley, R. (2001). Biogenic amines in vacuum packaged and carbon dioxide-controlled atmosphere-packaged fresh pork stored at − 1.50 degrees. *Journal of Food Protection*, 64, 220-227.

[155] Rokka, M., Eerola, S., Smolander, M., Alatomi, H. and Ahvenainen, R. (2004). Monitoring of the quality of modified atmosphere packaged boiler chicken cuts stored in different temperature conditions. B. Biogenic amines as quality- indicating metabolites. *Food Control*, 15, 601-607.

[156] González-Marco, A. and Ancín-Azpilicueta, C. (2006). Amine concentrations in wine stored in bottles at different temperatures. *Food Chemistry*, 99, 680-685.

In: Red Wine and Health
Editor: Paul O'Byrne

ISBN 978-1-60692-718-2
© 2009 Nova Science Publishers, Inc.

Chapter 7

SAFETY AND HEALTHINESS ENHANCEMENT OF RED WINES BY SELECTED MICROBIAL STARTERS

A. Caridi and R. Sidari

Unit of Microbiology, Department of "Scienze e Tecnologie Agro-Forestali e Ambientali" - DiSTAfA, Faculty of Agricultural Sciences, "Mediterranea" University of Reggio Calabria, Via Feo di Vito, I-89122 Reggio Calabria, Italy.

ABSTRACT

The modern consumer is remarkably health conscious; consequently, he searches for foods and beverages having positive biological properties, such as high contents in antioxidant and anticancer substances and low content in toxic compounds. Wine safety and healthiness depend on the interaction among various factors, several of which of microbial origin. In general, the effects of these factors on wine composition and safety are studied separately. This chapter explores scientific knowledge on the microbial role in the healthiness and safety enhancement of red wines. The following could give a good reason to propose a specific selection of microbial starters: (a) production of wines with low levels of sulphur dioxide using yeasts able to inhibit malolactic fermentation; (b) production of wines with low amounts of acetaldehyde using low-producing yeasts or acetaldehyde-removing lactic acid bacteria; (c) production of wines with low amounts of methanol using low-producing yeasts; (d) production of wines with low amounts of ethyl carbamate using yeasts low-producing urea during arginine degradation or lactic acid bacteria low-producing ethyl carbamate; (e) production of wines with low amounts of biogenic amines using low-producing yeasts or lactic acid bacteria; (f) production of wines with low amounts of medium-chain fatty acids using low-producing yeasts; (g) production of wines with high healthy phenolic compounds content using yeasts producing enzymes, reactive metabolites and/or parietal mannoproteins that interact with phenolic compounds; (h) production of wines with low amounts of ochratoxin A using yeasts or lactic acid bacteria able to remove it; (i) must detoxification by selected yeasts from pesticides, fungicides, and heavy metals originating from vineyard treatments. Genomic strategies could also be used to improve the useful microbial traits.

1. INTRODUCTION

Moderate consumers of wine, above all red wine, have been observed to have a reduced risk of cardiovascular disease compared to abstainers and heavy consumers [1]. The basic difference between red and white wines is their concentration of total phenolic compounds, which is generally 1.5 times higher in red grapes than in white grapes [2]. Phenolic compounds, but not only them, play a role in the reduction of cardiovascular disease risk similarly to certain fruits, grains and vegetables, which are core components of a traditional Mediterranean diet. Today, the consumer is remarkably health conscious; consequently, he searches for foods and beverages having positive biological properties, such as high contents in antioxidant and anticancer substances and low content in toxic compounds. Wine safety and healthiness depend on the interaction among various factors, several of microbial origin. In general, the effects of these factors on wine composition and safety are studied separately. This chapter explores scientific knowledge on the microbial role in the healthiness and safety enhancement of red wines.

2. PRODUCTION OF WINES WITH LOW LEVELS OF SULPHUR DIOXIDE USING YEASTS ABLE TO INHIBIT MALOLACTIC FERMENTATION

The ability of certain yeast strains to inhibit malolactic fermentation has been most commonly reported [3-10]; it has the potential to greatly impact on wine quality. In conventional winemaking processes, sulphur dioxide (SO_2) is added to white wines to control malolactic fermentation. However, SO_2 is harmful to humans [11] and, regarding the acute toxicity, it is included in the rank "highly toxic" by the Environmental Protection Agency of the United States [12]. Consequently, several methods have been proposed to decrease SO_2 use: selection of grape, soft crushing, must clarification with bentonite or gelatine before cold decantation, control of the temperature of winemaking and storage, pasteurization or filtration of wines, innovative technologies, addition of wine stabilisers, such as lysozyme [13] and bacteriocins [14]. Malolactic fermentability of wines differs according to the strain of *Saccharomyces cerevisiae* used [15]. Really, some yeast strains produce bacterial growth factors, such as amino acids, peptides and macromolecules, while others act as bacteria growth inhibitors by producing SO_2 and medium-chain fatty acids [16]. Cold-fermenting strains of *S. cerevisiae* possess a number of advantages compared to normal strains. In brewing, they are utilised for fermentation at low temperatures (6°C) and for production of qualitatively superior beers [17]. Cold-fermenting yeasts may be used as starters in winemaking from musts lacking in acidity since they synthesize malic acid rather than decomposing it, produce more glycerol, succinic acid and β-phenylethanol and less acetic acid and ethanol [18-19]. Succinic acid [20] and β-phenylethanol [21] inhibit lactic acid bacteria growth; they are greatly produced by some cold-fermenting *S. cerevisiae*. Wines produced by cold-fermenting strains of *S. cerevisiae* are less subjected to malolactic fermentation compared to those produced by normal strains. This system of microbiological stabilization of wine allows the reduction of SO_2 thus offering considerable advantages for consumer's health. Consequently, in order to stabilise wines with low levels of SO_2, the use of cold-fermenting *Saccharomyces* starters has been proposed [22]. Indeed, the wines so produced exhibit enhanced chemical and microbiological stability, and this contributes to a long-term maintenance of acidic freshness and to a notable limitation of ageing [23].

In addition, inhibition of lactic acid bacteria has also been considered to result from the depletion of nutrients by fermenting yeast [4,24]. After completion of alcoholic fermentation, it has been suspected that wine may be lacking nutrients, such as vitamins or amino acids that are essential for lactic acid bacteria. In support, it has been showed that during pure culture in a synthetic medium, yeast depleted certain amino acids, including arginine, to concentrations that may not have been sufficient for lactic acid bacteria growth [24]. Furthermore, there is a lack of information concerning the depletion by yeast of specific nutrients required by lactic acid bacteria.

3. PRODUCTION OF WINES WITH LOW AMOUNTS OF ACETALDEHYDE USING LOW-PRODUCING YEASTS OR ACETALDEHYDE-REMOVING LACTIC ACID BACTERIA

Acetaldehyde is one of the most important carbonyl compounds, originates from yeasts during alcoholic fermentation [25] or by ethanol oxidation [26-27]. It plays a role in colour development of red wines [28-29] and gives important sensory characteristics to wine since it is highly volatile [30]. With some exceptions, such as sherry type wines [31], acetaldehyde is considered undesirable at high concentrations; in fact, when present in excess it confers a green, grassy, apple-like aroma to wines [32]. Part of SO_2 bound to acetaldehyde tends to reduce the perception of the off spring flavour [33]; as consequence, it is required more SO_2, but this is a concern for health reasons.

Acetaldehyde has toxicological relevance and may cause mutagenesis and carcinogenesis [34] because it is able to react with amino groups of proteins, giving acetaldehyde-protein adducts [35-36]. It can also interact with DNA bases [37] producing a variety of adducts [38-39], prevalently N_2-ethyl-deoxyguanosine [40]. Consequently, it has been proposed as a carcinogenic agent behind ethanol-related oral cancers [41]. In addition, acetaldehyde can induce DNA base tandem mutations [42] that may be consequence of intra-strand crosslinks. Coexposure to ethanol and acetaldehyde contributes to cancers of the digestive tract [43]. Acetaldehyde is included in the following carcinogen lists: 1) International Agency for Research on Cancer, group 2b - possible carcinogen; 2) National Toxicology Program of the United States, reasonably anticipated to be a carcinogen; 3) State of California, proposition of 65 carcinogen list; 4) Environmental Protection Agency of the United States, Office of Pesticide Programs, category B2: probable human carcinogen with sufficient evidence of carcinogenicity from animal studies with inadequate or no data from epidemiologic studies in humans [44].

Freshly made wines usually have acetaldehyde concentrations below 75 mg/L [32], although wide ranges of values have been reported [45-47]. The initial values usually decline over time since acetaldehyde combines with polyphenols and other compounds in wine [48]. It has been found that the production of acetaldehyde during must fermentation depends on both grape cultivar and aromatic precursors in the must and technological factors such as pH, fermentation temperature, aeration and SO_2 concentration, and on the yeast strain involved

[49-50,46,51-52]. Generally, red wines show greater acetaldehyde concentration than white wines [52].

Some authors have reported that wines produced by spontaneous fermentations exhibit amount of acetaldehyde higher than those produced using selected yeasts [53,52].

In order to reduce acetaldehyde formation, so increasing wine safety, it is useful to control winemaking using specifically selected yeast strains [54-56]. Great variation in acetaldehyde production has been observed among different selected yeast strains; the acetaldehyde amount can range from 60 mg/L to more than 100 mg/L. However, acetaldehyde content can also vary according to must composition and fermentation conditions [52].

The use of immobilized yeast cells to carry out winemaking determines the production of wines with low amounts of acetaldehyde [57-59].

Lactic acid bacteria can decrease acetaldehyde content in wines during malolactic fermentation [29]. The genera *Lactobacillus* and *Oenococcus* are able to degrade SO_2-bound acetaldehyde slower than free acetaldehyde. This is probably attributable to the antimicrobial effect of the SO_2 released from SO_2-bound acetaldehyde [60-61]. It appears possible to decrease or even avoid acetaldehyde formation in wine by carrying out simultaneous alcoholic and malolactic fermentation [62]. Therefore, wines so produced could exhibit an enhanced safety due to the very low levels of acetaldehyde.

4. PRODUCTION OF WINES WITH LOW AMOUNTS OF METHANOL USING LOW-PRODUCING YEASTS

Methyl alcohol is produced in wine by pectinolytic enzymes splitting the methoxyl group from pectin present in crushed fruits such as grapes [63-65]. The International Office of Vine and Wine has proposed the limit of 150 mg of methanol/L for white and rose wines and of 300 mg/L for red wines [66]. It has been reported that red wines contain higher methanol levels than roses, while white wines contain even less [67]. In some cases, the methanol amount in wines was higher than the maximum limits indicated by International Office of Vine and Wine [68-69], in others, on the contrary, it was less than the maximum limits [70].

It is well known that methyl alcohol is a toxic and harmful substance to human health (when taken orally at 340 mg/kg of body weight) of whose ingestion or inhalation can cause blindness or death by lactic acidosis [71].

Methanol formation in wines depends on various factors, such as grape variety and quality, maceration treatment [72], fermentation temperature [73], and pectolytic enzymes used to facilitate must extraction or clarification [74-78]. Enzyme treatments can determine an increase in wine methanol content, even if other factors, among which the yeast strains used, can influence methanol production [79]. For example, it has been reported that the addition of gallic acid or coumaric acid during winemaking is a possible way to reduce methanol content in wines [80].

Different studies have reported that immobilized yeast cells produce wines with low amount of methanol improving, therefore, wine safety [73,57-59]. The presence of pectin methylesterase activity has been described also in *S. cerevisiae* [81-85]. It has been reported an inconsistent occurrence of the *PGU1* gene, encoding for endopolygalacturonase activity, in different strains of *Saccharomyces*, suggesting that this gene is not typical of *S. cerevisiae* [86]. Therefore, to produce wine exhibiting an enhanced safety, due to a very low methanol content, it is useful employing selected yeasts for none or low production of methanol because of lack of genes involved in pectinolytic enzymes expression and/or different levels of pectinolytic enzyme activity.

5. PRODUCTION OF WINES WITH LOW AMOUNTS OF ETHYL CARBAMATE USING YEASTS LOW-PRODUCING UREA DURING ARGININE DEGRADATION OR LACTIC ACID BACTERIA LOW-PRODUCING ETHYL CARBAMATE

Ethyl carbamate, also referred to urethane, can appears - due to the acidic pH of wine - by reaction of ethanol with the urea produced by yeasts when metabolise arginine, a major α-amino acid in grape juice [87-89], citrulline or carbamyl phosphate, both produced from arginine by lactic acid bacteria [90-91].

It is well known that ethyl carbamate is an animal carcinogen [92] found in fermented foods and beverages including wine [93-94]. Average amounts of ethyl carbamate found in wine are considered to increase the daily intake of this carcinogen significantly [95].

Diammonium phosphate has a regulatory effect on wine yeasts for ethyl carbamate production; consequently, it may be suitable to prevent the yeast utilisation of arginine and the subsequent formation of ethyl carbamate in wine [96].

Lactic acid bacteria can degrade arginine via arginine deaminase pathway; however, several strains do not degrade it completely and produce citrulline or carbamyl phosphate [97-98]; these compounds can later react with ethanol, yielding ethyl carbamate. The potential capacity for ethyl carbamate production and its precursors during malolactic fermentation has been investigated in different lactic acid bacteria showing that the strain *Lactobacillus hilgardii X1B* can use arginine via the arginine deaminase pathway; therefore, attention must be paid in the selection of lactic acid bacteria for malolactic fermentation [99]. Different concentrations of ethyl carbamate have been found in wines; in particular, red wines exhibit higher concentration than white wines. This variability depends on grape variety, nitrogen content of grape must, winemaking conditions and yeast strain used [100]. Excessive addition of inorganic nitrogen, to improve fermentative performance, often results in residual nitrogen that lead to microbial instability and ethyl carbamate accumulation in wine [101-103]. Moreover, the wine content in ethyl carbamate increases at high temperatures and for grape varieties containing high levels of arginine. It has been found that a high temperature during wine storage and transport [98] as well as the presence of lees during malolactic fermentation can give higher levels of this compound [88].

S. cerevisiae strains widely vary for the urea-forming ability [104] by arginine breakdown due to *CAR1*-encoded arginase. Therefore, certain yeast strains secrete urea into wine and may be unable to metabolise also the external urea [105].

It has been described the influence of ethanol and low pH on the ability of lactic acid bacteria strain to metabolise arginine and citrulline [106]. A close relationship between ethyl carbamate, ethyl lactate, and volatile acidity levels has been observed; aged wines are more likely to have significant levels of ethyl carbamate than young wines, in which the only precursor of ethyl carbamate appears to be the urea coming from yeast arginine metabolism [107].

To meet the consumer health concerns and the demand for ethyl carbamate-free wines, it may be possible to select strains of yeast and bacteria no producing or producing only traces of ethyl carbamate or its precursors [108]. Moreover, should be carried out malolactic bacteria selection for their ability to degrade arginine. In general, arginine degradation starts after the beginning or at the end of L-malic acid degradation. This has oenological importance, since it allows the winemaker to avoid arginine degradation removing cells or inhibiting cell activity after completion of L-malic acid degradation in wine. However, potential formation of ethyl carbamate is greater to higher wine pHs, condition that favours lactic acid bacteria growth and accelerates its metabolism. Another practicable way is to select lactic acid bacteria able to excrete citrulline from arginine degradation; the excreted citrulline could be reutilised by the same strain after depletion of arginine [90] or by other lactic acid bacteria becoming, thus, unavailable for formation of ethyl carbamate. Similarly, degradation of citrulline itself is an important lactic acid bacteria trait to select. It has been observed that some strains of *L. plantarum* are able to degrade arginine; also, some strains of *O. oeni* are able to degrade arginine and to excrete considerable amounts of citrulline when the malolactic fermentation occurs [104]. A great variability has been found in the ability of degrading arginine by different strains of *O. oeni*; most of the assayed heterofermentative lactobacilli are able to totally or partially degrade arginine, while the homofermentative strains did not. On the other hand, some *Pediococcus* are able to degrade arginine. Another criterion for selecting lactic acid bacteria strains is the high carbamate chinase activity to reduce the accumulation of citrulline or carbamyl phosphate [98].

6. PRODUCTION OF WINES WITH LOW AMOUNTS OF BIOGENIC AMINES USING LOW-PRODUCING YEASTS OR LACTIC ACID BACTERIA

Biogenic amines are organic bases mainly derived from amino acids decarboxylation often found in food and beverages. After uptake, they can cause allergy-like reactions in sensitive people and the undesirable physiological effects, such as headache, urticaria, rhinitis, respiratory and digestive problems, arise especially in presence of alcohol and acetaldehyde [109-113].

Biogenic amines have been found in musts and wines as documented in the literature [114-115]; the main of them in wine are histamine, tyramine, putrescine, cadaverine, and phenylethylamine [116-117]. Their production is influenced both by pedoclimatic characteristics and by winemaking conditions such as the presence of precursor amino acids, length of skin maceration, the contact between wine and yeast lees, the presence of microbial nutrients, wine pH and ethanol levels, growth of wild bacteria and yeasts [118,111,119-120]. Moreover, white wines, which show generally more acidic pH, contain lower biogenic amine amounts than red wines [121].

At present, the biogenic amine toxicological role in wine has not been established since the toxic threshold is difficult to determine. Although there are no biogenic amine limits established by regulations, it is advisable to prevent high biogenic amine levels and maintain them within recommended range whose upper limit for histamine is 2 mg/L in Germany, 5-9 mg/L in Belgium, 8 mg/L in France and 10 mg/L in Switzerland [116].

Although lactic acid bacteria responsible of malolactic fermentation are widely accepted as the main causative agents of amines formation, some studies referred that also wine yeast species are responsible for biogenic amine production [122-123]. In numerous wines, the biogenic amine concentration is low after alcoholic fermentation, and tends to increase during malolactic fermentation to a very variable extent [114].

Several lactic acid bacteria belonging to the *Lactobacillus*, *Leuconostoc*, and *Pediococcus* genera are proved capable of histamine formation [117] as well as *Pediococcus* strains are usually considered among the major ones responsible for histamine accumulation in wine [124]. Some authors demonstrated that also *O. oeni*, bacterial species commonly found in wines and associated with malolactic fermentation, might play a role in the production of histamine in wine [125-126]; another author reported that the ability of *O. oeni* to produce histamine is not a consistent characteristic of this species, and it seems to be strain-dependent [127]. It has been also studied the role of an *O. oeni* strain in putrescine production [128-129]. Putrescine content in wines aged with lees increases during ageing while it remains stable in those aged without lees [129]. Anyway, the values found are lower than the values reported for French [114] and Spanish wines [130].

It has been found that no spontaneous yeast species produce histamine, the main toxic amine, but produce other amines such as methylamine and agmatine, which can increase the toxic effect of histamine [111] by a mechanism of competition with amine oxidase enzymes. In particular, *Brettanomyces bruxellensis* strains produce phenylethylamine, *Metschnikowia pulcherrima* and *Kloeckera apiculata* produces, with a great strain variability, agmatine and phenylethylamine. *M. pulcherrima* also exhibited the ability to produce putrescine, while *Candida stellata* strains produces cadaverine. It has been reported that the ability of *S. cerevisiae* to produce biogenic amines is not a constant characteristic of this species, but it seems to be strain dependent.

In order to contribute to the safeguarding of consumer health, it is necessary to guide the fermentative processes - alcoholic and malolactic - and to eliminate or to minimise the activity of yeast spoilage strains. Alternative technologies include the use of *Schizosaccharomyces pombe* [131], high-density cell suspensions of yeasts [132], and immobilization of *O. oeni* and *Lactobacillus* species [133]. Moreover, considering the bacterial variability in decarboxylation capacity [134] and the high variability found among *S. cerevisiae* strains, it is possible to carry out different selection protocols with the aim to select: 1) strains of lactic acid bacteria that do not possess the decarboxylase genes [123] and may inhibit growth and activity of the endogenous decarboxylase-positive bacteria; 2) strains of *O. oeni* unable to produce biogenic amines [135]; 3) lactic acid bacteria species able to degrade amines by amino oxidases and strains of *S. cerevisiae* possessing little or no ability to produce amines [122].

7. PRODUCTION OF WINES WITH LOW AMOUNTS OF MEDIUM-CHAIN FATTY ACIDS USING LOW-PRODUCING YEASTS

Medium-chain fatty acids, such as hexanoic, octanoic, and decanoic acid, can inhibit both yeast and lactic acid bacteria, and their formation has been suggested to cause yeast-bacteria antagonism [136-138,16]. Yeast cells in the absence of oxygen always produce medium-chain fatty acid [139-141], while in aerobic or semi-aerobic conditions it has been observed a low production of medium-chain fatty acids and a high production of unsaturated fatty acids [142]. The medium-chain fatty acids are produced in different amounts during winemaking by the different strains of *S. cerevisiae* [143,137,141,144]. They have been associated to stuck and sluggish fermentation [145] because these fermentation by-products are toxic for yeast [146] since they act either as uncouplers [147] or as weak acid preservatives [148]. The toxicity of medium-chain fatty acids for yeasts increases as the ethanol concentration increases [149-150].

It is well known that hexanoic and octanoic acids are toxic for flies [151]. Regarding the acute toxicity, hexanoic acid is also included in the rank "not acutely toxic to moderately toxic" by the National Toxicology Program of the United States [152].

In order to reduce the amount of medium-chain fatty acid in wine it has been investigated the role of yeast lees. Effectively, parietal yeast mannoproteins have been associated with stimulation of malolactic bacteria growth in wine [153]. This could be due to the adsorption of the medium-chain fatty acids synthesised by *Saccharomyces* [154]. These compounds have been shown to inhibit bacterial growth and, therefore, their removal improves malolactic fermentation. Some authors reported that yeast lees could both determine a removal of the hexanoic, octanoic, and decanoic acids [155] by physical adsorption and act as oxygen substitutes, allowing the production of sterol and unsaturated fatty acid in yeast cell membrane [156]. The content of medium-chain fatty acid is dependent on the strain used in the fermentation, so this could be an important criterion when selecting yeast for oenological purposes [157].

8. PRODUCTION OF WINES WITH HIGH HEALTHY PHENOLIC COMPOUNDS CONTENT USING YEASTS PRODUCING ENZYMES, REACTIVE METABOLITES AND/OR PARIETAL MANNOPROTEINS THAT INTERACT WITH PHENOLIC COMPOUNDS

Many studies have been carried out to demonstrate the effects of yeast selection on the phenolic compounds of wines [158-162]. It has been shown that wine yeast influences concentration and composition of phenolic compounds in wine, since yeasts usually decrease the phenolic compounds [163]. Remarkable correlations between the yeast strain used for winemaking and phenolic compounds in wine have been reported, demonstrating that strain behaviour can somewhat modify chromatic properties, phenolic profile and antioxidant power of wine [160]. It is interesting to note that the interaction between grape cultivar and yeast is close and important, because grape variety, due to its phenolic composition, modulates yeast strain activity [164]. Wine yeasts affect the phenolic compounds in wine by the following different ways.

1) Yeast can interact with phenolic compounds in wines producing anthocyanin-β-D-glucosidase [165-167]. The use of a wine yeast strain with high β-glucosidase activity produces wine with a comparatively higher concentration of resveratrol than would conventional wine yeasts [168].

2) Yeast can interact with phenolic compounds in wines producing pyruvic acid [169-171], and acetaldehyde [172,27,170,173,171]. Acetaldehyde plays a role in colour development of red wines by polymerization between anthocyanins and catechins or tannins, forming stable polymeric pigments resistant to SO_2 bleaching [28-29]. Large amount of acetaldehyde, together with pyruvic acid, produced by selecting yeasts increase the formation of vitisins, which stabilise wine colour [170-171]. In fact, acetaldehyde and pyruvic acid accelerate polymerization reactions between anthocyanins and phenolics, or between phenolics, leading to different condensation products. Interaction between phenolics and pyruvic acid stabilises the phenolic compounds during aging of the wines [1].

3) Yeast can interact with phenolic compounds in wines producing and/or releasing mannoproteins and different polysaccharides [174-175,158,176-177]. The parietal adsorption of phenolic compounds responsible for wine colour [178-180,31] has important consequences for wine, because of the amount of pigment removed during winemaking [181-183]. In fact, there is a great diversity from yeast to yeast in the parietal adsorption activity [163,184-187,175,188-191]. Different studies have shown that anthocyanin adsorption increases with their esterification and methoxylation degree, suggesting that a hydrophobic interaction is involved in the adsorption mechanism [192-194]. Phenolic compounds interact with yeast mannoproteins that can be released in wine or retained on cell walls; the amount of mannoproteins released during winemaking depends on yeast strain and grape must [158]. To enhance the release of yeast mannoproteins, in some winemaking procedures wine is aged on lees with the addition of β-1,3 glucanase [177]. Mannoproteins can diminish the total polyphenol index of wine by weak and reversible interactions, mainly between anthocyanins and cell walls [195,179].

Wine yeast affects concentration and composition of phenolic compounds of red wines, so modifying also wine healthiness. Strategies can be employed to enhance a specific phenolic compound via choice of yeast strain producing different mannoproteins. It is useful to consider that also lactic acid bacteria could degrade anthocyanins when viable [196].

9. PRODUCTION OF WINES WITH LOW AMOUNTS OF OCHRATOXIN A USING YEASTS OR LACTIC ACID BACTERIA ABLE TO REMOVE IT

Ochratoxin A is a secondary metabolite of some species of storage fungi: *Aspergillus* species such as *A. ochraceus* produce ochratoxin A mainly in tropical climates and

Penicillium species such as *P. verrucosum* produce it in temperate climates [197]. Ochratoxin A is a strong nephrotoxic, carcinogenic, immunotoxic and teratogenic mycotoxin that can contaminate various foods and beverages, including wines [198-199]. Ochratoxin A is considered by the International Agency for Research on Cancer a possible human carcinogen (group 2B) based on sufficient evidence of carcinogenicity in experimental animals [200]. Various procedures have been developed to remove mycotoxins using yeasts [201-214], yeast cell walls [215-218], or yeast cell wall extracts [204,220,206,218]. Yeast mannoproteins play an important role in the ochratoxin A removal process, due to mycotoxin-binding capacity demonstrated for modified mannanoligosaccharide derived from the cell wall of *S. cerevisiae* [204]. Indeed, ochratoxin A removal depends on yeast macromolecules, such as mannoproteins [202], and corresponds to a spontaneous [218] adsorption mechanism [207] where mannoproteins act like a sponge, removing ochratoxin A. The toxin content of wines is greatly reduced by expressly selected yeasts. Remarkable differences among wine yeasts - both *Saccharomyces* [221] and non-*Saccharomyces* [222] - have been reported in the ochratoxin A sequestering activity during winemaking. This may depend on the different mannosylphosphate content in the mannoproteins of wine yeasts [223-224], but also on dissimilar fermentation and cell sedimentation dynamics, cell dimension, and flocculence. Hence, yeast strains that display enhanced binding of ochratoxin A may be selected for fermentation or added at some stage as a preparation of dead cells.

The action of lactic acid bacteria on ochratoxin A during malolactic fermentation varies according to strain; ochratoxin A appears to be removed by adsorption [225-226].

Much toxin can be removed during winemaking, and selected yeast strains and lactic acid bacteria may confer additional decreases in toxin concentration [227].

10. MUST DETOXIFICATION BY SELECTED YEASTS FROM PESTICIDES, FUNGICIDES AND HEAVY METALS ORIGINATING FROM VINEYARD TREATMENTS

The wide spread contamination of pesticide and fungicide residues in food is due to their extensive applications in agriculture. Because of their chemical nature, they may also be toxic [228-229] and non-biodegradable. Chemical residues can build up in the soil [230] and throughout the food chain [231]. Consumers worldwide are increasingly conscious of the potential environmental and health problems [232-234] associated with the build-up of toxic chemicals, also in must and wine [235]. Anyway, the impact of pesticide residues is still poorly understood; frequently it depends on the group the pesticide belongs to [236].

Many research workers have studied the dissipation of pesticides by yeast during must fermentation [237-243]. The presence of pesticide and fungicide residues in grape must showed negative effects over several yeasts (*Saccharomyces* and non-*Saccharomyces*) usually present in the fermentation process; the most described effect is a delay in the fermentation start. Each country has its own allowed maximal residue levels that reflect the agricultural practice followed, but fungicides employment should be controlled because of its toxicity effects [244].

The detoxification of wines from heavy metals, e.g. copper, originating from vineyard treatments is another interesting field of research [245-247]. Although copper is an essential element for all known living organisms, including humans and other animals, being a cofactor in numerous enzymatic processes, abnormally high levels of copper can be toxic to living cells [248-249].

Nowadays agricultural techniques for integrated pest management or biological production include the wide use of copper for chemical protection of plants. The increasing use of copper formulates in biological vineyards can be responsible, in some cases, of slow or stock fermentations. High concentrations of free copper ions in wine can be responsible for cellular alterations, because they can be rather dangerous, being involved in many undesirable reactions that would lead to the irreversible destruction of cellular components [250]. It is well known, in fact, that low amounts of copper play a key role on microbial activities, whereas elevated concentrations can be toxic to yeasts, affecting cell growth or causing the acquisition of tolerance to the metal. The copper resistance of wine strains of *S. cerevisiae* has been described as a potential discriminating strain characteristic [251]. Strain resistance, however, does not always result in an elevated accumulation of metals [252]. Repeated culture of a *S. cerevisiae* copper-resistant strain, grown in presence of elevated levels of copper and other metals, resulted in increased resistance, but in a decreased accumulation of the metals inside the cells [253,251]. Other authors showed that cells of *S. cerevisiae* strains that are resistant to Mn++ exhibited increased uptake of the metal [254] and studies on cadmium-tolerant cultures of yeast revealed a great increased proportion of cadmium bound in the cytosol [255].

11. GENOMIC STRATEGIES

Features such as fermentation performance, down-stream processing, alcohol content, and levels of desirable or undesirable chemical compounds are all dependant upon the yeast strain used [256]. Beside classical strategies to improve wine yeasts, alternative ways are to exploit yeast natural genetic diversity or even to genetically manipulate yeast strains in order to improve specific properties [257-258]. In developing wine yeast strains, it is therefore of the utmost importance to focus on health aspects and to develop yeasts that may reduce the risks and enhance the benefits with the goal to eliminate toxic and carcinogenic compounds eventually presents in wines.

The following are examples of modified microorganisms that could be used to improve wine healthiness and safety.

Regarding ethyl carbamate, a target for yeast improvement is to select or develop starter strains that are more nitrogen efficient for use in low nitrogen musts; therefore, a mutant containing an *ure2* recessive allele, which allows a more efficient proline utilising, has been constructed [259,101-103]. To reduce the formation of amino acid metabolism, it is possible the deletion of *car1* (arginase) or expression of *ure1* ethyl carbamate urea formation [257]. In a strain disrupted for the *car1* gene (encoding arginase) no urea or ethyl carbamate has been produced [260-262]. Another possibility is to express an acidic urease that degrades urea into ammonia and carbon dioxide in yeast [263]. Recently has been created a strain of *S. cerevisiae* with increases expression of urea amidolyase. This enzyme catalyses the hydrolysis of urea produced by *S. cerevisiae* during alcoholic fermentation. Since urea is a precursor of ethyl carbamate, the activity of urea amidolyase significantly reduces the potential for formation and accumulation of ethyl carbamate in the wine. The urease, from *Lactobacillus fermentum*, has successfully been expressed in *S. cerevisiae* [264].

Regarding biogenic amines production, a solution could be wine strains able to inhibit bacterial growth. The focus in wine research is on the development of wine yeasts that secrete bacteriocins or bacteriolytic enzymes to suppress growth of unwanted bacteria. In particular, the lysozyme gene (*hel1*), the *Pediococcus acidilactici* pediocin gene (*ped1*), the *Leuconostoc carnosum* leucocin gene (*lca1*) and the *Lactobacillus plantarum* plantaricin gene have been used to engineer bactericidal yeasts. These yeasts by secretion of lysozyme or bacteriocins are able to kill sensitive bacteria. Additional alternative is the expression of the *Aspergillus niger gox1* gene in yeasts that results in the production of hydrogen peroxide, which can lead to oxidation toxicity of bacteria. Moreover, the use of engineered wine yeasts that are capable of conducting malolactic fermentation should also circumvent the use of bacteria, which could be responsible of biogenic amines production [262]. In order to prevent the biogenic amines formation by lactic acid bacteria, a genetically stable industrial strain of *S. cerevisiae* has been created. A linear cassette containing the *S. pombe* malate permease gene (*mae1*) and the *O. oeni* malolactic gene (*mleA*) has been integrated, under control of the *S. cerevisiae pgk1* promoter and terminator sequences, into the *ura3* locus of an industrial wine yeast [265].

By inserting the gene that encodes the substrate 3 malonyl-CoA and the grapevine resveratrol synthase gene into conventional wine yeast, thus introducing the phenylpropanoid pathway into the yeast, the transformed yeast is able to synthesise resveratrol [266].

Although the huge range of possibilities offer by genetic engineering, a variety of factors, scientific, technical, economic, marketing, safety, legal and ethical issues has prevented the use of genetically improved yeasts on a commercial scale [262]. Therefore, a future introduction of genetically modified wine yeast requires, in agreement with current legislation, a detailed safety and environmental impact evaluation.

12. CONCLUSION

As a final point, scientific research in the last years has proposed a lot of way to enhance safety and healthiness of red wine by selected microbial starters but, probably, this is not the most important case. Perhaps it is more urgent to perform educating consumers about the benefits of regular and moderate red wine consumption, better if safety and healthiness enhanced.

13. REFERENCES

[1] Stockley, C. S. & Høj, P. B. (2005). Better wine for better health: fact or fiction? *Australian Journal of Grape and Wine Research, 11,* 127-138.
[2] Singleton, V. L. (1982). Grape and wine phenolics: background and prospects. In U. C. Davis, & V. L. Singleton (Eds.), *Proceedings of Symposium: Grape and wine centennial* (pp. 215-227). California, USA: University of California Press.
[3] Ribéreau-Gayon, J. & Peynaud, E. (1961). *Traité d'Oenologie* (II). Zwickau, Germany: Polytechnic Library Béranger.

[4] Fornachon, J. C. M. (1968). Influence of different yeasts on the growth of lactic acid bacteria in wine. *Journal of the Science of Food and Agriculture, 19*, 374-378.
[5] Boidron, A. M. (1969). Etude de l'antagonisme entre les levures et les bactéries du vin. *Connaissance de la Vigne et du Vin, 3*, 315-378.
[6] Lafon-Lafourcade, S. (1973). De la fermentescibilité malolactique des vins: interaction levures-bactéries. *Connaissance de la Vigne et du Vin, 7*, 203-207.
[7] Mayer, K. (1978). Progrès récents dans la connaissance des phénomènes microbiologiques en vinification. *Bulletin de l'Office International du Vin, 51*, 269-280.
[8] Lemaresquier, H. (1987). Inter-relationships between strains of *Saccharomyces cerevisiae* from the Champagne area and lactic acid bacteria. *Letters in Applied Microbiology, 4*, 91-94.
[9] Wibowo, D., Fleet, G. H., Lee, T. H. & Eschenbruch, R. E. (1988). Factors affecting the induction of malolactic fermentation in red wines with *Leuconostoc oenos*. *Journal of Applied Bacteriology, 64*, 421-428.
[10] Gilis, J.-F., Delia-Dupuy, M.-L. & Strehaiano, P. (1996). Etude qualitative et quantitative des interactions entre *Saccharomyces cerevisiae* et *Leuconostoc oenos*. *Journal International des Sciences de la Vigne et du Vin, 3*, 151-157.
[11] Yang, W. H. & Purchase, E. C. (1985). Adverse reactions to sulfites. *Canadian Medical Association Journal, 133*, 865-867.
[12] http://www.pesticideinfo.org/Detail_Chemical.jsp?Rec_Id=PC34503.
[13] Dell'Acqua, E. (1996). Lysozyme for improved wine quality control. *Trends in Food Science & Technology, 7*, 241.
[14] Dick, K. J., Molan, P. C. & Eschenbruch, R. (1992). The isolation from *Saccharomyces cerevisiae* of two antibacterial cationic proteins that inhibit malolactic bacteria. *Vitis, 31*, 105-116.
[15] Lafon-Lafourcade, S., Lonvaud-Funel, A. & Carre, E. (1983). Lactic acid bacteria of wines: stimulation of growth and malolactic fermentation. *Antonie van Leeuwenhoek, 49*, 349-352.
[16] Alexandre, H., Costello, P. J., Remize, F., Guzzo, J. & Guilloux-Benatier, M. (2004). *Saccharomyces cerevisiae-Oenococcus oeni* interactions in wine: current knowledge and perspectives. *International Journal of Food Microbiology, 93*, 141-154.
[17] Zambonelli, C., Giudici, P., Tini, V., Grazia, L., Caridi, A. & Castellari, L. (1994). Lieviti selezionati per la modifica della composizione di base dei vini. *Vignevini, 21*, 25-28.
[18] Castellari, L., Ferruzzi, M., Magrini, A., Giudici, P., Passarelli, P. & Zambonelli, C. (1994). Unbalanced wine fermentation by cryotolerant vs. non-cryotolerant *Saccharomyces* strains. *Vitis, 33*, 49-52.
[19] Bertolini, L., Zambonelli, C., Giudici, P. & Castellari, L. (1996). Higher alcohol production by cryotolerant *Saccharomyces* strains. *American Journal of Enology and Viticulture, 47*, 343-345.
[20] Amorim, H. V. (1996). An ecological reason for succinic acid formation by yeast. In *Anais XI SINAFERM, Simpósio Nacional de Fermentação* (II, pp. 724-729). São Carlos, Brazil.
[21] Guerzoni, M. E. & Gardini, F. (1988). Interazione tra lieviti e batteri lattici nella conversione dell'acido malico nei vini. *Industrie delle Bevande, 17*, 239-245.

[22] Caridi, A. & Corte, V. (1997). Inhibition of malolactic fermentation by cryotolerant yeasts. *Biotechnology Letters, 19,* 723-726.
[23] Caridi, A., Corte, V. & Zambonelli, C. (1998). Influence of the production yeast strain on the development of malolactic fermentation in white wine. *Food Technology and Biotechnology, 36,* 63-68.
[24] Beelman, R. B., Keen, R. M., Banner, M. J. & King, S. W. (1982). Interactions between wine yeast and malolactic bacteria under wine conditions. *Developments in Industrial Microbiology, 23,* 107-121.
[25] McCloskey, L. P. & Mahaney, P. (1981). An enzymatic assay for acetaldehyde in grape juice and wine. *American Journal of Enology and Viticulture, 32,* 159-162.
[26] Ebeler, S. E., & Spaulding, R. S. (1999). Characterization and measurement of aldehydes in wine. In A. L. Waterhouse, & S. E. Ebeler (Eds.), *Chemistry of Wine Flavor, ACS Symposium Series,* (pp. 166-179). Oxford, UK: Oxford University Press.
[27] Liu, S.-Q. & Pilone, G. J. (2000). An overview of formation and roles of acetaldehyde in winemaking with emphasis on microbiological implications. *International Journal of Food Science and Technology, 35,* 49-61.
[28] Timberlake, C. F. & Bridle, P. (1976). Interactions between anthocyanins, phenolic compounds, and acetaldehyde and their significance in red wines. *American Journal of Enology and Viticulture, 27,* 97-105.
[29] Somers, T. C. & Wescombe, L. G. (1987). Evolution of red wines. II. An assessment of the role of acetaldehyde. *Vitis, 26,* 27-36.
[30] Margalith, P. Z. (1981). *Flavour Microbiology.* Springfield, USA: Charles C. Thomas Publishers.
[31] Merida, J., Lopez-Toledano, A., Marquez, T., Millan, C., Ortega, J. M. & Medina, M. (2005). Retention of browning compounds by yeasts involved in the winemaking of sherry type wines. *Biotechnology Letters, 27,* 1565-1570.
[32] Zoecklein, B. W., Fugelsang, K. C., Gump, B. H., & Nury, F. S. (1995). *Wine analysis and production.* New York, USA: Chapman & Hall Enology Library.
[33] Burroughs, L. F. & Sparks, A. H. (1973). Sulphite-binding power of wines and ciders. II. Theoretical consideration and calculation of sulphite-binding equilibria. *Journal of the Science of Food and Agriculture, 24,* 199-206.
[34] Dellarco, V. L. (1988). A mutagenicity assessment of acetaldehyde. *Mutation Research, 195,* 1-20.
[35] Tuma, D. J. & Sorrell, M. F. (1985). Covalent binding of acetaldehyde to hepatic proteins. Role in alcoholic liver injury. *Progress in Clinical and Biological Research, 183,* 3-17.
[36] Niemela, O. (1999). Aldehyde-protein adducts in the liver as a result of ethanol-induced oxidative stress. *Frontiers in Bioscience, 4,* 506-513.
[37] Brooks, P. J. (1997). DNA damage, DNA repair, and alcohol toxicity - A review. *Alcoholism: Clinical and Experimental Research, 21,* 1073-1082.
[38] Hemminki, K. & Suni R. (1984). Sites of reaction of glutaraldehyde and acetaldehyde with nucleosides. *Archives of Toxicology, 55,* 186-190.
[39] Vaca, C., Nilsson, J. A., Fang, J. L. & Grafstrom, R. C. (1998). Formation of DNA adducts in human buccal epithelial cells exposed to acetaldehyde and methylglyoxal. *Chemico-Biological Interactions, 108,* 197-208.

[40] Fang, J. L. & Vaca, C. (1997). Detection of DNA adducts of acetaldehyde in peripheral white blood cells of alcohol abusers. *Carcinogenesis, 18,* 627-632.

[41] Tillonen, J., Homann, N., Rautio, M., Jousimies-Somer, H. & Salaspuro, M. (1999). Role of yeasts in the salivary acetaldehyde production from ethanol among risk groups for ethanol-associated oral cavity cancer. *Alcoholism, Clinical and Experimental Research, 23,* 1409-1415.

[42] Matsuda, T., Kawanishi, M., Yagi, T., Matsui, S. & Takebe, H. (1998). Specific tandem GG to TT base substitutions induced by acetaldehyde are due to intra-strand cross-links between adjacent guanine bases. *Nucleic Acids Research, 26,* 1769-1774.

[43] Blasiak, J., Trzeciak, A., Malecka-Panas, E., Drzewoski, J. & Wojewódzka, M. (2000). In vitro genotoxicity of ethanol and acetaldehyde in human lymphocytes and the gastrointestinal tract mucosa cells. *Toxicology in Vitro, 14,* 287-295.

[44] http://www.pesticideinfo.org/Detail_Chemical.jsp?Rec_Id=PC35597.

[45] Amerine, M. A., & Ough, C. S. (1980). *Methods for analysis of musts and wines.* New York, USA: John Wiley & Sons.

[46] Etiévant, P. X. (1991). Wine. In H. Maarse (Ed.), *Volatile compounds in foods and beverages* (483-532). New York, USA: Marcel Dekker Inc.

[47] Fleet, H. F., & Heard, G. M. (1993). Yeast growth during fermentation. In G. H. Fleet (Ed.), *Wine microbiology and biotechnology* (pp. 27-54). Newark, USA: Harwood Academic Publishers.

[48] Romano, P., & Suzzi, P. (1993). Sulfur dioxide and wine microorganisms. In G. H. Fleet (Ed.), *Wine microbiology and biotechnology* (pp. 373-393). Newark, USA: Harwood Academic Publishers.

[49] Millan, C. & Ortega, J. M. (1988). Fermentation of "Pedro Ximenez" grape must by different yeast races: correlation between fermented sugars, acetaldehyde, acetic acid and ethanol yielded. *Belgian Journal of Food Chemistry and Biotechnology, 43,* 79-81.

[50] Zambonelli, C. (1988). *Microbiologia e biotecnologia dei vini.* Bologna, Italy: Edagricole.

[51] Swiegers, J. H., Bartowsky, P. A., Henschke, P. A. & Pretorius, I. S. (2005). Yeast and bacterial modulation of wine aroma and flavour. *Australian Journal of Grape and Wine Research, 11,* 139-73.

[52] Regodón Mateos, J. A., Pérez-Nevado, F. & Ramírez Fernández, M. (2006). Influence of *Saccharomyces cerevisiae* yeast strain on the major volatile compounds of wine. *Enzyme and Microbial Technology, 40,* 151-157.

[53] Salvadores, M. P. & Cardell, E. (1995). Identificacíon de la flora levaduriforme asociada a vinificaciones en la denominacíon específica Abona-Sur de Tenerife. *Alimentaria, 264,* 37-40.

[54] Houtman, A. C. & Du Plessis, C. S. (1986). The grape cultivar and yeast strain on fermentation rate and concentration of volatile components in wine. *South African Journal of Enology and Viticulture, 7,* 14-20.

[55] García, M. J., Casp, A. & Alexandre, J. L. (1994). Influenza del ceppo di lievito e della temperatura di fermentazione sulla concentrazione di alcuni composti volatili. *Rivista di Viticoltura e di Enologia, 4,* 29-37.

[56] Fraile, P., Garrido, J. & Ancin, C. (2000). Influence of a *Saccharomyces cerevisiae* selected strain in the volatile composition of roses wines. Evolution during fermentation. *Journal of Agriculture and Food Chemistry, 48,* 1789-98.

[57] Kourkoutas, Y., Douma, M., Koutinas, A. A., Kanellaki, M., Banat, I. M. & Marchant, R. (2002). Continuous winemaking fermentation using quince-immobilized yeast at room and low temperatures. *Process Biochemistry, 39,* 143-148.

[58] Tsakiris, A., Bekatorou, A., Psarianos, C., Koutinas, A. A., Marchant, R. & Banat, I. M. (2004). Immobilization of yeast on dried raisin berries for use in dry white winemaking. *Food Chemistry, 87,* 11-15.

[59] Veeranjaneya Reddy, L., Harish Kumar Reddy, Y., Prasanna Anjaneya Reddy, L. & Vijaya Sarathi Reddy, O. (2008). Wine production by novel yeast biocatalyst prepared by immobilization on watermelon (*Citrullus vulgaris*) rind pieces and characterization of volatile compounds. *Process Biochemistry, 43,* 748-752.

[60] Fornachon, J. C. M. (1963). Inhibition of certain lactic acid bacteria by free and bound sulphur dioxide. *Journal of the Science of Food and Agriculture, 14,* 857-862.

[61] Hood, A. (1983). Inhibition of growth of wine lactic-acid bacteria by acetaldehyde-bound sulphur dioxide. *The Australian Grapegrower & Winemaker, 232,* 34-43.

[62] Osborne, J. P., Mira de Orduña, R., Pilone, G. J. & Liu, S.-Q. (2000). Acetaldehyde metabolism by wine lactic acid bacteria. *FEMS Microbiology Letters, 191,* 51-55.

[63] Cordonnier, R. (1987). Le méthanol et ses origines dans le vin. *Progrès Agricole et Viticole, 104,* 315-318.

[64] Ough, C. S., & Amerine, M. A. (1988). *Methods for analysis of musts and wines.* New York, USA: John Wiley & Sons.

[65] Ribéreau-Gayon, P., Glories, Y., Maujean, A., & Dubourdieu, D. (2000). *The chemistry of wine stabilization and treatments. Handbook of enology* (Vol. 2). New York, USA: John Wiley & Sons.

[66] Office International de la Vigne et du Vin (1990). Recueil des méthodes internationales d'analyse des vins et des moûts. Paris, France: Office International de la Vigne et du Vin.

[67] Ribéreau-Gayon, J., Peynaud, E., Sudraud, P. & Ribéreau-Gayon, P. (1982). *Sciences et techniques du vin: analyse et contrôle des vins.* Paris, France: Dunod.

[68] Lee, C. Y., Robinson, W. B., van Buren, J. P., Acree, T. E. & Stoewsand, G. S. (1975). Methanol in wines in relation to processing and variety. *American Journal of Enology and Viticulture, 26,* 184-187.

[69] Nykanen, L., & Suomalainen, H. (1983). *Aroma of beer wine and distilled alcoholic beverages.* London, UK: D. Reidel Publishing Company.

[70] Cabaroglu, T. (2005). Methanol contents of Turkish varietal wines and effect of processing. *Food Control, 16,* 177-181.

[71] Gnekow, B. & Ough, C. S. (1976). Methanol in wines and musts: source and amounts. *American Journal of Enology and Viticulture, 27,* 1-6.

[72] Silva, M. L. & Malcata, F. X. (1999). Effects of time of grape pomace fermentation and distillation cuts on the chemical composition of grape marcs. *Zeitschrift für Lebensmittel-Untersuchung und Forschung A. - Food Research and Technology, 208,* 134-143.

[73] Bardi, E., Koutinas, A. A., Psarianos, C. & Kanellaki, M. (1997). Volatile by-products formed in low-temperature wine-making using immobilized yeast cells. *Process Biochemistry, 32,* 579-584.

[74] Gnekow, B. & Ough, C. S. (1976). Methanol in wines and musts: source and amounts. *American Journal of Enology and Viticulture, 27,* 1-6.

[75] Brown, M. R. & Ough, C. S. (1981). Effects of two different pectic enzymes preparations, at several activity levels, on three pectin fractions of a white must. *American Journal of Enology and Viticulture, 32,* 272-276.

[76] Servili, M., Begliomini, A. L., Montedoro, G., Petruccioli, M. & Federici, F. (1992). Utilisation of a yeast pectinase in olive oil extraction and red wine making processes. *Journal of the Science of Food and Agriculture, 58,* 253-260.

[77] Bosso, A. & Ponzetto, L. (1994). Macerazione delle bucce in presenza di enzimi pectolitici del commercio: influenza sull'andamento della fermentazione alcolica dei mosti e sulle caratteristiche olfattive dei vini. *Rivista di Viticoltura e di Enologia, 3,* 45-66.

[78] Revilla, I. & González-SanJosé, M. L. (1998). Methanol release during fermentation of red grapes treated with pectolytic enzymes. *Food Chemistry, 63,* 307-312.

[79] Nicolini, G., Versini, G., Mattivi, F., Dalla Serra, A. (1994). Glicosidasi in mosti e vini. *Vignevini, 718,* 26-32.

[80] Hou, C.-Y., Lin, Y.-S., Wang, Y. T., Jiang, C.-M., Lin, K. T. & Wu M.-C. (2008). Addition of phenolic acids on the reduction of methanol content in wine. *Journal of Food Science, 73,* 432-437.

[81] McKay, A. M. (1990). Degradation of polygalacturonic acid by *Saccharomyces cerevisiae*. *Letters in Applied Microbiology, 11,* 41-44.

[82] Blanco, P., Sieiro, C., Díaz, A. & Villa, T. G. (1994). Production and partial characterization of an endopolygalacturonase from *Saccharomyces cerevisiae*. *Canadian Journal of Microbiology, 40,* 974-977.

[83] Gainvors, A., Frézier, V., Lemarasquier, H., Lequart, C., Aigle, M. & Belarbi, A. (1994). Detection of polygalacturonase, pectinlyase and pectin-esterase activities in a *Saccharomyces cerevisiae* strain. *Yeast, 10,* 1311-1319.

[84] Ubeda, J. F., Briones, A. I. & Izquierdo, P. (1998). Study of the oenological characteristics and enzymatic activities of wine yeasts. *Food Microbiology, 15,* 399-406.

[85] Blanco, P., Sieiro, C. & Villa, T. G. (1999). Production of pectic enzymes in yeasts. *FEMS Microbiology Letters, 175,* 1-9.

[86] Fernández-González, M., Úbeda, J. F., Vasudevan, T. G., Cordero Otero, R. R. & Briones, A. I. (2004). Evaluation of polygalacturonase activity in *Saccharomyces cerevisiae* wine strains. *FEMS Microbiology Letters, 237,* 261-266.

[87] Ingledew, W. M., Magnus, C. A. & Patterson, J. R. (1987). Yeast foods and ethyl carbamate formation in wine. *American Journal of Enology and Viticulture, 38,* 332-337.

[88] Ough, C. S., Crowell, E. A. & Gutlove, B. R. (1988). Carbamyl compounds reactions with ethanol. *American Journal of Enology and Viticulture, 23,* 61-70.

[89] Monteiro, F. F., Trousdale, E. K. & Bisson, L. F. (1989). Ethyl carbamate formation in wine: Use of radioactively labelled precursors to demonstrate the involvement of urea. *American Journal of Enology and Viticulture, 40,* 1-8.

[90] Liu, S.-Q., Pritchard, G., Hardman, M. & Pilone, G. J. (1994). Citrulline production and ethyl carbamate (urethane) precursor formation from arginina degradation by wine lactic acid bacteria *Leuconostoc oenos* and *Lactobacillus buchneri*. *American Journal of Enology and Viticulture, 45,* 235-242.

[91] Arena, M. E., Saguir, F. M. & Manca de Nadra, M. C. (1999). Arginine, citrulline and ornithine metabolism by lactic acid bacteria from wine. *International Journal of Food Microbiology, 52,* 155-161.

[92] Mirvish, S. S. (1968). The carcinogenic and metabolism of urethane and N-hydroxy urethane. *Advances in Cancer Research, 11,* 1-42.

[93] Ough, C. S. (1976). Ethyl carbamate in fermented beverages and foods. I. Naturally occurring ethyl carbamate. *Journal of Agriculture and Food Chemistry, 24,* 323-328.

[94] Ough C. S. (1993). Ethyl carbamate in foods and wine. *Bulletin of the Society of Medical Friends of Wine, 25,* 7-8.

[95] Zimmerli, B. & Schlatter, J. (1991). Ethyl carbamate: analytical methodology, occurrence, formation, biological activity and risk assessment. *Mutation Research, 259,* 325-350.

[96] Marks, V. D., van der Merwe, G. K. & van Vuuren, H. J. J. (2003). Transcriptional profiling of wine yeast in fermenting grape juice: regulatory effect of diammonium phosphate. *FEMS Yeast Research, 3,* 269-287.

[97] Kodama, S., Suzuki, T., Fujinawa, S., De la Teja, P. & Yotsuzuka, F. (1994). Urea contribution to ethyl carbamate formation in commercial wines during storage. *American Journal of Enology and Viticulture, 1,* 17-24.

[98] Bordons, A., Gil, J., Araque, I., Romero, S., Masquè M. C., Reguant, C., & Carretè, R. (2003). Study of arginina degradation by lactic acid bacteria in relation with possible appearance of ethyl carbamate in wines. In FEMS, *Abstracts of the 1° Congress of European Microbiologist.* Ljubljana, Slovenia, 29 June-3 July 2003.

[99] Arena, M. E., Manca de Nadra, M. C. & Muñoz, R. (2002). The arginine deaminase pathway in the wine lactic acid bacterium *Lactobacillus hilgardii X1B*: structural and functional study of the *arcABC* genes. *Gene, 301,* 61-66.

[100] Henschke, P. A., & Jiranek, V. (1993). Yeasts - metabolism of nitrogen compounds. In G. H. Fleet (Ed.), *Wine microbiology and biotechnology* (pp. 77-164). Newark, USA: Harwood Academic Publishers.

[101] Jiranek, V., Langridge, P. & Henschke, P. A. (1995). Regulation of hydrogen sulfide liberation in wine-producing *Saccharomyces cerevisiae* strains by assimilable nitrogen. *Applied Environmental Microbiology, 61,* 461-467.

[102] Jiranek, V., Langridge, P. & Henschke, P. A. (1995). Amino acid and ammonium utilization by *Saccharomyces cerevisiae* wine yeasts from a chemically defined medium. *American Journal of Enology and Viticulture, 46,* 75-83.

[103] Jiranek, V., Langridge, P. & Henschke, P. A. (1995). Validation of bismuth-containing indicator media for predicting H_2S producing potential of *Saccharomyces cerevisiae* wine yeast under enological conditions. *American Journal of Enology and Viticulture, 46,* 269-273.

[104] Ough, C. S., Huang, Z., An, D. & Stevens, D. (1991). Amino acid uptake by four commercial yeasts at two different temperatures of growth and fermentation: effects on urea excretion and readsorption. *American Journal of Enology and Viticulture, 41,* 26-40.

[105] Pretorius, I. S. (2000). Tailoring wine yeast for the new millennium: novel approaches to the ancient art of winemaking. *Yeast, 16,* 675-729.

[106] Arena, M. E. & Manca de Nadra, M. C. (2005). Influence of ethanol and low pH on arginine and citrulline metabolism in lactic acid bacteria from wine. *Research in Microbiology, 156,* 858-864.

[107] Uthurry, C. A., Varela, F., Colomo, B., Suárez Lepe, J. A., Lombardero, J. & García del Hierro, J. R. (2004). Ethyl carbamate concentrations of typical Spanish red wines. *Food Chemistry, 88,* 329-336.

[108] Uthurry, C. A., Suárez Lepe, J. A., Lombardero, J. & García Del Hierro, J. R. (2006). Ethyl carbamate production induced by selected yeasts and lactic acid bacteria in red wine. *Food Chemistry, 94,* 262-270.

[109] Maynard, L. S. & Schenker, V. J. (1962). Monoamine-oxidase inhibition by ethanol in vitro. *Nature, 196,* 575-576.

[110] Lehtonen, P., Saarimen, M., Vesanto, M. & Riekkola, M. L. (1992). Determination of wine amines by HPLC using automated precolumn derivatisation with o-phthaldehyde and fluorescence detection. *Zeitschrift für Lebensmittel Untersuchung und Forschung, 194,* 434-437.

[111] Bauza, T., Blaisse, A., Teissedre, P. L., Cabanis, J. C., Kanny, G. & Moneret-Vautrin, D. A. (1995). Les amines biogènes du vin: métabolisme et toxicité. *Bulletin de l'Office International du Vin, 68,* 42-67.

[112] Shalaby, A. R. (1996). Significance of biogenic amines to food safety and human health. *Food Research International, 29,* 675-690.

[113] Silla-Santos, M. H. (1996). Biogenic amines: their importance in foods. *International Journal of Food Microbiology, 29,* 213-231.

[114] Soufleros, E., Marie-Lyse, B. & Bertrand, A. (1998). Correlation between the content of biogenic amines and other wine compounds. *American Journal of Enology and Viticulture, 49,* 266-277.

[115] Landete, J. M., Ferrer, S., Polo, L. & Pardo, I. (2005). Biogenic amines in wines from three Spanish regions. *Journal of Agriculture and Food Chemistry, 53,* 119-1124.

[116] Lehtonen, P. (1996). Determination of amines and amino acids in wine. A review. *American Journal of Enology and Viticulture, 47,* 127-133.

[117] Lonvaud-Funel, A. (2001). Biogenic amines in wines: role of lactic acid bacteria. *FEMS Microbiology Letters, 199,* 9-13.

[118] Cilliers, J. D. & van Wyk, C. J. (1985). Histamine and tyramine content in South African wines. *South African Journal of Enology and Viticulture, 6,* 35-40.

[119] Gloria, M. B. A., Watson, B. T., Simon-Sarkadi, L. & Daeschel, M. A. (1998). A survey of biogenic amines in Oregon Pinot noir and Cabernet Sauvignon wines. *American Journal of Enology and Viticulture, 49,* 279-282.

[120] Soleas, G. J., Carey, M. & Goldberg, D. M. (1999). Method development of cultivar-related differences of nine biogenic amines in Ontario wines. *Food Chemistry, 64,* 49-58.

[121] Gerbaux, V. & Monany, C. (2000). Les amines biogènes dans les vins de Bourgogne. Teneurs, origine et maîtrise dans les vins. *Revue Française d'Oenologie, 183,* 25-28.

[122] Caruso, M., Fiore, C., Contursi, M., Salzano, G., Paparella, A. & Romano, P. (2002). Formation of biogenic amines as criteria for the selection of wine yeasts. *World Journal of Microbiology & Biotechnology, 18,* 159-163.

[123] Torrea, D. & Ancin, C. (2002). Content of biogenic amines in a Chardonnay wine obtained through spontaneous and inoculated fermentations. *Journal of Agriculture and Food Chemistry, 50,* 4895-4899.

[124] Aerny, J. (1985). Origine de l'histamine dans les vins. Connaissances actuelles. *Bulletin de l'Office International du Vin, 656-657,* 1016-1019.

[125] Lonvaud-Funel, A. & Joyeux, A. (1994). Histamine production by wine lactic acid bacteria: isolation of a histamine-producing strain of *Leuconostoc oenos*. *Journal of Applied Bacteriology, 77,* 401-407.

[126] Guerrini, S., Mangani, S., Granchi, L. & Vincenzini, M. (2002). Biogenic amine production by *Oenococcus oeni*. *Current Microbiology, 44,* 374-378.

[127] Moreno-Arribas, M. V., Polo, M. C., Jorganes, F. & Muñoz, R. (2003). Screening of biogenic amine production by lactic acid bacteria isolated from grape must and wine. *International Journal of Food Microbiology, 84,* 117-123.

[128] Mangani, S., Guerrini, S., Granchi, L. & Vincenzini, M. (2005). Putrescine accumulation in wine: role of *Oenococcus oeni*. *Current Microbiology, 51,* 6-10.

[129] Alcaide-Hidalgo, J., Moreno-Arribas, M. V., Martín-Álvarez, P. J. & Polo, M. C. (2007). Influence of malolactic fermentation, postfermentative treatments and ageing with lees on nitrogen compounds of red wines. *Food Chemistry, 103,* 572-581.

[130] Herbert, P., Cabrita, M. J., Ratola, N., Laureano, O. & Alves, A. (2005). Free amino acids and biogenic amines in wines and musts from the Alentejo region. Evolution of amines during alcoholic fermentation and relationship with variety, sub-region and vintage. *Journal of Food Engineering, 66,* 315-322.

[131] Gallander, J. F. (1977). Deacidification of eastern table wines with *Schizosaccharomyces pombe*. *American Journal of Enology and Viticulture, 28,* 65-68.

[132] Gao, C. & Fleet, G. H. (1995). Degradation of malic and tartaric acids by high density cell suspensions of wine yeasts. *Food Microbiology, 12,* 65-71.

[133] Maicas, S. (2001). The use of alternative technologies to develop malolactic fermentation in wine. *Applied Microbiology and Biotechnology, 56,* 35-39.

[134] Coton, E., Rollan, G. C., Bertrand, A. & Lonvaud-Funel, A. (1998). Histamine-producing lactic acid bacteria in wines: early detection, frequency and distribution. *American Journal of Enology and Viticulture, 49,* 199-204.

[135] Landete, J. M., Ferrer, S. & Pardo, I. (2007). Biogenic amine production by lactic acid bacteria, acetic bacteria and yeast isolated from wine. *Food Control, 18,* 1569-1574.

[136] Edwards, C. G. & Beelman, R. B. (1987). Inhibition of the malolactic bacterium *Leuconostoc oenos* (PSU-1) by decanoic acid and subsequent removal of the inhibition by yeast ghosts. *American Journal of Enology and Viticulture, 38,* 239-242.

[137] Edwards, C. G., Beelman, R. B., Bartley C. E. & McConnel A. L. (1990). Production of decanoic acid and other volatile compounds and the growth of yeast and malolactic bacteria during vinification. *American Journal of Enology and Viticulture, 41,* 48-56.

[138] Lonvaud-Funel, A., Joyeux, A. & Dessens, C. (1988). Inhibition of malolactic fermentation of wines by products of yeast metabolism. *Journal of the Science of Food and Agriculture, 44,* 183- 191.

[139] Lafon-Lafourcade, S., Geneix, C. & Ribéreau-Gayon, P. (1984). Inhibition of alcoholic fermentation of grape must by fatty acids produced by yeast. Their elimination by yeast ghosts. *Applied and Environmental Microbiology, 47,* 1246-1249.

[140] Hammond, J. R. M. (1993). Brewer's yeasts. In A.H., Rose, & J. S., Harrison (Eds.), *The Yeast. Yeast Technology* (5th, pp. 620). London, UK: Academic Press.
[141] Ravaglia, S. & Delfini, C. (1993). Production of MCFA and their ethyl esters by yeast strains isolated from musts and wines. *Italian Journal of Food Science, 1*, 21- 36.
[142] Suomalainen, H. & Lehtonen, M. (1979). The production of aroma compounds by yeast. *Journal of the Institute of Brewing, 85*, 149-156.
[143] Taylor, G. T., Thurston, P. A. & Kirsop, B. H. (1979). The influence of lipids derived from malt spent grains on yeast metabolism and fermentation. *Journal of the Institute of Brewing, 85*, 219-227.
[144] Bardi, L., Cocito, C. & Marzona M. (1999). *Saccharomyces cerevisiae* cell fatty acid composition and release during fermentation without aeration and in absence of exogenous lipids. *International Journal of Food Microbiology, 47*, 133-140.
[145] Malherbe, S., Bauer, F. F. & Du Toit, M. (2007). Understanding Problem Fermentations - A Review. *South African Journal of Enology and Viticulture, 28*, 169-186.
[146] Bisson, L. F. (1999). Stuck and sluggish fermentations. *American Journal of Enology and Viticulture, 50*, 107- 119.
[147] Steven, S. & Servaas Hofmayr, J.-H. (1993). Effects of ethanol, octanoic acids on fermentation and the passive influx of protons through the plasma membrane of *Saccharomyces cerevisiae*. *Applied Microbiology and Biotechnology, 38*, 656-663.
[148] Capucho, I. & San Romao, M. V. (1994). Effect of ethanol and fatty acids on the malolactic activity of *Leuconostoc oenos*. *Applied Microbiology and Biotechnology, 42*, 391-395.
[149] Henschke, P. A. (1997). Stuck fermentation: causes, prevention and cure. In M. Allen, P. Leske, & G. Baldwin, (Eds.), *Proceedings of the Seminar: Advances in Juice Clarification and Yeast Inoculation*, (pp. 30-41). Melbourne, Australia: Australian Society of Viticulture and Oenology.
[150] Viegas, C. A. & Sá-Correia, I. (1997). Effects of low temperatures (9-33 °C) and pH (3.3-5-7) in the loss of *Saccharomyces cerevisiae* viability by combining lethal concentrations of ethanol with octanoic and decanoic acids. *International Journal of Food Microbiology, 34*, 267-277.
[151] Legal, L., Moulin, B. & Jallon, J. M. (1999). The relation between structures and toxicity of oxygenated aliphatic compounds homologous to the insecticide octanoic acid and the chemotaxis of two species of *Drosophila*. *Pesticide Biochemistry and Physiology, 65*, 90-101.
[152] http://www.pesticideinfo.org/List_NTPStudies.jsp?Rec_Id=PC33719.
[153] Guilloux-Benatier, M., Guerreau, J. & Feuillat, M. (1995). Influence of initial colloid content on yeast macromolecule production and on the metabolism of wine microorganisms. *American Journal of Enology and Viticulture, 46*, 486-492.
[154] Guilloux-Benatier, M. & Feuillat, M. (1991). Utilisation d'adjuvants d'origine levurienne pour améliorer l'ensemencement des vins en bactéries sélectionnées. *Revue Française d'Oenologie, 132*, 51-55.
[155] Lafon-Lafourcade, S. (1984). Souches de levures. *Bulletin de l'Office International du Vin, 637*, 185-203.

[156] Munoz, E. & Ingledew, W. M. (1989). Effect of yeast hulls on stuck and sluggish wine fermentations: importance of the lipid component. *Applied and Environmental Microbiology, 55*, 1560-1564.

[157] Ravaglia, S. & Delfini, C. (1994). Inhibitory effects of medium fatty acids on yeast cells growing in synthetic medium and in sparkling Moscato wine "Asti Spumante". *Viticultural and Enological Sciences, 49*, 40- 45.

[158] Escot, S., Feuillat, M., Dulau, L. & Charpentier, C. (2001). Release of polysaccharides by yeast and the influence of polysaccharides on colour stability and wine astringency. *Australian Journal of Grape and Wine Research, 7*, 153-159.

[159] Riou, V., Vernhet, A., Doco, T. & Moutounet, M. (2002). Aggregation of grape seed tannins in model wine-effect of wine polysaccharides. *Food Hydrocolloids, 16*, 17-23.

[160] Caridi, A., Cufari, A., Lovino, R., Palumbo, R. & Tedesco, I. (2004). Influence of yeast on polyphenol composition of wine. *Food Technology and Biotechnology, 42*, 37-40.

[161] Sacchi, K. L., Bisson, L. F. & Adams, D. O. (2005). A review of the effect of winemaking techniques on phenolic extraction in red wines. *American Journal of Enology and Viticulture, 56*, 197-206.

[162] Bautista-Ortín, A. B., Romero-Cascales, I., Fernández-Fernández, J. I., López-Roca, J. M. & Gómez-Plaza, E. (2007). Influence of the yeast strain on Monastrell wine colour. *Innovative Food Science and Emerging Technologies, 8*, 322-328.

[163] Castino, M. (1982). Lieviti e polifenoli. *Rivista di Viticoltura e di Enologia, 34*, 333-348.

[164] Sidari, R., Postorino, S., Caparello, A. & Caridi, A. (2007). Evolution during wine aging of colour and tannin differences induced by wine starters. *Annals of Microbiology, 57*, 197-201.

[165] Delcroix, A., Günata, Z., Sapis, J. C., Salmon, J. M. & Bayonove, C. (1994). Glycosidase activities of three enological yeast strains during winemaking: effect on the terpenol content of muscat wine. *American Journal of Enology and Viticulture, 45*, 291-296.

[166] Sponholz, W. R. (1997). L'attività enzimatica dei lieviti e la stabilità del colore rosso dei vini. *Vignevini, 24*, 34-36.

[167] Manzanares, P., Rojas, V., Genoves, S. & Valles, S. (2000). A preliminary search for anthocyanin-β-D-glucosidase activity in non-*Saccharomyces* wine yeasts. *International Journal of Food Science & Technology, 35*, 95-103.

[168] Vrhovsek, U., Wendelin, S. & Eder, R. (1997). Effects of various vinification techniques on the concentration of *cis*- and *trans*-resveratrol and resveratrol glucoside isomers in wine. *American Journal of Enology and Viticulture, 48*, 214-219.

[169] Fulcrand, H., Benabdeljalil, C., Rigaud, J., Cheynier, V. & Moutounet, M. (1998). A new class of wine pigments generated by reaction between pyruvic acid and grape anthocyanins. *Phytochemistry, 47*, 1401-1407.

[170] Morata, A., Gómez-Cordovés, M. C., Colomo, B. & Suárez, J. A. (2003). Pyruvic acid and acetaldehyde production by different strains of *Saccharomyces cerevisiae*: relationship with visitin A and B formation in red wines. *Journal of Agricultural and Food Chemistry, 51*, 6475-6481.

[171] Morata, A., Gómez-Cordovés, M. C., Calderón, F. & Suárez, J. A. (2006). Effects of pH, temperature and SO_2 on the formation of pyranoanthocyanins during red wine

fermentation with two species of *Saccharomyces*. *International Journal of Food Microbiology, 106,* 123-129.

[172] Dallas, C., Ricardo-da-Silva, J. M. & Laureano, O. (1996). Interactions of oligomeric procyanidins in model wine solutions containing malvidin-3-glucoside and acetaldehyde. *Journal of the Science of Food and Agriculture, 70,* 493-500.

[173] Lopez-Toledano, A., Villano-Valencia, D., Mayen, M., Merida, J. & Medina, M. (2004). Interaction of yeasts with the products resulting from the condensation reaction between (+)-catechin and acetaldehyde. *Journal of Agricultural and Food Chemistry, 52,* 2376-2381.

[174] Saucier, C., Roux, D. & Glories, Y. (1995). Stabilité colloïdale des polymers catéchiques. Influence des polysaccharides. In A. Lonvaud-Funel (Ed.), *Oenologie '95: Symposium International d'Oenologie* (5th, pp. 395-400). Paris, France: Tec & Doc Lavoisier.

[175] Ferrari, S., Gheri, A., Rosi, I. & Trioli, G. (1997). Polisaccaridi del lievito e polifenoli. *Vignevini, 24,* 43-45.

[176] Feuillat, M., Escot, S., Charpentier, C. & Dulou, L. (2001). Élevage des vins rouges sur lies fines. Intérêt des interactions entre polysaccharides de levures et polyphénols du vin. *Revue des Oenologues, 98,* 17-18.

[177] Feuillat, M. (2003). Yeast macromolecules: origin, composition and enological interest. *American Journal of Enology and Viticulture, 54,* 211-213.

[178] Bourzeix, M. & Heredia, N. (1976). Etude des colorants anthocyaniques fixés par les levures de vinification. *Comptes Rendus de l'Académie d'Agriculture de France, 62,* 750-753.

[179] Vasserot, Y., Caillet, S. & Maujean, A. (1997). Study of anthocyanin adsorption by yeast lees. Effect of some physicochemical parameters. *American Journal of Enology and Viticulture, 48,* 433-437.

[180] Salmon, J. M., Fornairon-Bonnefond, C. & Mazauric, J. P. (2002). Interactions between wine lees and polyphenols: influence on oxygen consumption capacity during simulation of wine aging. *Journal of Food Science, 67,* 1604-1609.

[181] Mazauric, J.-P. & Salmon, J.-M. (2005). Interactions between yeast lees and wine polyphenols during simulation of wine aging. I. Analysis of remnant polyphenolic compounds in the resulting wines. *Journal of Agricultural and Food Chemistry, 53,* 5647-5653.

[182] Medina, K., Boido, E., Dellacassa, E. & Carrau, F. (2005). Yeast interactions with anthocyanins during red wine fermentation. *American Journal of Enology and Viticulture, 56,* 104-109.

[183] Mazauric, J.-P. & Salmon, J.-M. (2006). Interactions between yeast lees and wine polyphenols during simulation of wine aging. II. Analysis of desorbed polyphenol compounds from yeast lees. *Journal of Agricultural and Food Chemistry, 54,* 3876-3881.

[184] Cuinier, C. (1988). Influence des levures sur les composés phénoliques du vin. *Bulletin de l'Office International du Vin, 61,* 596-601.

[185] Delteil, D. (1995). Les macérations en rouge: l'art du détail. *Revue des Oenologues, 77,* 23-25.

[186] Conterno, L., Tortia, C., Minati, J. L. & Trioli, G. (1997). La selezione di un ceppo di lievito per il Barolo. *Vignevini, 24,* 30-33.

[187] Cuinier, C. (1997). Ceppi di lievito e composizione fenolica dei vini rossi. *Vignevini, 24*, 39-42.

[188] Girard, B., Yuksel, D., Cliff, M. A., Delaquis, P. & Reynolds, A. G. (2001). Vinification effects on the sensory, colour and GC profiles of Pinot noir wines from British Columbia. *Food Research International, 34*, 483-499.

[189] Boisson, R., Lempereur, V. & Berger, J. L. (2002). Sélection d'une souche de levure extractrice des composés phénoliques du raisin, issue du terroir Beaujolais: L1515. *Revue des Oenologues, 104*, 38-41.

[190] Eglinton, J. & Henschke, P. (2003). Winemaking properties of *Saccharomyces bayanus* - initial observations of the potential for red winemaking. *Australian and New Zealand Grapegrower and Winemaker, 473*, 18-20.

[191] Malacrinò, P., Tosi, E., Caramia, G., Prisco, R. & Zapparoli, G. (2005). The vinification of partially dried grapes: a comparative fermentation study of *Saccharomyces cerevisiae* strains under high sugar stress. *Letters in Applied Microbiology, 40*, 466-472.

[192] Boivin, S., Feuillat, M., Alexandre, H. & Charpentier, C. (1998). Effect of must turbidity on cell wall porosity and macromolecule excretion of *Saccharomyces cerevisiae* cultivated on grape juice. *American Journal of Enology and Viticulture, 49*, 325-331.

[193] Morata, A., Gómez-Cordovés, M. C., Suberviola, J., Bartolomé, B., Colomo, B. & Suárez, J. A. (2003). Adsorption of anthocyanins by yeast cell walls during the fermentation of red wines. *Journal of Agricultural and Food Chemistry, 51*, 4084-4088.

[194] Morata, A., Gómez-Cordovés, M. C., Colomo, B. & Suárez, J. A. (2005). Cell wall anthocyanin adsorption by different *Saccharomyces* strains during the fermentation of *Vitis vinifera* L. cv Graciano grapes. *European Food Research and Technology, 220*, 341-346.

[195] Chatonnet, P., Dubourdieu, D. & Boidron, J. N. (1992). Incidence des conditions de fermentation et d'élevage des vins blancs secs en barriques sur leur composition en substances cédées par le bois de chêne. *Sciences des Aliments, 12*, 665-685.

[196] Vivas, N., Lonvaud-Funel, A. & Glories, Y. (1997). Effect of phenolic acids and anthocyanins on growth, viability and malolactic activity of a lactic acid bacterium. *Food Microbiology, 14*, 291-300.

[197] Ringot, D., Lerzy, B., Chaplain, K., Bonhoure, J.-P., Auclair E. & Larondelle Y. (2007). In vitro biosorption of ochratoxin A on the yeast industry by-products: Comparison of isotherm models. *Bioresource Technology, 98*, 1812-1821.

[198] Galvano, F., Ritieni, A., Piva, G., & Pietri, A. (2005). Mycotoxins in the human food chain. In D. Diaz (Ed.), *Mycotoxins Blue Book* (pp. 187-224). Nottingham, United Kingdom: Nottingham University Press.

[199] Varga, J. & Kozakiewicz, Z. (2006). Ochratoxin A in grapes and grape-derived products. *Trends in Food Science & Technology, 17*, 72-81.

[200] International Agency for Research on Cancer (1993). Monographs on the evaluation of carcinogenic risks to humans: some naturally occurring substances, food items and constituents, heterocyclic aromatic amines and mycotoxins (56, pp. 489-521). Lyon, France: International Agency for Research on Cancer.

[201] Stanley, V. G., Ojo, R., Woldesenbet, S. & Hutchinson, D. H. (1993). The use of *Saccharomyces cerevisiae* to suppress the effects of aflatoxicosis in broiler chicks. *Poultry Science, 72*, 1867-1872.

[202] Bauer, J. (1994). Möglichkeiten zur Entgiftung mykotoxinhaltiger Futtermittel. *Monatshefte fur Veterinärmedizin, 49,* 175-181.
[203] Scott, P. M., Kanhere, S. R., Lawrence, G. A., Daley, E. F. & Farber, J. M. (1995). Fermentation of wort containing added ochratoxin A and fumonisins B1 and B2. *Food Additives and Contaminants, 12,* 31-40.
[204] Devegowda, G., Aravind, B. I. R., & Morton, M. G. (1996). *Saccharomyces cerevisiae* and mannanoligosaccharides to counteract aflatoxicosis in broilers. In *Proceedings of the Australian Poultry Science Symposium* (8th, pp. 103-106). Sydney, Australia.
[205] Devegowda, G., Raju, M. V. L. N. & Swamy, H. V. L. N. (1998). Mycotoxins: novel solutions for their counteraction. *Feedstuffs, 70,* 12-15.
[206] Baptista, A. S., Horii, J., Calori-Domingues, M. A., Micotti da Glória, E., Salgado, J. M. & Vizioli, M. R. (2004). The capacity of manno-oligosaccharides, thermolysed yeast and active yeast to attenuate aflatoxicosis. *World Journal of Microbiology & Biotechnology, 20,* 475-481.
[207] Bejaoui, H., Mathieu, F., Taillandier, P. & Lebrihi, A. (2004). Ochratoxin A removal in synthetic and natural grape juices by selected oenological *Saccharomyces* strains. *Journal of Applied Microbiology, 97,* 1038-1044.
[208] Caridi, A., Cufari, A., Galvano, F., Geria, M., Postorino, S., Tafuri, A., & Ritieni, A. (2004). New microbiological approach to reduce ochratoxin levels in alcoholic beverages. In *Abstracts of the International ICFMH Symposium Food Micro 2004* (19th, p. 264). Portorož, Slovenia, 12-16 September 2004.
[209] Caridi, A., Galvano, F., Tafuri, A., & Ritieni, A. (2005). Ochratoxin A removal during alcoholic fermentation. In *Abstracts of the International Conference on Environmental, Industrial and Applied Microbiology BioMicroWorld2005* (1st, p. 518) Badajoz, Spain, 15-18 Mars 2005.
[210] Caridi, A., Galvano, F., Tafuri, A., & Ritieni, A. (2005). Yeast selection for ability to remove ochratoxin A during winemaking. In *Abstracts of the International Workshop on Advances in Grapevine and Wine Research* (1st, p. 74) Venosa, Italy, 14-17 September 2005.
[211] Garcia Moruno, E., Sanlorenzo, C., Boccaccino, B. & Di Stefano, R. (2005). Treatment with yeast to reduce the concentration of ochratoxin A in red wine. *American Journal of Enology and Viticulture, 56,* 73-56.
[212] Caridi, A., Galvano, F., Tafuri, A. & Ritieni, A. (2006). In-vitro screening of *Saccharomyces* strains for ochratoxin A removal from liquid medium. *Annals of Microbiology, 56,* 135-137.
[213] Leong, S. L., Hocking, A. D., Varelis, P., Giannikopoulos, C. & Scott, E. S. (2006). Fate of ochratoxin A during vinification of Semillon and Shiraz grapes. *Journal of Agricultural and Food Chemistry, 54,* 6460-6464.
[214] Péteria, Z., Térenb, J., Vágvölgyia, C. & Varga, J. (2007). Ochratoxin degradation and adsorption caused by astaxanthin-producing yeasts. *Food Microbiology, 24,* 205-210.
[215] Huwig, A., Freimund, S., Käppeli, O. & Dutler, H. (2001). Mycotoxin detoxification of animal feed by different adsorbents. *Toxicology Letters, 122,* 179-188.
[216] Santin, E., Paulillo, A. C., Maiorka, A., Satiko, L., Nakaghi, O., Macari, M., Fischer da Silva, A. V. & Alessi, C. (2003). Evaluation of the efficacy of *Saccharomyces cerevisiae* cell wall to ameliorate the toxic effects of aflatoxin in broilers. *International Journal of Poultry Science, 2,* 341-344.

[217] Yiannikouris, A., Poughon, L., Cameleyre, X., Dussap, C.-G., François, J., Bertin, G. & Jouany, J.-P. (2003). A novel technique to evaluate interactions between *Saccharomyces cerevisiae* cell wall and mycotoxins: application to zearalenone. *Biotechnology Letters, 25,* 783-789.

[218] Ringot, D., Lerzy, B., Bonhoure, J. P., Auclair, E., Oriol, E. & Larondelle, Y. (2005). Effect of temperature on in vitro ochratoxin A biosorption onto yeast cell wall derivatives. *Process Biochemistry, 40,* 3008-3016.

[219] Zaghini, A., Roncada, P., Anfossi, P. & Rizzi, L. (1998). Aflatoxin B1 oral administration to laying hens: effects on hepatic MFO activities and efficacy of a zeolite to prevent aflatoxicosis B1. *Revue de Medecine Veterinaire, 6,* 668-669.

[220] Raju, M. V. L. N. & Devegowda, G. (2000). Influence of esterified-glucomannan on performance and organ morphology, serum biochemistry and haematology in broilers exposed to individual and combined mycotoxicosis (aflatoxin, ochratoxin and T-2 toxin). *British Poultry Science, 41,* 640-650.

[221] Caridi, A., Galvano, F., Tafuri, A. & Ritieni, A. (2006). Ochratoxin A removal during winemaking. *Enzyme and Microbial Technology, 40,* 122-126.

[222] Cecchini, F., Morassut, M., Garcia Moruno, E. & Di Stefano, R. (2006). Influence of yeast strain on ochratoxin A content during fermentation of white and red must. *Food Microbiology, 23,* 411-417.

[223] Caridi A. (2006). Enological functions of parietal yeast mannoproteins. *Antonie van Leeuwenhoek, 89,* 417-422.

[224] Caridi A. (2007). New perspectives in safety and quality enhancement of wine through selection of yeasts based on the parietal adsorption activity. *International Journal of Food Microbiology, 120,* 167-172.

[225] Fernandes, A., Venâncio, A., Moura, F., Garrido, J. & Cerdeira, A. (2003). Fate of ochratoxin A during a vinification trial. *Aspects of Applied Biology, 68,* 73-80.

[226] Fernandes, A., Ratola, N., Cerdeira, A., Alves, A. & Venâncio, A. (2007). Change in ochratoxin A concentration during winemaking. *American Journal of Enology and Viticulture, 58,* 92-96.

[227] Hocking, A. D., Leong, S. L., Kazi, B. A., Emmett, R. W. & Scott, E. S. (2007). Fungi and mycotoxins in vineyards and grape products. *International Journal of Food Microbiology 119,* 84-88.

[228] Radice, S., Marabini, L., Gervasoni, M., Ferraris, M. & Chiesara, E. (1998). Adaptation to oxidative stress: effects of vinclozolin and iprodione on the HepG2 cell line. *Toxicology, 129,* 183-191.

[229] Gray Jr., L. E., Wolf, C., Lambright, C., Mann, P., Price, M., Cooper, R. L. & Ostby, J. (1999). Administration of potentially antiandrogenic pesticides (procymidone, linuron, iprodione, chlozolinate, p,p0-DDE, and ketoconazole) and toxic substances (dibuthyl- and diethylhexylphtalan PCB 169, and ethane dimethane sulphonate) during sexual differentiation produces diverse profiles of reproductive malformations in the male rat. *Toxicology and Industrial Health, 15,* 94-118.

[230] Athiel, P., Alfizar, Mercadier, C., Vega, D., Bastide, J., Davet, P., Brunel, B. & Cleyet-Marel, J. C. (1995). Degradation of iprodione by a soil *Arthrobacter*-like strain. *Applied and Environmental Microbiology, 61,* 3216-3220.

[231] Radice, S., Ferraris, M., Marabini, L., Grande, S. & Chiesara, E. (2001). Effect of iprodione, a dicarboximide fungicide, on primary cultured rainbow trout (oncorhynchus mykiss) hepatocytes. *Aquatic Toxicology, 54,* 51-58.

[232] Rankin, G. O., Teets, V. J., Nicoll, D. W. & Brown, P. I. (1989). Comparative acute renal effects of three N-(3,5-dichlorophenyl)-carboximide fungicides: N-(3,5-dichlorophenyl)succinimide, vinclozolin and iprodione. *Toxicology, 56,* 263-272.

[233] Bruynzeel, D. P., Tafelkruijer, J. & Wilks, M. F. (1995). Contact dermatitis due to a new fungicide used in the tulip bulb industry. *Contact Dermatitis 33,* 8-11.

[234] Draper, A., Cullinan, P., Jones, M. & Newman Taylor, A. (2003). Occupational asthma from fungicides fluazinam and chlorothalonil. *Occupational and Environmental Medicine, 60,* 76-77.

[235] Cabras, P., Diana, P., Meloni, M., Pirisi, F. M. & Pirisi, R. (1983). Reversed-phase high-performance liquid chromatography of pesticides. VII. Analysis of Vinclozolin, Iprodione, Procymidone, Dichlozolinate and their degradation product 3,5-dichloroaniline on white must and wine extracts. *Journal of Chromatography, 256,* 176-181.

[236] Navarro, S., Oliva, J., Navarro, G. & Barba, A. (2001). Dissipation of Chlorpyrifos, Fenarimol, Mancozeb, Metalaxyl, Penconazole, and Vinclozolin in grapes. *American Journal of Enology and Viticulture, 52,* 35-40.

[237] Fatichenti, F., Farris, G. A., Deiana, P., Cabras, P., Meloni, M. & Pirisi, F. M. (1983). A preliminary investigation into the effect of *Saccharomyces cerevisiae* on pesticide concentration during fermentation. *European Journal of Applied Microbiology and Biotechnology, 18,* 323-325.

[238] Farris, G. A., Fatichenti, F., Cabras, P., Meloni, M. & Pirisi, F. M. (1989). Flour-yeast and fungicide interactions. *Sciences des Aliments, 9,* 553-560.

[239] Cabras, P., Angioni, A., Garau, V. L., Melis, M., Pirisi, F. M., Farris, G. A., Sotgiu, C. & Minelli, E. V. (1997). Persistence and metabolism of folpet in grapes and wine. *Journal of Agriculture and Food Chemistry, 45,* 476-479.

[240] Cabras, P., Angioni, A., Garau, V. L., Pirisi, F. M. & Brandolini, V. (1998). Chromatographic determination of azoxystrobin, fluazinam, kresoxim methyl, mepanipyrim and tetraconazole, in grapes, must and wine. *Journal of AOAC International, 81,* 1185-1189.

[241] Cabras, P., Angioni, A., Garau, V. L., Pirisi, F. M., Farris, G. A., Madau, G. & Emonti, G. (1999). Pesticides in fermentative process in wine. *Journal of Agriculture and Food Chemistry, 47,* 3854-3857.

[242] Cabras, P. & Angioni, A. (2000). Pesticide residues in grapes, wine, and their processing products. *Journal of Agriculture and Food Chemistry, 48,* 967-973.

[243] Čuš, F. & Raspor, P. (2008). The effect of pyrimethanil on the growth of wine yeasts. *Letters in Applied Microbiology, 47,* 54-59.

[244] Calhelha, R. C., Andrade, J. V., Ferreira, I. C. & Estevinho, L. M. (2006). Toxicity effects of fungicide residues on the wine-producing process. *Food Microbiology, 23,* 393-398.

[245] Olasupo, N. A., Scott-Emuakpor, M. B. & Ogunshola, R. A. (1993). Resistance to heavy metals by some Nigerian yeast strains. *Folia Microbiologica, 38,* 285-287.

[246] Johnston, J. R., Baccari, C. & Mortimer, R. K. (2000). Genotypic characterization of strains of commercial wine yeasts by tetrads analysis. *Research in Microbiology, 151,* 583-590.

[247] Dunn, B., Levine, R. P. & Sherlock, G. (2005). Microarray karyotyping of commercial wine yeast strains reveals shared, as well as unique, genomic signatures. *BMC Genomics, 6,* 53-73.

[248] Nagasue, N., Kohno, H., Chang, Y. C. & Nakamura, T. (1989). Iron, copper and zinc levels in serum and cirrhotic liver of patients with and without epatocellular carcinoma. *Oncology, 46,* 293-296.

[249] Wilson, J. D., Braunwald, E., Isselbacher, K. J., Petersdorf, R. G., Martin, J. B., Fauci, A. S. & Root, J. R. (1991). Harrison's Principles of Internal Medicine. New York, USA: McGraw Hill.

[250] Felix, K. & Weser, U. (1988). Release of copper from yeast copper-thionein after S-alkylation of copper-thiolate clusters. *Biochemical Journal, 252,* 577-581.

[251] Brady, D., Glaum, D. & Duncan, J. R. (1994). Copper tolerance in *Saccharomyces cerevisiae*. *Letters in Applied Microbiology, 18,* 245-250.

[252] Brandolini, V., Tedeschi, P., Capece, A., Maietti, A., Mazzotta, D., Salzano, G., Paparella, A. & Romano, P. (2002). *Saccharomyces cerevisiae* wine strains differing in copper resistance exhibit different capability to reduce copper content in wine. *World Journal of Microbiology & Biotechnology, 18,* 499-503.

[253] White, C. & Gadd, G. M. (1986). Uptake and cellular distribution of copper, cobalt and cadmium in strains of *Saccharomyces cerevisiae* cultured on elevated concentrations of these metals. *FEMS Microbiology Ecology, 38,* 277-283.

[254] Bianchi, M. E., Carbone, M. I., Lurchial, G. & Magni, G. E. (1981). Mutants resistant to manganese in *Saccharomyces cerevisiae*. *Current Genetics, 4,* 215-220.

[255] John, M., Imai, M. & Murayama, T. (1985). Different distribution of Cd^{++} between Cd-sensitive and Cd-resistant strains of *Saccharomyces cerevisiae*. *Journal of General Microbiology, 131,* 51-56.

[256] Slezen, R. J. (2008). Wine Genomics. *Microbial Biotechnology, 1,* 97-103.

[257] Rainieri, S. & Pretorius, I. S. (2000). Selection and improvement of wine yeasts. *Annals of Microbiology, 50,* 15-31.

[258] Giudici, P., Solieri, L., Pulvirenti, A. M. & Cassanelli, S. (2005). Strategies and perspectives for genetic improvement of wine yeasts. *Applied Microbiology and Biotechnology, 66,* 622-628.

[259] Henschke, P. A. (1997). Wine yeast. In F. K. Zimmermann, & K.-D. Entian (Eds.), *Yeast Sugar Metabolism* (pp. 527-560). Lancaster, USA: Technomic Publishing.

[260] Kitamoto, K., Oda, K., Gomi, K. & Takahashi, K. (1991). Genetic engineering of a sake yeast producing no urea by successive disruption of arginase gene. *Applied Environmental Microbiology, 57,* 301-306.

[261] Dequin, S. (2001). The potential of genetic engineering for improving brewing, wine-making and baking yeasts. *Applied Microbiology and Biotechnology, 56,* 577-588.

[262] Pretorius, I. S., De Barros Lopes, M. A. & Høj, P. B. (2004). Development of superior wine yeast: current status and future opportunities to meet the consumer challenge. *Bulletin de l'Office International du Vin, 77,* 389-421.

[263] Ough, C. S. & Trioli, G. (1988). Urea removal from wine by an acid urease. *American Journal of Enology and Viticulture, 39,* 303-307.

[264] Visser, J. J., Coton, E. P. N., Bauer, F., Viljoen, M. & van Vuuren, H. J. J. (1999). Engineering an acid urease for heterologous expression in *Saccharomyces cerevisiae*. *Current Genetics, 35,* 321.

[265] Husnik, J. I., Volschenk, H., Bauer, J., Colavizza, D., Luo, Z. & van Vuuren, H. J. J. (2006). Metabolic engineering of malolactic wine yeast. *Metabolic Engineering, 8,* 315-323.

[266] Becker, J. V. W., Armstrong, G. O., van der Merwe, M. J., Lambrechts, M. G., Vivier, M. A. & Pretorius, I. S. (2003). Metabolic engineering of *Saccharomyces cerevisiae* for the synthesis of the wine-related antioxidant resveratrol. *FEMS Yeast Research, 4,* 79-85.

In: Red Wine and Health
Editor: Paul O'Byrne

ISBN 978-1-60692-718-2
© 2009 Nova Science Publishers, Inc.

Chapter 8

SUGARS, ORGANIC ACIDS AND GLYCEROL METABOLISM OF LACTIC ACID BACTERIA FROM FRUITS AND FERMENTED BEVERAGES: INFLUENCE ON THE PRODUCTS QUALITY

María Cristina Manca de Nadra[5], Fabiana María Saguir and Ana María Strasser de Saad

Facultad de Bioquímica, Química y Farmacia - Universidad Nacional de Tucumán, Ayacucho 471 and Centro de Referencia para Lacobacilos (CERELA)- Chacabuco 145. 4000 Tucumán. Argentina

ABSTRACT

Growth and metabolism of lactic acid bacteria (LAB) are essential in the quality of many fermented beverages like cider and wine. In these cases, they convert L-malic acid into L-lactic acid during the malolactic fermentation (MLF). In addition to malic acid, some other organic acids, sugars and carbon sources as glycerol may be utilized by LAB modifying the sensory quality of these products. In fruits juice and related product, they are considered spoilage microorganisms.

Carbohydrates metabolism by LAB follows the homofermentative or heterofermentative pathways with formation of lactate, or lactate, acetate, ethanol and CO_2, respectively. Studies on tomatoes microflora demonstrate that it is mainly constituted by obligatory heterofermentative LAB. D, L-lactic and acetic acids, CO_2, ethanol and diacetyl formed from glucose and fructose by LAB, affect the sensory properties of tomato purée by producing undesirable buttermilk and fermented flavor. In *Oenococcus oeni* strains from Argentinian wines growing in synthetic medium with acetate, equimolecular amount of D-lactate and ethanol in molar relation higher than 1 are produced from glucose. In deficient nutritional condition, glucose is diverted to the cysteine biosynthesis with decreased D-lactate recovery. In these strains the favorable effect of L-malic acid on the growth in synthetic medium and without essential amino acids is correlated with the energy gain associated with MLF.

---

[5]Correspondence to e-mail: mcmanca@fbqf.unt.edu.ar

Heterofermetative LAB from wine can metabolize citrate mainly to acetate, lactate, and carbon dioxide. Cells of *O. oeni* co-metabolizing citrate-glucose increase rate and molar yield growth. End products from glucose change: ethanol decreases and acetate is formed with ATP production via acetate kinase. It have been also demonstrated in this bacterium that citrate avoid essential amino acids requirement for growth. Fermentation balances indicate that part of citrate is diverted to the amino acids synthesis derived from aspartic acid.

Glycerol, produced during alcoholic fermentation in beverages, brings desirable properties (body, softness). But if it is used by LAB, depending on the pathway involved, the products formed can affect the product quality. Apparently the pathways to degrade glycerol in the species *Pediococcus pentosaceus* are variable. In the wine *Ped. pentosaceus* N_5p strain, glycerol is incorporated by an energy-dependent mechanism. It is degraded by the glycerol kinase (GK) pathway producing D-lactate, acetate and aroma compounds which can alter the flavor balance. *Ped. pentosaceus* CAg from beer degrade glycerol simultaneously by GK and glycerol dehydratase pathways producing high volatile acidity and aroma compounds that confer unacceptable flavors.

INTRODUCTION

Lactic acid bacteria (LAB) comprise an ecologically diverse group of microorganisms united by formation of lactic acid as the primary metabolite of sugar metabolism by either homo- or heterofermentative pathways. (Kandler, 1983, Davis et al., 1985; Lonvaud-Funel, 1999; Carr et al., 2002; Liu, 2002). LAB are fastidious microorganisms as regards their nutritional requirements, especially in growth factors such as amino acids, vitamins, purines and pyrimidines (Amoroso et al., 1993, Aredes Fernandez et al., 2004; Saguir and Manca de Nadra, 1997, 2007). Makarova et al. (2006) reported that the LAB have small genomes encoding a range of biosynthetic capabilities that reflect both prototrophic and auxotrophic characters.

LAB species are indigenous to food-related habitats, including plants (fruits, vegetables, and cereal grains) and milk environments. In addition, they are naturally associated with the mucosal surfaces of animals, e.g., small intestine, colon, and vagina.

Historically the genera Lactobacillus, Leuconostoc, Pediococcus and Streptococcus form the core of the group (Wood and Holzapfel, 1995; Stiles and Holzapfel 1997, Axelsson 1998). Taxonomic revision of these genera and the description of new genera mean that LAB could comprise, in their broad physiological definition, around 20 genera.

Metabolism of LAB has been exploited throughout history for the preservation of foods and beverages in nearly all societies dating back to the origins of agriculture (Miller and Wetterstrom, 2000). In addition to preservation, LAB also contribute to other product characteristics, such as flavor, texture and nutritional value (Carr et al., 2002; Welman and Maddox, 2003; Adolfsson et al., 2004).

Today, LAB play a prominent role in the world food supply, performing the main bioconversions in fermented dairy products, meats, and vegetables (Liu, 2003). LAB also are critical for the production of wine, cider, coffee, silage, cocoa, sourdough, and numerous indigenous food fermentations (Wood, 1998). Increased knowledge of LAB physiology such as metabolism, nutrient utilization, etc., is one way to achieve more controlled processes. Modern genetic techniques are also used in this way.

LAB can multiply in fruits and derivate products, which could be attributed to their metabolic diversity and tolerance to high acid environments. This fact may affect their quality both, positively and negatively (Liu 2002). Whereas in certain fermented beverages their growth and metabolism are desirable, in fresh fruits juice can lead to spoilage. Tajchakavit, (1998) demonstrated that *Lactobacillus* and *Leuconostoc* spp. can multiply in apple juice producing an undesirable buttermilk flavor caused by diacetyl production, a fermented flavor caused by organic-acid production and the swelling of packages caused by production of carbon dioxide from sugar and organic acids metabolism.

In fermented beverages, LAB are important mainly for L-malic acid degradation (Malolactic fermentation, MLF) which follows the alcoholic fermentation (AF) by yeasts (Davis et al. 1985). MLF produces the deacidification of wines and contributes to biological stability and flavor complexity (Fig. 1). Citric acid is other organic acid generally utilized by wine LAB in the natural medium. Some wine lactobacilli are known to degrade glycerol and mannitol, two of the main polyols in wine. All these transformation greatly influence the sensory and hygienic quality of wines.

Other metabolic activities of LAB of importance with regard to fermented beverages and juice fruits production are the proteolytic activity (Manca de Nadra et al., 1999, 2005; Aredes Fernandez et al., 2006, Savijoki, 2006), volatile aromatic compounds formation and aroma precursors (D'Incecco et al., 2004, Grimaldi et al., 2005), arginine metabolism, one of the major amino acids found in citrus, grapes juices and wines and amine production (Arena et al., 1999, 2002, 2005, Spano et al., 2007), anti-microbial compounds (Strasser de Saad et al., 1995) and exopolysaccharides production (Manca de Nadra and Strasser de Saad, 1995).

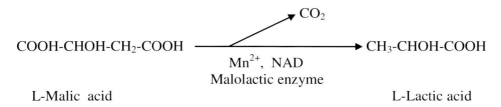

Figure 1. Malolactic fermentation by lactic acid bacteria from wines

The primary focus of this chapter is to evaluate the current knowledge of the sugars, organic acids and glycerol metabolism of LAB from fruits and fermented beverages, with a view to improve our understanding about their influences on the quality and manufacture of related food products.

SUGARS METABOLISM IN LACTIC ACID BACTERIA

The wide application of LAB in the production of fermented foods depends to a great extent on the unique features of sugar metabolism in these organisms. These bacteria produce mainly lactic acid from sugar, providing an effective method of preserving fermented products (Ehrmann and Vogel, 2005). The well established status of LAB as food organisms together with a relatively simple physiology make them suitable targets for metabolic engineering strategies aimed at the improvement of food quality and human health (Renault, 2002).

Two main sugar fermentation pathways can be distinguished among LAB to form lactic acid either the homo-or heterofermentative pathway (Fig. 2). The homofermentative pathway, results in the transformation of glucose to pyruvate, though Embden-Meyerhof-Parnas pathway (glycolsis) in which lactic acid is almost exclusively produced under standard condition. NADH formed by the oxidation of glyceraldehyde-3-phosphate to 1,3-bisphosphoglycerate is reoxidized to NAD^+ in the formation of lactate from pyruvate through the action of lactate dehydrogenases (LDH). The LDH enzymes vary in their stereospecificity and can yield D- or L-lactic acid or the racemic mixture (DL). Thus, 1 mole of glucose should produce 2 moles of lactic acid and energetically, glycolysis yields 2 moles ATP per mole glucose. Examples of lactobacilli that are obligate homofermenters are *Lactobacillus delbrueckii* and *Lactobacillus jensenii* (Hemme and Foucaud-Scheunemann, 2004).

In the heretofermentative pathway the microorganisms lack aldolase and must divert the flow of carbon through a different series of reaction, the pentose phosphate or phosphoketolase pathway in which significant amounts of other end products in addition to lactic acid are produced (Cocaign-Bousquet et al., 1996; Neves et al., 2005). From 1 mole of glucose, heterofermentative bacteria produce 1 mole each of lactate, CO_2, and either acetic acid and/or ethanol. Unlike homofermentative microorganisms, these bacteria possess phosphoketolase, the enzyme responsible for the cleavage of xylulose-5-phosphate to form glyceraldehyde-3-phosphate and acetyl phosphate. As consequence that only half of the carbon from glucose is converted to glyceraldehyde-3-phosphate only 1 mole of ATP is formed per mole glucose. However, heterofermentative bacteria can gain additional energy though conversion of acetyl-phosphate to acetate (Fig. 2).The LAB wine *Oenococcus oeni* (formely *Leuconostoc oenos,* Dick et al, 1995) is a heterofermentative bacterium (Kunkee, 1991).

Homo and heterofermentative metabolism differ fundamentally with respect to the requirement for regeneration of the reduced cofactors, NADH or NADPH.

Various growth conditions may alter the end product formation by some LAB. In lactobacilli, metabolites other than lactate may be the major end products of hexose metabolism at conditions of glucose limitation or in the presence of oxygen as electron acceptor (Cocaign-Bousquet et al., 1996; Axelsson, 2004). In *Lactococcus lactis* subsp. *lactis* MG1363 a shift in products formation by increasing aeration resultes in the formation of acetate, CO_2, and acetoin replacing formate and ethanol as end products (Nordkvist et al., 2003). When oxygen is present in the medium, the tight coupling of catabolic carbon fluxes that is needed to satisfy the redox balance is alleviated, since NAD^+ can be regenerated by the activity of NADH oxidases.

Besides obligate homo- and heterofermentative bacteria, Kandler and Weiss (1986) also described a third group of bacteria known as the facultative heterofermenters. Although these bacteria utilize hexoses through the homofermentative pathway, they also possess an inducible phosphoketolase with pentoses acting as inducers. Examples of wine bacteria belonging to this group are *Lac. casei* and *Lact. plantarum*.

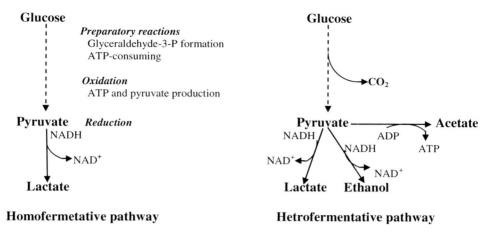

Figure 2. Glucose fermentation pathways in LAB from fruits and fermented beverages

Diacetyl is an important metabolite from the technology point of view that can be also formed from glucose catabolism. This is synthesized as an intermediary in the reductive decarboxylation of the pyruvic acid to 2,3-butanediol (Fig. 3) (Cogan, 1987; Ramos et al., 1995), and diacetyl is the product resulting from the chemical decarboxylation of a-acetolactate (Veringa et al., 1984; Hugenholtz and Starrenburg, 1992). Pyruvic acid is also derived essentially from the citric acid metabolism, and the formation of 2,3-butanediol may contribute to the redox balance of cellular metabolism. Diacetyl is an unstable end product and like other carbonyl compounds, such as acetaldehyde, it is further reduced to the corresponding alcohol, in this case 2,3-butanediol. The ability to utilize diacetyl by *O. oeni* has been demonstrated (Bartowsky and Henschke, 2004). Diacetyl imparts a buttery aroma and flavour to many fermented foods and beverages, being a key flavour compound of most fermented dairy products such as butter. Diacetyl is present in wine, cider and brandy. It is also found in beer, however in this beverage, it is considered to be spoilage characteristic. In wine, the diacetyl concentration is generally low relative to its flavour threshold and appears to be important to determining wine style (Bartowsky and Henschke, 2004).

Sugar metabolism, as well as the effects derived from the presence of mixed substrates, has been widely studied in strains of both homofermentative and heterofermentative LAB relevant to the dairy industry, such as *L. lactis*, *Leuconostoc mesenteroides*, and *Leuconostoc lactis*, mainly because of the importance of diacetyl as a flavor compound in dairy products (Cogan et al., 1981; Cogan, 1987, Starrenburg and Hugenholtz, 1991; Schmitt et al., 1992., Ramos et al., 1994; Vaningelgem et al., 2006). These studies have reported on growth stimulation, alterations in the substrate uptake rates, and molar ratios of the end products caused by the additional presence of citrate. Moreover, of all LAB *L. lactis* is by far the most extensively studied organism. The relative simplicity of its metabolism that converts sugars via the homofermentative pathway to pyruvate, generating energy mainly through substrate level phosphorylation, makes it an attractive target for the development of effective cell factories. On the other hand the availability of a large number of genetic tools (de Vos, 1999) and the complete genome sequence (Bolotin, 2001) consolidated its status as a model for LAB and offers the opportunity of adopting global approaches that could provide a comprehensive picture of how cellular components interact to produce a functional organism (Kuipers, 1999).

As regards to sugar metabolism in non-dairy LAB, such as fruits and fermented beverages less attention has been devoted.

Sugar Metabolism in Lactic Acid Bacteria from Fermented Beverages

Fermented beverages such as wine contain a range of monosaccharides (pentoses and hexoses) and disaccharides, with arabinose, glucose, fructose and trehalose being the major sugars (Liu, 2002). After completion of alcoholic fermentation, low concentrations of hexose sugars may remain in the wine.

The utilization of sugars by wine LAB as carbon and energy sources during MLF has been demonstrated in a number of studies and there exist species and strain differences in sugar utilization (Davis et al., 1986a, b; Fourcassie et al., 1992; Salou et al., 1994; Liu et al., 1995). Glucose and trehalose are generally preferred over other sugars (Liu et al., 1995). However, glucose remains the most frequently employed catabolic substrate providing energy necessary for growth of *O. oeni* from wines. Saguir and Manca de Nadra (1996) studied the effect of varying glucose concentrations in synthetic medium on biomass formation by a strain of *O. oeni* (Fig. 4).

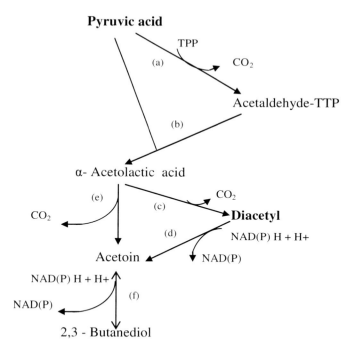

Figure 3. Pathway for diacetyl formation by LAB from pyruvate. Pyruvate decarboxylase (a), a-acetolactate synthase (b), non-enzymatic decarboxylation of α-acetolactic acid, diacetyl reductase (d), a-acetolactate decarboxylase (e), acetoin reductase (f), TTP thiamine PPi.

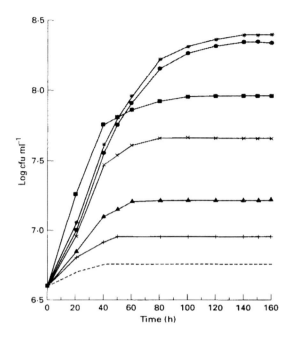

Figure 4. Effect of varying glucose on the growth of O. oeni m. Synhtetic medium without glucose (--) and with glucose (−) g/l: + 0.25; ▲ 0.5; x 1; ■ 4; * 10; • 20. (From Saguir and Manca de Nadra, 1996)

They demonstrated that no growth occurred when glucose was omitted. 0.5 g/l was the growth-limiting concentration and it was stimulated when glucose was increased to 4 g/l. Higher concentrations from 4 to 10 g/l did not modify the growth. With 20 g/l glucose, a slight stimulation of growth was observed during the first 30 h incubation but the final biomass was lower (Fig. 4). The authors established that one g/l sugar was completely used by this organism and that in the presence of 4 g/l glucose, between 40 and 50% was consumed by the end of growth. This explains why higher concentrations of glucose did not modify the growth of O. oeni M as shown in Figure 4. Saguir and Manca (1996) studied the metabolism of glucose at different concentrations, measuring the growth products after 150 h incubation of O. oeni m at 30°C. A synthetic medium without glucose was also analyzed. In order to measure the production of acetate, cells were cultivated in the basal synthetic medium with glucose, without potassium acetate. According to the theoretical stoichiometry of heterofermentative glucose metabolism 1 mmol of D-lactic acid was produced per mmol of glucose consumed and it was directly proportional to the growth. The ethanol produced in the medium was higher than 1 mmol per mmol of glucose and it could be derived from glucose and acetate. The additional 0.21, 0.64, 1.39 and 2.14 mmol/l produced in the presence of 0.25, 0.5, 1 and 4 g/l of glucose respectively (Table 1) could come from the potassium acetate of the medium.

However, the low percentage recovery of carbon from acetate to ethanol indicated that the rest of the acetate consumed could be incorporated as biomass, as reported by Schmitt et al., (1992). None of the L-lactic and acetic acids, diacetyl, acetoin or 2,3-butanediol were produced from glucose. These results indicate that the O. oeni strain from wine in synthetic medium ferments glucose via the heterolactic pathway to D-lactic acid, ethanol and CO_2, as ilustrated in the Figure 5, without acetate production from it. Ethanol can also be formed from some other substance than glucose as acetate, which also could be incorporated as biomass.

Table 1. Potassium acetate consumption and metabolite production in basal synthetic medium at different glucose concentrations

Glucose (mmol/l)	Potassium acetate (mmol/l)	Etanol produced (mmol/l)
1.39	1.49	1.60
2.77	3.02	3.41
5.55	6.60	6.94
22.22	10.21	17.54

Initial level of acetate: 166.5 mmol/l.
Potassium acetate consumption was measured after 150 h incubation at 30°C. (From Saguir and Manca de Nadra, 1996).

As mentioned above reports on the alteration of the pattern of fermentation products in LAB as a result of mixotrophic conditions are common in the literature (Cogan 1987; Lindgren et al., 1990.; Veiga-da-Cunha and Foster, 1992a). According to Saguir and Manca de Nadra, (1996, 2002) the addition of citrate showed a change in the analytical balance of the end products of glucose metabolism in the strain m of *O. oeni*: Ethanol concentration from glucose diminished from 1:1 to 1:0.6 and acetic acid was produced with an enhancement of ATP production via acetate kinase. As ATP production from glucose was more efficient in the presence of citric acid, the citrate + glucose-grown cells metabolized less glucose than glucose-grown cells. Cogan, (1987) reported that in *O. oeni* strains co-metabolizing glucose + citrate, little or no ethanol was produced. Gänzle et al,. (2007) described that lactate, ethanol and CO_2 are the major products of hexose metabolism unless co-substrates are present that enable the regeneration of reduced cofactors. Thus, under reductive conditions, cells experience a shortage of NAD^+ and so acetyl phosphate is converted to ethanol rather than acetate. Conversely, in the presence of electron-acceptors, acetyl-phosphate can be converted to acetate with the yield of an additional molecule of ATP as indicated in Figure 2 and increased volatile acidy.

Given the prominence of sugar metabolism and energy conversion systems in *Lactobacillales*, Makarova et al., (2006) examined the evolution of these systems through phyletic patterns, reflecting the presence or absence of genes in individual genomes in a manner similar to that described by Kooning and Galperin, (2003). Most of the genes involved in these functions are represented in all that species of LAB. These genes include those coding for the downstream part of glycolysis, from glyceraldehyde-3P to pyruvate and pyruvate conversion to lactate and 2,3-butanediol; acetate formation from acetyl-CoA; several reactions of the pentose–phosphate pathway; and the mannose-specific phosphotransferase system. The authors also demonstrated that these enzymes are insufficient to completely define the metabolism of any individual species, and several reactions are specific to individual lineages. The presence or absence of key enzymes involved in lactate fermentation poorly correlates with the phenotypes of the *Lactobacillales*. However, it has been shown that under certain conditions *Lactobacillales* can switch between sole production of lactic acid and the production of mixed end products, including acetic acid, lactic acid, ethanol, and CO_2 (Liu 2003; Hemme and Foucaud-Scheunemann, 2004).

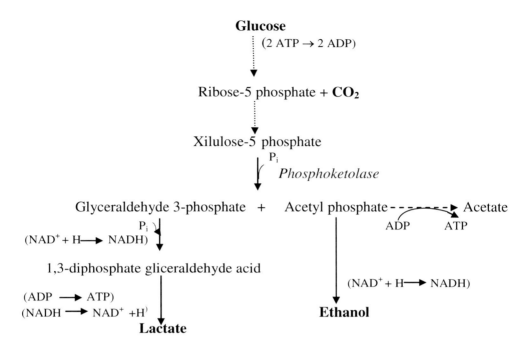

Figure 5. Heterofermentative metabolism of glucose in O. oeni from wines. According to Saguir and Manca de Nadra (1996) in O. oeni growing in synthetic medium glucose was recovered as CO2, ethanol and D-lactic acid. In presence of citric acid ethanol from glucose diminished and acid acetic was produced.

Glycerol and erythritol are alternative metabolites of LAB from glucose (Korakli et al., 2002). In *O. oeni* erythritol formation is likely to be governed by comparable mechanisms as in *Lact. sanfranciscensis*. Erythritol formation occurs only after panthotenic acid starvation (Richter et al., 2001). Panthotenic acid is required for the biosynthesis of coenzyme A, a cofactor in the phospho transacetylase reaction, and a reduced phospho transacetylase activity prevents cofactor recycling from acetyl-phosphate.

On the other hand, Saguir and Manca de Nadra (2002) demonstrated in the strain of *O. oeni* m from argentinian wine that it could be able to obtain carbon source for the synthesis of some essential amino acids through the catabolism of glucose. Specifically they reported that glucose could be involved in the cysteine formation under the studied conditions. This was related with the fact that when analyzed the fermentation balances from glucose in the synthetic culture medium where one essential amino acid was omitted in turn, in absence of asparagine, isoleucine or tyrosine approximately equimolecular amounts of D-lactic acid and ethanol were formed according to the theoretical stoichiometry of glucose metabolism (Fig. 6). Only the absence of cysteine was able to reduce the recovery of glucose as D-lactic acid, from 96% to 72%. In bacteria, cysteine is synthesized from serine by incorporation of sulphide or thiosulphate (Kitabatake et al. 2000) and serine is synthesized from 3-phosphoglycerate (Fig. 7). This late compound is an intermediate in the glucose metabolism.

The general assumption is that biomass synthesis in LAB is predominantly from building blocks present in the culture medium. However, this dissociation between catabolism of the energetic substrates (glucose, organic acids) and carbon assimilation from organic nitrogen sources (amino acids) may be less complete in deficient nutritional conditions, with some exchange of carbon flux between the different types of carbon substrates.

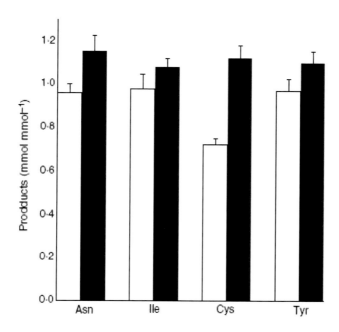

Figure 6. D-lactic acid (□) and ethanol (■) production from glucose by O. oeni m. Results are the ratio of amount of D-glucose consumed and D-lactic acid or ethanol produced in each basal synthetic medium deficiente in one essential amino acid (indicated at the bottom).(From Saguir and Manca de Nadra ,2002).

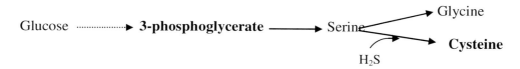

Figure 7. Cysteine formation from intermediary of glycolysis, 3-phosphoglycerate. According to Saguir and Manca de Nadra (2002) in deficient synhtetic medium, glucose could be involved in the cysteine formation.

Sugars Metabolism in Lactic Acid Bacteria from Fruits and Fruit Juices

In fresh fruits juice LAB are considered spoilage organisms. In the microbiological spoilage of fruit juices have been implicated yeasts, molds, and acetic and lactic bacteria causing formation of slime, gas, off flavor, turbidity, and changes in acidity by sugar and/or organic acids catabolism (Murdock and Hatcher, 1975; Juven, 1976). *Lac. plantarum* is a bacterial species that is frequently involved in several processes such as plant, meat and fish fermentations. As a spoilage agent *Lact. plantarum* can cause increasing volatile acidity and, in some cases, the degradation of tartaric acid leading to a depreciation of juice fruits. Its characterization is difficult because it is genotypically closely related and phenotypically highly similar to *Lact. pentosus* and *Lact. paraplantarum* (Curk et al. 1996). It has been demonstrated a PCR based-method that uses short recA gene sequences to perform a clear distinction among *Lact. plantarum*, *Lact. pentosus* and *Lact. paraplantarum* (Torriani et al., 2001,). Arena et al., (1996, 1999) identified from oranges surface *Lact. plantarum* strains and studied their amino acids and glucose utilization pattern in complex medium. They demonstrated that *Lact. plantarum* N8 and N4 strains co-metabolized glucose with arginine, citrulline or ornithine and that the utilization of arginine or citrulline reduced the glucose consumption rate (Table 2), presumably by providing an additional energy source from amino acids catabolism.

Table 2. Glucose consumption by *Lact. plantarum* N8 and N4 strains in BM and in BM with added arginine, citrulline or ornithine at 1 g/l*

Growth (h)	Glucose consumption (mmol/l)							
	Lact. plantarum N8				*Lact. plantarum* N4			
	BM	BM+Arg	BM+Cit	BM+Orn	BM	BM+Arg	BM+Cit	BMOrn
6	1.66	1.55	1.45	1.47	1.46	1.22	1.25	1.50
12	3.40	3.20	3.20	3.42	3.50	2.70	3.25	3.40
18	5.10	4.91	4.81	5.20	5.12	4.60	4.80	5.20
24	5.55	5.55	5.55	5.55	5.55	5.55	5.55	5.55

*BM, basal medium; Arg, arginine; Cit, citrulline; Orn, ornithine. Initial concentrations (mmol/ l): glucose, 5.55; arginine, 5.74; citrulline, 5.75; ornithine, 7.57. Means of three replicates, no significant difference (P50.05). (From Arena et al., 1999).

On the other hand Saguir et al., (2008) demonstrated in the N4 strain of *Lact. plantarum* from oranges that glucose utilization increased in the media containing dipeptides compared with the medium containing free amino acid in stress nutritional conditions. *Lact. plantarum* N4 consumed 20% of the initial glucose concentration at the end of exponential growth in a deficient basal medium containing a amino acid mixture. When Gly-Gly, Leu-Leu or both dipeptides replaced the respective free amino acids in this medium, sugar utilization increased from 4 to 6.2, 7.2 and 8.5 g/l, respectively (Fig. 8). This fact was related with the higher growth production in presence of dipeptides than free amino acids but not with a higher utilization for dipeptide uptake. The authors conclude that the ability of *Lact. plantarum* to use dipeptides efficiently could satisfy its nitrogen requirements in spoilage of orange juice, which is naturally low in amino acids.

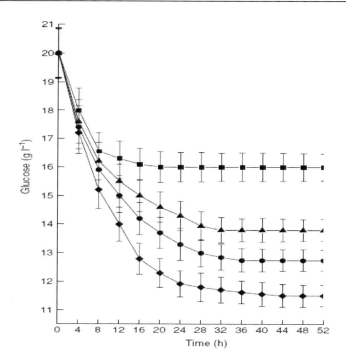

Figure 8. Changes in concentrations of residual glucose in cultures of Lact. plantarum N4. (■) Deficient basal medium with the amino acid mixture, control medium; (▲) control medium with Gly-Gly in place of glycine; (●) control medium with Leu-Leu in place of leucine; (◆) control medium with Gly-Gly and Leu-Leu in place of the respective amino acids. (From Saguir et al., 2008).

A study on tomato surface by Sajur et al., (2007) found that numbers of LAB of approximately $\log_{10} 4.5$ cfu/ml was in accordance with the results reported by Brackett (1988) and Drosinos et al. (2000). Enterobacteriaceae and yeasts were also isolated from tomatoes surface in similar way as that reported by Drosinos et al. (2000). Among isolates *Leuc. mesenteroides* ssp. *mesenteroides*, identified by FISH technique according to Blasco et al., (2003) was the predominant microflora, which might be related to better adaptation to tomato conditions and be able to initiate growth more rapidly than other LAB. *Leuc.* spp. predominance, and more particularly *Leuc. mesenteroides* in unprocessed vegetables had been reported by Nguyen-the and Carlin (2000). Sajur et al., (2007) further investigated the effect of the growth and metabolism of the strain Tsc of *Leuc. mesenteroides* subsp. *mesenteroides* on autochthonous microflora evolution on tomato purée during storage at temperature abusive. They showed the microbial population evolution in tomato purée medium inoculated with the strain Tsc stored at 30 °C for 26 d, and in uninoculated tomato purée medium as control (Fig. 9). In control medium, the initial microflora (1.6×10^1 cfu/g), constituted 75% by bacteria belonging to LAB group and 25% by bacteria identifed as *Staphylococcus* sp. on the basis that they were positive for gram staining, catalase activity and DNAse and coagulase tests, increased significantly reaching a maximum value of 10^6 cfu/g at 4 d. After 8 d it began to decrease progressively to reach a final cell concentration of 1.8×10^3 cfu/g at 16 d. Yeasts count was positive (3×10^4 cfu/g) just at 2 d and most at 12 d. Yeasts did not decreased at anytime during the tomato purée storage period. When the tomato purée was inoculated with *Leuc. mesenteroides* subsp. *mesenteroides* Tsc the initial bacterial population corresponding to 5.3×10^6 cfu/g increased by about 2 log cycles in 48 h, the inoculated organism being isolated. On the other hand, at 2d storage, yeasts count was approximately 2 log cycle lower than that obtained in uninoculated medium. Yeasts continued growing to reach the same cell density as that observed in control medium. After 8 d incubation in inoculated tomato purée medium, the bacterial count also began to decrease but at a lower rate than that obtained in the uninoculated one (Fig. 9). Samples of uninoculated tomato purée medium were sensorially unacceptable at 8 d storage (odor and visual signs of alteration) whilst this effect was just observed in the inoculated medium at 19 d storage. These results demonstrate that the growth and metabolism of *Leuc. mesentroides* subsp. *mesenteroides* inhibit natural bacterial development and delaying the growth of yeasts in tomato purée.

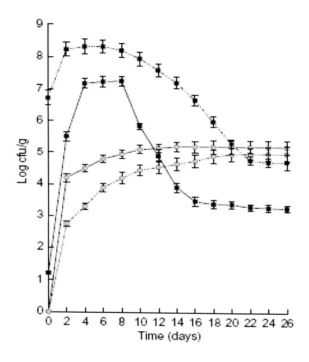

Figure 9. Evolution of bacteria and yeasts in tomato purée media. Uninoculated medium (—) and inoculated medium with Leuc. Mesenteroides ssp. mesenteroides Tsc (- - -) stored at 30 °C. Bacteria cfu/g (■), yeasts cfu/g (○). (From Sajur et al., 2007)

These authors also demonstrated that native tomato purée microflora utilized glucose and fructose producing D, L-lactic and acetic acids and ethanol for growth, which is relate with a heterofermentative metabolism. The amount of end products by native microflora occurred in a higher extent than inoculated microorganism (Fig. 10a,b), especially in the case of fructose consumption and L-lactic acid formation (80 and 98% higher in control medium than in inoculated medium, respectively). So the autochthonous bacterial microflora from tomato purée was not mainly composed by the predominant microorganism from tomatoes surface, even when heterofermentative microorganisms were present. This fact could be related with the low pH of internal tissue of tomato which would favor the growth of other LAB, such as Lactobacilli. On the other hand tomato composition could be an important factor in enabling the growth of LAB requiring growth factors. Babu et al., (1992) reported the stimulatory effect of tomato juice on the growth of *Lactobacillus* sp. Metabolism of natural microflora was correlated with the changes in sensory properties of tomato purée medium producing undesirable buttermilk and fermented flavor by the high diacetyl and organic acids concentration, respectively. The inhibition of natural microflora delayed these changes in the medium. Simsek et al., (2004) reported in sourdough process the importance of role of the lactic and acetic acids on the aroma profile. Sajur et al., (2007) described that in tomato purée *Leuc. mesenteroides* ssp. *mesenteroides* Tsc preferred as main carbon and energy source glucose rather than fructose for growth (Fig. 10b). A similar result was reported by Gardner et al., (2001) in *Leuc. mesenteroides* growing in vegetable juice medium. By contrast, in *Lact. sanfranciscensis* from sourdough, maltose is the preferred carbon source for growth (Gänzle et al., 2007). It is internalized by a maltose/H^+ symporter and cleaved to glucose and glucose-1-phosphate by maltose phosphorylase (Stolz et al., 1996). The obligate heterofermentative organisms *Lact. brevis*, *Lact. pontis*, *Lact. reuteri* and *Lact. fermentum* also exhibit this enzymatic activity (Stolz et al., 1996).

Sajur et al., (2007) demonstrated that the D-lactic acid, CO_2, etanol and acetic acid were formed from sugars heterofermentative metabolism by *Leuc. mesenteroides* subsp. *mesenteroides* Tsc in tomato purée (Fig. 10b). However the amount of D-lactic acid was lower than expected theoretical value indicating that sugars metabolism could be involved in biosynthesis reactions. Similar result was reported in *O. oeni* as mentioned above (Saguir and Manca de Nadra, 2002). In inoculated medium the changes in organoleptic properties were evident 11 d later than in uninoculated medium and this fact was related to the quantities of the metabolites produced (specially organic acids) in the different uninoculated/inoculated media during storage.

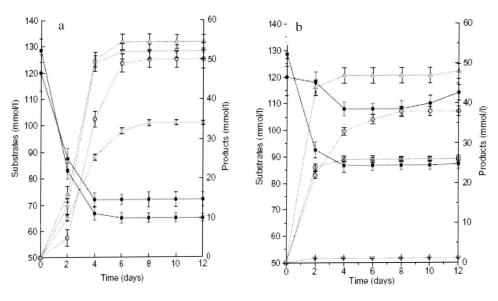

Figure 10. Substrates consumption and metabolites production in uninoculated (a) and inoculated (b) tomato purée medium during storage at 30 °C. Substrates: glucose (■), fructose (●). Products: D-lactic acid (□), L-lactic acid (∇), acetic acid (Δ), ethanol (O). (From Sajur et al., 2007).

The faster production of organic acids during the first 48 h incubation in inoculated tomato purée medium with respect to control medium explained the rapid pH diminution (Fig. 11). This may contribute to the inhibitory effect of inoculated microorganism growth on natural microflora of tomato purée. *Leuc. mesenteroides* subsp. *mesenteroides* could be considered to help to control the contaminates proliferation on tomato purée during storage at abusive temperature.

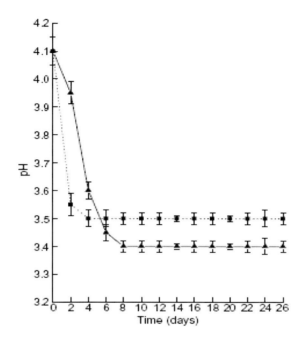

Figure 11. Variation of pH in tomato purée media during storage time at 30 °C. Uninoculated medium (▲) and inoculated medium (■). (From Sajur et al., 2007).

ORGANIC ACIDS METABOLISM BY LACTIC ACID BACTERIA FROM FRUITS AND BEVERAGES

Because of the complexity of the media in which natural fermentations occurs strong metabolic interactions between the multiple substrates are expected.

L-malic and citric acids are certainly the organic acids that LAB from wine degrades most frequently in their natural environment. *O. oeni* is the major species responsible for the conversion of L-malic acid to L-lactic acid though MLF (Fig. 1) (Kunkee, 1991). On the other hand, citrate metabolism is widespread among LAB. The breakdown of citrate results in the production of acetate, formate, ethanol, acetaldehyde, acetoin, 2,3-butanediol, diacetyl, and carbon dioxide. Some of these compounds such as diacetyl contribute to the flavor development in fermented foods including fermented beverages (Ramos et., 1994; De Figueroa et al., 1998; Nielsen and Richelieu, 1999, Augagneur et al., 2007). The ability to metabolize citrate is dependent on the presence of the enzyme citrate permease (CitP), which has been characterized in strains belonging to the genera *Oenococcus, Leuconostoc* and

Lactococcus (Ramos et al., 1994; Bandell et al., 1998; García-Quintáns et al., 1998). Citrate and malate uptake are electrogenic process, which together with the formation of a pH gradient across the cell membrane, results in the formation of a proton motive force and hence generation of metabolic energy (Bandell et al., 1998). In *O. oeni* both organic acids are internalized by an electrogenic uniport mechanism generating the membrane potential $\Delta\psi$ (Ramos et al., 1996).

Saguir and Manca de Nadra (1996) demonstrated that the growth of wines *O. oeni* strains was greatest in synthetic medium with L-malic and/or citric acids. Organic acids (Fig. 12), especially citric acid, increased the growth of the strain of *O. oeni* m, but neither L-malic nor citric acid alone or in combination supported the growth in the absence of sugar, confirming that under the experimental conditions, glucose was the main or sole carbon source. The maximum specific growth rates the strain m of *O. oeni* were 0.094 h⁻ for cells growing in basal medium with 4 g/l glucose, 2.5 g/l L-malic acid and 0.7 g/l citric acid during the early stage of growth. This could be related with the fact that organic acids could avoid both carbon flux and energy limitations Enhanced growth rate was obtained for other *O. oenos* strains when L-malic or citric acids were used in addition to glucose (Schmitt and Divies 1992; Loubière et al.. 1992; Salou et al 1994; Augagneur et al. 2007).

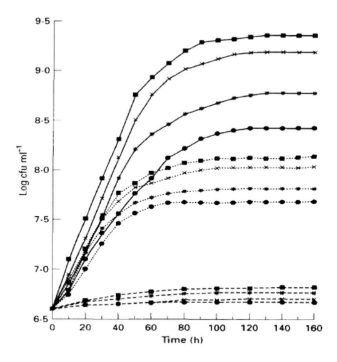

Figure 12. Effect of 2.5 g/l of L-malic acid and 0.7 g/l of citric acid on the growth of O. oeni m. Basal medium without glucose (---); with 1 g/l of glucose (...); and with 4 g/l glucose (—).Without organic acids (•); with L-malic acid (*);with citric acid (x); with both organic acids (■). (From Saguir and Manca de Nadra, 1996).

Saguir and Manca de Nadra (1996) also demonstrated that glucose, L-malic and citric acids were simultaneously consumed by the *O. oeni* strain as illustrated in Figure 13. As soon as growth began glucose, L-malic and citric acids were simultaneously utilized. The L-malic acid was metabolized at a higher rate than glucose and citric acid. L-malic and citric acids were completely consumed after 40 and 80 h incubation at 30°C respectively. Consumption of the triple substrate could explain the maximum growth rate found in the early stage of *O. oeni* m growth with both organic acids. Similar results were reported by Tracey and Van Roogen, (1988) for *O. oeni* growing on glucose + malate. Radler, (1975) found that L-malic acid was utilized before sugar but Pimentel et al., (1994) showed that L-malic acid was simultaneously consumed with glucose when *O. oeni* was incubated at 37°C, pH 4.0 or 4.5, and that citrate was consumed more slowly than malate. Miranda et al., (1997) reported that the co-metabolism of sugar with L-malate is strain and pH dependent.

In *O. oeni*, citric acid was consumed only when the glucose concentration was 1 g/l or higher. Possibly this concentration was necessary for citrate uptake (Saguir and Manca de Nadra, 1996).

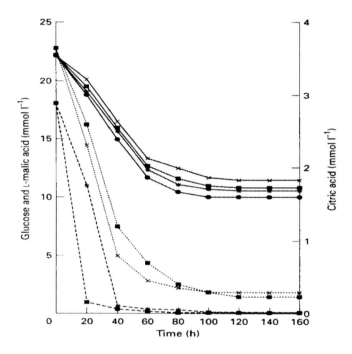

Figure 13. Glucose, L-malic and citric acids consumption by O. oeni m metabolism in the presence of 4 g/l glucose. Glucose (—); L-malic acid (---) and citric acid (. . .). Without organic acids (●); with L-malic acid (*); with citric acid (x); with both organic acids (■). (From Saguir and Manca de Nadra, 1996).

Saguir and Manca de Nadra (2002) studied the time course of L-malic acid utilization and L-lactic acid formation in basal media lacking an essential amino acid for the *O. oeni* m growth, in presence of 2.5 g/l of L-malic acid (Fig. 14). They demonstrated that the L-malic acid utilization began immediately growth began in the basal medium without asparagine, isoleucine or tyrosine and it was consumed more rapidly after 40 h incubation. In these conditions after 80 h incubation *O. oeni* m degraded nearly all of the initial L-malic acid, especially in absence of tyrosine and it was accompanied by a corresponding increase in concentration of L-lactic acid. When cysteine was omitted from basal medium, *O. oeni* m began to use the dicarboxylic acid at 40 h incubation at 30°C coinciding with the end of lag growth phase. In this condition, L-malic acid was consumed at a lower rate than those observed when asparagine, cysteine or tyrosine were individually eliminated from basal medium and this could be related with the lower growth rate reached by this strain in absence of cysteine. L-Lactic acid continued to accumulate into the medium throughout the period of L-malic acid degradation and accounted for approximately 100% L-malic acid consumed. The production of L-lactic acid from L-malic acid by *O. oeni* m in the cited media could explain why the final pH values were higher (about 0.15 unit) than initial pH value. These results exclude any possibility of some incorporation of L-malic acid into biomass. However, the biochemical energy gain by proton motive force associated with MLF (Fig. 1) must be taken into account as additional advantage to carry out anabolic reactions and cellular processes. Salema et al., (1996) reported that the intracellular L-malate decarboxylation leads to the consumption of a proton yielding a pH gradient (ΔpH) and efflux of lactic acid. Similarly, the decarboxylation of oxaloacetate into pyruvate during citrate metabolism generates a ΔpH (Ramos et al., 1994; Lolkema et al., 1995; Salema et al., 1996; Marty-Teysset et al., 1996; Konings, 2002).

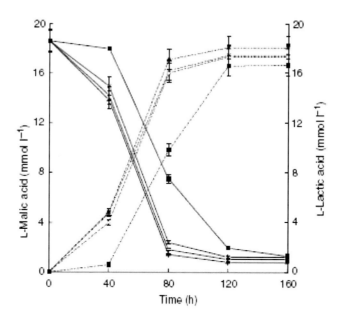

Figure 14. L-malic acid consumption (—) and L-lactic acid production (----) by *O. oeni* m metabolism in each basal medium deficient in one essential amino acid. Without: Aspn (O); Ile (X); Cys (■); Tyr (▲). (From Saguir and Manca de Nadra, 2002).

The effects of L-malic and citric acids on the growth, the ΔpH, the $\Delta\psi$ and the expression of carboxylic acids transporters were investigated under several pH conditions by Augagneur et al., (2007). At pH 5.3, the results obtained were in agreement with previous studies for which a stimulating effect of organic acids was observed at pH 4.8 or above (Saguir and Manca de Nadra 1996, 2002; Versari et al. 1999). In addition the L-malate and citrate consumption contributed to the generation of a high ΔpH. The stimulating effect of L-malate for the biomass formed increased at low pH, whereas the addition of citrate in the medium resulted in a strong inhibition. Despite this inhibition of the growth, *O. oeni* was able to maintain a pH gradient close to 2 units in PM-citrate buffer at pH 3.2. Consequently, the negative impact of citrate observed during growth at pH 3.2, did not significantly affect the maintenance of the pH gradient. This suggested that citrate did not act as a direct inhibitor of growth, but probably one of its end products, such as acetate, played this role. Acetate is a weak acid presenting a pKa of 4.75 that is produced during the first step of citrate breakdown. Thus, when the pH is equal or below 4.5, most of the acetate present in the medium is protonated and can re-enter the bacterium. Moreover, at pH 4.5 and 3.2, acetate is quickly accumulated in media containing citrate. The addition of acetate during the growth or during ΔpH and Δψ measurements showed that it played a significant role in the inhibition of the growth and to a lesser extent to the alteration of the pH gradient and membrane potential. Thus, it appears that citrate metabolism has a stimulating or inhibitory effect as a function of the external pH. Study of the genes expression involved in the organic acids metabolism showed that at pH 4.5 and 3.2 the presence of L-malate led to an increased amount of mRNA of mleP encoding a malate transporter (Augagneur et al., 2007). This suggests that mleP encodes a carrier protein responsible for L-malate uptake by *O. oeni* as previously described (Labarre et al., 1996).

Saguir and Manca de Nadra (1996) studying the utilization of citric acid in a basal synthetic medium wih with glucose and citrate, determined that acetic and D-lactic acids and CO_2 were produced from citric acid as illustrated in Figure 15. No aroma compounds were detected.

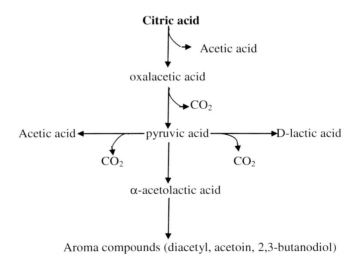

Figure 15. End-products from citric acid metabolism in LAB. According to Saguir and Manca de Nadra (1996) in O. oeni growing in synthetic medium citric acid was completely recovered as CO2, and D-lactic and acetic acids. In absence of isoleucine or asparagine an imbalance from citrate to D-lactic acid was observed (Saguir and Manca de Nadra, 2002).

The time course of citric acid utilization and metabolic products formation in basal media lacking an essential amino acid for *O. oeni* M growth in presence of 0.7 g/l of citric acid, respectively (Fig. 16 and Table 3) was also investigated by Saguir and Manca de Nadra (2002). The citric acid utilization was faster when isoleucine was omitted from culture medium than in absence of tyrosine, asparagine or cysteine. This result coincided with the higher growth rate reached by *O. eni* m in the basal medium without isoleucine in presence of citric acid. When cysteine, tyrosine or asparagine were individually eliminated from basal medium, the final consumption of citric acid was 85.7, 78.6 and 77.1%, respectively, at 120 h incubation at 30°C (Fig. 16). At this time, 120 h (Table 3), a 100% recuperation of glucose–citrate utilization as D-lactic acid was observed only when tyrosine was omitted from the complete medium, in the same way as for basal medium. The recovery of glucose–citrate as D-lactic acid was 27, 21 and 18% lower than in the complete basal medium with citric acid, when asparagine, isoleucine or cysteine were removed from culture medium, respectively. Ethanol and acetate production from glucose- citrate metabolism by *O. oeni* m was not affected by the omission of asparagine, isoleucine, cysteine or tyrosine from culture medium and no diacetyl, acetoin or 2,3- butanediol were produced. The lower recovery of glucose-citrate as D-lactic acid only observed when citrate was present in the synthetic medium lacking asparagine or isoleucine, indicated that part of it metabolism was diverted by *O. oeni* for the synthesis of asparagine or isoleucine amino acids (both derivate from aspartic acid), via oxalacetate (Fig.15). Moreover, the amount of D-lactic acid recovered from glucose-citrate metabolism was 5% higher in the absence of isoleucine than in the medium without asparagine, supporting the idea that citric acid utilization would be involved primarily in the asparagine biosynthesis.

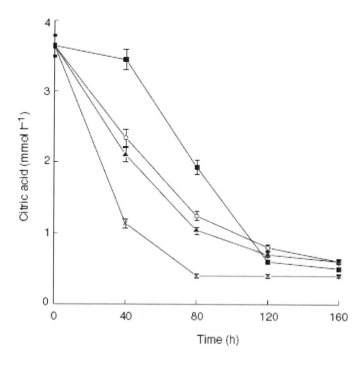

Figure 16. Citric acid consumption by *O. oeni* m metabolism in each basal medium deficient in one essential amino acid. Aspn (O); Ile (X); Cys (■); Tyr (▲). (From Saguir and Manca de Nadra, 2002).

Table 3. Product stoichiometries of *O. oeni* strain growing on glucose + citric acid in each basal medium deficient in one essential amino acid.

Amino acid omitted in the medium	D-lactate (mmol/mmol of glu+cit)	Ethanol (mmol/mmolglu)	Acetate (mmol/mmol of glu+cit)
L-Asparagine	0.73±0.03	0.76±0.03	0.43±0.02
L-Isoleucine	0.79±0.04	0.71±0.02	0.46±0.02
L-Cysteine	0.82±0.03	0.61±0.03	0.53±0.03
L-Tyrosine	1.03±0.04	0.65±0.03	0.49±0.02

(From Saguir and Manca de Nadra, 2002).

Thus, citric acid catabolism in nutritional stress condition in *O. oeni* can be involved in the biosynthesis of aspartate-derived amino acids: asparagine and isoleucine. Ramos et al., (1995) demonstrated in *O. oeni* isolated from wine, that at least 10% of the citric acid supplied was converted to aspartate that was not excreted to the extracellular medium. Marty-Teysset et al., (1996) have reported that the citrate pathway in *Leuc. mesenteroides* subsp. *mesenteroides*, under certain culture conditions, was directed towards the formation of aspartate.

Saguir and Manca de Nadra, (1998) demonstrated that *O. oeni* was able to produce L-asparagine in synthetic medium deprived of asparagine supplemented with a tenfold higher concentration of L-aspartic acid. This production increased in presence of L-malic and citric acids and ammonium sulphate. The stimulant effect of ammonium ion suggested that the number of amino acids retained in the medium could not supply the entire nitrogen requirement of the cell to carry out anabolic reaction. Different results were reported by Cocaign-Bousquet et al., (1995), which observed that the growth of two *Lactococcus* strains from vegetable and dairy origin, in minimal synthetic medium was not perturbed by the suppression of ammonium ion indicating that the amino acid and nucleotide content of the medium satisfies the nitrogen requirement for biomass synthesis.

The shift to an alternative pathway of citrate breakdown in different conditions for the production of other end products such as acetoin was also described. Ramos et al., (1995) showed that in *O. oeni*, 94% of pyruvate was converted into acetoin at pH 4.0. This orientation, under low pH conditions, could tend to a lower production of weak acids and thus lesser perturbation of intracellular pH.

Utilization of acetic acid as biosynthetic precursor for cellular component synthesis was also demonstrated in LAB. Collins and Bruhn (1970) reported that exogenous acetate and acetate from citrate metabolism was incorporated into cell lipids of *L. lactis* subsp. *lactis* var. *diacetylous*. Similar result was demonstrated in this bacterium by Nordkvist (2003) since the addition of extracellular acetate increased the sizes of the pools of intracellular acetyl-phosphate and acetyl-CoA at which fatty acids could be synthesized. However, Saguir ad Manca de Nadra (2002) concluded in *O. oeni* that acetic acid derived from citric acid was not involved in the biosynthesis reactions.

On the other hand Sajur et al. (2007) investigated the utilization of L-malic and citric acids and their metabolic products during the natural microflora growth in control tomato purée during storage at 30 °C. The same experience was carry out in the natural medium inoculated with *Leuc. mesenteroides* subsp *mesenteroides* Tsc, where the natural bacterial growth was inhibited as mentioned above (Fig. 17).

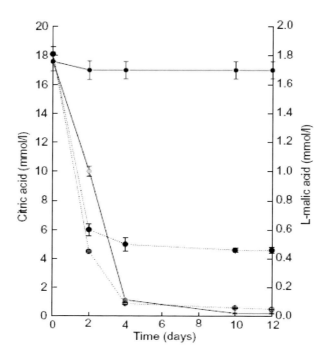

Figure 17. Citric and L-malic acids consumption in tomato purée media during storage at 30 °C. Citric acid (—), L-malic acid (- - -). Uninoculated medium (O), inoculated medium (●).

Initial concentrations of citric and L-malic acids were 17.59 and 1.79 mmol/l, respectively. These results coincided with those reported for San Marzano tomato varieties from Italy (Loiudice et al., 1995). Forty-seven percentage and 87.5% of initial citric acid concentration was utilized at 2 and 4d incubation, respectively. Natural microflora consumed 88.8% of initial L-malic acid at 2d incubation and almost 100% at 4d. Considering the low initial concentration of the dicarboxylic acid, only a very small amount of L-lactic acid could have been formed from its catabolism, this product being mainly formed from sugar metabolism. It was noticeable that in inoculated tomato purée citric acid was not utilized although 56% of initial L-malic acid was utilized (Fig. 17). L-lactic acid was accumulated into the medium throughout the period of L-malic acid degradation and accounted for approximately 100% L-malic acid consumed. Thus Citric and L-malic acids were consumed in control medium but in inoculated medium with the strain of *Leuc. mesenteroides* subsp *mesenteroides* citric acid was not utilized.

Starrenburg and Hugenholtz, (1991) reported in *L. lactis* and *Leuc.* sp. that the activity of the citrate permease has an optimum pH between 5.5 and 6.0. In tomato purée the pH of the natural medium, lower than 5.0, could explain the inability of the strain of *Leuc. mesenterides* to utilize it. In *Leuconostoc* and *Lactococcus*, only a stimulating effect was reported and explained by the action of citrate as an external electron acceptor, resulting in additional acetate and ATP production (Schmitt et al., 1990; Starrenburg and Hugenholtz, 1991), or by its implication in mechanisms against lactate toxicity (Magni et al., 1999). In *Leuconostoc* and *Lactococcus*, the transporter involved in the uptake of citrate acts as a divalent citrate/monovalent lactate antiporter, whereas in *O. oeni* the transporter catalyzes uniport of monoanionic citrate (Ramos et al. 1994; Marty-Teysset et al. 1996; Bandell et al., 1998). Analysis of citrate consumption in *Leuc. paramesenteroides* J1 showed that its citrate permease and its citrate lyase are induced by the presence of citrate in the growth medium. Southern blot analysis demonstrated that the citMCDEFGRP cluster is located in a plasmid. Homology of the inferred gene products with characterized enzymes reveals that citP encodes the citrate permease P, citC the citrate ligase and citDEF the subunits of the citrate lyase of *Leuconostoc* (Drider et al., 2004).

GLYCEROL METABOLISM IN LACTIC ACID BACTERIA

Glycerol is quantitatively the most important by-product produced by yeast during alcoholic fermentation besides ethanol and carbon dioxide. It is a non-volatile compound which has not aromatic properties, but which significantly contributes to fermented beverages quality by providing sweetness and fullness (Ribereau Gayon et al., 1972; Eustace and Thornton, 1987).

Even when wine LAB play an important role in the MLF (Kunkee, 1991; Lonvaud-Funel, 1999), after alcoholic fermentation, when sugars are exhausted, glycerol can be used by LAB to maintain their viability and, depending on the way used for degrading it, they can be responsible for alterations of wine quality. Bacteria belonging to the genera *Lactobacillus* and *Pediococcus* that degrade glycerol are associated with the spoilage of wine (Beneduce et al., 2004). Different metabolic ways implied in the degradation of glycerol have been described in bacteria and little information exist referred to LAB in general and particularly in those species involved in the fermented beverages.

The LAB from wine has not the same ability to use glycerol and two catabolic pathways are mainly involved: the Glycerol dehydratase (reductive) and the Glycerol kinase (oxidative) pathways but Glycerol dehydrogenase pathway can also be involved.

When glycerol is metabolized by Glycerol dehydratase pathway (Fig. 18), they could be responsible for the development of bitterness. Through this way, glycerol is transformed into β- hydroxypropanal by means of the action of the enzyme glycerol dehydratase β-hydroxypropanal can follow different ways: it can be reduced to 1.2 or 1,3-propanediol by action of the corresponding propanediol dehydrogenase. β- hydroxypropanal can undergo spontaneous intramolecular dehydration and give rise to acrolein whose formation is favored by the acid conditions and heat, which explains its presence in spirits fermented and distilled beverages (Serjak et al, 1954; Sovolob and Smyley, 1960). The last product combined with wine polyphenols is responsible for bitterness (Smiley and Sobolov, 1962; Rankine and Bridson, 1971). For that reason, its formation is undesirable in wines and other fermented drinks.

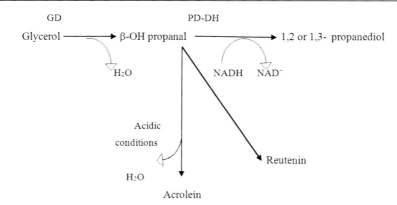

Figure 18. Glycerol dehydratase pathway. Glycerol dehydratase (GD), Propanediol dehydrogenase (PD-DH).

Among LAB, this pathway is present in some wine strains of *Lact. brevis*, *Lact. buchneri*, that use glycerol in co-fermentation with fructose or glucose (Sobolov and Smiley, 1960; Schutz and Radler, 1984 a,b; Talarico and Dobrogosz, 1990). Both strains can also co-ferment glycerol with ribose or lactate (Veiga da Cunha and Foster, 1992 a,b)

Glycerol dehydratase pathway is also demonstrated in *Lact. collinoides* and *Lact. diolivorans* isolated from bitter tasting ciders in which glycerol was partially removed (Claisse and Lonvaud-Funel, 2000; Sauvageot et al., 2000; Garai-Ibabe et al., 2008) *Lact. collinoides* uses glycerol in the presence of fructose producing always 1,3-propanediol as the main end-product in all environmental conditions assayed except with 5.55 mM fructose, where equimolar amounts of 1,3-propanediol and 3-hydroxypropionic acid were found. The β- hydroxypropanal was transitorily accumulated in the culture medium under almost all culture conditions, but no disappearance of β- hydroxypropanal occur at pH 3.6, a usual value in cider making. After sugar exhaustion, *Lact. collinoides* strain oxidated lactic acid and/or mannitol to obtain energy and these oxidations were accompanied by the removal of the toxic β- hydroxypropanal increasing the 1,3-PDL, 3-hydroxypropionic acid and acetic acid contents.

The second involved metabolic way in the catabolism of glycerol constitutes the Glycerol kinase pathway (Fig. 19), by which glycerol is phosphorilated to glycerol 3-phosphate by a glycerol kinase using ATP and magnesium. The glycerol 3-phosphate formed is oxidized to dihydroxyacetone phosphate by a glycerol 3-P dehydrogenase that can be NAD-dependent, FAD- dependent or NAD - independent being these last those that uses an external electron acceptor different from the NAD, like nitrate, succinate, etc (Lin, 1976). Later the generated metabolites arrive until pyruvate to originate their products of fermentation, like in the oxidative way. The enzymes of this metabolic way widely were studied and are members of regulon *glp*.

This pathway is present among homofermentative wine LAB (Lonvaud-Funel, 1986; Salado and Strasser de Saad, 1995; Pasteris and Strasser de Saad, 1997; Pasteris and Strasser de Saad 1998; Pasteris and Strasser de Saad, 2005). High volatile acidity and aroma compounds are produced from glycerol, conferring unacceptable flavor to wine.

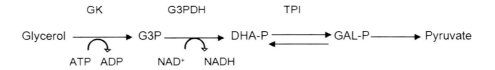

Figure 19. Glycerol kinase pathway. Glycerol kinase (GK), Glycerol-3P-dehydrogenase (G3PDH), Triose phosphate isomerase (TPI).

The third implied metabolic way in the use of glycerol is represented by the oxidative pathway (Fig. 20), by which glycerol is oxidized to dihydroxyacetone by NAD - dependent glycerol dehydrogenase and the product is then phosphorilated by the dihydroxyacetone kinase. The dihydroxyacetone phosphate generated, is in balance with 3-phosphate glyceraldehyde, through a triose-P isomerase. These last ones are substrates of the glycolitic way, through which the products derived from the pyruvate metabolism will be synthesized: lactate, acetate, ethanol and aroma compounds (diacetyl, acetoin, 2,3-butanediol), depending on the involved microorganism and the functionality of the enzymatic systems.

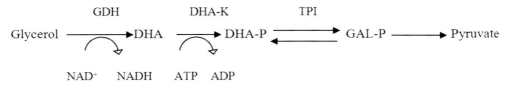

Figure 20. Glycerol dehydrogenase pathway. Glycerol dehydrogenase (GDH), Dihydroxyacetone phosphate kinase (DHA-K), Triose phosphate isomerase (TPI).

It is important to emphasize that this metabolic route has not been deciphers in lactic bacteria until our works in *Ped. pentosaceus* (Pasteris and Strasser de Saad, 2005).

Glycerol Metabolism in Pediococcus Pentosaceus

From Wine

Previous information about glycerol utilization by *Ped. pentosaceus* was that referred to a strain isolated from silage. Dobrogosz and Stone (1962) reported that glycerol is oxidized to pyruvate, producing lactate, acetate acetoin and CO_2 in a molar ratio 1:1:1:3. The enzymes involved are glycerol kinase and FAD dependent α-glycerophosphate dehydrogenase that use oxygen as electron aceptor. The hydrogen peroxide is them degraded by a catalase activity. The aerobic growth on glycerol and the existence of a catalase activity suggest the presence of citocroms in this group of microorganisms.

Considering the importance of glycerol in wine, your excessive consumption is regarded as undesirable. Being *Ped. pentosaceus* the predominant species in same argentine wines (Manca de Nadra and Strasser de Saad, 1987; Strasser de Saad and Manca de Nadra, 1987), if the strains possess the ability to use glycerol they can be responsible of wine spoilage. In the aim of know the contribution of this specie to the composition and the quality of the wine, Salado and Strasser de Saad (1995) begin the study of glycerol metabolism in wine strains.

Among the strains of *P. Pentosaceus* isolated from argentinian wines,only two of them are capable to growth on glycerol as sole carbon source E$_{13}$p and N$_5$p. The last strain was selected for studies since it produce a bacteriocin that was demonstrated useful for wine microflora control (Strasser de Saad et al., 1995)

Ped. pentosaceus N$_5$p degrade glycerol in microaerophilic conditions, producing D-lactate, acetate and diacetyl. Among these products, diacetyl at very low levels and acetate at certain concentrations are undesirable compounds in alcoholic beverages because its involvement in the production of off flavor. For this reason, the study of the effect of factors involved in vinification as ethanol, SO$_2$ and malate was considered useful for the understanding the influence of these strains on the composition and qualyty of wine (Salado and Strasser de Saad,1996).The addition of malate inhibits partially glycerol utilization. Ethanol inhibits the growth of this strain and the consumption of glycerol and malate. Moreover, lactate and acetate production decrease and diacetyl production is abolished. SO$_2$ stimulate the bacterial growth and glycerol consumption but in the presence of malate it is reduced. Lactate and acetate production are not modified but diacetyl production is inhibited. These results we permit to conclude that, in the wine conditions, N$_5$p strain has not a potential responsibility neither on glycerol degradation nor wine spoilage.

In the aim to explain the pathway of glycerol consumption and the end products formed by *Ped. pentosaceus* N$_5$p, all possible enzyme activities involved were determined cell free extracts (Pasteris and Strasser de Saad,1997).

In this strain, the pathway of Glycerol kinase is present, involving glycerol kinase and a NAD-independent glycerol-3-phosphate dehydrogenase. The levels of these activities suggest a probable role of glycerol in the induction the enzymes mainly of G3PDHi and a repressor effect of glucose . This pathway is present in *Lact. casei* Cog 812 (Lonvaud-Funel, 1986) strain that use glycerol but only when glucose is absent producing lactate and aroma compounds. In this strain degradation of glycerol occur by a glycerol kinase and a NAD$^+$-dependent glycerol 3-P dehydrogenase. The products of the metabolism are lactate, acetoin and diacetyl.

The pathway of Glycerol dehydratase detected in heterofermentative lactobacilli (Schutz and Radler, 1984a and b;Talarico and Dobrogosz, 1990) is absent in *Ped. pentosaceus* N$_5$p.

The enzymes related to lactate formation are NAD- dependent and NAD-independent lactate dehydrogenases (LDH). The levels of NAD-dependent D-LDH are always higher than that of NAD-dependent L-LDH, that is activated by fructose1,6-diphosphate, whereas the opposite ratio is observed in NAD-independent LDHs that degrade lactate. These results explain the absence of L-lactate from glycerol.

In glycerol medium, the sugar is absent and NAD independent L-LDH activity is 3-fold higher that the NAD dependent L-LDH favouring the transformation of L-lactate to pyruvate and this lactate isomer was not detected. Pyruvate is derived by pyruvate dehydrogenase to acetaldehyde-TPP and from this compound, acetate and aroma compounds were formed. The enzyme activities related to aroma compounds formation are α-acetolactate synthetase, diacetyl reductase and acetoin reductase. The presence and levels of acetate kinase and acetaldehyde dehydrogenase explain the formation of acetate.

The presence of glycerol kinase pathway in this strain was confirmed by the isolation and characterization of the enzymes involved: glycerol kinase and NAD-independent glycerol-3-phosphate dehydrogenase.(Pasteris and Strasser de Saad, 1998).

These studies constituted de first demonstration of Glycerol kinase pathway in the genus *Pediococcus* and the second enzyme activity, NAD-independent G-3-P dehydrogenase is reported by the first time in lactic acid bacteria.

The regulatory aspects of the glycerol catabolism pathway in *Ped. pentosaceus* N5p were determined by Pasteris and Strasser de Saad (2005). The expression of enzymatic activities is regulated by glycerol concentration and oxygen availability. The highest levels of the activities of this pathway are expressed in aerobic conditions and at the lowest concentration of glycerol, decreasing with the increase in glycerol concentration in the growth media (Fig. 21). The activities of glycerol dehydrogenase pathway are also detected in these conditions but the levels demonstrated allow to establish that glycerol is mainly degraded by glycerol kinase pathway.

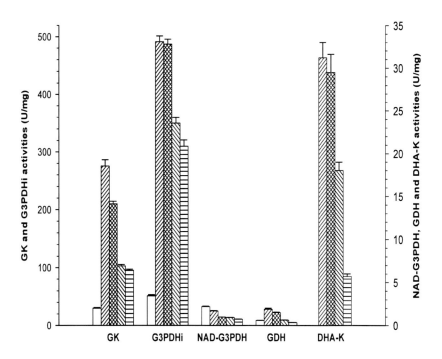

Figure 21. Enzymatic activities involved in glycerol degradation when *P. pentosaceus* N$_5$p was grown in (☐) 5.5 mM glucose or different glycerol concentrations: (▨) 5.7 mM, (▧) 10.3 mM, (▩) 21.6 mM, (▤) 42.6 mM. GK, glycerol kinase; G3PDHi, NAD-independent glycerol 3-P dehydrogenase; NAD-G3PDH, NAD-dependent glycerol 3-P dehydrogenase; GDH, glycerol dehydrogenase; DHA-K, dihydroxyacetone kinase.(From Pasteris and Strasser de Saad, 2005).

In aerobiosis, glycerol is transformed in D-lactate, acetate and a low proportion of glycerol (5.2 to 15%) produce acetoinic compounds like diacetyl and 2,3-butanediol (Table 4). The products obtained from glycerol in aerobiosis, differ according to the balances obtained for other LAB such as *Ped. pentosaceus* (Dobrogosz and Stone, 1962) and *Lact. casei* Cog 812

(Lonvaud-Funel, 1986) in which, besides lactate and acetate, the acetoin production was informed. The last product is not formed by *Ped. pentosaceus* N₅p under these conditions. Aerobic degradation of glycerol by Glycerol kinase pathway is observed in other LAB such as *Streptococcus faecium* (Esders and Michrina, 1979) and *Streptococcus faecalis* (Jacobs and Van Demark, 1960).

Table 4. Glycerol and glucose utilization by *Pediococcus pentosaceus* N₅p, growing in aerobic conditions: substrates and products at the end of growth

Carbon source (mM)	Substrates consumption (mM) Glucose	Glycerol	Products (mM) D-lactate	Acetate	Diacetyl	2,3-BD	CO₂	C.R
Glucose 5.5	5.5	---	5.4	3.5	0.90	0.115	5.52	99.4
Glycerol 5.7	---	5.7	0.70	3.2	0.75	0.115	4.99	98.8
Glycerol 10.6	---	9.8	1.7	5.9	0.90	0.130	7.96	98.6
Glycerol 21.3	---	14.4	2.60	9.8	0.92	0.135	11.91	99.4
Glycerol 42.6	---	16.1	5.2	9.2	0.70	0.130	10.86	99.7

CO₂ concentration was calculated considering its generation by pyruvate dehydrogenase and α-acetolactate decarboxylase: 1 mol CO₂/mol acetate and 2 mol CO₂/mol diacetyl or 2,3-Butanediol (2,3-BD). C.R, carbon recovery as percentage. (From Pasteris and Strasser de Saad, 2005).

The enzymatic activities (Figs. 22 and 23) related to product formation are also modulated by glycerol. NAD-dependent lactate dehydrogenases are not affected by glycerol. Diacetyl reductase and acetoin reductase are inhibited by glycerol whereas NAD-independent lactate dehydrogenases, NADH oxidase as CoA-independent acetaldehyde dehydrogenase, and acetate kinase are stimulated.

The behaviour of lactate dehydrogenases could be correlated with the lower production of lactate in glycerol than in glucose media. The low levels of L-LDH and the high levels of L-LDHi are probably related to the absence of L-lactate in fermentation balances of *Ped. pentosaceus* N₅p.

The enzymatic activities behaviour is in conformity with the fermentation balances; we proposed a pathway for glycerol catabolism in *Ped. pentosaceus* N₅p (Fig. 24).

Being no information about the transport of glycerol neither in LAB from wine nor in the genus *Pediococcus* from other ecological areas, the mechanism of glycerol uptake was determined in *Ped. pentosaceus* N₅p, the species of the genus *Pediococcus* in which the glycerol catabolism has been better studied (Pasteris and Strasser de Saad, 2008).

Contrary to what happens in most of the microorganisms whose transport system is inducible, the glycerol transport system in *Ped. pentosaceus* is constitutively expressed as reported in *Saccharomyces cereviciae* strains where the intracellular concentration of glycerol provide a basis for both osmo- and halotolerance (Ferreyra et al., 2005).

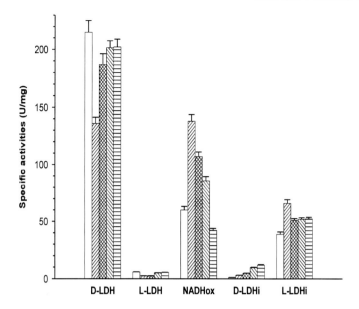

Figure 22: Enzymatic activities involved in the production and degradation of lactate and NADH oxidase activity when P. pentosaceus N5p was grown in (☐) 5.5 mM glucose or different glycerol concentrations: (▨) 5.7 mM, (▩) 10.3 mM, (▩) 21.6 mM, (▤) 42.6 mM.. D and L- LDH, NAD-dependent D and L-lactate dehydrogenases; D and L- LDHi, NAD-independent D and L-lactate dehydrogenases; NADHox, NADH oxidase. (From Pasteris and Strasser de Saad, 2005).

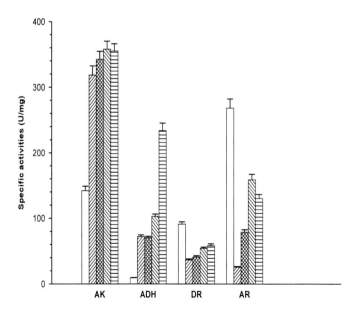

Figure 23. Enzymatic activities involved in acetate and aroma compounds synthesis when P. pentosaceus N5p was grown in (☐) 5.5 mM glucose or different glycerol concentrations: (▨) 5.7 mM, (▩) 10.3 mM, (▩) 21.6 mM, (▤) 42.6 mM. AK, acetate kinase; ADH, NAD-acetaldehyde dsehydrogenase; DR, diacetyl reductase; AR, acetoin reductase. (From Pasteris and Strasser de Saad, 2005).

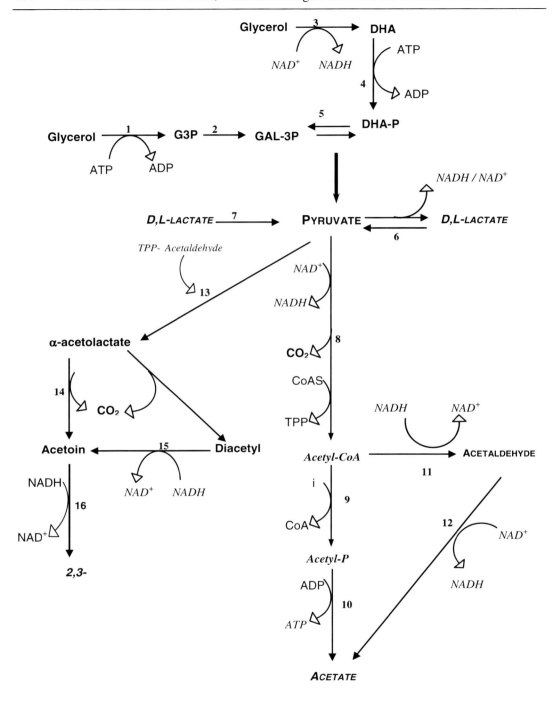

Figure 24. Metabolic pathway scheme for aerobic glycerol catabolism in Pediococcus pentosaceus N5p. 1, glycerol kinase; 2, NAD-independent glycerol 3-P dehydrogenase; 3, glycerol dehydrogenase; 4, dihydroxyacetone kinase; 5, triose phosphate isomerase; 6, NAD-dependent lactate dehydrogenases; 7, NAD-independent lactate dehydrogenases; 8, pyruvate dehydrogenase; 9, phosphotransacetylase; 10, acetate kinase; 11, CoA-dependent acetaldehyde dehydrogenase; 12, CoA-independent acetaldehyde dehydrogenase; 13, α-acetolactate synthase; 14, α-acetolactate decarboxylase; 15, diacetyl reductase; 16, acetoin reductase (From Pasteris and Strasser de Saad, 2005).

Many of the bacterial species investigated have been reported to take up glycerol by facilitated diffusion, e.g. Enterobacteriaceae (Sanno et al., 1968; Richey and Lin, 1972; Lin, 1976) and some LAB (Charrier et al., 1997; Froger et al. 2001; Álvarez et al., 2004).

Several lines of evidence were presented to indicate that glycerol uptake in *Ped. pentosaceus* is an energy-dependent carrier transport system (Pasteris and Strasser de Saad, 2008). The presence of uptake when resting cells were treated with $HgCl_2$ and the absence of counterflow indicate that facilitated diffusion is not involved in glycerol transport. On the other hand, glycerol uptake is inhibited by the metabolic poisons that affect ATP availability by acting on either electron transport or ATPase activity, and by the proton-conducting uncouplers without any effect on Glycerol kinase activity. The restoration of uptake in de-energized cells by the glucose addition of and low concentration of cyanide-*m*-chlorophenyl hydrazone is achieved. On the basis of these results, the first in the genus *Pediococcus*, we provide evidence for an energy-dependent uptake of glycerol involving proton motive force directly or coupled to ATP synthesis.

From Beer

Beer is a rather unfavorable growth medium for most microorganisms because of its low pH, lack of nutrients and the presence of hop-derived compounds and alcohol (Simpson, 1991).

It has been shown that many bacterial strains retain their viability for extended periods in beer, but as long as they are not able to grow in the product they are not harmful and should not be considered as beer spoilage organisms (Lawrence and Priest, 1981).

LAB in breweries may play also two distinct roles. On the one hand, they are generally regarded as a hazard for modern breweries and on the other hand, as one of the latest improvements in brewing technology when used as starter cultures to acidify malt or wort (Linko et al.,1998)

The bacteria generally regarded as most hazardous for modern breweries are bacteria belonging to the genera *Pediococcus* and *Lactobacillus* (Simpson and Fernandez, 1992. They can be found in malt, wort, pitching yeast (Rainbow, 1981; Priest, 1987), fermenting must and beer. *Pediococcus* are generally considered to be the most undesirable contaminant (Priest, 1987; Rainbow, 1971; Tsuchiya et al., 2000) with *Ped. damnosus* being the species responsible for the majority (90%) of all *Pediococcus*-induced beer spoilage (Lawrence and Priest, 1981). Pediococci are well known producers of diacetyl and its reduced forms: acetoin and 2,3-butanediol from sugars. Furthermore, they produce certain viscosity, a thixothrophic mucus that disappears with vigorous agitation. In consequence, they produce acidity, affect clarity and produce off- odorous compounds. Both genera *Pediococcus* and *Lactobacillus* have been related to the amine buildup in beers (Chen et al., 1979; Zee et al., 1981; Izquierdo-Pulido et al., 1995).

However, certain *Lact. plantarum* and *Ped. pentosaceus* strains may be used as starter cultures in malting, offering interesting possibilities to ensure balanced enzyme activities and to avoid harmful *Fusarium* contaminations (Linko et al.,1998).

Traditionally, brewers have viewed the sensitivity of a beer to bacterial spoilage as an important character. Indeed, many studies have been directed at measuring and controlling beer spoilability.

The ability of LAB to grow in beer was correlated with parameters such as attenuation level, pH, beer colour and contents of ethanol, free aminoacids, soluble nitrogen, a range of individual aminoacids, total or individual fermentable sugars and the undissociated forms of SO_2 and hop bitter acids (Pfenninger et al., 1979; Dolezil and Kirsop, 1980; Simpson and Fernandez, 1992).

During alcoholic fermentation by yeast, glycerol is produced and it could be a carbon source for the bacteria present in a medium where the fermentable sugars has been exhausted. However, the possible utilization of this carbon source has not been studied in lactic acid bacteria from beer to correlate it with beer spoilage. This study was carried out by Vizoso Pinto et al. (2004)

Among the LAB isolated from beer at different stages of elaboration, *Ped. pentosaceus* was the predominant species and the only that used glycerol as sole carbon source. Its utilization was studied in CAg strain growing on glycerol or on glycerol and limited concentration of glucose.

Table 5. Enzymatic activities degrading glycerol during the growth of Pediococcus pentosaceus CAg.

Carbon source	Enzymatic Activity (U/mg)			
	GK	NADi-G3PDH	GDA	1,3-PDH
Glu 48 h	0.0	1.16	3.06	8.33
Glu+Gly 48 h	0.0	0.0	32.34	11.44
Glu+Gly 96 h	246	3.85	23.94	3.48
Gly 48 h	115	14.37	62.19	42.49
Gly 96 h	251	17.40	32.19	14.74

Carbon source: Glu, glucose (5.5 mM); Gly, glycerol (42.6 mM). Enzyme activities: GK, glycerol kinase; NADi-G3PDH, NAD-independent glycerol 3-P dehydrogenase; GDA, glycerol dehydratase; 1,3-PDH, 1,3-propanediol dehydrogenase. (From Vizoso Pinto et al., 2004)

In this strain, Glycerol kinase and Glycerol dehydratase pathways were responsible for glycerol degradation.

In glycerol medium, strain CAg degraded it by two different pathways, 71% and 29% of glycerol by the Glycerol kinase and Glycerol dehydratase pathways respectively. The enzymatic activity of these pathways inversely varies after 48 h of growth (Table 5).

This behaviour is supported not only by the evolution of glycerol consumption but also by the evolution of product formation and pH (Fig. 25). Higher levels of Glycerol kinase pathway activities towards the end of growth could be related to the increase in acetate. Furthermore, the conversion of lactate into acetate via pyruvate is evidenced by the fact that lactate, mainly the D-isomer, was consumed and afterwards remained constant in parallel with the increasing acetate levels. 29% glycerol is transformed in 1,3-propanediol by the glycerol dehydratase pathway. This reaction and the formation of 2,3-butanediol from pyruvate may supply the NAD required to oxidize lactate and to transform pyruvate in acetyl CoA (Table 6).

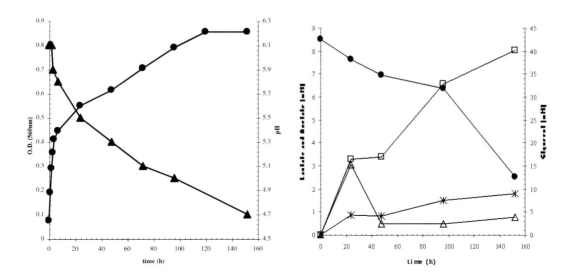

Figure 25. Evolution of growth (●) and pH (▲) of culture of P. pentosaceus CAg in glycerol medium (1 a). Glycerol consumption (●), D-lactate (△), L-lactate (✻) and acetate (□) production (1 b). (From Vizoso Pinto et al., 2004).

Table 6. Glycerol and glucose utilization by *Pediococcus pentosaceus* CAg: substrates and products at the end of growth.

Carbon source	Substrates (mM) Glu	Gly	Products (mM) D-Lac	L-Lac	Acetate	Diac	2,3-BD	1,3-PD	CO_2	CR
Glu	5.5	---	3.85	3.70	1.30	0.1	0.82	0	3.14	97.03
Glu+Gly	5.5	41.47	7.00	4.11	5.06	0.90	8.50	14.50	23.86	94.28
Gly	---	30.60	0.76	1.76	8.04	0.11	5.50	8.00	19.26	97.30

Carbon source: Glu, glucose (5.5 mM); Gly, glycerol (42.6 mM). Products: D-Lac, D-Lactate; L-Lac, L-Lactate; 2,3-BD, 2,3-butanediol; 1,3-PD, 1,3-propanediol. CO_2 concentration was calculated considering its generation by pyruvate dehydrogenase and α-acetolactate decarboxylase: 1mol CO_2/ mol acetate and 2 mol CO_2/ mol diacetyl (Diac) or 2,3-BD. CR, carbon recovery as percentage (From Vizoso Pinto et al., 2004).

According to our results D-lactate is only degraded in glycerol medium. Perhaps this difference with the glucose- glycerol medium could be correlated to requirement of energy .In glycerol medium, the extra carbon source (glucose) is absent and glycerol consumption is lower than in glycerol-glucose medium. In the later, only 12.5% glycerol was recovered as acetate whereas in glycerol medium about 25% of glycerol was transformed in acetate. Then, this suggests that strain CAg needs to produce more acetate to obtain ATP in glycerol medium what is possible by degrading lactate.

In glucose and glycerol medium, the sugar is rapidly consumed and the acids formed in the first hours correspond to its degradation (Fig. 26). Glycerol (35%) is firstly degraded by Glycerol dehydratase pathway since enzymatic activities from the Glycerol kinase pathway were absent at this point (Table 5).

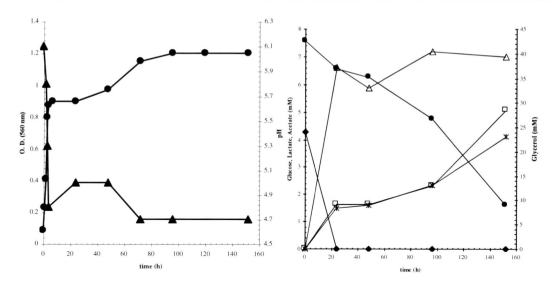

Figure 26. Evolution of growth (●) and pH (▲) of culture of P.pentosaceus CAg in glycerol and glucose medium (2 a). Glycerol (●) and glucose (♦) consumption, D-lactate (△), L-lactate (✻) and acetate (□) production (2 b). (From Vizoso Pinto et al., 2004)

These results are in coincidence with the lag period in acid production. As long as glucose is present, NAD is provided by the reaction that leads to the formation of 1,3-propanediol. But, when glucose has been consumed, Glycerol kinase way is expressed to produce ATP and regenerate NAD. ATP could be produced via acetate and the oxidation of NADH could be coupled to the reaction that forms 2,3-butanediol(Table 5)

In this condition, although the enzymatic activities of Glycerol dehydratase pathway are important, the function of Glycerol kinase pathway would be even more important since it can supply energy (ATP) and NAD. This could be the reason why no further 1,3- propanediol formation is needed. Glycerol dehydratase pathway metabolises glycerol to 1,3- propanediol in two steps. The intermediary product of this pathway is β-hydroxypropanal, which is a toxic metabolite and needs to be reduced 1,3- propanediol in order to detoxify the cell. β-hydroxypropanal, combined with polyphenols is responsible of an undesirable bitter taste in fermented beverages. On the other hand, under acidic conditions, it is dehydrated to acrolein, a lachrymatory agent considered an undesirable component for public health and responsible for peppery flavours (Smiley and Sobolov, 1962; Sauvageot et al, 2000; Claise and Lonvaud, 2000).

The intermediary of the Glycerol dehydratase pathway has not been detected in any condition, suggesting that in strain CAg it is used as hydrogen acceptor and efficiently transformed into 1,3-propanediol This finding agrees with that reported by Claisse and Lonvaud-Funel (2000) in *L. collinoides* IOEB 9527 from cider. In contrast, the cider strain LMG 18850 of *L. collinoides*, converts glycerol in β- hydroxypropanal, a precursor of acrolein (Sauvageot et al., 2001).

Glycerol kinase pathway of CAg strain involved a NAD-independent glycerol-3-phosphate dehydrogenase as that reported in *P. pentosaceus* N_5p from wine (Pasteris and Strasser de Saad 1997).

Considering the basal activities of the enzymes of the reductive pathway detected in the cell-free extracts and the ability of *Ped. pentosaceus* CAg to use glycerol independently of the prior growth history of the cells, it seems reasonable to assume that the enzymes involved are constitutive. Though, the presence of glycerol in the media would increase their expression. In contrast, the enzymes involved in the Glycerol kinase pathway may appear be inducible.

In our experimental conditions, the enzymatic activities of the Glycerol dehydrogenase pathway were absent in *Ped. pentosaceus* CAg.

These results constitute the first evidence of the Glycerol dehydratase pathway in the genus *Pediococcus* and its relation to the Glycerol kinase pathway. Apparently the pathways to degrade glycerol in this genus are variable. According to the strain it may depend both on the presence or absence of genes encoding specific enzymes and on the conditions of their expression.

Finally, we may conclude that in beer, even if a good attenuation is obtained, the glycerol produced during alcoholic fermentation could be used as carbon source by *Ped. pentosaceus* CAg. Therefore, another reason why *Ped. pentosaceus* should be considered a spoilage species is its capacity of producing high volatile acidity and aroma compounds from glycerol, conferring unacceptable flavor to beer. Hence, the ability to degrade glycerol should be correlated with the sensitivity of a particular beer to bacterial spoilage and considered as a selection criterion to exclude a strain of LAB from the starter cultures to acidify malt or wort.

REFERENCES

Adolfsson, O., Meydani, S.N. and Russell, R.M. (2004) Yogurt and gut function. *American Journal of Clinical Nutrition*, 80, 245-256.

Álvarez, F., Medina, M., Pasteris, S.E., Strasser de Saad, A.M., and Sesma, F. (2004). Glycerol metabolism of *Lactobacillus rhamnosus* ATCC 7469: cloning and expression of two glycerol kinase genes. *Joural of Molecular Microbiology and Biotechnology* ,7, 170-181.

Amoroso, M.J., Saguir, F.M. and Manca de Nadra, M.C. (1993) Variation of nutritional requirements of *Leuconostoc oenos* by organic acids. *Journal International des Science Vigne et du Vin*, 27, 135–144

Aredes Fernandez, P.A., Saguir, F.M. and Manca de Nadra, M.C. (2004) Effect of dipeptides on the growth of *Oenococcus oeni* in synthetic medium deproved of amino acids. *Current Microbiology*, 49, 361–365

Aredes Fernandez, P.A. and Manca de Nadra, M.C. (2006). Growth response and modifications of organic nitrogen compounds in pure and mixed cultures of lactic acid bacteria from wines. *Current Microbiology*, 52, 86–91.

Arena, M.E., Seguir, F.M. and Manca de Nadra, M.C. (1996). Inhibition of growth of *Lactobacillus plantarum* from citrus fruits in the presence of organic acids. *Microbiology- Aliment- Nutrition*, 14, 219-226.

Arena, M.E., Saguir, F.M. and Manca de Nadra, M.C. (1999) Arginine dihydrolase pathway in Lactobacillus plantarum from orange. *International Journal of Food Microbiology*, 4, 203–209.

Arena M. E., Manca de Nadra M.C. and Muñoz R. (2002). The arginine deiminase pathway in the wine lactic acid bacterium *Lactobacillus hilgardii* X1B: structural and functional study of the arcABC genes. *Gene*, 301, 61-66.

Arena M.E. and Manca de Nadra M.C. (2005). Influence of ethanol and low pH on arginine and citrulline metabolism in lactic acid bacteria from wine. *Research Microbiology*, 156, 858-864.

Augagneur, Y., Ritt, J.F., Linares, D.M., Remize, F., Tourdot-Maréchal, R., Garmyn, D. and Guzzo, J. (2007). Dual effect of organic acids as a function of external pH in *Oenococcus oeni*. *Archives of Microbiology*, 188, 147-157 .

Axelsson, L. (1998). Lactic acid bacteria: classification and physiology. In: Lactic Acid Bacteria: *Microbiology and Functional Aspects, 2nd ed*. Salminen, S., von Wright, A. (Eds.), pp. 1 –72. Marcel Dekker, New York Ya está

Axelsson, L. (2004) Lactic acid bacteria: classification and physiology. In: Lactic Acid Bacteria. *Microbiological and Functional Aspects, third ed*. pp. 1-66., Salminen, S., von Wright, A., Ouwehand, A. (Eds.), Marcel Dekker, New York.

Babu, V., Mital, B. K. and Garg, S. K. (1992). Effect of tomato juice addition on the growth and activity of *Lactobacillus acidophilus*. Internacional Journal of Food Microbiology, 17, 67-70.

Bandell, M., Lhotte, M. E., Marty-Teysset, C., Veyrat, A., Prévost, H., Dartois, V., Divie`s, C., Konings, W. N. and Lolkema, J. S. (1998). Mechanism of the citrate transporters in carbohydrate and citrate cometabolism in *Lactococcus* and *Leuconostoc* species. *Applied and Environmental Microbiology*, 64, 1594-1600.

Bartowsky, E.J. and Henschke, P.A. (2004). The 'buttery' attribute of wine-diacetyl-desirability, spoilage and beyond. International *Journal of Food Microbiology*, 96 235-252.

Beneduce, L., Spano, G., Vernile, A., Tarantino, D., and Massa, S. (2004). Molecular characterization of lactic acid populations associated with wine spoilage. *Journal of Basic Microbiology*, 44 (1), 10-6.

Blasco, L., Ferrer, S. and Pardo, I. (2003). Development of specific fluorescent oligonucleotide probes for in situ identiWcation of wine lactic acid bacteria. *FEMS Microbiology Letters*, 225, 115-123.

Bolotin, A., Wincher, P., Mauger, S., Jaillon, O., Malarme, K., Weissenbach, J., Ehrlich, S.D. and Sorokin, A. (2001). The complete genome sequence of the lactic acid bacterium *Lactococcus lactis* ssp. *lactis* IL1403. *Genome Research*, 2001, 11, 731-753.

Brackett, R. E. (1988). Changes in the microXora of packaged fresh tomatoes. *Journal of Food Quality*, 11, 89-105.

Carr, F.J., Chill, D. and Maida, N. (2002) The lactic acid bacteria: a literature survey. *Critical Review Microbiology*, 28, 281-370.

Charrier, V., Buckley, E., Parsonage, D., Galinier, A., Darbon, E., Jaquinod, M., Forest, E., Deutscher, J. and Claiborne, A. (1997). Cloning and sequencing of two enterococal glpK genes and regulation of the encoded glycerol kinases by phosphoenolpyruvate dependent, phosphotransferase system-catalysed phosphorilation of a single hystidin residue. *Journal of Biological Chemistry*, 272 (22), 14166-14174.

Chen, E. and Van Gheluwe, G. (1979). Analysis of histamine in beer. *Journal of American Society of Brewery Chemists*, 37, 91-95.

Claisse, O. and Lonvaud-Funel, A. (2000). Assimilation of glycerol by a strain of *Lactobacillus collinoides* isolated from cider. *Food Microbiology*, 17, 513-519.

Cocaign-Bousquet, M., Garrigues, C., Novak, L., Lindley, N.D. and Loubiere, P. (1995). Rational development of a simple synthetic medium for the sustained growth of *Lactococcus lactis*. *Journal of Applied Bacteriology*, 79, 108-116.

Cocaign-Bousquet, M., Garrigues, C., Loubiere, P., Lindley, N.D. (1996). Physiology of pyruvate metabolism in *Lactococcus lactis*. *Antonie van Leeuwenhoek*, 70, 253– 267.

Cogan, T. M., O'Dowd M. and Mellerick, D. (1981). Effects of pH and sugar on acetoin production from citrate by *Leuconostoc lactis*. *Applied Environmental Microbiology*, 41, 1-8.

Cogan, T. M. (1987). Co-metabolism of citrate and glucose by *Leuconostoc* spp.: effects on growth, substrates, and products. *Journal of. Applied Bacteriology*, 63, 551-558.

Collins, E. B. and Bruhn, J. C. (1970). Roles of acetate and pyruvate in the metabolism of *Streptococcus diacetilactis*. *Journal of Bacteriology*, 1970, 103, 541-546.

Curk, M.C., Hubert, J.C. and Bringel, F. (1996). *Lactobacillus paraplantarum* sp. now., a new species related to *Lactobacillus plantarum*. *International Journal Systematic Bacteriology*, 2, 595-598.

Davis, C.R., Wibowo, D., Eschenbruch, R., Lee, T.H. and Fleet, G.H. (1985) Practical implications of malolactic fermentation: a review. American *Journal of Enology and Viticulture*, 36, 290-301.

Davis, C.R., Wibowo, D., Fleet, G.H. and Lee, T.H. (1986a) Growth and metabolism of lactic acid bacteria during and after malolactic fermentation of wines at different pH. *Applied and Environmental Microbiology*, 51, 539–545.

Davis, C.R., Wibowo, D., Fleet, G.H. and Lee, T.H. (1986b) Growth and metabolism of lactic acid bacteria during fermentation and conservation of some Australian wines. *Food Technology in Australia*, 38, 35-40.

De Figueroa, R. M., Cerutti de Guglielmone, G.I., Betino de Cardenas, L. and Oliver, G. (1998). Flavour compound production and citrate metabolism in *Lactobacillus rhamnosus* ATCC 7469. *Milchwissenschaft*, 53, 617-619.

de Vos, W.M. (1999). Safe and sustainable systems for food-grade fermentations by genetically modified lactic acid bacteria. *International Dairy Journal*, 9, 3 -10.

D'Incecco, N., Bartowsky, E.J., Kassara, S., Lante, A., Spettoli, P. and Henschke, P.A. (2004). Release of glycosidically bound flavour compounds from Chardonnay by *Oenococcus oeni* during malolactic fermentation. *Food Microbiology*, 21, 257- 265.

Dobrogosz, W.J. and Stone, R.W. (1962). Oxidative metabolism in *Pediococcus pentosaceus*. *Journal of Bacteriology*, 84, 716-723.

Dolezil, L. and Kirsop, B.H. (1980). Variations amongst beers and lactic acid bacteria relating to beer spoilage. *Journal of the Institute of brewing*, 86, 122-124.

Drider, D., Bekal, S. and Prévost, H.(2004). Genetic organization and expression of citrate permease in lactic acid bacteria. Mini-Review. *Genetics and Molecular Research*, 2, 273-281.

Drosinos, E. H., Tassou, C., Kakiomenou, K.and Nychas, G. J. E. (2000). Microbiological, physico-chemical and organoleptic attributes of a country tomato salad and fate of *Salmonella enteriditis* during storage under aerobic or modiWed atmosphere packaging conditions at 4 °C and 10 °C. *Food Control*, 11, 131-135.

Ehrmann, M.A., Vogel, R.F., 2005. Molecular taxonomy and genetics of sourdough lactic acid bacteria. *Trends Food Science Technology* 16, 31-42.

Esders, T.W. and Michrina, C.A. (1979). Purification and properties of L-∝-glycerophosphate oxidase from *Streptococcus faecium* ATCC 12755. *Journal of Biological Chemistry*, 254, 2710-2715.

Eustace, R., and Thornton, R.J. (1987). Selective hybridization of wine yeast for higher yields of glycerol. *Canadian Journal of Microbiology*, 33, 112-117.

Ferreyra, C., Van Voorst, F., Martins, A., Neves, L., Oliveira, R., Kielland-Brandt, M., Lucas, C., and Brandt, A. (2005). A member of the sugar transporter family, Stl1p is the glycerol/H$^+$ symporter in *Saccharomyces cerevisiae*. *Molecular Biology Cell*, 16, 2068-2076.

Fourcassie, P., Makaga-Kabinda-Massard, E., Belardi, A. and Maujean, A. (1992). Growth, glucose utilization and malolactic fermentation by Leuconostoc oenos strains in 18 media deficient in one amino acid. *Journal of Applied Bacteriology*, 73, 489-496.

Froger, A., Rolland, J.P., Bron, P., Lagrée, V., Le Cahérec, F., Deschamps, S., Hubert, J.F., Pellerin, I., Tomas, D., and Delamarche, C. (2001). Functional characterization of a microbial aquaglyceroporin. *Microbiology*, 147, 1129-1135.

Garai-Ibabe G., Ibarburu I., Berregi I., Claisse O. Lonvaud-Funel A., Irastorza A. and Dueñas M.T. (2008). Glycerol metabolism and bitterness producing lactic acid bacteria in cidermaking. *Bioprocess Biosystematics Engineering*, 31(2), 127-135.

García-Quintáns, N., Magni, C., de Mendoza, D. and P. López. (1998). The citrate transport system of *Lactococcus lactis* subsp. *lactis* biovar diacetylactis is induced by acid stress. *Applied and Environmental Microbiology*, 64, 850-857.

Gardner, N. J., Savard, T., Obermeier, P., Caldwell, G. and Champagne, C.P. (2001). Selection and characterization of mixed starter cultures for lactic acid fermentation of carrot, cabbage, and onion vegetable mixtures. *International Journal of Food Microbiology*, 64, 261-275.

Gänzle M.G., Vermeulen, N. and Vogel, R. F. (2007). Carbohydrate, peptide and lipid metabolism of lactic acid bacteria in sourdough. *Food microbiology*, 24,128-138.

Grimaldi, A., Bartowsky, E. and Jiranek, J. (2005). A survey of glycosidase activities of commercial wine strains of *Oenococcus oeni*. *International Journal of Food Microbiology*, 105, 233– 244.

Hemme D. and Foucaud-Scheunemann C (2004). *Leuconostoc*, Characteristics, use in dairy technology and prospects in functional foods. *Inernational Dairy Journal*, 14, 467-94.

Hugenholtz, J. and Starrenburg, M.J.C. (1992). Diacetyl production by different strains of *Lactococcus lactis* subsp. *lactis* var. *diacetylactis* and *Leuconostoc* spp. *Applied Microbiology and Biotechnology*, 38, 17- 20.

Izquierdo-Pulido M., Font-Fabregas J., Carceller-Rosa J. M., Marine-Font A. and Vidal-Carou C. (1995). Biogenic amine changes related to lactic acid bacteria during brewing. Journal of *Food Protection*, 59 (2), 175-180.

Jacobs, N.J. and Van Demark, P.J. (1960) Comparisons of the mechanism of glycerol oxidation in aerobically and anaerobically grown *Streptococcus faecalis*. *Journal of. Bacteriology*, 79, 532-538.

Juven, B.J. (1976). Bacterial spoilage of citrus products at pH lower than 3.5. *Journal of Food Protectection*, 39, 819-822.

Kandler, O. (1983). Carbohydrate metabolism in lactic acid bacteria. *Antonie van Leeuwenhoek*, 49, 209-224.

Kandler, O. and Weiss, N.(1986). Regular, nonsporing Gram-positive rods. In: Bergey's manual of systematic bacteriology, vol. 1, pp. 1208-1234. Sneath, P.H.A., Mair, N.S., Sharpe, M.E. and Holt, J.G. (Eds). *Williams and Wilkins*. Baltimore, MD.

Kitabatake, M., So, M.W., Tumbula, D.L. and Soll, D. (2000). Cysteine biosynthesis pathway in the archaeon Methanosarcina barkeri encoded by acquired bacterial genes? *Journal of Bacteriology*, 182, 143-145.

Kooning, E. and Galperin, M. (2003). Sequence–Evolution–Function: Computacional Approaches in Comparative Genomics. *Kluwer Academic*, London.

Konings ,W.N. (2002) The cell membrane and the struggle for life of lactic acid bacteria. Antonie Van Leeuwenhoek, 82, 3-27.

Korakli, M., Gänzle, M.G., Knorr, R., Frank, M., Rossmann, A. and Vogel, R.F. (2002). Metabolism of Lactobacillus sanfraniscensis under high pressure: investigations using stable carbon isotopes. In: *Trends in High Pressure Bioscience and Biotechnology*, pp. 287-294. Hayashi, R. (Ed.), Elsevier, Amsterdam.

Kuipers, O.P. (1999) Genomics for food biotechnology: prospects of the use of high-throughput technologies for the improvement of food microorganism. *Current Opinion Biotechnology*, 10, 511–516.

Kunkee, R.E. (1991). Some roles of malic acid in malolactic fermentation in winemaking. *FEMS Microbiology Review*, 88, 55-72.

Labarre, C., Guzzo, J., Cavin J.F. and Divies, C. (1996b) Cloning and characterization of the genes encoding the malolactic enzyme and the malate permease of *Leuconostoc oenos*. *Applied and Environmental Microbiology*, 62, 1274-1282.

Lawrence, D.R. and Priest, F.G. (1981). Identification of brewery cocci. *Proceedings of the European Brewing Convention*, Copenhagen.pp. 217-227.

Lin, E.C.C. (1976). Glycerol dissimilation and its regulation in bacteria. *Annual Review of Microbiology*, 36, 535-578.

Lindgren, S. E., Axelsson, L. T. and McFeeters, R. F. (1990). Anaerobic L-lactate degradation by *Lactobacillus plantarum*. *FEMS Microbiology Letters*, 66, 209–214.

Linko, M., Haikara, A., Ritala, A. and Penttila, M. (1998). Recent advances in the malting and brewing industry. *Journal of Biotechnology*, 65, 85-98.

Liu, S.-Q., Davis, C.R. and Brooks, J.D. (1995) Growth and metabolism of selected lactic acid bacteria in synthetic wine. *American Journal of Enology and Viticulture*, 46, 166-174.

Liu, S.-Q. (2002). Review: Malolactic fermentation in wine – beyond deacidification. Journal of *Applied Microbiology*, 92, 589–601.

Liu, S.-Q. (2003). Practical implications of lactate and pyruvate metabolism by lactic acid bacteria in food and beverage fermentations. *International Journal of Food Microbiology*, 83, 115– 131.

Loiudice, R., Impembo, M., Laratta, B., Villari, G., Lo Voi, A., Siviero, P., et al.(1995). Composition of San Marzano tomato varieties. *Food Chemistry*, 53, 81-89.

Lolkema, J.S., Poolman, B. and Konings, W.N. (1995). Role of scalar protons in metabolic energy generation in lactic acid bacteria. *Journal of Bioenergetics and Biomembranes*, 27, 467-473.

Lonvaud-Funel A. (1986). Recherches sur les bactéries lactiques du vin. Fonctions métaboliques, croissance, génétique plasmidique. *Thèse Université de Bordeaux II*, France.

Lonvaud-Funel, A. (1999). Lactic acid bacteria in the quality improvement and depreciation of wine. *Antonie van Leeuwenhoek*, 76, 317-331.

Loubière, P., Salou, P., Leroy, M.J., Lindley, N.D. and Pareilleux, A. (1992) Electrogenic malate uptake and improved growth energetics of the malolactic bacterium *Leuconusroc oenos*. Growth on glucose-malate mixtures. *Journal of Bacteriology*, 174, 5302-5308.

Makarova, K., Slesarevb, A., Wolfa, Y., Sorokina, A., Mirkinc, B., Koonina, E., Pavlovb, D.A., Pavlovab. N. et al. (2006). Comparative genomics of the lactic acid bacteria. *pPNAS*, 103,. 42, 15611-15616.

Magni, C., de Mendoza, D., Konings, W.N. and Lolkema, J.S. (1999). Mechanism of citrate metabolism in *Lactococcus lactis*: Resistance against lactate toxicity at low pH. *Journal of Bacteriology*, 181, 1451-1457.

Manca de Nadra M.C. and Strasser de Saad A.M. (1987). Evolution of lactic acid bacteria during the different stages of vinification of Cafayate (Argentina) wine. *Microbiologie- Aliments- Nutrition*, 5, 235-240.

Manca de Nadra M.C. and Strasser de Saad A.M. (1995). Polysaccharide production by *Pediococcus pentosaceus* from wine.International *Journal of Food Microbiology*, 27,101-106.

Manca de Nadra, M.C., Farias, M.E., Moreno-Arribas, V., Pueyo, E. and Polo, M.C. (1999). A proteolitic effect *Oenococcus oeni* on the nitrogenous macromolecular fraction of red wine. *FEMS Microbiology Letters*, 174, 41 - 47.

Manca de Nadra M.C, Farías M.E., Pueyo E. and Carmen Polo M.C. (2005). Protease activity of *Oenococcus oeni* viable cells on red wine nitrogenous macromolecular fraction in presence of SO_2 and ethanol. *Food Control*, 16:851-854.

Marty-Teysset, C., Posthuma, C., Lolkema, J.S., Schmitt, P., Divies, C. and Konings, W.N. (1996) Proton motive force generation by citrolactic fermentation in Leuconostoc mesenteroides. *Journal of Bacterioaogy*, 178, 2178–2185.

Miller, N. and Wetterstrom, W. (2000). In: The Cambridge *World History of Food., Vol 2,* pp 1123-1139. Kiple, K. and Ornelas, K. (Eds). *Cambridge University Press*, Cambridge, UK.

Miranda, M., Ramos, A., Veiga-da-Cunha, M., Loureiro-Dias, M.C. and Santos, H. (1997). Biochemical basis for glucose-induced inhibition of malolactic fermentation in Leuconostoc oenos. *Journal of Bacteriology*, 179, 5347-5354.

Murdock, D.J and Hatcher,W.S. (1975). Growth of microorganisms in chilled orange juice. Journal of Milk and *Food Technology*, 38, 393-396.

Neves, A.R., Pool, W.A., Kok, J., Kuipers, O.P., Santos. H. (2005). Overview on sugar metabolism and its control in *Lactococcus lactis*– The input from in vivo NMR. *FEMS Microbiology Reviews*, 29, 531–554.

Nguyen-the, C. and Carlin, F. (2000). Fresh and processed vegetables. In The microbiological safety and quality of food, pp. 620-684. Lund, B. M., Baird-Parker, T. C. and Gould, G. W. (Eds.). *Aspen Publishers, Inc.*, Gaithersburg, Maryland.

Nielsen, J. C. and Richelieu, M. (1999). Control of flavor development in wine during and after malolactic fermentation by *Oenococcus oeni*. *Applied and Environmental Microbiology*, 65,740-745.

Nordkvist, M., Siemsen Jensen, N.B., and Villadsen, J. (2003). Glucose metabolism in *Lactococcus lactis* MG1363 under different aeration conditions: Requirement of acetate To sustain growth under microaerobic conditions. *Applied and Environmental Microbiology*, 69, 3462-3468.

Pasteris, S.E. and Strasser de Saad, A.M. (1997) Enzymatic activities involved in glycerol utilization by *Pediococcus pentosaceus* from argentinian wine. *Microbiologie- Aliments- Nutrition*, 15, 139-145.

Pasteris, S.E., Strasser de Saad, A.M.(1998). Characterization of glycerol kinase and NAD-independent glycerol-3-phosphate dehydrogenase from *Pediococcus pentosaceus* N$_5$p. *Letters in Applied Microbiology*, 27, 93-97.

Pasteris, S.E. and Strasser de Saad, A.M. (2005). Aerobic glycerol catabolism by *Pediococcus pentosaceus* from wine. *Food Microbiology*, 22, 399- 407.

Pasteris, S.E. and Strasser de Saad, A.M. (2008). Transpor of glycerol by *Pediococcus pentosaceus* from wine. *Food Microbiology*, 25, 545-549.

Pfenninger, H.B., Schur, F., Anderegg, P. and Schlienger, E. (1979). Veranderung der Kohlenhydrat- und Aminosaurenzusammensetzung von Bier durch Lactobacillen und Pediococcen. Proceeding of the European Brewery *Convention, West Berlin*, pp. 491-504.

Pimentel, M.S., Silva, M.H. Cortes, I. and Mendes Faia, A. (1994). Growth and metabolism of sugar and acids of *Leuconostoc oenos* under different conditions of tcmpcraturc and pH. *Journal of Applied Bacteriology,* 76, 42- 46.

Priest, F.G. (1987). Gram-positive brewery bacteria,. In: Brewing Microbiology. F.G. Priest and I. Campbell (Eds). pp. 121-154, *Elsevier Applied Sciences*, New York.

Rainbow, C. (1971). Spoilage organisms in breweries. *Proceeding of Biochemistry*. 6, 15-17,31.

Rainbow, C. (1981). Beer spoilage organisms. *In Brewing Sciences, vol 2*, Pollock, J.R.. (Ed). Chapter 9, pp. 491-550. Academic Press, London.

Radler, F. (1975) The metabolism of organic acids by lactic acid bacteria. In *Lactic acid Bacteria in Beverages and Food* . pp. 17-27. Carr, J.G., Cutting, C.V. and Whiting, G.C.(Eds). Academic Press. London.

Ramos, A., Jordan, K. N., Cogan, T. M. and Santos, H. (1994). 13C nuclear magnetic resonance studies of citrate and glucose cometabolism by *Lactococcus lactis. Applied and Environmental Microbiology*, 60, 1739-1748.

Ramos, A., Lolkema, J.S., Konings, W.N. and Santos, H. (1995). Enzyme basis for pH regulation of citrate and pyruvate metabolism by *Leuconostoc oenos. Applied and Environmental Microbiology*, 61,1303-1310.

Ramos, A and Santos, H. (1996). Citrate and sugar co-fermentation in Leuconosctoc oenos, a 13C nuclear magnetic resonance study. *Applied and Environmental Microbiology*, 62, 2577-2585.

Rankine, B.C. and Bridson, D.A. (1971). Glycerol in Australian wines and factors influencing its formation. *American Journal of Enology and Viticulture*, 22, 6-12.

Renault, P. (2002). Genetically modified lactic acid bacteria: applications to food or health and risk assessment. Biochimie, 84, 1073-1087.

Ribereau-Gayon, J., Peynaud, E. , Sudrau, P. and Ribereau-Gayon, P. (1972). Traité d' Oenologie. *Sciences et Techniques du Vin*, pp.353-361. Dunod , Paris.

Richter, H., Vlad, D. and Unden, G. (2001). Significance of pantothenate for glucose fermentation by Oenococcus oeni and for suppression of the erythritol and acetate production. *Archives of Microbiology*, 175, 26- 31.

Richey, D.P., Lin, E.C.C.(1972). Importance of facilitated diffusion for effective utilization of glycerol by *Escherichia coli*. *Journal Bacteriology*, 112, 784-790.

Salado, A.I.C. and Strasser de Saad, A.M. (1995) Glycerol utilization by *Pediococcus pentosaceus* strains isolated from argentinian wines. *Microbiologie-Aliments-Nutrition*, 13, 319-325.

Salado, A.I.C., Strasser de Saad, A.M.(1996). Effect of ethanol and sulfur dioxide on glycerol utilization by *Pediococcus pentosaceus* strains from wine. *Microbiologie-Aliments-Nutrition*, 14, 263-269.

Salema, M., Lolkema, J.S., San Romao, M.V. and Loureiro Dias, M.C. (1996). The proton motive force generated in *Leuconostoc oenos* by L-malate fermentation. *Journal of Bacteriology*, 178, 3127-3132.

Salou, P., Loubiere, P. and Pareilleux, A. (1994) Growth and energetics of *Leuconostoc oenos* during cometabolism of glucose with citrate or fructose. *Applied and Environmental Microbiology*, 60, 1459-1466.

Saguir, F.M. and Manca de Nadra, M.C. (1996). Organic acids metabolism under different glucose concentrations of Leuconostoc oenos from wine. *Journal of Applied Bacteriology*, 81, 393-397.

Saguir, F.M. and Manca de Nadra, M.C. (1997). Growth and metabolism of Leuconostoc oenos in synthetic media. *Microbiologie-Aliments-Nutrition*, 15, 131-138.

Saguir, F.M. and Manca de Nadra M.C. (1998). Influence of L-malic and citric acids on the L-asparagine biosynthesis by *Leuconostoc oenos*. *Microbiologie-Aliments-Nutrition*, 16, 91-99.

Saguir, F.M. and Manca de Nadra, M.C. (2002) Effect of L-malic and citric acids metabolism on the essential amino acid requirements for *Oenococcus oeni* growth. *Journal of Applied Microbiology*, 93, 295-301.

Saguir, F.M. and Manca de Nadra, M.C. (2007) Improvement of a chemically defined medium for the sustained growth of *Lactobacillus plantarum*: nutritional requirements. *Current Microbiol*, 54, 414-418.

Saguir, F.M., Loto Campos, I.E and Manca de Nadra, M.C. (2008) Utilization of amino acids and dipeptides by *Lactobacillus plantarum* from orange in nutritionally stressed conditions. *Journal of Applied Microbiology*, in press.

Sajur S.A., Saguir F.M. and Manca de Nadra M.C. (2007). Effect of dominant species of lactic acid bacteria from tomato on natural microflora development in tomato puree. *Food Control*, 18 (5), 594-600.

Sanno, Y., Wilson, T.H., Lin, E.C.C. (1968). Control of permeation to glycerol in cells of *Escherichia coli*. *Biochemistry Biophysic Research Communications*, 32, 344-349.

Sauvageot, N., Gouffi, K. , Laplace, J.M. and Auffray, Y. (2000). Glycerol metabolism in *Lactobacillus collinoides*: production of 3-hydroxypropionaldehyde, a precursor of acrolein. *International Journal of Food Microbiology*, 55, 167-170.

Savijoki, K., Ingmer, H. and Varmanen, P. (2006) Proteolytic systems of lactic acid bacteria. Mini-review. *Applied Microbiology Biotechnology*, 71, 394-406.

Schmitt, P., Divies, C. and Merlot, C. (1990). Utilization of citrate by *Leuconostoc mesenteroides* subsp. *cremoris* in continuous culture. *Biotechnology Letters*, 12, 127-130.

Schmitt P., Diviès, C., and R. Cardona. 1992. Origin of end-products from the co-metabolism of glucose and citrate by *Leuconostoc mesenteroides* subsp. *cremoris*. *Applied Microbiology and Biotechnology* 36, 679-683.

Schutz H. and Radler F. (1984a). Propanediol dehydratase and metabolism of glycerol of *Lactobacillus brevis*. *Archives of Microbiology*, 139, 366-370.

Schutz H., Radler F. (1984b). Anaerobic reduction of glycerol to 1,3-propanediol by *Lactobacillus brevis* and *Lactobacillus buchneri*. *Systematic Appliel Microbiology*, 5, 169-178.

Serjak, W.C., Day, W.H.,Vantanen, J.M. and Boruff, C.S. (1954). Acrolein production by bacteria found in distillery grain mashes. *Applied Microbiology*, 2, 14-20.

Simpson, W. J. (1991) Molecular structure and antibacterial function of hop resin materials. Ph.D. Thesis, *Council for National Academic Awards*, UK.

Simpson, W.J. and Fernandez, J.L. (1992). Selection of beer-spoilage lactic acid bacteria and induction of their ability to growth in beer. *Letters in Applied Microbiology*, 14, 13-16.

Simsek, Ö., Con, A. H. and Tulumoglu, S. (2004). Isolating lactic starter cultures with antimicrobial activity for sourdough processes. *Food Control*, 17, 263–270.

Smiley, K.L. and Sobolov, M. (1962). A cobamide-requiring glycerol dehydratase from an acrolein-forming Lactobacillus. *Archives Biochemistry Biophysic*, 97, 538-543.

Sobolov, M. and Smiley, K.L. (1960) Metabolism of glycerol by an acrolein forming *Lactobacillus*. *Journal of Bacteriology*, 79, 261-266.

Spano G., Massa S. Arena M.E. and Manca de Nadra M.C. (2007). Arginine metabolism in wine Lactobacillus plantarum: in vitro activities of the enzymes arginine deiminase (ADI) and ornithine transcarbamilase (OTCase). *Annals of Microbiology*, 57(1), 67-70.

Starrenburg, M. J. C. and Hugenholtz, J. (1991). Citrate fermentation by *Lactococcus* and *Leuconostoc* spp. *Applied and Environmental Microbiology*, 57, 3535-3540.

Stiles, M.E. and Holzapfel, W.H. (1997). Review article: lactic acid bacteria of foods and their current taxonomy. *International Journal of Food Microbiology*, 36, 1 - 29.

Stolz, P., Hammes, W.P., and Vogel, R.F. (1996). Maltose-phosphorylase and hexokinaxse activity in lactobacilli from traditionally prepared sourdoughs. *Advances in Food Sciencs*, 18, 1-6.

Strasser de Saad, A.M. and Manca de Nadra M.C.(1987). Isolation and identification of lactic acid bacteria from Cafayate (Argentina) wines. *Microbiologie- Aliments- Nutrition*, 5, 45-49.

Strasser de Saad, A.M., Pasteris, S.E. and Manca de Nadra, M.C.1(1995.). Production and stability of Pediocin N_5p in grape juice medium. *Journal of Applied Bacteriology*, 78, 473-476.

Talarico T.L. and Dobrogosz W.J.(1990). Purification and characterization of glycerol dehydratase from *Lactobacillus reuteri*. *Applied Environmental Microbiology*, 56,1195-1197.

Tajchakavit, S., Ramaswamy, H. S. and Fustier, P. (1998). Enhanced destruction of spoilage microorganisms in apple juice during continuous flow microwave heating. *Food Research International*, 31, 713-722.

Torriani, S., Clementi, F., Vancanneyt, M., Hoste, B., Dellaglio, F. and Kersters, K. (2001). Differentiation of *Lactobacillus plantarum*, *L. pentosus* and *L. paraplantarum* species by RAPD-PCR and AFLP. *Systematic Applied Microbiology*, 4, 554-560.

Tracey, R.P. and Van Roogen, T.J. (1988) Utilization of glucose, fructose and malic acid by malolactic bacteria: effect of ethanol and formation of mannitol and volatile acids. *Journal of Applied bacteriology*, 65, 113-118.

Tsuchiya, Y., Nakakita, Y., Watari, J. and Shinotsuka, K. (2000). Monoclonal antibodies specific for the beer-spoilage ability of lactic acid bacteria. *Journal of American Society of Brewing Chemists*, 58, 89-93.

Vaningelgem, F., Ghijsels, V., Tsakalidou, E. and De Vuyst, L. Cometabolism of citrate and glucose by *Enterococcus faecium* FAIR-E 198 in the absence of cellular growth. *Applied and Environmental Microbiology*, 2006, 72, 319-326

Veiga-da-Cunha, M., and M. A. Foster. (1992a). Sugar-glycerol co-fermentations in lactobacilli: the fate of lactate. *Journal Bacteriology*, 174, 1013-1019.

Veiga da Cunha, M. and Foster, M.A. (1992b). 1,3-propanediol: NAD$^+$ oxidoreductases of *Lactobacillus brevis* and *Lactobacillus buchnerii*. *Applied and Environmental Microbiology*, 58, 2005-2010.

Veringa, H.A., Verburg, E.H. and Stadhouders, J. (1984). Determination of diacetyl in dairy products containing a-acetolactic acid. *Netherlands Milk Dairy Journal*, 38, 251-263.

Versari A, Parpinello GP, Cattaneo M (1999) Leuconostoc oenos and malolactic fermentation in wine: a review. *Ournal of Industrial Microbiology Biotechnology*, 23, 447-455.

Vizoso Pinto, M.G., Pasteris, S.E. and Strasser de Saad, A. M. (2004). Glycerol catabolism by *Pediococcus pentosaceus* isolated from beer. *Food Microbiology*, 21, 111-118.

Welman, A.D. and Maddox, I.S. (2003) Exopolysaccharides from lactic acid bacteria: perspectives and challenges. *Trends Biotechnology*, 21, 269-274

Wood, B.J.B. and Holzapfel, W.H. (1995). *The genera of lactic acid bacteria*; Chapman and Holl: London.

Wood, B. (1998). *Microbiology of Fermented Foods, Second edition, vol 2*, B.J. Wood (Ed.).Blackie Academic and Professional, London.

Zee, J. A. Simard R. E., Vaillancourt R. and Boudrareau A. (1981). Effect of *Lactobacillus brevis*, *Sacharomyces uvarum* and grist composition on amine formation in beer. *Journal of Canadian Institute of Food Sciences and Technology*, 14, 321-325.

In: Red Wine and Health
Editor: Paul O'Byrne

ISBN 978-1-60692-718-2
© 2009 Nova Science Publishers, Inc.

Chapter 9

LEVELS OF PESTICIDE RESIDUES IN RED WINE AND HEALTH RISK ASSESSMENT

José Oliva, Paula Payá[6] and Alberto Barba
Dept. Agricultural Chemistry, Geology and Pedology. Faculty of Chemistry,
University of Murcia. Campus Espinardo, s/n. 30100, Murcia, Spain.

ABSTRACT

The control of pests and diseases of the vine (insects, mites, nematodes and fungi) along with pruning and fertilization are the pillars which should underlie a profitable wine production. The emergence of pesticide residues is a direct result of the various treatments with phytosanitary products during the growing period of the vine and especially among the veraison and maturing and their concentration depends on factors such as: active materials, formulations and doses used, time elapsed between application and harvest, pre-harvest interval of the pesticide and environmental factors (sunlight, rain, etc.). The choice of the proper pesticide and application under good agricultural practice criteria (GAP) reduce the presence of residues in grapes and wine to the utmost.

Available data indicate that there are substantial losses of pesticide residues in the transformation of grape to must and this to wine. It is imperative to note the importance of residue dissipation rates in the crop for their possible presence in wine. The oenological processes commonly used in winemaking as crushing, pressing, racking, clarification and filtration are very important in the disappearance of pesticide residues in wine. Lastly, the art of winemaking including or not maceration, adding of tannins, cryomaceration, etc., influence the disappearance of pesticide residues as well. Also, it should be noted that the characteristics of wine preservation (oak age, time in bottle, temperature, etc.) may influence on their disappearance.

This chapter will discuss experimental data on the disappearance and final levels of insecticides, fungicides and herbicides, such as organophosphates, growth regulators, phthalimide, dicarboximide, benzimidazoles, triazoles, dithiocarbamates, strobirulinas, dinitroanilines, urea derivatives, etc., in wine.

The presence of pesticide residues in wine due to the incorrect use of the phytosanitary products on crops and their possible transfer to must and wine greatly

---

6 Correspondence to: paulapp@um.es, Phone 0034968367473.

concerned the consumer, since there are no maximum residue levels (MRL) for wine established in the European legislation at the moment.

Finally, an approximation of the estimated daily intake (EDI), obtained from the experimental data, will be reported to set comparison with the acceptable daily intake (ADI). In addition, *in vitro* bioavailability trials of some insect growth regulators will be exposed for complementary assessment of health risks due to pesticides residues in red wine.

INTRODUCTION

In recent years, the theme of nutrition and health relating to the moderate consumption of wine in general and the red one in particular has acquired major importance particularly since the publication of the famous article on the "French Paradox" in 1992. This referred to the fact that under similar fat intakes, in France, where wine has been part of the usual diet, there was 60% fewer heart attacks than in England or the United States where consumption of wine was not so frequent [Renaud and Lorgeril, 1992].

The Mediterranean diet broadly speaking is nothing more than the consumption of fresh fruits and vegetables, meat without fat, olive oil and wine of course. All these amounts ingested in a moderate and balanced way that makes this diet beneficial to avoid miscellaneous types of cardiovascular diseases. The term of Mediterranean diet was devised by Ancel Keys and Margaret in the 50's in a cookbook entitled "How to eat well and stay well, the Mediterranean way", long before the first reports of the Seven Countries Study came to light. The Mediterranean countries participating in this study were: Greece, Yugoslavia and Italy. The study focused their hypothesis on the role of fats providing that the total fat ranged 25% and 37% of the total energy in these countries and saturated fats were between 7% and 11%. Also, the relationship between polyunsaturated fatty acids/saturated ones ranged from 0.39 to 0.45. Nowadays, the term Mediterranean diet is not confined only to a diet low in total fat and low saturated fatty acids but also to other nutrients and non-nutrients present in vegetables and processed products which have important antioxidant properties. Wine is one of the main pillars of the Mediterranean diet which supplement its nutritional benefits regarding the quality of fats in the diet. All this is giving a new dimension to the concept of Mediterranean diets [Criqui et al., 1987; Gaziano et al., 1993].

Among the various dietary factors that have been studied in the epidemiology of the cardiovascular disease, the most consistent association has been an inverse relationship with moderate consumption of wine or alcohol, resulting in a reduction of 20-40%. Moderate amounts of alcohol raise levels of HDL-cholesterol, although it may have other beneficial effects unexplained by this increase. Studies in France suggested that wine could have a greater protective effect than other alcoholic beverages, given its antioxidant content capable of reducing the oxidation of LDL-cholesterol. However, this has not been revealed in all epidemiological studies probably due to different patterns of consumption of wine that can be observed in the Mediterranean off the Anglo-Saxon countries, in which these studies are mostly carried out. It seems true that moderate consumption of wine has less harmful effects on diseases than the rest of alcoholic beverages for its consumption pattern and characteristics. It is also possible that there is some interaction between the consumption of wine, alcohol and other components of the diet as fat [Potter and Beeves, 1984; Criqui et al.,

1987; Morgan and Levine, 1988; Rimm et al., 1991; Gaziano et al., 1993; Maclura, 1993; Gronback et al., 1995; Willet and Lenart, 1996; Polychronopoulou and NASK, 1999; Serra-Majid, 1999].

Undoubtedly, wine has a decisive role for the benefit of Mediterranean diets on health. Nevertheless, its effect is limited to the Northern countries of the Mediterranean, since its consumption is nil in the South. The promotion of a Mediterranean diet implies the recommendation to consume wine regularly but sparingly, as many epidemiological studies reported consistently that regular moderate consumption of alcoholic beverages and wine in particular can have protective cardiovascular effect and even a protective effect on total mortality.

For a long time, wine has been used as an appetite stimulant and digestive aid. The alcohol content in wine can be considered as a primary source of calories (1 g alcohol provides 7 Kcal). Alcoholic beverages also provide some micronutrients such as iron, although high alcohol consumption could displace other foods and therefore nutrients, thus causing serious nutritional deficiencies in the diet of non-moderate drinkers [Morgan and Levine, 1988; Soria, 1997; Wamhoff et al., 1998; Polychronopoulou and NASK, 1999]. But, it is also very true that alcohol consumption causes diseases, adverse situations and attitudes (liver cirrhosis; traffic accidents; unintentional injuries; family-, social- and working- changes for alcoholism, criminal behavior and suicide, etc.). Prolonged and high intake of alcohol cause adverse effects on the left ventricular function and the relationship between high consumption of alcohol and cardiomyopathy has been widely recognized. Excessive consumption of alcohol also increases the risk of hypertension and stroke [Aluestad and Haugen, 1999; Huonker et al., 1999].

However, recent investigations regarding the effects of alcohol consumption in general and of red wine in particular have focused on the beneficial aspects rather than the negatives. Therefore, the most important thing is that other perspectives have been opened in which the role of wine offers some very attractive hopes. No longer speaking of cardiovascular disease but also extending the range to cancer, senile dementia, Alzheimer's disease class, inflammatory diseases, senile degeneration of the retina of the elderly, degenerative diseases, signs of old age, etc. The latter aspect is extremely interesting in a world where the longevity of the population is increasing and where offering a better quality for life is imperative [Escrich, 1997; Miura et al., 1997; Koch, 1997; Clement et al., 1998; Draczynska et al., 1998; Lin and Tsai, 1999; Elattar and Virji, 1999; Jang and Pezzuto, 1999).

Two consequences directly derive from these facts. On the one hand, wine components are investigated and studied to explain the positive and hopeful results in relation to the benefits that moderate consumption leads on health in general and particularly on cardiovascular diseases. On the other hand, consumers are more demanding than before and so, stricter controls are asked for wine components including those of exogenous character as pest and disease control in grapes during their cultivation, seeing that residues can be cause of chronic toxicity in humans.

Reviewing the current situation of wine-making, it is observed that wine is part of the active and open trade. The globalization of its sales is a historical constant. Since the Roman Empire (Italy) and its colonies, the Romans established commercial networks in Europe, Africa and Asia, thus developing demand for wines. Throughout the 20th and 21st centuries, production and trade in wine have been subjected to a process of change supported by technological innovation. This process has multiplied due to the amazing increase in communication systems, tourism and globalization of markets. Thus, after the strong growth in the global wine production experienced during the 70's, in which over 10 million hectares of vineyards were reached, a throwback in the implanted surface took place in the 80's mainly due to the excess of wine on the market. Consequently there has been an eradication of vineyards leaving only about 8 million hectares cultivated and Italy, Russia, France, Turkey and Spain cover the 80% of the total eradication. Even though, the largest surface area devoted to growing grapes remains in the European Union (EU) with the 45% of the world vine production area [Dutruc-Rosset, 2005].

Despite the uprooting of vineyards, the contrast of the evolution of global production and consumption of wine continues reflecting a situation of structural surplus production in the market at the moment. This situation determines high competitiveness in the international arena. World wine production, supposing around 270 million hl, is heavily concentrated in countries with strong wine tradition such as France, Italy and Spain. In fact, Europe produces 70% of the total world wine-making. Although, the late 20th century brought new wine-producing countries that are reaching increasing influence on the market by less rigid-productive models than the Europe's designations of origin (D.O.). Moreover, global consumption of wine had slight upward trends in the second half of the 90s, standing at around 220 million hl in 2002. The main areas of consumption are generally the same as the producer ones, perhaps influenced by a more widespread culture of wine [Dutruc-Rosset, 2005].

To achieve this production and also with adequate yields, the use of pesticides in agriculture is an irrefutable fact and of course viticulture is not an exception to this rule. Even the integrated control, which considers wild useful fauna, application limits and doses, among other resources, provides for the use of synthetic pesticides. Therefore, their use is still necessary to obtain qualitatively and quantitatively correct vintages [Giraudon et al., 2000].

However, the use of plant protection involves a series of consequences to consider. Perhaps the greatest concern in this regard rests with the problems of toxicological nature, either directly because they carry risks to consumers or indirectly by the environmental damage [Cormis, 1991]. But, it is also true that the short persistence in soil and low mobility of pesticides used in the vineyard allow us to infer that the chances of contamination of soil and subsoil aquifers are minimal as long as they are applied under criteria of good agricultural practices. But, this is not the case when considering the risk to consumers. During the growing season of the vine and especially among the ripening and maturing, farmers employ a range of products like insecticides, fungicides and herbicides. Those which have penetrating or systemic characteristics are more likely to be found in the grape must and thereafter in wine. Those products of contact stay on the surface of berries and can leave residues especially when used shortly before the harvest. This is why the authorities impose pre-harvest intervals (time that must elapse between treatment and harvest) depending on the persistence of the product. In other words, the detection of pesticide residues at a greater or lesser concentration in grapes in particular and crops in general depends crucially on the characteristics of the pesticide used (nature, formulation, dose, etc.). Although, the influence of other less controllable factors such as climate does also exist [Seib, 1985; Liu et al., 1996; Roberts and Hudson, 1999; Ebbert et al., 1999; South et al., 2000; Sckidmore and Ambrus, 2004; Reynolds et al. 2005; Henrieta et al., 2005 and 2006; Cabizza et al., 2007].

Recently, there have been many investigations on the evolution occurred in pesticide residues along the stages of technological transformation of grapes into wine, as we can see in this chapter. In fact, the currently available experimental data show that if such products are used under proper agricultural practices, residues should not appear at the time of harvest, and therefore in wine, exceeding the established maximum residue limits (MRLs).

As examples of the foregoing, we find the following studies: (i) The study conducted by Goats and Conte in 2001 showed that for 201 pesticides (84 fungicides, 88 insecticides and herbicides 29) recorded in Italy for use in grapes, it have been recently established MRLs for 16 fungicides and 5 insecticides in wine. However, the bibliographic data show that considering the MRLs for future wines was not consistent with the corresponding values in grapes [Goats and Conte, 2001]; (ii) A study intended to control the presence of pesticide residues in 92 wines from Greece and Yugoslavia for 2 consecutive years revealed that only one wine from Greece had 0.3 mg/l of irpodione and six wines from Yugoslavia contained vinclozolin residues in all the samples tested. The rest of the samples tested contained residues at not quantifiable levels [Avramides et al., 2003]; (iii) There have been also controls for specific plant protection products such as the determination of the content of propamocarb in 72 red wines, being all resulting values below 0.1 mg/kg [Taylor et al., 2004]. Therefore, it seems that when grapes are managed under good agricultural practices, final pesticide levels in or on them are minimal.

As stated above, pesticide dissipation on the surface of grapes depends on factors such as: capability of the active ingredient to accede to the grape surface, physico-chemical properties of the pesticide, the amount of pruina in the grape skin, etc., and obviously the weather conditions [Garcia-Cazorla and Xirau- Vayreda, 1994; Papadopoulou-Mourkidou et al., 1995; Cabras et al., 1998; Tsiropoulos et al., 1999; Marin et al., 2003 ; Lentza-Rizos et al., 2006].

Once the grapes are in the winery, the next step will be the obtaining of the wine from them. The process of transformation from grapes to wine comprises the following stages: mechanic treatment of the grapes (crushing and destemming), correction of musts if necessary, encubing (alcoholic fermentation and maceration), separation of wine (descubing and pressing), malolactic fermentations, racking, stabilization (clarification and filtration), vintage and bottling [Zoecklein et al., 1995; Boulton et al., 1996]. All these processes can vary the concentration of pesticide residues present in the grapes, concentrating their levels with a corresponding risk to the consumer or reducing them to safety. Even some studies have proposed the creation of equations based on kinetic analysis that would allows us to predict the concentration of certain substances such as ethyl carbamate in wine after a period of storage at a given temperature. It can predict the time for consumption when concentration of ethyl carbamate do not exceed certain levels capable of producing chronic toxicity in consumers [Hasnip et al., 2004].

This chapter sets out various studies on the effect of different oenotechnological processes to eliminate residues of fungicides, insecticides and herbicides. The aim is to prove that mostly there are great reductions of the levels found in grapes. Therefore, the consumption of wine does not have toxicological risks for consumers from the view point of exogenous pollutants such as pesticides, even when grapes are treated under unfavourable agricultural conditions. Finally, a study conducted on the *in vitro* bioavailability and estimated daily intake of four insect growth regulators (IGR) from grapes and wine is shown.

STUDY ON THE ELIMINATION OF FUNGICIDES IN RED WINE

As commented in the introduction, the variation of pesticide residue levels during the wine-making processes depends on the initial concentration of these in grapes as well as on the nature of the active ingredients and the process followed for the wine-making [García-Cazorla and Xirau-Vayreda, 1994; Navarro et al., 1997, 1999 and 200; Flori et al., 2000; Goats and Angioni, 2000; Fernández et al., 2005a and 2005b; Oliva et al., 2006, 2007a and 2007b]. Thus, in a work on the evolution of the residues of propineb, vinclozolin, procymidone and iprodione in Tempranillo grape cultivated in La Rioja (Spain), it was found that the decline in of the fungicide concentration from grape juice to wine was: 51.4% for propineb, 61% for vinclozolin, 41.1% for procymidone and 17.24% for iprodione [Zaballa et al., 1992].

Studying the ratio of decline during the vinification for famoxadone, recently applied fungicide to vines that belongs to the family oxazolidinedione, it is found that there is an elimination of 100% of the fungicide, both with and without wine-making maceration because from grapes harvested at levels near its MRL (2 mg/kg), a level below the limit of quantification of the product (0.05 mg/kg) is reached in wine [De Melo et al., 2006].

For spiroxamine, a new fungicidal active substance belonging to the spiroketalamine class of substances with protective, curative and eradicative effects against mildews, we note that the elimination from grapes to wine is affected by performing or not maceration. So, when the wine-making is performed without maceration, the elimination is between 20-27%, whereas for wines produced with maceration, the elimination increases to 45-62%. The transfer factor between grapes and grape juice was 0.55 and therefore half of the fungicide was removed together with the solid parts of grapes. And in the process from grape to wine, the transfer factor was 0.26. In general, the elimination of spiroxamine residues from grapes to wine ranges 23-56% depending on the wine-making technique used. And there are no residues more than 10% of MRL of the product in wine after a treatment with GAP (Good Agricultural Practices), so there is no toxicological risks in wines obtained from grapes treated with spiroxamine [Tsiropoulos et al., 2005].

When we do monitor the behavior of quinoxyfen, we observe that after four applications in field, there was a residue level of 0.38 mg/kg in grapes and a half-life time average of 7.24 days. During the wine-making without maceration, less than 50% of the residue was transferred from the grapes to must. Separating the less from the must performed by the must centrifugation caused the total disappearance of the residue. After fermentation with or without maceration no residues were detected in wine [Cabras et al., 2000]. Also, the fate of four new fungicides (cyprodinil, fludioxonil, pyrimethanil and tetraconazole) from the treatment on vine to the production of wine was studied. The influence of clarifying agents (bentonite, charcoal, potassium caseinate, gelatine and polyvinylpolypyrrolidone) on residue concentrations in wine was also studied. Grape processing into wine caused considerable residue reduction with cyprodinil (ca. 80%), fludioxonil (ca. 70%) and tebuconazole (ca. 50%) and no reduction with pyrimethanil. The two wine-making techniques employed (whit and without maceration) had the same influence on the residue concentrations in wine, except for fludioxonil which showed maximum residue reduction with vinification with maceration. Among the clarifying agents tested, only charcoal showed effective action on the elimination of residue content in wine, proving complete elimination, or almost, of fungicide residues [Cabras et al., 1997].

Another study reported the behavior of fenhexamid in grapes, during wine-making and the effect of the microflora of the alcoholic and malolactic fermentation on in its disappearance. The elimination of this fungicide during the wine-making depends on whether the process is carried out with or without maceration by the grape skin. So, when no maceration was performed, an elimination of 49% occurred. But, the elimination was 62% with maceration. Therefore, the presence of the peel in contact with the fungicide for some time produced an increase in the elimination of the fungicide studied. No effect of yeasts and bacteria involved in the wine-making was found for fenhexamid disappearance [Cabras et al., 2001]. Also, a study of our research group on this fungicide leaded to similar results [Oliva et al., 2006]. It is also important to study the degradation of certain fungicides and their transformation into other products with toxic action. One example is the pesticide captan. This degraded in must, even to 100% of tetrahydrophtalimide (THPI) at the end of the fermentation and thus, only THPI can be determined in wine. The degradation from captan to THPI in must and wine is due to the acidity. The metabolite was present at low levels in grapes and the dissipation model showed that the mechanism was mainly due to photo-degradation and codistillation [Angioni et al., 2003].

Also, the evolution of residual levels of four fungicides (cyprodinil, fludioxonil, pyrimethanil and quinoxyfen) during elaboration of three types of wine with maceration (traditional red wine, carbonic maceration red wine and red wine of long maceration and prefermentation at low temperature) has been studied [Fernández et al., 2005a]. The disappearance curves of each fungicide have been analyzed during the period of time of each wine-making process (21 days) and during the different oenological steps involved in the elaborations. To ascertain the dissipation rate of residues in each wine-making procedure, the experimental data have been fitted to the follow mathematic model [Gunther and Blinn, 1955; Timme and Freshe, 1980; Timme et al., 1986]:

$R_t = R_0 \bullet e^{-kt}$ (a)
$Ln\ R_t = Ln\ R_0 - Kt$ (b)

(a) R_t is the residue concentration at time t (mg/kg).
R_0 is the theoretical initial residue concentration at t=0 (mg/kg).
K is the fungicide decay constant.
t is the time elapsed since the phytosanitary treatment.

(b) $Ln\ R_0$ and K are constants.
$Ln\ R_t$ and t are variables; the second one depends on the first.

This type of analysis allows the behaviour of fungicide residues during the wine-making procedures to be known, by showing the correlation that exists between the residual levels and the time, and also the fungicide decay constants. These values of K represent the tendency of the residues of each fungicide to be reduced to a greater or lesser degree during overall wine-making procedures and depending on factors like: degradation, adsorption on skins and lees or on clarifying agents used to clean the must and wine, variety of grape and wine-making method, among others [Navarro et al., 1997, 1999 and 200; Flori et al., 2000;

Cabras and Angioni, 2000; Fernández et al., 2005a and 2005b; Oliva et al., 2006, 2007a and 2007b]. In addition, it is also possible to study if the correlation existing between variables is more or less significant from the statistical point of view, through a statistical demonstration with the number of pairs of values used in the coefficient calculus. To do this, we can use the following equation [Miller and Miller, 1993]:

$$t = |r| \sqrt{(n-2)} / \sqrt{(1-r^2)} \quad (c)$$

It allows to us obtain a value of distribution t-Student that can be compared to t tabulated values. If t calculated is superior to t tabulated the correlation between both variables is statistically significant. In equation (c), r represents the correlation coefficient and n the liberty grades.

The study based on the time employed in the transformation from grape to wine begun with the crushing of grapes (first day) and concluded 21 days later (clarified wine). The results of the fit are presented in Table I.

Table 1. Statistical parameters derived from the linear fit of the data during the time employed in each vinification (21 days).

Fungicide	Traditional method			Carbonic maceration			Long maceration		
	r	|k|	t	r	|k|	T	R	|k|	T
Cyprodinil	0.879	0.211	3.684*	0.940	0.238	4.751*	0.869	0.242	3.505*
Fludioxonil	0.890	0.688	1.947	0.975	0.210	7.605**	0.746	0.252	1.586
Pyrimethanil	0.829	0.142	2.965*	0.919	0.136	4.020*	0.910	0.160	4.390*
Quinoxyfen	0.906	0.533	2.145	0.896	0.181	2.850	0.808	0.096	1.942

r = correlation coefficient; |k| = absolute value of constant rate; t = calculated value of t-distribution for $P<0.05$, significant grade of the correlation between variables: *$P< 0,05$, **$P<0,01$, ***$P<0,001$.

As can be seen from these data, the linear correlation between Ln R_t and the time was not good in all assays, with correlation coefficients inferior to 0.8 for fludioxonil in the wine-making of long maceration, being the most unfavourable coefficient calculated. The rest of correlation coefficient values oscillated between 0.808 and 0.975, values that correspond, respectively, to quinoxyfen in the elaboration of long maceration and fludioxonil in the elaboration by carbonic maceration. In relation to fungicide decay constant values, we can establish a dissipation rate for the four fungicides. For each wine-making procedure it was as follows:

Traditional wine-making procedure (maceration of four days):
Fludioxonil > Quinoxyfen > Cyprodinil > Pyrimethanil.
Long maceration wine-making procedure (four days at 5 °C and six at room temperature):Fludioxonil > Cyprodinil > Pyrimethanil > Quinoxyfen.
Carbonic maceration wine-making procedure (maceration of ten days in CO_2 atmosphere): Cyprodinil > Fludioxonil > Quinoxyfen > Pyrimethanil.

For all wine-making methods, except carbonic maceration, fludioxonil was the fungicide that showed the highest constant value (K). For maceration carbonic wine-making the highest value of K corresponded to cyprodinil. Pyrimethanil decay constants were the lowest in all vinifications with the exception of the long maceration wine-making procedure, where the lowest was presented for quinoxyfen.

The second study was made taking into account the steps of wine-making procedures. For this purpose 4-5 wine-making steps for each elaboration were established as follows:

Traditional wine-making procedure to obtain red wines: crushing grapes (phase 0), maceration period (phase 1), must (phase 2), racked wine (phase 3) and clarified wine (phase 4).

Wine-making procedure to obtain red wines of long maceration and prefermentative process at low temperature: crushing grapes (phase 0), freeze maceration (phase 1), room temperature maceration (phase 2), must (phase 3), racked wine (phase 4) and clarified wine (phase 5).

Carbonic maceration wine-making to obtain red wine: grape (phase 0), half maceration period (phase 1), must (phase 2), racked wine (phase 3) and clarified wine (phase 4).

In this case, the linear fit of results was performed taking into consideration the oenological steps of each wine-making procedure, i.e., the relationship between each phase and the preceding phase was based not on the time elapsed, but on the residual values connected of the stage in question. To do, the time (t) was substituted for the steps in equations (a) and (b). The results of the study are shown in Table II.

Table 2. Statistical parameters derived from the linear fit of the data during the steps envolved in each vinification.

Fungicide	Traditional method			Carbonic maceration			Long maceration method		
	r	|k|	t	r	|k|	t	r	|k|	T
Cyprodinil	0.974	1.236	7.509**	0.947	1.254	5.511*	0.936	1.021	5.533**
Fludioxonil	0.890	1.374	1.947	0.979	1.104	8.404**	0.834	0.968	2.135
Pyrimethanil	0.957	0.858	5.679*	0.926	0.711	4.235*	0.942	0.683	5.596**
Quinoxyfen	0.906	1.064	2.144	0.895	0.907	2.843	0.883	0.361	2.661

r = correlation coefficient; |k| = absolute value of constant rate; *t* = calculated value of t-distribution for *P<0.05*, significant grade of the correlation between variables: *P< 0,05, **P<0,01, ***P<0,001.

The correlation between the residues of cyprodinil and the different steps of all wine-making procedures was statistically very significant. The contrary was observed for quinoxyfen, for which the disappearance of its residues during the steps of wine-making procedures was not significant in any of the cases.

As regards the calculated values of the constant rate, the following dissipation rate was found for each vinification:

Traditional wine-making procedure (maceration of four days):
Fludioxonil > Cyprodinil > Quinoxyfen > Pyrimethanil.
Long maceration wine-making procedure (four days at 5 °C and six at room temperature):
Cyprodinil > Fludioxonil > Pyrimethanil > Quinoxyfen.

Carbonic maceration wine-making procedure (maceration of ten days in CO_2 atmosphere): Cyprodinil > Fludioxonil > Quinoxyfen > Pyrimethanil.

In general, the results obtained were very similar to those observed in the other study (for time). Fludioxonil showed the highest decay constant values in wine-making procedures without maceration and in the traditional wine-making, and pyrimethanil presented the lowest in all cases with the exception of long maceration wine-making procedure.

In this study differences existed between wine-making procedures with and without maceration for cyprodinil and fludioxonil. In vinifications with maceration cyprodinil showed higher constant rates than in vinifications without this maceration phase. However, decay constant values of fludioxonil were superior in procedures with maceration phase. The tendency of pyrimethanil and quinoxyfen to decay in the transition from one step to the next in the context of overall vinification methods (with or without maceration) was very similar. The constant rates calculated for these fungicides ranged from 0.565 to 0.858 for pyrimethanil in white wine-making and traditional procedure respectively, and from 0.683 to 1.064 for quinoxyfen in the same vinifications as the previous case. The only important difference for quinoxyfen was appreciated between long maceration wine-making procedure and rosé vinification.

At the end of both studies we can affirm that in wine-making procedures with maceration the relationships between the residue concentrates and the steps found were more significant than those calculated between residue levels and the time. Correlation coefficients were superior in the study performed by steps for all fungicides. The major difference between studies, time or step appeared in the wine-making without maceration procedures.

Therefore, depending on the type of wine-making that takes place, we will find greater or lesser elimination of pesticides, which implies that the health and hygiene quality and possible toxicity for pesticide residues to consumers will be affected by the type of wine-making performed.

Another study by Flori et al. (2000) also used an exponential equation based on the different oenotechnological stages involved in the elimination of various fungicide residues [Flori et al., 2000]. The purpose of this study was to determine the final residues in wine and the percentage of elimination from grapes to wine so that the toxicological risk to consumers was assessed.

Table 3 shows the percentage of elimination of some fungicide residues studied after the four wine-making processes were carried out to transform the grapes into wine (crushing the grapes, clarifying the must, fermentation and running of the wine) and also includes the rate of degradation (K) and the correlation between the amount removed and the operations or steps performed. As pointed, most of the fungicides studied suffered more than 80% of elimination and even some reached the total elimination during the wine-making process. In addition, the correlation factors between the amount removed and the various stages of the wine process were higher than 0.90 for most of the fungicides. This indicates that there is good correlation between the dissipation of fungicides and the various oenotechnological stages involved by the wine-making. The values found are indicative of a high elimination of fungicide residues during the wine-making process, which supposes residues well below the MRL in wines and therefore no influence from the toxicological point of view on the consumer health.

Table 3.- Percentage of elimination of fungicides during the wine-making process.

Active ingredient	% elimination	K	R^2
Thiophanto methyl	49.6	0.195	0.844
Copper	86.7	0.368	0.620
Metalaxyl	77.7	0.368	0.980
Penconazole	89.3	0.404	0.730
Fenarimol	85.4	0.434	0.803
Triadimenol	75.4	0.495	0.846
Furalaxyl	84.8	0.504	0.952
Iprodione	89.9	0.588	0.979
Myclobutanil	91.5	0.737	0.522
Procymidone	94.5	0.791	0.946
Propyconazole	95.5	0.846	0.652
Benomyl	95.5	0.846	0.927
Benalaxyl	96.7	0.850	0.994
Vinclozolin	97.9	1.022	0.966
Mancozeb	99.0	1.222	0.912
Metiram	99.3	1.384	0.850
Dichlofluanid	99.8	1.649	0.906
Folpet	99.9	1.737	0.985
Cymoxanil	99.9	1.768	0.776

Another point is the use of clarifying agents and filtration to remove residues of fungicides. Thus, the effects of six clarification agents (egg albumin, blood albumin, bentonite + gelatine, charcoal, PVPP and silica gel) on the removal of residues of three fungicides (famoxadone, fluquinconazole and trifloxystrobin) applied directly to a racked red wine, elaborated from Monastrell variety grapes from the D.O. Region of Jumilla (Murcia, Spain) are studied. The clarified wines were filtered with 0.45 µm nylon filters to determine the influence of this winemaking process in the disappearance of fungicide residues. In general, trifloxystrobin was the lesser persistent fungicide in the wines, except for the assay egg albumin. On the contrary, fluquinconazole was the most persistent. The elimination depended on the product nature, although the water stability and light presence seemed to be more influencing within this than the solubility and polarity of the compound. The best fining substances were charcoal and PVPP. Silica gel and bentonite plus gelatine were ineffective to reduce considerably the residues levels in the wine clarified by them. In general, filtration was not an effective step in the elimination of wine residues. The greatest elimination after filtration was obtained in wines clarified by egg albumin and bentonite plus gelatine and the lowest one in those clarified by PVPP [Oliva et al., 2007a]

Another study with the same fining agents and four fungicides (cyprodinil, fludioxonil, pyrimethanil and quinoxyfen) reported that in general, and for all fungicides except for quinoxyfen, albumin blood was the most effective fining agent in eliminating residues, while the silica gel was ineffective for all pesticides except fludioxonil. The fungicide quinoxyfen was the lesser persistent one in clarified wines and appeared in the highest percentage in the lees. Generally, the filtration was not an effective step to eliminate the residues from the wine.

The greatest reduction after the filtration was obtained for wines clarified by charcoal and the lowest one for those clarified by PVPP [Fernández et al., 2005b].

Another factor to consider is the effect that the yeast responsible for the fermentation may have on the disappearance of some fungicides. Particularly, some influence has been found for two yeasts (*Saccharomyces cerevisiae* and *Kloeckera apiculata*) and two lactic acid bacteria (*Leuconostoc oenos* and *Lactobacillus plantarum*) on the degradation of six fungicides (azoxystrobin, cyprodinil, fludioxonil, mepanipyrim, pyrimethanil and tretraconazole) during the alcoholic and malolactic fermentation. The results showed that the degradation occurred only during the alcoholic fermentation for the fungicide pyrimethanil (decline of 20-40% compared to the control concentration after 10 days of fermentation). For the other five fungicides, the alcoholic fermentation did not produce elimination by any of the possible mechanisms (i.e. pesticide degradation by yeast or pesticide adsorption on yeast). None of the bacteria studied showed any effect on the fungicide degradation during the malolactic fermentation [Cabras et al., 1999].

Also, the effect of red wine malolactic fermentation on the fate of seven fungicides (carbendazim, chlorothalonil, fenarimol, metalaxyl, oxadixyl, procymidone and triadimenol) was investigated. After malolactic fermentation using *Oenococcus oeni*, the concentrations of chlorothalonil and procymidone diminished only slighty [Ruediger et al., 2005].

Other studies based on the potential toxicology of grapes and wine related to the presence of exogenous pollutants indicated the effect that pesticide treatments may have on the presence of heavy metals in grapes and wine. Some fungicides may have effect on heavy metals present in the vineyard by changing its usual content of them. A study conducted by Salvo et al. in 2003 found that levels of Cu (II), Pb (II) and Zn (II) were below the toxicological limits for wines obtained from vineyards either treated or not and that Cd (II) was not detected for them. However, contents of heavy metals were increased in those treated with pesticides respect for the treated grapes with water. Particularly, quinoxyfen, a mixture of dinocap and penconazole, and dinocap significantly raised the Cu (II) and Zn (II) content in white and red wines. Pb levels were increased significantly by the treatment with azoxystrobin and sulphur [Salvo et al., 2003]. In another case, by studying the influence of the fungicides mancozeb, zoxamide, copper oxychloride on the concentration of manganese, copper, lead and cadmium in red wines from Sicily, it was found that wines from treated plots with zoxamide and mancozeb showed levels of manganese and zinc three times higher than those observed in controls. The wines from grapes treated with copper oxychloride, showed significant increases for Cu (II) (up to 50%). Also moderated increases were observed for Pb (II) and Cd (II) (La Pera et al., 2008). Also, another study was focused on the variation of the content of some metals that could come or not from pesticide applications on crops in order to assess the toxicological risks to consumers. Authors concluded that the presence of copper and its transfer from grapes to juice and wine was influenced by the number of applications, the period between application and harvest, and the amount of copper applied. Of the total samples tested in 16 wine cellars in Italy, 18% exceeded the MRL established (20 mg/kg). It was therefore recommended that the time between treatment and harvest was extended from 20 days to 40-50 days. In addition, this study reflected that the copper content did not depend on the strategy of pest control (conventional, integrated or organic). Among the three above factors, the most important was the amount of copper applied since this was the reason for the 44% concentration phenomena registered between grapes and wines [García-Esparza et al., 2006].

Finally, the possible effect of the processes of alcoholic fermentation on the total level of arsenic and its inorganic species [As (III) and As (V)] and the organic ones (monomethyl arsonic acid [MMA] and dimethyl acid arsinic [DNA]) in 45 wines from southern Spain was examined. The total levels of arsenic were very similar for the different types of wines studied. The levels of arsenic in the wine samples analyzed ranged between 2.1 and 14.6 µg/l. The results suggested that the consumption of these wines should not suppose significant contribution to the intake of total and inorganic arsenic when in the diet of a moderate drinker [Herce-Pagliai et al., 2002].

Besides that, the presence of pesticide residues in wine does not depend on being used in plant control as conventional programs or integrated pest management (IPM) since a screening of pesticide residues carried out on 47 samples of wine grapes grown according to IPM revealed that 2.1% of the samples did not contain any residues above the limit of quantification; 59.6% contained the same or less than their MRLs, and the other 38.3% exceeded the MRLs for cyprodinil and fludioxonil. Therefore, obtaining these wines with grapes grown under IPM did not present any toxicological problem in 60% of the cases. The samples that violated the MRL could generate problems in the wines derived from them considering that there was no decline of the residues during the fermentation process [Basa et al., 2008].

STUDY ON THE ELIMINATION OF INSECTICIDES IN RED WINE

Insecticides commonly used in vineyards keep pseudo first order kinetics for dissipation with half-life time of a few days and hence, often have very low initial deposits. In addition, if the pre-harvest intervals are respected, we can observe that that residues found in the grapes harvested are much lower and even undetectable in some cases. But, not always GAP are met. This is why studies on the disappearance of some insecticides during the wine-making have been conducted.

In this sense, Cabras et al. (1995) conducted a study with various insecticides. Among all, methyl chlorpyrifos was the one which presented a smaller deposit in grapes (0.16 ppm). The residue found in must was considerably lower than found in grapes indicating the affinity of this insecticide for the suspended matter. This fact was corroborated by the corresponding reduction occurred when lees were separated from must by centrifugation. The wines produced with and without maceration had the same residues (0.03 ppm) being 5 times lower than those found in grapes. No residues were detected in wines clarified by charcoal in comparison with the more moderate effectiveness achieved by other clarifying agents. Fenthion showed a high rate of disappearance since 7 days after the treatment the residue declined to 0.06 ppm. During the wine-making, the residue remained in the liquid phase confirmed by the fact that no disappearance was observed in must when the lees were separated by centrifugation. After fermentation, the residue in wine was the same as in grapes. Its behavior during the clarification was similar to methyl chlorpyrifos. Methidation showed moderate persistence, although its residue decreased up to 0.02 ppm in seven days. During the wine-making, about half of the initial concentration was transferred to the must and no disappearance was observed during the fermentation. There were no significant reductions in residue levels during the clarifications except for the case of charcoal, which achieved by reduction of 75% of the initial concentration. Parathion methyl presented the greatest rate of disappearance in grapes. During the wine-making, the transfer from grapes to wine leaded to reductions of 65% in the residue level. Performing or not maceration proved similar influence on residue reduction being in both cases 86% of declining. In the clarification of the pesticides tested, only charcoal offered great efficiency achieving the complete absorption of the residue. Quinalphos behavior was similar to that of methyl parathion during the phases of wine-making and clarification [Cabras et al., 1995]. Seeing these results, it can be stated that there was very significant decline for the main organophosphate insecticides during the winemaking process, for which the elimination ranged 60-100%, except for the case of fenthion where it was nil.

Years later (2000), a compilation done by Goats and Angioni compared the disappearance of several insecticides applied to vineyard for the wine-making [Goats and Angioni, 2000]. It was found that azinphos methyl decreased until almost 16 times its initial value in the grapes when wine was undergone with maceration and reaching a level of 0.04 ppm in the beverage [Goodwin and Ahmad, 1998]. Quinalphos declined until more than 5 times its initial level. Chlorpyrifos reached levels of residues in wine between 24 and 185 times lower than those initially presented grapes, depending on the initial amount (the larger initial residue, the higher disappearance) and no differences were observed between the wines obtained with and without maceration. In all cases, the greatest disappearance occurred in the process of descubing, pressing and racking [Cabras et al., 1994; Hall et al., 1996; Navarro et al., 1999]. Chlorpyrifos methyl maintained a behavior similar to earlier, presenting a lower decrease (5 times) in the finished wine [Cabras et al., 1995]. Dimethoate and fenthion insecticides were more persistent in the wine, virtually maintaining the same concentration during the vinification (i.e. 0.28 ppm-initial to 0.20 ppm-final and 0.06-initial to 0.04 ppm-final for dimethoate and fenthion respectively) and observing very slight differences between the wines obtained with or without maceration [Cabras et al., 1994, 1995]. Fenitrothion decreased 19 times, reaching 34 times less, when the wine-making was performed without maceration [Hall et al., 1996]. Methidation only fell to half its initial value while methyl parathion declined more than 7 times its value and up to 28 times depending on their initial concentration. There were no differences between both with and without maceration [Cabras et al., 1995; Hall et al., 1996].

Work carried out at the University of Murcia (SE Spain) revealed the disappearance of four insecticides included in the group of insect growth regulators and inhibitors (fenoxycarb, flufenoxuron, lufenuron and pyriproxyfen). In micro-vinifications conducted on grapes treated with them, we could observe that no residues exceeding their limit of quantification (LOQ = 0.05 mg/l) in the immediate products for consumer (musts, clarified wine and filtered wine) were detected. This was probably due to the separation of the solid and semi-solid by-products by the practice of the pressing and racking processes. The transfer of these residues from must to wine was nil and all the residues were found in the crushed grapes and by-products (pomace and lees). The pomace was predominantly where the residues of these products were transferred in the wine-making. This allows us to say that these pesticides were removed linked to the solid parts of the grapes (i.e. peel and seeds), which are the common elements of the by-products. Among the four insecticides, the greatest dissipation during the wine-making was found for flufenoxuron, while lufenuron, fenoxycarb, and pyriproxyfen showed lower levels throughout the process and their dissipations were less intense. Finally, the bottled wine would have come into the market without quantifiable residues (LOQ = 0.05

mg/kg). Among the samples for which residues were found, we can establish the following order according to their concentration: pomace> crushing > lees. The presence of the residues in the pomace (average 0.36 mg/kg) and lees (average 0.13 mg/kg) should be considered in obtaining industrially spirits, alcohols, feed, grape seed oil and food additives such as calcium tartrate, which are the principal derivatives from these products, because the starting material would be contaminated with pesticide residues and could suppose health risks [Payá, 2008]. The transfer factors among the three types of samples mentioned were studied for each pesticide as well. Values of the factor greater than 1 indicated concentration of residues, while values less than 1 represented an elimination of the pesticide. We found that the average transfer factor in pomace was 2.54 and 1.92 when the grape treatments were performed under GAP or critical agricultural practices (CAP), respectively. In the lees, there was no transfer of flufenoxuron or lufenuron, while there was maintenance of the level of fenoxycarb and pyriproxyfen under GAP because the transfer factor was 1.06 on average and even we found dissipation under CAP since their transfer factor was 0.56 on average. In the crushing, it was observed maintenance of the levels regarding the harvest both under GAP and CAP, with transfer factors of 1.44 and 0.80 on average, respectively but being the transference nil in the the case of lufenuron under GAP.

In an study on the effect of red wine malolactic fermentation on the fate of three insecticides (carbaryl, chlorpyrifos and dicofol), it was found that after malolactic fermentation using Oenococcus oeni, the concentrations of the active compounds chlorpyrifos and dicofol were the most significantly reduced [Ruediger et al., 2005].

In the above study, which was conducted in Italy in 2000, researchers also set out the percentages of elimination of some insecticides after the four oenotechnological processes carried out to transform the grapes into wine (crushing the grapes, clarifying the must, fermentation and running of the wine) and included the rate of degradation (K) and the correlation between the amount removed and the operations or steps performed as well (Table IV).

Table 4.- Percentage of elimination of insecticides in the wine-making process.

Active ingredient	% elimination	K	R^2
Fenthion	69.6	0.243	0.796
Methidathion	78.5	0.432	0.814
Parathion methyl	87.6	0.590	0.879
Tetradifon	90.2	0.616	0.793
Dicofol	90.7	0.734	0.930
Diazinon	100	0.835	0.566
Quinalphos	96.6	0.930	0.934
Chlorpyrifos methyl	96.8	0.930	0.955
Deltametrhin	100	1.630	1.000

Considering the figures outlined in the table above, it can be concluded that high reductions take place during the wine-making process, since the dissipation rates were from 70% to the total elimination of the product. Also, it appears that the residue data for the insecticides studied had good correlations to their degradation kinetics, with the exception of diazinon.

STUDY ON THE ELIMINATION OF HERBICIDES IN RED WINE

In some geographical areas, persistent herbicides are used in growing grapes with the possibility that the grapes and subsequently wine become contaminated with their residues, especially if the plant protection product is systemic. However, works on this topic are scarce, unlike the existing ones on the disappearance of other pesticides such as insecticides and fungicides.

However, the behavior of some herbicides as norflurazon, oxadiazon, trifluralin and oxyfluorfen in Shiraz and Doradillo grapes were investigated in Southern Australia. The results indicated slow dissipation of herbicides on the surface of the Shiraz grapes. Moreover, it was found that oxyflurorfen and trifluralin were no longer found in grapes after 4 days of the pesticide treatment, while norflurazon and oxadiazon persisted after a month of the application. Norflurazon was the product more significantly persistent in grapes. About 14% of norflurazon and 0.24% of oxadiazon penetrated grape flash in white grapes but only 1.47% of norflurazon and nothing for oxadiazon penetrated the red grapes. The residues of the herbicides in the must were degraded more rapidly during the first fermentation. Oxyfluorfen disappeared completely on the second day while trifluralin degraded after 24 days added to wine (in experiences of wine fortifications). With regard to the clarification, the cellulose pad and diatomaceus hearth showed no influence on norflurazon or oxadiazon while presented moderate influence on trifluralin and oxifluorfen. The cellulose pad got to reduce by 23.52% and 58.95% of the initial amounts of trifluralin and oxyfluorfen in the wine respectively. The diatomaceus Herat only reduced these two pesticide residues in 55.15% and 74.22% of the initial concentration in the wine. The mixture of the two clarifying agents significantly increased the elimination of the residues in the red wine. Charcoal completely removed the herbicide residues in wine [Ying and Williams, 1999].

All the works analyzed show high eliminations of the pesticide residues present in grapes for wine-making. Therefore, the residue levels in wines would be well below the limits set out for residues in grapes, which means additional safety for consumers. This allows us to say that moderate consumption of wine would be beneficial for its natural components (phenolic compounds with antioxidant activity) but would not introduce hazards related to exogenous pollutants.

IN VITRO BIOAVAILABILITY AND INTAKE ESTIMATION OF PESTICIDE RESIDUES IN RED WINES

Studying the bioavailability of substances for humans have been primarily used in pharmaceutical development and monitoring, although this term is not exclusively related to us. Briefly, it defines the grade in which exogenous compounds can penetrate and be used by any living organism determining then compound's influence on these. The reality is that there are many limitations to block the pathway to the target. Very different are the exposure possibilities to exogenous agents in organisms and for all of them the bioavailability can potentially be studied. In human oral exposure, many are the causes which can lower or prevent the availability of compounds such us drugs, food supplements or pollutants (e.g. application form, other medications, sex, age, health status, foods, physiological processes)

[Fait and Colosio, 1998; Ramírez and Lacasaña, 2001]. But overall, the particular commodity in which residues are can be pointed as the most relevant factor among the external causes to restrict the potential availability and effectiveness of pesticides in humans [Johnson, 1997; Hodgson and Smart, 2001; Ross et al., 2001]. At present, very few jobs relate pesticide bioavailability with food. Most of the trials are focused on the bioavailability from soils for species such as shrimps, earthworms or cells. However, our research group "Chemistry and Action of Pesticides" has begun studying this feature in miscellaneous foods at the University of Murcia (SE Spain) in order to assess real food risks related to pesticide residues. The *in vitro* bioavailability of different insecticides belonging to the group IGR (e.g. fenoxycarb, pyriproxyfen, lufenuron and flufenoxuron) have been investigated in fresh and processed products of citrus, stone fruits, leafy and fruiting vegetables, and grapes. The trials simulated *in vitro* human gastrointestinal conditions for digestion measuring the dialyzed amount that passed through the semipermeable cellulose derived tubing commercially and specifically designed for these tests [Payá et al., 2006 and 2007; Payá, 2008]. As results, no *in vitro* bioavailability was detected for these insecticides when samples of grapes and wine were spiked at the levels found after the PHI and food transformation (0.05-1 µg/g). The pesticides dialyzed at spiking levels ranging 70-100 µg/g in wine but 50-100 µg/g in grapes. In any case, these levels were much higher than those left by these pesticides in the agricultural products after the crop application. Therefore, we can say that *in vitro* the residue levels found in these foods did not overpass the first and foremost biological barrier for oral income of xenobiotics, thus preventing their arrival to a place of systemic action in the human body. In all cases, it was noted that according to their characteristics for the dialysis, the pesticides could be ordered as: fenoxycarb > pyriproxyfen > lufenuron > flufenoxuron. Therefore, the most dialyzable pesticides were fenoxycarb and pyriproxyfen and the lesser ones were the two benzoylphenylureas (i.e flufenoxuron and lufenuron). The different commodities could also be sorted according to the matrix effect they present against the dialysis: red grapes > red wine > solvent standards. Therefore, at equal initial concentrations, there is greater dialysis when the pesticides were: solvent > red wine > red grapes. The results indicate that the bioavailability of pesticides is influenced by their physicochemical nature, concentration in the sample, characteristics of the matrix where they are studied and the selectivity of the dialysis membrane [Payá, 2008].

Nowadays, the assessment of human exposure to pesticides in foods is mainly performed according to deterministic or probabilistic approaches. Although the deterministic point of view is based on the worst case situation and many are the contradictions that can be claimed, it continues being the official way of determination for the EU organisms involved in this field [Lambe, 2002; Tomerlin, 2003; Verdonck et al., 2006]. In studies conducted by our research group using the wine intake data provided by the Spanish National Statistics Institute (INE) for the adult population classified with regard to the different living area in Spain (nationally, Region of Murcia or locally, rural and non-rural) we overall found that at least there was a safety factor of 883 between our estimated daily intake (EDI) and the legally acceptable daily intake (ADI) for the residues of the insecticides mentioned above. Our EDI set hypothetical pesticide concentrations of 0.05 mg/l (i.e. LOQ) in red wine although previous experiments had shown that no residues above this level could be found in the beverage due to the wine-making practices. Considering the same concentration but with frequency food consumption surveys representatively conducted by us among locally youth-, adult- and elder population, this value raised to 1407, slightly different from the previous one due to the methodological differences between the consumption figures (Payá, 2008). We can conclude that even in the worst-case calculation there were very broad safety factors between the daily ingestion of these products and consequent chronic toxicity hazards for consumers living in all classes of residence area in Spain and belonging to the principal red wine drinking groups in our Region.

REFERENCES

Ajuestad, M; Haugen, OA. Death behind the wheel. *Tidsskz Nor Laegeforen,* 1999 119 (7), 966-968.

Angioni, A; Garau, VL; Aguilera, A; Melis, M; Minelli, EV; Tuberoso, C; Cabras, P. GC-ITMS determination and degradation of captan during winemaking. *Journal of Agricultural and Food Chemistry,* 2003 51, 6761-6766.

Avramides, EJ; Lentza-Rizos, C; Mojasevic, M. Determination of pesticide residues in wine using gas chromatography with nitrogen-phosphorus and electron capture detection. *Food Additives & Contaminants,* 2003 20, 699-706.

Basa, H; Gregorcic, A; Cus F. Pesticide residues in grapes from vineyards included in integrated pest management in Slovenia. *Food Additives & Contaminants,* 2008 25, 438-443.

Boulton, RB; Singleton, VL; Bisson, LF; Kunkee, RE. Principles and practices of winemaking. New York: Champman & Hall; 1996.

Cabizza, M; Satta, M; Falcón, S; Onano, M; Uccheddu, G. Degradation of cyprodinil, fludioxonil, cyfluthrin and pymetrozine on lettuce alter different application methods. *Journal of Environmental Science and Health, Part B,* 2007 42, 761-766.

Cabras, P; Garau; VL; Melis, M; Pirisi, FM; Cubeddu, M; Cabitza, F. Residui di dimetoato e clorpirifos nell´uva e nel vino. *Attiche Giornate Fitopatologiche,* 1994 1, 27-32.

Cabras, P; Angioni, A; Garau, VL; Melis, M; Pirisi, FM; Minelli, EV; Cabitza, F; Cubeddu, M. Fate of some new fungicides (cyprodinil, fludioxonil, pyrimethanil and tebuconazole) from vine to wine. *Journal of Agricultural and Food Chemistry,* 1997 45, 2708-2710.

Cabras, P; Angioni, A; Garau, VL; Pirisi, F; Espinoza, J; Mendoza, A; Cabitza, F; Pala, M; Brandolini, V. Fate of azoxystrobin, fluazinam, kresoxim-methyl, mepanipyrim and tetraconazole from vine to wine. *Journal of Agricultural and Food Chemistry,* 1998 46, 3249-3251.

Cabras P; Angioni A; Garau VL; Pirisi FM; Farris, GA; Madau G; Emonti, G. Pesticides in fermentative processes of wine. *Journal of Agricultural and Food Chemistry,* 1999 47, 3854-3857.

Cabras, P; Angioni, A. Pesticide residues in grape, wine and their processing products. *Journal of Agricultural and Food Chemistry,* 2000 48(4), 967-973.

Cabras, P; Angioni, A; Garau, VL; Pirisi, FM; Cabitza, F; Pala, M; Farris, G.A. Fate of quinoxyfen residues in grapes, wine, and their processing products. *Journal of Agricultural and Food Chemistry,* 2000 48, 6128-6131.

Cabras, P; Angioni, A; Garau, VL; Pirisi, FM; Cabitza, F; Pala, M; Farris, GA. Fenhexamid residues in grapes and wine. *Food Additives & Contaminants,* 2001 18, 625-629.

Cabras, P; Conte, E. Pesticide residues in grapes and wine in Italy. *Food Additives & Contaminants*, 2001 18, 880-885.

Cabras, P; Garau, VL; Pirisi, FM; Cubeddu, M; Cabitza, F; Spanedda, L. Fate some insecticidas from vine to wine. *Journal of Agricultural and Food Chemistry*, 1995 43, 2613-2615.

Clement, MV; Hirpara, JL; Chawdhury, SH; Pervaiz, S.Chemopreventive agent resveratrol, a natural product derived from grapes, triggers CD95 signaling-dependet apoptosis in human tumor cells. *Blood,* 1998 92(3), 996-1002.

Criqui, MH; Cowan, LD; Tyroler, HA. Lipoproteins as mediators for the effects of alcohol consumption and cigarette smoking on cardiovascular mortality: results from the Lipid Research Clinics Follow-up Study. *American Journal of Epidemiology,* 1987 126, 629-637.

De Cormis, L. Produits homologués: Quelles garanties pour l'elaborateur de vins et les consommateurs?. *Revue Française d'Oenologie,* 1991 129, 19-23.

De Melo, S; Caboni, P; Pirisi, FM; Cabras, P; Alves, A; Garau, VL. Residues of the fungicide famoxadone in grapes and its fate during wine production. *Food Additives & Contaminants*, 2006 23, 289-294.

Draczynska-Lusiak, B; Doung, A; Sun, AY. Oxidized lipoproteins may play a role in neuronal cell death in Alzheimer disease. *Molecular Chemical Neuropathology,* 1998 33(2), 139-148.

Dutruc-Rosset, G. Situación y estadísticas del sector vitivinícola mundial en 2002. Informe de la Oficina Internacional de la Vid y del Vino. *Semana Vitivinícola,* 2005 3076/77, 2582-2656.

Ebbert, TA; Taylor, RAJ; Downer, RA; Hall, FR. Deposit structure and efficacy of pesticide application. I: Interaction between deposit size, toxicant concentration and deposit number. *Pesticide Science*, 1999 55, 783-792.

Elattar, TMA; Virji, AS. Modulating effect of resveratrol and quercetin on oral cancer cell growth and proliferation. *Anti-Cancer Drugs,* 1999 10(2), 187-193.

Escrich, E. La prevención del cancer y el vino. *Semana Vitivinicola* 1997 2678(79), 4324-4329.

Fait, A; Colosio, C. Recent advances and current concepts in pesticide hazards. In: Emmet EA, Frank AL, Gochfeld M, Hez SM editors. Year book of occupational and environmental medicine. St. Louis: Elsevier Science, Health Science Division; 1998; 15-29.

Fernández, MJ; Oliva, J; Barba, A; Cámara, MA. Effects of clarification and filtration processes on the removal of fungicide residues in red wines (var. Monastrell). *Journal of Agricultural and Food Chemistry*, 2005a 53, 6156-6161.

Fernández, MJ; Oliva, J; Barba, A; Cámara, MA. Fungicide dissipation curves in wine-making process with and without maceration step. *Journal of Agricultural and Food Chemistry*, 2005b 53, 804-811.

Flori, P; Frabboni, B; Cesari, A. Pesticide decay models in wine-making process and wine storage. *Italian Journal of Food Science,* 2000 12, 279-289.

García-Esparza, MA; Capri, E; Pirzadeh, P; Trevisan, M. Copper content of grape and wine from Italian farms. *Food Additives & Contaminants*, 2006 23, 274-280.

García-Cazorla, J; Xirau-Vayreda, M. Persistence of dicarboximidic fungicide residues in grapes, must and wine. *American Journal of Enology and Viticulture*, 1994 45(3), 338-340.

Gaziano, JM ; Buring, JE ; Breslow, JL ; Goldhaber, SZ ; Rosner, B ; Van Denburgh, M; Willet, W; Hennekens, CH. Moderate alcohol intake, increased levels of high density lipoprotein and its subfractions and decreased risk of myocardial infarction. *New England Journal of Medicine,* 1993 329, 1829-1834.

Giraudon, S; Medina, B; Merle, MH; Tusseau, D. Análisis y controles. In: Flanzy C editor. *Enología: Fundamentos científicos y tecnológicos.* Madrid: Mundi-Prensa and AMV Ediciones; 2000; 232-242.

Goodwin, S; Ahmad, N. Relationship between azinphos methyl usage and residues on grapes and in wine in Australia. *Pesticide Science,* 1998 53, 96-100.

Gronback, M; Deis, A; Sorensen, TIA; Becker, U; Schnohr, P; Jensen, G. Mortality associated with moderate intakes of wine, beer or spirits. *British Medical Journal,* 1995 310, 1165-1169.

Gunther, FA; BLINN, RC. Analysis of insecticides and acaricides. New York; Interscience Publ. Inc.; 1955.

Hasnip, S; Caputi, A; Crews, C; Brereton, P. Effects of storage time and temperature on the concentration of ethyl carbamate and its precursors in wine. *Food Additives & Contaminants*, 2004 21, 1155-1161.

Henriet, F; Deloy, S; Pigeon, O; Moreau, JM. Fate of epoxiconazole and Kresoxim-methyl in wheat according to time of application. *Communications in Agricultural and Applied Biological Sciences*, 2005 70(4), 1013-1022.

Henriet, F; Pigeon, O; Moreau, JM. Influence of the spraying system on fungicides distribution on wheat plants. *Communications in Agricultural and Applied Biological Sciences*, 2006 71(2-pt-A), 193-195.

Herce-Pagliai, C; Moreno, I; González, G; Repetto, M; Cameán, AM. Determination of total arsenic, inorganic and organic arsenic species in wine. *Food Additives & Contaminants*, 2002 19, 542-546.

Hodgson, E, Smart, R. Introduction to biochemical toxicology. 3rd Edition. Connecticut: Appleton & Lange; 2001.

Hounker, M; Schumacher, YO; Ochs, A; Sorichter, S; Keul, J; Rossle, M. Cardiac function and haemodynamics in alcoholic cirrhosis and effects of the transjugular intrahepatic portosystemic stent shunt. *Gut,* 1999 44 (5), 743-748.

Jang, M; Pezzuto, JM. Cancer chema preventive activity of resveratrol. *Drugs Experimental Clinical Research,* 1999 25(2-3), 65-77.

Johnson, LR. Gastrointestinal physiology. 5th Edition. St Louis: Mosby; 1997.

Koch, A. Red wine. Resveratrol for a longer life. *Deutsche Apotheker Zeitung,* 1997 137(46), 4155-4157.

Lambe, J. The use of food consumption data in assessments of exposure to food chemicals including the application of probabilistic modeling. *Proceedings of the Nutrition Society*, 2002 61, 11-18.

La Pera, L; Dugo, G; Rando, R; Di Bella, G; Maisano, R; Salvo, F. Statistical study of the influence of fungicide treatments (mancozeb, zoxamide, copper oxychloride) on heavy metal concentrations in Sicilian red wine. *Food Additives & Contaminants*, 2008 25, 302-313.

Lentza-Rizos, C; Avramides, AJ; Kokkinaki, K. Residues of azoxystrobin from grapes to raisins. *Journal of Agricultural and Food Chemistry*, 2006 54, 138-141.

Lin, JK; Tsai, SH. Chemoprevention of cancer and cardiovascular disease by resveratrol. *Proccedings of the National Science Council, Republic of China, Part B,* 1999 23(3), 99-106.

Liu, SH; Campbel, RA; Studens, JA; Waner, RG. Adsortion and traslocation of glyphosate in aspen as influenced by droplet size, droplet number and herbicide concentration. *Weed Science*, 1996 44, 482-488.

Maclure, M. A demostration of deductive, metaanalysis: ethanol intake and risk of myocardial infarction. *Epidemiologic Reviews,* 1993 15, 328-351.

Marín, A; Oliva, J; García, C; Navarro, S; Barba, A. Dissipation rates of cyprodinil and fludioxonil, in lettuce and table grape under cold storage condition. *Journal of Agricultural and Food Chemistry,* 2003 51, 4708-4711.

Miller, JC; Miller, JN. Estadística para química analítica. Delawere, USA: Addison-Wesley Iberoamerican, S.A.; 1993.

Miura, Y. Dietary precaution against cancer. *Igaku no Ayumi,* 1997 183(8), 530-536.

Morgan, MY; Levine, JA. Alcohol and nutrition. *Actes Nutrition Society*, 1988 47, 85-98.

Navarro, S; García, B; Navarro, G; Oliva, J; Barba, A. Effect of wine-making practices on the concentrations of fenarimol and penconazole in rose wines. *Journal of Food Protection*, 1997 60, 1120-1124.

Navarro, S; Barba, A; Oliva, J; Navarro, G; Pardo, F. Evolution of residual levels of six pesticides during elaboration of red wines. Effect of winemaking process in their disappearance. *Journal of Agricultural and Food Chemistry*, 1999 47, 264-270.

Navarro, S; Oliva, J; Barba, A; Navarro, G; García, MA; Zamorano, M. Evolution of chlorpyrifos, fenarimol, metalaxyl, penconazole and vinclozolin in red wines elaborated by carbonic maceration of Monastrell grapes. *Journal of Agricultural and Food Chemistry*, 2000 48, 3537-3541.

Oliva, J; Barba, A; Payá, P; Cámara, MA. Disappearance of fenhexamid residues during wine-making process. *Communications in Agricultural and Applied Biological Sciences*, 2006 71/2, 65-74

Oliva, J; Payá, P; Cámara, MA; Barba, A. Removal of famoxadone, fluquinconazole and trifloxystrobin residues in red wines: Effects of clarification and filtration processes. *Journal of Environmental Science and Health, Part B*, 2007a 42, 775-781.

Oliva, J; Payá, P, Cámara, MA; Barba, A. Removal of pesticides from white wine by the use of fining agents and filtration. *Communications in Agricultural and Applied Biological Sciences*, 2007b 72/2, 171-180.

Papadopoulos-Mourkidou, E; Kotopoulou, A; Papadopoulos, G. Dissipation of cyproconazole and quinalphos on/in grapes. *Pesticide Science*, 1995 45(2), 111-116.

Payá, P; Mulero, J; Oliva, J; Barba, A; Morillas, J; Zafrilla, P. In vitro availability of insect growth regulators from vegetables. *Communications in Agricultural and Applied Biological Sciences*, 2006 71(2B), 549-553.

Payá, P.; Mulero, J.; Oliva, J.; Cámara, M.A.; Zafrilla, P., Barba, A. Bioavailability of insect growth regulators in citrus and stone fruits. *Communications in Agricultural and Applied Biological Sciences*, 2007 72(2), 151-159.

Payá, P. Persistence, degradation and bioavailability of insect growth inhibitors and regulators in plant origin foods, PhD Dissertation. Murcia: University of Murcia editor; 2008.

Polychronopoulou, A; Naska, A. Vino y nutrición. *Semana Vitivinicola,* 1999 2782/83, 4171-4172.

Potter, JF; Beeves, DG. Pressor effect of alcohol in hypertension. *The Lancet,* 1984 1, 119-122.

Renaud, S; De Lorgeril, M. Wine, alcohol, platelets, and the French paradox for coronary heart disease. *The Lancet,* 1992 339, 1523-1526.

Reynolds, SL; Fussell, RJ; Mcarthur, R. Investigation into the validity of extrapolation in setting maximum residue levels for pesticides in crop of similar morphology. *Food Additives & Contaminants,* 2005 22, 31-38.

Rimm, EB; Giovanucci, EL; Willett, WC. Prospective study of alcohol consumption and risk of coronary disease in men. *The Lancet,* 1991, 338, 464-468.

Roberts, T; Hudson, D. Metabolic pathways of agrochemicals. Part two: Insecticides and fungicides. Cambridge: The Royal Society of Chemistry; 1999.

Ramírez, JA; Lacasaña, M. Plaguicidas: clasificación, uso, toxicología y medición de la exposición. *Archivos de Prevención de Riesgos Laborales,* 2001 4(2), 67-75.

Ross, JH, Driver, JH, Cochran, RC, Thongsinthusak, T, Krieger, RI. Could pesticide toxicology studies be more relevant to occupational risk assessment?. *Annals of Occupational Hygiene,* 2001 45, S5-S17.

Ruediger, GA; Pardon, KH; Sas, AN; Godden, PW; Pollnitz, AP. Fate of pesticides during the winemaking process in relation to malolactic fermentation. *Journal of Agricultural and Food Chemistry,* 2005 53, 3023-3026.

Sal, C; Fort, F; Busto, O; Zamora, F; Arola, L; Guash, J. Fate of some common pesticides during vinification process. *Journal of Agricultural and Food Chemistry,* 1996 44, 3668-3671.

Salvo, F; La Pera, L; Di Bella, G; Nicotina, M; Dugo, G. Influence of different mineral and organic pesticide treatments on Cd(II), Cu(II), Pb(II) and Zn(II) contents determined by derivative potentiometic stripping análisis in Italian white and red wines. *Journal of Agricultural and Food Chemistry,* 2003 51, 1090-1094.

Sckidmore, MW; Ambus, A. Pesticide metabolism in crops and livestock. In Hamilton D, Crossley S editors. *Pesticide residues in food and drinking water: Human exposure and risks.* West Sussex, UK: Wiley and Sons; 2004; 63-120.

Seiber, JN. General principles governing the fate of chemicals in the environment. In: Hilton JL editor. *Agricultural chemical of the future.* Belltsville, USA: Symposium on Agricultural Research no. 8; 1985.

Serra-Majen, L. El vino en el contexto de las Dietas Mediterráneas. *Semana Vitivinicola,* 1999 2782/83, 4174-4175.

Soria, P. El vino como alimento: la cara y la cruz. *Semana Vitivinicola,* 1997 2678/79, 4437-4444.

Sur, N; Pal, S; Banerjee, H; Adityachaudhury, N; Bhattacharyya, A. Communication to the editor photodegradation of fenarimol. *Pest Management Science,* 2000 56, 289-292.

Taylor, JC; Hird, SJ; Sykes, MD; Startin, JR. Determination of residues of propamocarb in wine by liquid chromatography-electrospray mass spectrometry with direct injection. *Food Additives & Contaminants,* 2004 21, 572-577.

Timme, G; Frehse, H; Laska, V. Statistical interpretation and graphic representation of the degradational behaviour of pesticide residues II. *Planzenschutz-Nachrichten Bayer,* 1986 39, 187-203.

Timme, G; Freshe, H. Statistical interpretation and graphic representation of the degradational behaviour of pesticide residues I. *Pflanzenschutz-Nachrichten Bayer*, 1980 33, 47-60.

Tomerlin, JR. A comparison of dietary exposure and risk assessment methods in US and EU. In: Voss G, Ramos G editors. Chemistry of crop protection: **progress and prospects in science and regulation**. Massachusetts, USA: **Wiley-VCH**; 2003; 355-370.

Tsiropoulos, NG; Aplada-Sarlis, P; Miliadis, GE. Evaluation of teflubenzuron residue levels in grapes exposed to field treatments and in the must and wine produced from them. *Journal of Agricultural and Food Chemistry*, 1999 47, 4583-4586.

Tsiropoulos, NG; Miliadis, GE; Likas, DT; Liapis, K. Residues of spiroxamine in grapes following field application and their fate from vine to wine. *Journal of Agricultural and Food Chemistry*, 2005 53, 10091-10096.

Verdonck, FAM; Sioen, I, Baert, K; Van Thuyne, N; Bilau, M; Matthys, C; De Henauw, S; De Meulenaer, B; Devlieghere, F; Van Camp, J; Vanrolleghem, PA; Van Sprang, P; Verbeke, W; Willems, J. Uncertainty and variability modelling of chemical exposure through food. *Archives of Public Health*, 2006 64, 159-173.

Wamhoff, H. Wine and health. *Chemie Unserer Zeit,* 1998 32(2), 87-93.

Willet, WC; Lenart, EB. Dietary factors. In: Manson JE, Ridker PM, Gaziano JM, Hennekens CH editors. *Prevention of Myocardial Infarction.* New York, USA: Oxford University Press; 1996; 351-383.

Ying, GG; Williams, B. Herbicide residues in grapes and wine. *Journal of Environmental Science and Health, part B*, 1999 34(3), 397-411.

Zaballa, O; Iñiguez, M; Ayala, R; Puras, PM. Estudio de residuos de fungicidas desde la uva al vino. *Enología Profesional*, 1992 23, 82-92.

Zoecklein, BW; Fugelsang, KC; Gump, BH; Nury, FS. Wine analysis and production. New York: Chapman & Hall; 1995.

Reviewed by:

Prof. Dr. Jorge Mataix (Dept. Agrochemistry and Environment, University Miguel Hernández, Elche, Spain).

Prof. Dr. Antonio Valverde (Dept. Physical Chemistry, Biochemistry and Inorganic Chemistry, University of Almería, Almería, Spain).

Chapter 10

SULPHUR DIOXIDE IN WINES: AUTOMATED DETERMINATION USING FLOW INJECTION ANALYSIS

Constantinos K. Zacharis, Paraskevas D. Tzanavaras, Demetrius G. Themelis and John A. Stratis

Laboratory of Analytical Chemistry, Department of Chemistry,
Aristotelian University of Thessaloniki, GR-54124, Greece

ABSTRACT

Sulphur dioxide (SO_2) is one of the most debated chemical components used in enology. Its important antioxidant, preservative and antiseptic properties are indispensable for the health, stability and quality of wine. Despite the fact that sulphur dioxide is among the most detested chemical components used in enology, up to now no alternative components were found able to have comparable effective antiseptic and preservative action combined with low toxicity. As sulphur dioxide has toxic effects on humans, the World Health Organization (WHO) has defined the maximum daily intake of sulphur dioxide as 0.7 mg kg^{-1} of body weight, whereas the lethal intake is defined as 1.5 g kg^{-1} of body weight. On this basis, the European Union has established maximum allowed concentrations in wines which are 160 mg L^{-1} for red wines and 210 mg L^{-1} for white and rose wines. It is therefore recommended to limit the use of sulphur dioxide.

Automation is a key demand in modern Analytical Chemistry, especially when it comes to quality control of pharmaceutical, food, and environmental samples which have the most profound effects on human activity and life. In the majority of the cases, a lot of samples have to be analyzed and it is critical to produce reliable analytical information in the minimum of time. Flow injection analysis offers great potentials on the field of automation in terms of high sampling rate, precision, accuracy and cost effectiveness.

The present study reviews automated flow injection methods for the determination of sulphur dioxide in wines, including several detection systems such as UV-Vis spectrophotometry, fluorimetry, chemiluminescence, amperometry, conductivity etc.

INTRODUCTION

Chemical Properties of Sulphur Dioxide

Sulphur dioxide is a colorless gas. It smells like burnt matches. It can be oxidized to sulphur trioxide (SO_3), which in the presence of water vapor is readily transformed to sulphuric acid (H_2SO_4) mist. SO_2 can be oxidized to form acid aerosols and it is a precursor to sulphates, which are one of the main components of respirable particles in the atmosphere [1, 2].

Sulphur dioxide takes part in a number of equilibria including:

$$2H_2O + SO_{2\,(aq)} \leftrightarrow H_3O^+ + HSO_3^-{}_{(aq)} \leftrightarrow 2H_3O^+ + SO_3^{2-}$$

The molecular sulphur SO_2 is most toxic to yeasts and bacteria. As it can be seen from the above equilibrium, the proportion of molecular sulphur will depend on the concentration of H_3O^+ ion. The more acidic the environment, the smaller the total amount of sulphur dioxide needed to get the required quantity of molecular sulphur dioxide. The actual percentage of SO_2 present in molecular form depends on pH and typically varies from 6 to 0.5% at a pH value of 3.0 to 4.0, respectively. Moreover, ionic "sulphur dioxide" HSO_3^- is most effective as an antioxidant.

Sulphur dioxide binds with aldehydes and other chemicals. In this bound state it is unable to act as an antioxidant or germicide and will not neutralize NaOH.

Natural sources of SO_2 include releases from volcanoes, oceans, biological decay and forest fires. The most important man-made sources of SO_2 are fossil fuel combustion, smelting, manufacture of sulphuric acid, conversion of wood pulp to paper, incineration of refuse and production of elemental sulphur. Coal burning is the single largest man-made source of sulphur dioxide accounting for about 50% of annual global emissions, with oil burning accounting for a further 25 to 30%.

The major health concerns associated with exposure to high concentrations of sulphur dioxide include effects on breathing, respiratory illness, alterations in pulmonary defenses, and aggravation of existing cardiovascular disease. In the atmosphere, sulphur dioxide mixes with water vapor producing sulphuric acid. This acidic pollution can be transported by the wind over many hundreds of miles, and deposited as acid rain [1, 3].

Sulphur Dioxide in Wines

Sulphur protects damage to the wine by oxygen, and again helps prevent organisms from growing in the product. This also allows the wine to "last longer", which lets it age and develop all of those complex flavors we all love and enjoy so much. If sulfites were not added, the wine would turn into vinegar in a few months. The year of 1487 marked a turning point in the history of good winemaking. In that year, a Prussian royal decree officially permitted the use of sulphur dioxide (SO_2) as a wine additive for the first time. To help preserve their wines during transport, Dutch and English wine traders regularly burnt sulphur candles inside barrels before filling them. It was a trick that they learned from the Romans who conducted the same practice over millennia ago [4]. As stated previously, although the antiseptic qualities of sulphur and SO_2 have been known for more than two thousand years, the association of sulphur compounds and their biological effect on bacteria and yeast began to be understood in the 18th century. Today, the use of the additive SO_2 is an almost universally accepted winemaking practice.

Sulphur dioxide is best known as the food additive 220 or 202. Although it is naturally produced in small amounts by wine yeast during alcoholic fermentation, most of the SO_2 found in wines added by the winemaker. It is added at most stages of the white winemaking process, from crushing through to bottling. It is used less liberally during red winemaking, but with an almost mandatory addition being made following the completion of the malolactic fermentation of these wines. SO_2 is added in the form of a powder, or is directly fed into the wine as a gas from a dosing gun [5, 6].

Sulphur dioxide provides three important properties in winemaking:

1. Its antiseptic qualities stun if not kill wild yeast and bacteria that are present in or on the fruit.
2. It has anti-oxidative properties, that is, it helps protect wine from the deleterious effects of oxygen.
3. It destroys the enzyme that causes enzymatic browning in juice. In the absence of SO_2, wine would likely be brown or amber in color, smell oxidized (or have a sherry-like aroma), and probably be ruined by bacterial spoilage.

Home winemakers should strive to keep the total SO_2 added to any wine (from fermentation to bottling) under 100 mg L^{-1}. Recipes that call for initial SO_2 dosages of 120 mg L^{-1} or more can be reduced to between 30 mg L^{-1} and 50 mg L^{-1} and, depending upon the wine's pH, still provide the required protection. A sensitive palate can detect over 50 mg L^{-1} of SO_2 and too much SO_2 can destroy the bouquet of a wine, eliminate delicate flavors and add a chemical taste as well. Finally, the total amount of SO_2 in a finished, bottled wine should be the least amount required.

Sulphur dioxide that is initially added to must or juice becomes chemically bound to various compounds present in the juice and pulp or formed during fermentation. These compounds settle as lees following fermentation and are separated from the wine by being siphoned off during the first racking. Following the first racking, it's not unusual to find very little if any SO_2 present in the wine. Generally, a wine that contains 200 – 450 mg L^{-1} total SO_2 typically 20 – 40 mg L^{-1} of it is free to protect the wine from spoilage [4].

In the United State, the law states that [7,8]:

1. Wines cannot contain more than 350 mg L^{-1} sulfites.
2. Wines with more than 10 mg L^{-1} must have a "contains sulfites" warning label.
3. Producers must show levels below 10 mg L^{-1} by analysis to omit the label.
4. Wines must have less than 1 mg L^{-1} to have a label that says "no sulfites".
5. This level must be shown by analysis.
6. All wines must carry the label whether made in the US or abroad.

FLOW INJECTION ANALYSIS

Principles

Flow injection analysis (FI) is a well-established automated technique with numerous and widespread applications in quantitative chemical analysis. It is characteristic that more than 12,000 FI papers have been published in scientific journals since 1975 – when it was originally proposed by Ruzicka and Hansen [9]. A simplified definition of flow injection analysis might be: "FI is an automated, continuous flow approach to perform chemical analysis". It is based on injecting a small, well-defined volume of sample, into a continuously flowing carrier stream to which appropriate auxiliary reagent streams can be added, whereby a concentration gradient of the sample is created.

All of the virtually innumerable concentrations represented in the gradient can potentially be exploited for the readout. Thus, in contrast to conventional continuous flow procedures (and all batch methods), FI does not rely on complete mixing of sample and reagent(s) (physical homogenization). Combined with the inherent exact timing of all events it is neither necessary to wait until all chemical reactions have proceeded to equilibrium (chemical homogenization). These features, that allow transient signals to be used as the readout, do not only permit the procedures to be accomplished within a very short time (typically in less than 30 s), but have open new and novel avenues to perform an array of chemical analytical assays, which are either very difficult and in many cases directly impossible to implement by traditional means [10]. Thus, in FI it is feasible to base the principles of an analytical assay on the measurement of unstable intermediate compounds, which might exhibit particularly interesting analytical characteristics; to exploit extremely fast detection principles relying on bio- or chemiluminescence; to develop assays based on kinetic discrimination-based schemes by taking advantage of the reaction rates of the individually occurring reactions in methods comprising a series of reactions; to perform so-called *stopped-flow* measurements, where an sample/reagent segment is stopped within the detector, and where the signal recorded directly can be related to the concentration. Such approaches are especially valuable in slow reactions and enzymatic assays [11].

The most common manifold configurations are what are often called *single-stream*, *two stream*, and *three stream* manifolds. A single-stream manifold is depicted schematically in the following Fig. 1a [12].

In this scheme, a stream containing reagent is pumped through the system. A certain volume of sample is injected into the stream, and dispersion causes mixing of the carrier/reagent with the sample zone leading to chemistry between analyte and reagent as the zone passes through the reaction coil and the flow through cell of the detector.

The two-stream manifold (see Fig. 1b) can be used in two different modes depending on the complexity of the chemical systems. The first is with single-stage chemistry, similar to that described for the single-stream application. In the two-stream approach, the sample is injected into a non-reacting carrier, and the reagent stream is merged with it downstream. This provides a more uniform mixing of the reagent with sample over the whole length of the sample zone, and often provides better sensitivity and performance compared to the single-steam approach. For this reason, the two-stream manifold is often preferred over the single-stream manifold for simple chemistries. In multi-stage chemistries, the sample is injected into the first stream containing a reagent. The analyte reacts with the reagent, generating an intermediate. On merging with the second stream, the intermediate reacts with another reagent, forming the product that is finally measured by the detector [13]. Three stream manifolds are generally used for two stage or three stage chemistries in an analogous way as described above.

FI is generally a simple and inexpensive technique employing common instrumentation such as peristaltic pumps and low-pressure injection valves. Compared to batch methods it offers increased sampling rate, lower reagents consumption, better precision and high versatility.

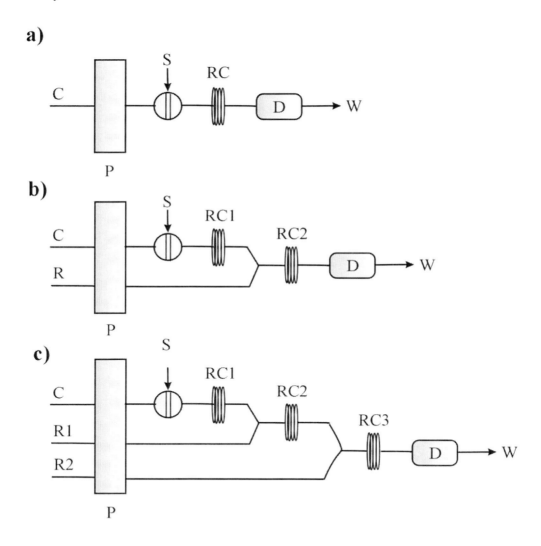

Figure 1. Typical FIA single (a), two (b) and three (c) streams manifolds. Where C = carrier, S = sample, R, R1, R2 = reagents, RC1, RC2, and RC3 = reaction coils, P = pump, D = detector and W = waste.

FIA – Gas Diffusion

Membrane sampling devices (MSD) can be used not only for dilution, but also for other sample processing operations, such as matrix modification or elimination, sampling of gas streams, solvent extraction, and analyte enrichment. Because they are so versatile, it is deserved to be briefly discussed [13-15].

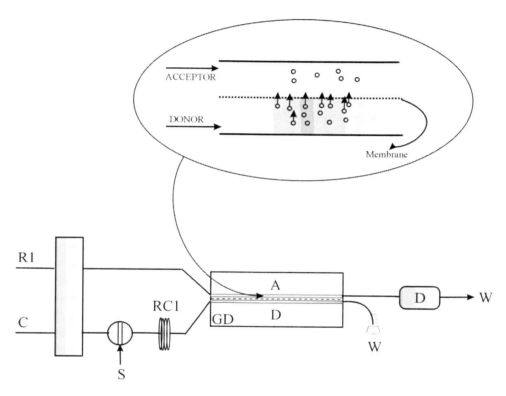

Figure 2. A typical FI - gas diffusion manifold. The cycles represent the gaseous analyte molecules.

The principle of FI – gas diffusion technique is schematically shown in Fig. 2. One of the streams is called the donor stream, which can be either a liquid or gas stream. The other is the receiving stream. The donor stream contains the analyte, and can either be a dispersed sample zone injected into a carrier stream, or the sample stream itself. When the donor stream containing the analyte flows past the membrane, a defined portion or fraction of the analyte will be transferred by mass transport across the membrane to the receiving solution. Generally, only a fraction will be transferred, but with fixed, reproducible conditions, the fraction will be constant. This allows calibration for quantitative analysis [15].

In the case of sulphur dioxide determination, a simple configuration consists of two liquid streams, a strong acidic donor solution (D) and an acceptor (A) solution containing a reagent (R1), separated by a gas-permeable membrane [12, 15]. The role of the membrane does not restrict to the separation of the donor and acceptor solutions but also to form a barrier for potential interfering compounds that co-exist in the sample. When a sample is injected in the strong acidic donor solution, the liberated sulphur dioxide diffuses through the membrane and dissolves into the acceptor solution. Then, the dissolved SO$_2$ reacts with the reagent (R1) and form a colored product which it finally monitored by the detector.

FI Wine Analysis

Wine is a product with a very complex composition. Among the large number of substances found in wine, many are at very low concentrations even though they play a main role in wine characteristics, evolution, and/or quality. A complete analysis of wine is a time-consuming process, but it yields the necessary information for both elaboration of a quality product and conservation under proper conditions. Usually, the number of parameters to be analyzed is simplified to fulfil the knowledge of the evolution of the process or the food laws. Therefore, only a few parameters are periodically checked. The most common are: soluble solids, reducing sugars, alcoholic degree, pH, total and volatile acidity, sulphur dioxide, color, polyphenol index, iron, and organic acids. For monitoring wine composition most of the analytical methods recognized by the international community as official methods of analysis are manual methods with high robustness and precision, even though more recent methods may be based on modern automated instrumental techniques. Nevertheless, the manual methods are slow, tedious, and require a high level of human participation. The new faster methods, which usually have the appropriate sensitivity, selectivity, and precision, can circumvent the problem created by the large number of samples to be analyzed in order to guarantee proper monitoring of wine production [16].

Due to its automation potentialities flow injection analysis has been widely used in wine quality control for the determination of various analytes (e.g metals, ethanol, urea, acetic acid, biogenic amines, etc). It is worth to mention that in many circumstances FI is employed as sample introduction technique prior to a separation technique (e.g. capillary electrophoresis). This coupling combines the unique and advantageous features of both techniques and can be applied when multi-component analysis is needed. A compilation of selected recent applications of FI to wine analysis can be found in Table 1.

APPLICATIONS

The FI analytical methods for the determination of sulphur dioxide in wines can be classified in three main sub-sections depending on the detection principles:

1. spectrophotometric & spectrofluorimetric
2. chemiluminometric
3. electroanalytical

The analytical procedures were considered in terms of analytical methodology, figures of merit and analyses of real samples. Additional information considered significant on sampling strategies and sample pretreatment were also included.

Table 1. Selected FI applications in wine analysis.

Analyte	Method principle	Sampling rate (samples h^{-1})	c_L	Ref.
Acetic acid	Tri-enzyme sensor using amperometric detection.	20	50 nM	[17]
Anthocyanins	On-line solid phase extraction (SPE) and evaporation followed by HPLC	–	0.2 mg L^{-1}	[18]
Biogenic amines	Capillary electrophoresis (CE) coupled to mass spectrometry (MS) after on-line sample introduction with FI	–	18-90 ng mL^{-1}	[19]
Cadmium	Preconcentration of the analyte in a knotted reactor and measurement by inductively coupled plasma (ICP)	–	5 ng L^{-1}	[20]
Calcium	Color-complex formation with methylthymol blue (MTB) and detection at 610 nm	90	1.7 mg L^{-1}	[21]
Calcium and magnesium	On-line masking of Mg^{2+} and direct photometric measurement of Ca^{2+} with MTB. Mg^{2+} is calculated by subtraction from the total signal without the masking process.	–	2.1 mg L^{-1} (Ca^{2+}) 1.8 mg L^{-1} (Mg^{2+})	[22]
Catechins and procyanidins	Reaction of vanillin in acid medium to yield a coloured product with maximum absorption at 500 nm.	23	4.5 mg L^{-1}	[23]
Ethanol	A membraneless gas diffusion unit was used for the isolation of the analyte from the sample prior its spectrophotometric detection after reaction with K$_2$Cr$_2$O$_7$.	–	0.27 v/v (%)	[24]
Gluconic acid	FI coupled to amperometric biosensor was employed for the analyte detection.	–	190 nM	[25]
Glycerol	Monitoring the rate of formation of NADH from the reaction of glycerol and NAD+ catalyzed by the enzyme glycerol dehydrogenase in solution.	54	–	[26]
Histamine	Spectrofluorimetric determination of histamine by its reaction with o-phthaldehyde.	24	30 μg L^{-1}	[27]

Table 1. (Continued)

Analyte	Method principle	Sampling rate (samples h^{-1})	c_L	Ref.
Iron	Extraction with MIBK of the complex formed between Fe(III) and thiocyanate. The extraction is performed using an on-line device for gravimetric analysis. Total iron analysis is accomplished by sending a small sample aliquot directly to the FAAS nebulizer.	18.5	30 µg L^{-1}	[28]
Lead	Sorption of Pb(II) on polyurethane column and determination of the eluted plug by FAAS. Total Pb(II) content was measured after digestion with HNO$_3$	48	1 µg L^{-1}	[29]
Malic acid	Spectrophotometric determination of malic acid based on the detection of NADH, formed after oxidation of l-malate to oxaloacetate, catalysed by l-malate dehydrogenase	22	9 mg L^{-1}	[30]
Polyphenols and anthocyans	FI coupled to diode-array detector (DAD) was used for the quantification of total polyphenol and total anthocyans at 280 and 520nm, respectively.	25-30	0.229 mg L^{-1} (polyphenol) 0.543 mg L^{-1} (anthocyan)	[31]
Proline	Reaction of the analyte with tris(2,2'-bipyridyl)ruthenium(II) and chemiluminescence detection	20 (red wines) 60 (white wines)	10 nM	[32]
Reducing sugars	An unsegmented liquid/vapor phases flow injection system for determining reducing sugars in wines using a focalized poly(tetrafluoroethylene) (PTFE) coiled reactor positioned at a microwave oven.	54	9 µM	[33]
Resveratrol	A C$_{18}$ mini column was utilized for the preconcentration of analyte prior to its chemiluminescent detection after reaction with KMnO$_4$ and HCHO.	–	3.3 nM	[34]

Table 1. (Continued)

Analyte	Method principle	Sampling rate (samples h^{-1})	c_L	Ref.
Tartaric acid	Spectrophotometric FI method based on the reaction of tartaric acid with sodium vanadate.	28	–	[35]
Urea	Spectrofluorimetric measurement of ammonia released by the enzymatic hydrolysis of urea.	–	–	[36]

Spectrophotometric and Spectrofluorimetric Detection

Spectrophotometry is the most widely applied technique for the determination of SO_2 in wines. This detection mode itself offers simplicity, cost-effective instrumentation readily available in all laboratories and low operational costs. The variety of existing suitable reagents for spectrophotometric analyses has led to the publication of a considerable number of FI procedures [37-48].

A gas-diffusion FI assay with spectrophotometric detection has been proposed by Decnop-Weever et al. [37] for the quantification of sulphur dioxide in wine samples. The proposed method was based on the change of the absorbance of an indicator solution (bromocresol green) due to the pH shifting, when sulphur dioxide diffused via a permeable membrane into the indicator solution. Satisfactory linearity in the range of 1 –20 mg L^{-1} was achieved while the limit of detection was equal to 0.1 mg L^{-1}. The reproducibility of the method was good within the range between 0.7 – 1.5 %. The main drawback of this work is that the samples and reagents should be flushed with nitrogen before their use. The results obtained with the proposed method were in good agreement with those from reference standard method (iodometric titration).

Another gas-diffusion FI method has been proposed by Bartroli et al. [38] where free and total sulphur dioxide were assayed. The sample was injected into the carrier and then merged with a stream which provided a sufficiently acidic medium for the free SO_2 to diffuse across the membrane. The acceptor stream, a mixture of p – aminoazobenzene and formaldehyde, collected the analyte and transported the resulting reaction product formed in a reaction coil to the detector, where its absorbance was monitored at 520 nm. In the case of total SO_2 determination, the sample was hydrolyzed by NaOH in order to release all bound SO_2 prior to injection in the FI manifold. The method was validated in terms of linearity, sensitivity, accuracy and precision. The calibration curves were linear in the ranges of 5 – 300 mg L^{-1} and 2 – 35 mg L^{-1} for the analysis of total and free sulphur dioxide, respectively. The limits of detection were 2 and 0.2 mg L^{-1} and the sampling rates were 20 and 50 h^{-1} respectively.

In a similar fashion, Mataix et. al. [39] developed a FI method for the determination of SO_2 in wines after pervaporation. The proposed approach was based on the spectrophotometric (at 578 nm) determination of sulphur dioxide after its reaction with p – rosaniline and formaldehyde. The gaseous analyte was liberated from the liquid phase after acidification into the pervaporation unit and collected in the acceptor solution containing the p – rosaniline and formaldehyde reagent mixture. The calibration curve was ranged between 2.0 and 20 mg L^{-1} while the relative standard deviation was < 3.0%.

A comparative study with and without gas – diffusion using various FI manifolds have been carried out by Mana et. al. [40] for the determination of total species of sulphite, hydrogen sulphite and sulphur dioxide. The principle of the method lays on the reaction of the analytes with o- phthalaldehyde (OPA) in the presence of ammonium ion at pH = 6.5 to produce fluorescent derivatives monitored at $\lambda_{ext.}$ = 330 nm and $\lambda_{em.}$ = 390 nm. The gas – diffusion unit was used to improve selectivity when sulphite is determined in the presence of thiosulphate, thioglycolate, tetrathionate, cysteine and ascorbate. The developed FI – GD assay was applied to the determination of SO_2 in red and white wines.

In the same fashion, a FI – GD approach has been developed by Atanassov et. al. [41] for the determination of SO_2 and CO_2 in table wines. The determination of analyte was based on the decolorization of malachite green by SO_2. The calibration curve ranged from 50 to 300 mg L^{-1}, while the relative standard deviation was lower than 4.5 %. The same reagent was also employed by Melo et. al. [42] for the quantification of sulphite after gas – diffusion through a concentric tubular membrane. The derivative was monitored at 620 nm while the injected sample volume was 400 μL. The assay allows a sampling throughput of 30 samples h^{-1}, while the precision of the method was < 0.015 at concentrations of 1 and 20 mg L^{-1}.

Another spectrophotometric approach was proposed by Silva et. al. [43] in which the gaseous SO_2 passed through the GD membrane and reacted with Mn(II) ion in acetate buffer at pH = 5.5. The oxidation of Mn(II) took place proportionally to the free S(IV) content and the oxidized species formed reacted with iodide to form iodine which finally was measured spectrophotometrically at 352 nm. The method enables the determination of both free and total sulphite in wines. The calibration curve was linear up to 26 mg L^{-1} with a limit of detection of 1 mg L^{-1}. A previous sample treatment step is required to eliminate the hydrogensulfite/aldehyde adducts. This step was carried out by the addition of tris(hydroxymethylaminomethane) and EDTA into the sample prior to analysis.

An alternative GD – FI method has been proposed by the research group of M. Korn [44]. Free and total sulfite was determined indirectly in wines and fruit juices. The assay was based on the reduction of the analyte by metallic zinc forming H_2S. The produced H_2S diffuses through the membrane and finally reacts with N,N-dimethylphenylene diamine (DMPD) and Fe^{3+}. The reaction product was detected at 665 nm. Analytical parameters such as flow rates, pH and concentration of reagents, affecting the sensitivity of the method were studied and optimized to gain maximum peak height. The proposed method showed a high analytical throughput (40 runs h^{-1}), an adequate limit of detection (0.12 and 0.25 mg L^{-1} for free and total sulfite respectively) and a relatively wide linear range between 1 and 25 mg L^{-1}.

A different FI method for the determination of sulfite in wines using the stopped-flow approach has been published by Perez-Ruiz et. al. [45]. The method was based on the decrease of the catalytic activity of formaldehyde to the oxidation of p – phenylenediamine by hydrogen peroxide. The method was validated in terms of linearity, precision and accuracy and limit of detection. The linear working range was 5 – 60 mg L^{-1} with a sampling rate of 25 samples h^{-1}.

Recently, a batch and FI spectrophotometric method has been developed by Hassan et al. [46] for the quantification of sulfite in beverages. The method is based on the reaction of the analyte with diaquacobyrinic acid heptamethyl ester (diaquacobester) in acidic medium (pH = 3) forming a highly stable sulfite cobester complex (SO_3Cbs). In the presence of sulfite, absorption bands at 313, 425, 349 and 525 nm were used for the analyte quantification. Analytical parameters such as flow rate, sample volume, pH of the reaction, etc were studied and optimized. A limit of detection of 10 ng mL^{-1} was achieved while the linear range of the calibration curve was 0.03 – 25 μg mL^{-1}. Finally, the proposed method was applied successfully to determine the sulfite content of some beverages.

Fatibello-Filho et. al. [47] proposed a spectrophotometric method for the determination of sulfite in white wine, vinegars and juices. The method was based on the inhibitory effect of the analyte on the activity of the enzyme polyphenol oxidase. The enzyme catalyzes the oxidation of cathecol to o-quinone which coupled to each other producing a melalin-like colour detected at 410 nm. Interferences such as ascorbic acid were eliminated by passing the sample through a glass column packed with ascorbate oxidase. The method exhibits good linearity in the range of 40 to 600 μmol L^{-1} while the limit of detection was equal to 2.2 μmol

L^{-1}. The sampling frequency was 26 samples h^{-1} and the results obtained were confirmed by a batch iodimetric method.

A flow – through optical sensor was fabricated by Richter, et. al [48] for the automated determination of sulfite in wines. The principle of the method was that the reaction product of the analyte with *p*-rosaniline and formaldehyde was transiently immobilized on an ion – exchange support packed in a flow cell. Finally, the retained analyte was eluted by HCl. The chemical and the instrumental parameters were studied and optimized in terms of method sensitivity. The signal obtained was proportionally to the analyte concentration in the range of $0.16 - 6.0$ μg mL^{-1} with a limit of detection of 49 ng mL^{-1}.

An alternative FI approach has been proposed by Maquieira, A. et. al. [49] for the quantification of total and free SO_2. The authors developed a continuous flow micro-distillation unit where the nitrogen carrier stream propels the volatilized SO_2 to an absorption module. In this module, SO_2 reacts with 2,2'-dinitro-5,5'-dithiodibenzoic acid in phosphate buffer medium (pH = 6) yielding a yellow product which is finally detected at 410 nm. To determine total SO_2, a previous hydrolysis step of the sample was carried out using NaOH. The results obtained were in good agreement with those found from the reference distillation method.

Chemiluminometric Detection

Flow injection analysis coupled to chemiluminescence (CL) detection offers significant advantages in terms of automation and ability to capture the maximum light emission during the reaction. Compared to spectrophotometry, CL generally provides higher sensitivity and extended linearity.

A FI – chemiluminometric method has been proposed by Liang Huang et. al. [50] for the determination of free and total sulfite in wine samples. The developed method was based on the suppression of luminol CL by sulfite after gas diffusion. EDTA was used to enhance the inhibitory effect of the analyte. Linearity was obeyed in the range of 10 to 800 μmol L^{-1} with a relative standard deviation of 2 %.

Rhodamine 6G was used as chemiluminescent reagent for the determination of total sulfite in wines [51]. The oxidation reaction of the analyte by Rhodamine 6G was accompanied by weak CL emission. Therefore, a surfactant such as Tween 20 or 80 was used by the authors to enhance the CL intensity. The method provided linear response against sulfite concentration in the range of 0.05 to 10 mg L^{-1}. The achieved limit of detection was 0.03 mg L^{-1}.

A micro – flow FI method has been developed by He et. al. [52] where a CL signal was produced after the reaction of Ce(IV) and sulfite sensed by rhodamine 6G. The surfactant Tween 80 was used to improve the weak CL emission. The method responded linearly in the range of $1 - 60$ mg L^{-1} with a limit of detection of 0.5 mg L^{-1}. The relative standard deviation was 3 % at the concentration level of 20 mg L^{-1}.

A FI – GD apparatus with chemiluminescence detection was exploited for the determination of sulfite in wines [53]. The method was based on the reaction of Na_2CO_3 – Cu(II) with the analyte while the intensity of the emitted CL was monitored by a home – made CL detector. The calibration curve was linear in the range of $1 - 500 \times 10^{-6}$ mol L^{-1}. The limit of detection was 5×10^{-7} mol L^{-1}. The sample was diluted 100 – 500 fold prior to its injection. The concentration of sulfite in French and Chinese red and white wines was found to be in the range of 72 to 189 mg L^{-1}.

Electrochemical Detection

Electrochemical is one of the most sensitive detection modes and it is used when the analyte compounds contain an electrochemical active group.

A chemically modified glassy electrode has been utilized in a FI apparatus by Casella, et al. [54] for the determination of sulphur-containing compounds (sulphite, sulphide, thiosulphate, cysteine, cystine, etc). The method was based on the electro-oxidation of the analytes. The FI parameters were studied and optimized in terms of linearity and sensitivity. The calibration curve was linear in the studied range of 0.2 – 1000 μmol L^{-1} while the limit of detection was 0.2 μmol L^{-1}. Finally, the data obtained from wine analyses were evaluated and compared with those obtained from anion – exchange chromatography.

An amperometric detector was incorporated in a FI apparatus for the determination of sulfite in beverages [55]. The method was based on the detection of the analyte at a copper surface in an alkaline medium. A gas – diffusion manifold was exploited for the flow extraction of sulfite as SO_2 through a membrane. The method was validated in terms of linearity (1.0 to 5.0 mmol L^{-1}), precision (RSD = 4%), selectivity and limit of detection (0.04 mmol L^{-1}). The sampling rate was 50 samples h^{-1}. The positive interference produced by volatile ethanol was taken into account on the final determination results. Finally, the proposed method was applied to the analysis of sulfite in alcoholic and non – alcoholic beverages.

A similar approach has been proposed by Azevedo et. al. [56] for the determination of total and free SO_2 in wines using a FI - GD manifold. The novelty of the method was the use of an amperometric detector consisting of a glassy carbon electrode modified with a tetraruthenated porphyrin film. The limit of detection achieved was 3 μmol L^{-1}. The method was successfully applied on the quantification of analyte in dry red and white wines. In addition, the results obtained were compared with those obtained with the reference iodometric method.

A dual – channeled electrochemical detector has been constructed by Cardwell et. al. [57] for the simultaneous determination of SO_2 and ascorbic acid in wines and fruits. In addition, a gas diffusion unit was employed to improve the selectivity of the method. Ascorbic acid was detected on a glassy carbon electrode at a voltage of + 0.42 V while SO_2 on a platinum electrode at + 0.90 V, using a Ag/AgCl reference electrode in both cases. In order to eliminate interferences from the matrix of red and sweet wines, the samples were cleaned – up with quaternary amine SAX solid phase extraction cartridges prior to analysis. The method provided a linear response for the determination of SO_2 ranging from 0.25 – 15 mg L^{-1} with a limit of detection of 0.05 mg L^{-1}. The obtained results were confirmed by ion – exclusion chromatography.

Chen et. al [58] used a FI manifold coupled to a coulometric detector based on porous carbon felt working electrode. Sulphur dioxide was used as electro active compound in order to evaluate the detector characteristics (selectivity, linear response range, detection limit, etc). The linear determination range was 1.6×10^{-5} - 1.6×10^{-4} mol L^{-1} with a 10 μL injected volume. The flow rate towards to the detector was 0.4 mL min^{-1} with a limit of detection of 2

× 10^{-8} mol L^{-1}. The performance of the coulometric flow cell was also evaluated by the determination of the analyte in wine samples.

A conductimetric FI method has been developed by Tavares Araujo et. al. [59] for the determination of sulfite in wines and fruit juices. In brief, the formed gaseous SO_2 from acidification of sulfite was passed through a membrane and was trapped in alkaline medium. The change of conductivity of the acceptor stream was measured as a peak corresponding to the analyte concentration. The determination range was 1 - 50 mg L^{-1} sulfite with a limit of detection of 0.03 mg L^{-1}. The precision and the accuracy of the method were evaluated giving a relative standard deviation of 0.2% ($n = 10$). The method provides good accuracy with a recovery ranging from 97.3% to 99.3%. A quite similar approach has been proposed by Kuban et. al [60] for the determination of free and total of SO_2. A GD manifold was used to improve the selectivity of the method. Bound SO_2 was quantitated after alkaline hydrolysis of wine samples with NaOH and determined conductometrically. The achieved detection limit was 1 mg L^{-1} while the relative standard deviation was less than 0.8 % at the 10 mg L^{-1} concentration level.

A biosensor has been fabricated by Groom et. al. [61] for the determination of sulfite in wine, beer and dried fruit samples. Tetrathiafulvalene and tetracyanoquinodimethane were selected to form a biosensor for the analyte detection. Also, a dialysis membrane with a molecular weight cut-off between 6 and 8 KDa was used to cover the sensing area of a vitreous carbon electrode. The biosensor was incorporated into a FI apparatus. The calibration curve was linear up to 5 µmol L^{-1}. A potential drawback of the method is that a time period of 10 min was required for baseline stabilization. The biosensor was active up to 55 repeated analyses during 26 hours. The results obtained were in a good agreement with those from the pararosalinine reference method.

An indirect amperometric method has been proposed by Alipazaga, et. al. [62], for the quantification of sulfite in wine samples. The method was based on the measurement of Cu(III) chemically generated by the S(IV) induced oxidation of Cu(II) − tetraglycine complex by dissolved oxygen. The method was validated in terms of linearity (5 − 100 µmol L^{-1}), precision and accuracy (R.S.D. 1.4 %) and limit of detection (1 µmol L^{-1}).

A bulk acoustic wave impedance sensor coupled to a FI − GD manifold has been exploited by Su et. al. [63] for the determination of SO_2 in wines. The method was based on an on-line membrane separation of the analyte released from a stream of H_2SO_4 into a solution of $H_2O_2 - H_2SO_4$. The conductance increase due to the oxidation of SO_2 to H_2SO_4 was monitored by a bulk acoustic wave impedance sensor. Analytical parameters (flow rate, injected volume, temperature, composition of acceptor stream, etc) affecting the sensitivity of the method were studied and optimized. A sample frequency of 78 samples h^{-1} was achieved with a linear determination response up to 1 mmol L^{-1}. The limit of detection was 5 µmol L^{-1} while a good reproducibility was obtained with a R.S.D. ranging from 0.57 to 1.23 %.

FI − gas diffusion methods for the determination of SO_2 in wines are summarized in Table 2.

Table 2. FI – gas diffusion methods for the determination of SO$_2$ in wine analysis.

Method principle	Linearity	Detection	Sampling rate (samples h^{-1})	c_L	Ref.
Change on absorbance of bromocresol green	1 – 20 mg L^{-1}	spectrophotometry	–	0.1 mg L^{-1}	[37]
A mixture of p – aminoazobenzene and formaldehyde was used for the analyte reaction	5 - 300 mg L^{-1} * 2 – 35 mg L^{-1} **	spectrophotometry	20 * 50 **	2 mg L^{-1} * 0.2 mg L^{-1} **	[38]
Reaction of the analyte with o- phthalaldehyde in the presence of ammonium ion	2.5 mmol L^{-1} – 5 μmol L^{-1}	spectrofluorimetry	–	–	[40]
Decolorization of malachite green in the presence of the analyte.	50 – 300 mg L^{-1}	spectrophotometry	–	–	[41]
Use of a concentric tubular membrane and reaction of the analyte with malachite green	1 – 20 mg L^{-1}	spectrophotometry	30	–	[42]
Oxidation of Mn(II) by S(IV) and the oxidized species formed react with iodide to form iodine	0 – 26 mg L^{-1}	spectrophotometry	–	1 mg L^{-1}	[43]
Reduction of SO$_2$ by metallic Zn. The produced H$_2$S reacts with N,N-dimethylphenylene diamine (DMPD) and Fe^{3+}.	1 – 25 mg L^{-1}	spectrophotometry	40	0.25 mg L^{-1} * 0.12 mg L^{-1} **	[44]
Suppression of luminol CL by SO$_3^-$.	10 – 800 μmol L^{-1}	chemiluminescence	–	10 μmol L^{-1}	[50]
Reaction of Na$_2$CO$_3$ – Cu(II) with SO$_2$.	1 – 500 μmol L^{-1}	chemiluminescence	–	0.5 μmol L^{-1}	[53]
Use of a copper surface as working electrode.	1 – 5 mmol L^{-1}	amperometry	50	0.04 mmol L^{-1}	[55]
An amperometric detector was used consisting of a glassy carbon electrode modified with a tetraruthenated porphyrin film.	–	amperometry	–	3 μmol L^{-1}	[56]
A dual – channeled detector was used for the determination of the analyte on a platinum working electrode.	0.25 – 15 mg L^{-1}	electrochemical	–	0.05 mg L^{-1}	[57]
Change of conductivity of the acceptor stream in the presence of SO$_2$	1 – 50 mg L^{-1}	conductivity	–	0.03 mg L^{-1}	[59]
A conductimetric detector was employed for the analyte detection	–	conductivity	–	1 mg L^{-1}	[60]
The on-line membrane separation of the analyte released from a stream of H$_2$SO$_4$ into a solution of H$_2$O$_2$ – H$_2$SO$_4$ was exploited. The conductance increase was monitored by a bulk acoustic wave impedance sensor.	0 – 1 mmol L^{-1}	acoustic wave sensor	78	5 μmol L^{-1}	[63]

* Total SO$_2$
** Free SO$_2$

REFERENCES

[1] http://en.wikipedia.org, Free electronic encyclopedia.
[2] Holleman, A. F.; Wiberg, E. *Inorganic Chemistry*, Academic Press, San Diego, 2001.
[3] United States Environmental Protection Agency (EPA) http://www.epa.gov/oar/urbanair/so2
[4] Amerine, M.A.; Ough, C.S.; *Methods for Analysis of Musts and Wines*, Wiley, New York, 1980.
[5] Godden, P. W.; Francis, I. L.; Field, J. B. F.; Gishen, M.; Coulter, A. D.; Valente, P. J.; Hoj, P. B.; Robinson, E. M. C. An evaluation of the technical performance of wine bottle closures. (2002) Proceedings of the 11th Wine Industry Technical Conference. pp. 44-52.
[6] Usseglio-Tomasset, L. Properties and use of sulphur dioxide, *Food Additives and Contaminants*, 1992, *9*, 399-404.
[7] http://www.themorethanorganic.com
[8] World Health Organization website, http://www.who.int
[9] Ruzicka, J; Hansen, E.H. Flow injection analyses. Part I. A new concept of fast continuous flow analysis, *Anal. Chim. Acta*, 1975, *78*, 145-157.
[10] Hansen, E.H. The impact of flow injection on modern chemical analysis: Has it fulfilled our expectations? And where are we going? *Talanta*, 2004, *64*, 1076-1083.
[11] Bendtsen, A.B.; Hansen, E.H., Spectrophotometric flow injection determination of trace amounts of thiocyanate based on its reaction with 2-(5-bromo-2-pyridylazo)-5-diethylaminophenol and dichromate: Assay of the thiocyanate level in saliva from smokers and non-smokers *Analyst*, 1991, *116*, 647-651.
[12] Ruzicka, J.; Hansen E. H. *Flow Injection Analysis*, J. Wiley and Sons, 1981.
[13] Karlberg B.; Pacey, G.E. *Flow Injection Analysis. A Practical Guide*, Elsevier, 1989.
[14] Van der Linden, W.E. The optimum composition of pH-sensitive acceptor solution for membrane separation in flow injection analysis, *Anal. Chim. Acta*, 1983, *155*, 273-277.
[15] Van der Linden, W.E. Membrane separation in flow injection analysis – Gas diffusion, *Anal. Chim. Acta*, 1983, *153*, 359-369.
[16] Luque de Castro, M.D.; Gonzalez-Rodriguez, J.; Perez-Juan, P. Analytical methods in wineries: Is it time to change? *Food Rev. Intern.* 2005, *21*, 231-265.
[17] Mizutani, F.; Hirata, Y.; Yabuki, S.; Iijima, S. Flow injection analysis of acetic acid in food samples by using trienzyme/poly(dimethylsiloxane)-bilayer membrane-based electrode as the detector, *Sensors and Actuators B*, 2003, *91*, 195-198.
[18] Mataix, E.; Luque de Castro, M. D. Determination of anthocyanins in wine based on flow-injection, liquid–solid extraction, continuous evaporation and high-performance liquid chromatography–photometric detection, *J. Chromatogr. A*, 2001, *910*, 255-263.
[19] Santos B.; Simonet, B.M.; Ríos A.; Valcárcel M. Direct automatic determination of biogenic amines in wine by flow injection - capillary electrophoresis - mass spectrometry, *Electrophoresis*, 2004, *25*, 3427-3433.
[20] Lara, R.F.; Wuilloud, R.G.; Salonia, J.A.; Olsina, R.A.; Martinez, L.D. Determination of low cadmium concentrations in wine by on-line preconcentration in a knotted reactor coupled to an inductively coupled plasma optical emission spectrometer with ultrasonic nebulization, *Fresenius J Anal Chem*, 2001, *371*, 989-993.

[21] Themelis, D. G.; Tzanavaras, P. D.; Anthemidis, A. N.; Stratis, J. A. Direct, selective flow injection spectrophotometric determination of calcium in wines using methylthymol blue and an on-line cascade dilution system. *Anal. Chim. Acta*, 1999, *402*, 259-266.

[22] Themelis, D. G.; Tzanavaras, P. D.; Trellopoulos, A. V.; Sofoniou, M. C. Direct and selective flow-injection method for the simultaneous spectrophotometric determination of calcium and magnesium in red and white wines using on-line dilution based on "zone sampling", *J. Agric. Food Chem.*, 2001, *49*, 5152-5155.

[23] Gonzalez-Rodrıguez, J.; Perez-Juan, P.; Luque de Castro, M.D. Flow injection determination of total catechins and procyanidins in white and red wines, *Innovative Food Science & Emerging Technologies*, 2002, *3*, 289-293.

[24] Choengchan, N.; Mantima, T.; Wilairat, P.; Dasgupta, P.K.; Motomizu, S.; Nacapricha, D.; A membraneless gas diffusion unit: Design and its application todetermination of ethanol in liquors by spectrophotometric flow injection, *Anal. Chim. Acta*, 2006, *579*, 33-37.

[25] Campuzano, S.; Gamella, M.; Serra, B.; Reviejo, A. J.; Pingarron, J. M. Integrated electrochemical gluconic acid biosensor based on self-assembled monolayer-modified gold electrodes. Application to the analysis of gluconic acid in musts and wines. *J. Agric. Food Chem.* 2007, *55*, 2109-2114.

[26] Oliveira, H. M.; Segundo, M. A.; LIMA, J. L. F. C.; Grassi, V.; Zagatto, E. A. G.; Kinetic enzymatic determination of glycerol in wine and beer using a sequential injection system with spectrophotometric detection, *J. Agric. Food Chem.* 2006, *54*, 4136-4140.

[27] Del Campo, G.; Gallego, B.; Berregi, I. Fluorimetric determination of histamine in wine and cider by using an anion-exchange column-FIA system and factorial design study, *Talanta*, 2006, *68*, 1126-1134.

[28] De Campos Costa, R. C.; Araújo, A. N.; Determination of Fe(III) and total Fe in wines by sequential injection analysis and flame atomic absorption spectrometry, *Anal. Chim. Acta*, 2001, *438*, 227-233.

[29] Lemos V. A.; De la Guardia, M.; Ferreira, S. L.C. An on-line system for preconcentration and determination of lead in wine samples by FAAS. *Talanta*, 2002, *58*, 475-480.

[30] Segundo, M. A.; Rangel, A. O. S. S.; Kinetic determination of L(−) malic acid in wines using sequential injection analysis, *Anal. Chim. Acta*, 2003, *499*, 99-106.

[31] Gonzalez-Rodrıguez, J.; Perez-Juan, P.; Luque de Castro, M. D. Method for the simultaneous determination of total polyphenol and anthocyan indexes in red wines using a flow injection approach, *Talanta*, 2002, 53-59.

[32] Costin, J. W.; Barnett, N. W.; Lewis, S. W. Determination of proline in wine using flow injection analysis with tris(2,2'-bipyridyl)ruthenium(II) chemiluminescence detection, *Talanta*, 2004, *64*, 894-898.

[33] Oliveira, A. F.; Fatibello-Filho, O.; Nobrega, J. A., Focused-microwave-assisted reaction in flow injection spectrophotometry: a new liquid-vapor separation chamber for determination of reducing sugars in wine, *Talanta*, 2001, *55*, 677-684.

[34] Ren, J. J.; Liu, H. Y.; Hao, Y. H., He, P. G.; Fang, Y. Z. Determination of resveratrol in red wine by solid phase extraction-flow injection chemiluminescence method, *Chinese Chemical Letters*, 2007, *18*, 985-988.

[35] Fernandes, E. N.; Reis, B. F. Automatic spectrophotometric procedure for the determination of tartaric acid in wine employing multicommutation flow analysis process, *Anal. Chim. Acta,* 2006, *557,* 380-386.

[36] Iida Y.; Ikeda, M.; Aoto, M.; Satoh, I. Fluorometric determination of urea in alcoholic beverages by using an acid urease column-FIA system. *Talanta,* 2004, *64,* 1278-1282.

[37] Decnop-Weever, L.G.; Kraak, J.C. Determination of sulphite in wines by gas-diffusion flow injection analysis utilizing spectrophotometric pH-detection. *Anal. Chim. Acta,* 1997, *337,* 125-131.

[38] Bartroli, J.; Escalada, M.; Jorquera, C. J.; Alonso, J. Determination of total and free sulphur dioxide in wine by flow injection analysis and gas-diffusion using p - aminoazobenzene as the colorimetric reagent, *Anal. Chem.,* 1991, *63,* 2532-2535.

[39] Mataix, E; Luque de Castro, M. D. Determination of total and free sulphur dioxide in wine by pervaporation–flow injection, *Analyst,* 1998, *123,* 1547-1549.

[40] Mana, H.; Spohn, U. Sensitive and selective flow injection analysis of hydrogen sulfite/sulphur dioxide by fluorescence detection with and without membrane separation by gas diffusion, *Anal. Chem.* 2001, *73,* 3187-3192.

[41] Atanassov, G. T.; Lima, R. C.; Mesquita, R. B. R.; Rangel, A. O. S. S.; Toth, I. V. Spectrophotometric determination of carbon dioxide and sulphur dioxide in wines by flow injection. *Analusis,* 2000, *28,* 77-82.

[42] Melo, D.; Zagatto, E.A.G.; Mattos, I.L.; Maniasso, N.; Spectrophotometric flow-injection determination of sulphite in white wines involving gas diffusion through a concentric tubular membrane. *J. Brazil. Chem. Soc,* 2003, *14,* 375 – 379.

[43] [43]Silva, R. L. G. N. P.; Silva, C. S.; Nobrega, J. A.; Neves, E. A. Flow injection spectrophotometric determination of free and total sulfite in wines based on the induced oxidation of manganese(II). *Anal. Lett.* 1998, *31,* 2195-2208.

[44] Caldas Santos, J. C.; Korn, M. Exploiting sulphide generation and gas diffusion separation in a flow system for indirect sulphite determination in wines and fruit juices. *Microchim. Acta,* 2006, *153,* 87-94.

[45] Perez-Ruiz, T.; Martinez-Lozano, C.; Tomas, V.; Carrion, F. J. Flow injection analysis of formaldehyde and sulphite using the oxidation of p-phenylenediamine by hydrogen peroxide, *Int. J. Environ. An. Ch.* 1993, *53,* 195-203.

[46] Hassan, S. S. M.; Hamza, M. S. A.; Mohamed, A. H. K. A novel spectrophotometric method for batch and flow injection determination of sulfite in beverages, *Anal. Chim. Acta,* 2006, *570,* 232-239.

[47] Fatibello-Filho, O.; Da cruz Vieira, I. Flow injection spectrophotometric determination of sulfite using a crude extract of sweet potato root (*Ipomoea batatas* (L.) Lam.) as a source of polyphenol oxidase. *Anal. Chim. Acta,* 1997, *354,* 51-57.

[48] Richter P.; Luque de Castro, M. D.; Valcarcel, M. Spectrophotometric flow-through sensor for the determination of sulphur dioxide, *Anal. Chim. Acta,* 1993, *283,* 408-413.

[49] Maquieira, A.; Casamayor, F.; Puchades, R. Determination of total and free sulphur dioxide in wine with a continuous-flow microdistillation system, *Anal. Chim. Acta,* 1993, *283,* 403-407.

[50] Liang Huang, Y.; Kim, J. M.; Schmid, R. D. Determination of sulphite in wine through flow-injection analysis based on the suppression of luminol chemiluminescence, *Anal. Chim. Acta,* 1992, *266,* 317-323.

[51] Huang, Y.; Zhang, C.; Zhang, X.; Zhang, Z., Chemiluminescence of sulfite based on auto-oxidation sensitized by rhodamine 6G, *Anal. Chim. Acta*, 1992, *391*, 95-100.

[52] He, D.; Zhang, Z.; Huang, Y. Chemiluminescence microflow injection analysis system on a chip for the determination of sulfite in food, *Anal. Lett.*, 2005, *38*, 563-571.

[53] Lin, J.-M.; Hobo, T. Flow-injection analysis with chemiluminescent detection ofsulphite using $Na_2CO_3 - NaHCO_3 - Cu^{2+}$ system. *Anal. Chim. Acta,* 1996, *323*, 69-74.

[54] Casella, I. G.; Contursi, M.; Desimoni, E.; Amperometric detection of sulphur-containing compounds in alkaline media, *The Analyst*, 2002, *127*, 647-652.

[55] Corbo, D.; Bertotti, M. Use of a copper electrode in alkaline medium as an amperometric sensor for sulphite in a flow-through configuration, *Anal. Bioanal. Chem.* 2002, *374*, 416-420.

[56] Azevedo, C. M. N.; Araki, K.; Toma, H. E.; Angnes, Lucio, Determination of sulphur dioxide in wines by gas-diffusion - flow injection analysis utilizing modified electrodes with electrostatically assembled films of tetraruthenated porphyrin, *Anal. Chim. Acta*, 1999, *387*, 175-180.

[57] Cardwell, T. J.; Christophersen, M. J. Determination of sulphur dioxide and ascorbic acid in beverages using a dual channel flow injection electrochemical detection system, *Anal. Chim. Acta*, 2000, *416*, 105-110.

[58] [58]Chen, G. N.; Liu, J. S.; Duan, J. P. Chen, H. Q. Coulometric detector based on porous carbon felt working electrode for flow injection analysis, *Talanta*, 2000, *53*, 651-660.

[59] Tavares Araujo, C.S.; Lira de Carvalho, J.; Ribeiro Mota, D.; de Araujo, C.L.; Coelho, N.M.M. Determination of sulphite and acetic acid in foods by gas permeation flow injection analysis. *Food Chem.* 2005, *92*, 765-770.

[60] Kuban, P.; Janos, P.; Kuban, V. Gas diffusion-flow injection determination of free and total sulphur dioxide in wines by conductometry, *Collect Czech Chem C*, 1998, *63*, 770-782.

[61] Groom, C.A; Luong, J.H.T.; Masson, C, Development of a flow injection analysis mediated biosensor for sulfite, *J. Biotechn.*, 1993, *27*, 117-127.

[62] Alipazaga, M.V.; Kosminsky, L.; Coichev, N.; Bertotti, M. S(IV) induced autoxidation of Cu(II)/tetraglycine complexes in the presence of aldehydes: mechanistic considerations and analytical applications, *Talanta*, 2002, *57*, 375-381.

[63] Su, X.; Wei, W.; Nie, L.; Yao, S. Flow injection determination of sulfite in wines and fruit juices by using a bulk acoustic wave impedance sensor coupled to a membrane separation technique, *The Analyst*, 1998, *123*, 221-224.

Reviewed by

Dr. Anastasios Economou[*], Assistant Professor, Laboratory Of Analytical Chemistry, Department Of Chemistry, University Of Athens, Athens 157 71, Greece..

---

[*] Tel: + 30 210 7274298, Fax: +30 210 7274557 , E-Mail: Aeconomo@chem.uoa.gr

In: Red Wine and Health
Editor: Paul O'Byrne

ISBN: 978-1-60692-718-2
© 2009 Nova Science Publishers, Inc.

Chapter 11

DOES OAK AGING IMPROVE THE ANTIOXIDANT ACTIVITY OF RED WINES?

Pedro Rodríguez-Rodríguez[1], Patrick Rabión[2], Gaspar Ros-Berruezo[1] and Encarna Gómez-Plaza[1]*

[1]Departamento de Tecnología de Alimentos, Nutrición y Bromatología. Facultad de Veterinaria, Universidad de Murcia. Campus de Espinardo, Murcia, España
[2]Finca Omblancas. Carretera de Jumilla-Ontur km 3, Jumilla, Murcia, España

ABSTRACT

Antioxidant activity (AOA) is currently considered to be one of the most significant characteristics of red wines. The beneficial influence of the moderate consumption of red wine on human health is generally thought to be due to the AOA of wine polyphenols. An important part of the winemaking process, especially for high quality wines, is aging in oak barrels. Aging affects the chemical characteristics of wines, especially the polyphenol profile and concentration. Some compounds are degraded, new ones are formed. Moreover, some compounds may be incorporated into the wine from the oak wood of the barrels. Some authors claim that younger red wines are more beneficial for health than aged wines but little information exists on the correlation of AOA and wine age.

We have studied the evolution of AOA and the total phenol content of wines obtained from different varieties (Cabernet Sauvignon, Petit Verdot and Monastrell) during twelve months of aging in stainless steel tanks or oak barrels to check how this parameter changes with aging and whether it is related with the variety or type of aging.

In general, it was observed that AOA decreases with age. However, the use of oak barrels leads to wines with higher AOA when comparing the results with the control wines stored in tanks for the same period of time.

Keywords: wine, antioxidant activity, phenolic compounds, aging

---
* Correspondence to: Tel. 34 968 367323, e-mail: encarnag@um.es

1. INTRODUCTION

The antioxidant activity of wines has been confirmed in numerous experimental assays and epidemiological studies [1, 2, 3, 4 and 5]. AOA is currently considered to be one of the most significant characteristics of red wines and is associated with the antioxidant activity of wine polyphenols. These phenolic compounds, which include phenolic acids and flavonoids, are extracted from grapes during the maceration process. The AOA of red wines has been correlated with their flavonol [6 and 7], anthocyanin [8] and tannin [9] content, although it is believed that AOA is linked with total phenol concentration rather than with individual compounds. Not all phenolic compounds display the same antioxidant activity and the phenolic composition of wine can be strongly affected, not only qualitatively but also quantitatively, by cultivation methods, grape varieties, maturity, enological techniques and the aging process [10, 11, 12, 13, 14 and 15]. Phenolic compounds undergo chemical transformations during winemaking and aging. It is probably during aging that the greatest number of polymerization and condensation reactions occur, which strongly modify the composition of a wine [16 and 17] and its quality attributes.

High quality wines are aged in oak barrels for several months. During oak maturation diffusion between the wine and barrel compounds contributes to the formation and development of the sensorial characteristics of aged wines. The amount of phenolics extracted into wine depends on aging time, oak type and barrel size [18 and 19]. The effect of aging on AOA is not clear and, indeed, contradictory studies can be found. The results found by [20, 21 and 22] showed that aging increased the antioxidant potential of wines, leading to higher 1,1-diphenyl-2-picrlhydrazyl (DPPH), superoxide radical (SRSA) and 2,2´-azobis-(2-amidinopropane) dihydrochloride-lipid peroxidation (ABAP-LP) indices. In contrast [23, 24 and 25] claimed that young wines had a greater antioxidant effect, with a higher 2,2'-azino-bis-3-ethylbenzothiazoline-6-sulphonic acid (ABTS) index and greater ability to inhibit lipidic peroxidation in a methyl-linoleate medium. This lack of consensus has called into question the effect of ageing on the antioxidant potential of wine, whether aged in oak barrels or in tanks.

2. MATERIALS AND METHODS

Red wines from Monastrell, Cabernet Sauvignon and Petit Verdot varieties were studied. Wines were matured in two different conditions: in oak barrels for 12 months or in stainless steel tanks for the same period of time. In the case of the Monastrell wines, barrels of different volumes (300, 400 and 500 litres), oak origin (French or American oak) and toasting degree (medium, medium plus and one toasting degree intermediate between medium and medium plus) were also used to check the effect of the type of the barrel on the wine characteristics.

2.1. Total Phenol Content Determination

Total phenol contet was determined using the Folin-Ciocalteu reagent [26].

Wine samples were diluted (1:50 in Monastrell wines and 1:100 in Cabernet Suvignon and Petit Verdot wines) and 7.5 mL of water and 0.3 mL of the Folin-Ciocalteu reagent (dilution 1:1) were added to 1 mL of diluted wine. After 3 minutes, 1mL of a saturated solution of sodium carbonate was added. After 20 minutes, the sample absorbance at 760 nm was measured in a UV/vis spectophotometer (Evolution 300, Thermo Scientific). The concentration of phenolic compounds was calculated using gallic acid as standard.

2.2. Total Antioxidant Capacity Determination

This assay is based on the decoloration that occurs when the radical cation ABTS•+ is reduced to ABTS (2,2'-azinobis-3-ethylbenzothiazoline-6-sulfonic acid). The radical was generated by reaction of a solution of ABTS in tampon phosphate salin (pH 7.4) with MnO_2. This solution was filtered with filter of 0.2 µm and it was kept into fridge. The assay was made up with 1000 µL of ABTS•+ solutions and 100 µL of the sample and carried out in darkness at room temperature. Absorbance measurements at 734 nm were made after 2 minutes of reaction time. The results were expressed in mM of Trolox, using the relevant calibration curve (Trolox equivalent antioxidant capacity, TEAC).

2.3. Determination of Chromatic Parameters

Total anthocyanins [27], total phenol index [28], total tannins [29] and polymeric anthocyanins [30] were determined.

3. RESULTS AND DISCUSSION

- Determination of the Antioxidant Activity

The ABTS radical has been extensively used to evaluate the AOA of wines, and other foods and beverages [31, 32, 33 and 34]. The radical cation of the 2,2'-azino-bis-(3-ethylbenzothiazoline-6-sulphonic acid) has a characteristic absorption spectrum, with maxima at 414, 645, 734 and 815 nm [35 and 36]. However, red wine samples have other compounds that absorb at 414 nm, which is why 734 nm was chosen for the measurement of TEAC in this study. ABTS enables determinations to be performed easily and quickly, allowing a considerable number of samples to be processed together, and provides very reliable results. The radical can be generated from ABTS in various systems: enzymatically using myoglobin [37] or horseradish peroxidase [38]; chemically with MnO_2 [31], potassium persulfate [39] or peroxide radicals [34]; or even electrochemically [40]. In our study the method was adapted according to [41] using a reaction time of 2 minutes. This modification allows to know the "fast antioxidant activity" to be ascertained since the free radical reacts rapidly with the polyphenols during the first step of the reaction. Using a reaction of only 2 minutes also prevents false results due to the generation of other compounds with a capacity to capture the free radical [42].

Different studies have shown significant correlations between different methods to evaluate AOA, especially for oxygen radical absorbance capacity assay (ORAC), ABTS, DPHH and cupric reducing antioxidant capacity (CUPRAC). Each can be considered as a relevant and reliable characteristic of the AOA of wines [43]. High TEAC values indicate that the mechanisms of the antioxidant action of extracts was as H donor and it could terminate the oxidation process by converting free radicals to stable forms.

- Correlation of Antioxidant Activity with the Phenolic Compounds of Wine

Several studies have provided strong evidence that phenolic compounds are the main responsible for the antioxidant activity of wines. The AOA of red wine has been correlated with their flavonol, anthocyanin and tannin contents although it is more probably linked with total phenols rather than individual ones.

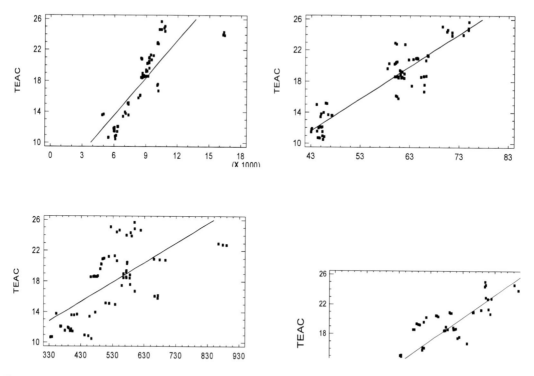

Figure 1, 2, 3 and 4: Regression Analysis of TEAC values with different chromatic characteristics. A: TEAC vs PC; B: TEAC vs OD280; C: TEAC vs Total tannins; D: TEAC vs Total Anthocyanins. TEAC: Trolox Equivalent Antioxidant Capacity (mM); PC: Phenolic Compound (mg/L, gallic acid equivalents); OD280: Total Phenolic Index, measure at 280 nm.

Figures 1, 2, 3 and 4 show the correlations between the antioxidant activity of the wines and the different chromatic parameters in the studied wines. We found a high correlation between the antioxidant activity and OD 280 ($r^2=0.85$), and with total phenolic compounds ($r^2=0.69$), correlations that are similar to the results obtained by other authors [44, 2, 45, 46 and 7].

A high correlation was also found with total anthocyanins ($r^2=0.83$) and the correlation was also significant with total tannins ($r^2=0.44$). Other investigations have indicated that the total phenol, flavonoid and flavanol contents of wines are strongly correlated with antioxidant properties whereas a weak correlation was found for anthocyanins [25 and 9].

- Effects of Variety, Aging Time and Aging Method on the Antioxidant Activity

Quantitatively, Monastrell wines are the most important wines in the D.O. Jumilla. Together with Monastrell, other varieties are being introduced in this area and vinified. Among these varieties, Cabernet Sauvignon and Petit Verdot are very well adapted to this area and are being used to improve Monastrell wines but also to obtain monovarietal wines. The chromatic characteristics of these wines before aging, together with their TEAC values are shown in Table 1. Petit Verdot and Cabernet Sauvignon wines showed a higher phenolic content than Monastrell wines (principally due to a larger concentration of anthocyanins and tannins) and almost doubled the antioxidant activity of Monastrell wines.

Table 1. Antioxidant capacity (TEAC) of the different wines before aging.

Wine sample	TEAC	PC	OD280	TT	TA	PA
PETIT VERDOT	27.72c	9910.42b	76.66c	697.01b	697.69c	70.39c
CABERNET SAUVIGNON	27.01b	9792.36b	67.60b	718.13b	521.95b	52.71b
MONASTRELL	16.24a	7472.92a	47.13a	461.07a	263.15a	30.37a

TEAC: Trolox Equivalent Antioxidant Capacity (mM); PC: Phenolic Compound (mg/L, gallic acid equivalents); OD280: Total Phenolic Index, TT: Total Tannin (mg/L), TA: Total Anthocyanin, PA: polymeric Anthocyanin (mg/L).

Our objective was to study how the aging process affects the antioxidant activity of these wines and whether differences can be found between wines from the different varieties and according to the different methods of aging. To this end, Monastrell, Cabernet Sauvignon and Petit Verdot wines were matured in medium toasted new American oak barrels. Samples were taken at 3, 6, 9 and 12 months. The analysis of the data was conducted with a multivariate analysis of the variance (MANOVA). Three factors were considered: grape variety, length of aging and aging system. The results of the MANOVA analysis (Table 2) indicated that variety was the factor that promoted the greatest differences in antioxidant and chromatic characteristics, much more than length of aging time or the aging system. Similarly, some authors have concluded that the age of a wine is not a crucial factor in determining AOA and other factors such as grape variety, cultivars and winemaking protocol are probably more significant [25].

The differences observed in the wines before aging can also be found during aging. Petit Verdot and Cabernet maintained the differences with Monastrell wines, in which AOA was almost 40% lower. This lower AOA could be attributed to the lower phenolic content including total and polymeric anthocyanins and total tannins. As stated above, the correlation between phenolic compounds and AOC has been described by many authors [44, 2, 45 and 46]. AOA decreased during aging, differences being close to 10% on average with respect to initial values, as found by other authors [47 and 48]. This decrease correlated with the decrease in phenolic compounds. During wine aging, part of the phenolic compounds may be degraded, oxidized or increase their degree of polymerization until they precipitate, which could explain the decrease in OD280. It should also be noted that aging led to differences in the anthocyanin composition. Total anthocyanis decreased by aproximatively 42% in all the wines, whereas polymeric anthocyanins increased by around 40%. These large changes in anthocyanin composition were not reflected in the AOA of wines (as mentioned, changes due to aging were around 10%). The AOA of anthocyanins is related to the number of hydroxyl groups, catechol moiety in the ring B, hydroxylation and methylation pattern and acylation. Since most anthocyanin condensations do not affect the number of hydroxyl groups of the involved polyphenols, this could explain why polymerisation reactions do not always produce a substantial modification of the AOA [47]. The fact that polymerization of the anthocyanins does not affect TEAC is also observed in the studies of [47 and 48] when microoxygenated and control wines were compared. Micro-oxygenation promotes the polymerization of phenolic compounds similar to that observed in barrels, and no differences in TEAC were observed.

Table 2. Results for the multivariate analysis of variance for the aging of Petit Verdot, Cabernet Sauvignon and Monastrell wines.

FACTOR		TEAC	OD280	PC	TT	TA	PA
Variety	Petit Verdot	20.40b	65.60c	10.13c	580.10b	414.50c	108.09c
	Cabernet Sauvignon	20.40b	62.90b	9.40b	582.30b	365.60b	76.44b
	Monastrell	12.40a	45.10a	6.30a	416.72a	181.50a	35.52a
Months	3	20.40c	62.70b	10.00b	521.49b	431.50d	55.87a
	6	18.60b	56.30a	8.50a	591.80c	327.60c	57.35a
	9	15.70a	56.00a	8.10a	526.30b	270.90b	87.43b
	12	16.30a	56.40a	7.90a	465.90a	252.10a	92.75b
Aging system	Oak barrel	18.00b	58.70b	8.50b	562.00b	328.80b	69.45a
	Control	17.50a	56.9a	8.70a	490.80a	312.20a	77.24b

TEAC: Trolox Equivalent Antioxidant Capacity (mM); PC: Phenolic Compound (g/L, gallic acid equivalents); OD280: Total Phenolic Index, TT: Total Tannin (mg/L), TA: Total Anthocyanin, PA: polymeric Anthocyanin (mg/L).

The interaction plots help to check whether the different varieties behaved similarly or not during aging (Figure 5). It can be that the TEAC of the three wines evolved similarly, decreasing from 0 to 9 months of aging and stabilizing for the last 3 months. The plot shows that the profile of evolution of the AOA of wines with aging time is similar independently of the variety.

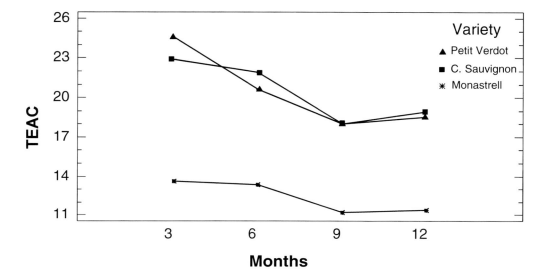

Figure5. Variety x Month interaction plot.

As regards the aging systems used (tanks or oak barrels) the AOA of oak-aged wines was higher than that of tank-aged wines. The former wines showed a higher phenolic compound content probably due to phenolic compounds being extracted from wood. The higher concentration of total tannins is also of note. Wine may extract ellagitannins, tannic compounds with antioxidant characteristics, from the wood [49]. These compounds could be the reason why oak-aged wines showed higher AOA compared with tank aged wines [50, 51 and 52].

-Influence of the Characteristics of the Barrel on the Antioxidant Activity

Given that oak-aged wines seem to present higher antioxidant properties than tank aged wines, the influence of the characteristics of the barrel was also studied on Monastrell wines to check whether if affected the AOA.

Effect of Barrel Volume

Monastrell wine was aged in French oak barrels (same tonelery and toasting degree) with different volumes of 300, 400 and 500 litres. The results were also compared with the control wine aged in tank (Table 3), which was found to decrease its AOA with time, especially from 3 to 6 months. The AOA of oak-aged wines on the other hand, increased up to six months, falling slightly after that (Figure 6). The sustantial extraction of phenolic compounds from wood probably contributed to this observed increase in AOA. There is a greater transfer of ellagitannins from wood to wine during the early stages of aging and it is known that these compounds regulate the oxidation mechanism in wines [48]. [25] stated that maturation in oak barrels may contribute to the capacity of the resultant wines to maintain AOA for a longer time. After six months, the oxidation of some phenolic compounds and their precipitation led to a decrease phenolic compound levels. The greatest differences with the control wine in this respect were observed at 6 months, when the wine aged in the smaller barrels showed the largest phenolic content and higher AOA. The highest surface/volume ratio of smaller barrels speeds up the transfer reactions between wood and wine [18 an 53].

At 9 and 12 months the highest AOA was found in wines aged in the largest barrels. The oxidation and condensation of phenolic compounds, including the disappearance of ellagitannins, is considered to take place faster in smaller barrels and slower in large barrels [18 an 53]. If compounds such as the ellagitannins are maintained for longer time, they may contribute to maintaining the AOA by two different mechanisms, their own antioxidant potential and the fact that they contribute to stabilising wine phenolic compounds, protecting them from oxygen and favouring condensation reactions.

Table 3. Evolution of chromatic characteristics of Monastrell wines during 12 months of aging in French oak barrels with three different volumes: 500, 400 and 300 litres.

Sample	months	PC	OD280	TT	TA	PA
FR 500L		7279.17b	46.59b	351.32a	230.80	31.97c
FR 400L	3	5418.06a	46.66b	339.27a	223.96	31.56b
FR 300L		8236.81c	46.19b	482.87c	216.49	33.09d
Control		7001.39b	45.18a	461.50b	229.56	30.30a
FR 500L		7334.72c	44.84b	558.67b	193.79b	32.92b
FR 400L	6	6876.39b	44.91b	572.00b	202.81b	32.41b
FR 300L		8373.61d	46.59c	625.33c	216.18c	33.84b
Control		6112.50a	43.13a	398.01a	164.24a	19.76a
FR 500L		7158.33c	46.56b	467.47b	161.44b	45.23c
FR 400L	9	6855.56b	46.73b	493.33c	151.51a	43.53b
FR 300L		6138.89a	47.38b	489.33c	156.96ab	43.56b
Control		6038.89a	44.71a	388.00a	166.41b	36.69a
FR 500L		6029.17c	46.91c	342.40a	153.50c	43.41c
FR 400L	12	6077.78c	46.51b	394.67c	166.54b	40.91b
FR 300L		5704.17b	46.76c	372.40b	148.37ab	44.43d
Control		5485.72a	44.59a	336.80a	143.71a	38.31a

TEAC: Trolox Equivalent Antioxidant Capacity (mM); PC: Phenolic Compound (mg/L, gallic acid equivalents); OD280: Total Phenolic Index, TT: Total Tannin (mg/L), TA: Total Anthocyanin, PA: polymeric Anthocyanin (mg/L). FR: French oak

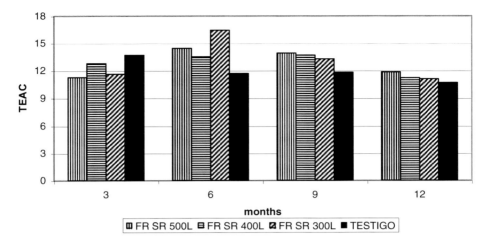

Figure 6. Evolution of TEAC of Monastrell wines during 12 months of oak aging in French oak barrels with three different volumes: 500, 400 and 300 litres.

Toasting Degree of the Barrel

The toasting process deeply influences the morphology and chemical composition of wood. High temperatures promote changes in the macromolecular structure (facilitating the access of wine to wood components) followed by chemical reaction, leading to the formation of new compounds, such as furfuryl or guaiacyl compounds [54, 55 and 56]. Toasting intensity affects the extent of these changes. On the other hand, high temperatures can degrade certain wood components, such as ellagitannins. The more pronounced the heating treatment, the more severe the effects, and ellagitannins may disappear from the most superficial layers of the wood [57].

In this study, Monastrell wine was aged in barrels with the same characteristics but with different toasting degrees. The behaviour of a control wine was also followed (Table 4). Results showed that, after 12 months, the highest AOA was observed in the wine aged in barrels with the lowest degree of toasting (medium toasting)(Figure 7).

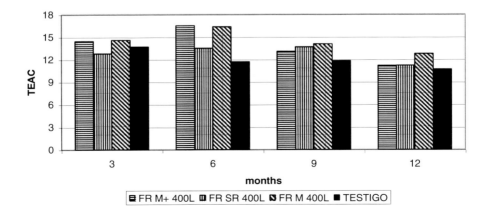

Figure 7. Evolution of TEAC of Monastrell wines during 12 months of aging in French oak barrels with three different toasting degrees.

These wines also showed the highest phenolic content (more extractable compounds were transferred from wood), the highest tannin content (probably due to the greater presence of ellagitannins) and more polymeric anthocyanins.

Table 4. Evolution of chromatic characteristics of Monastrell wines during 12 months of aging in French oak barrels with three different toasting degrees.

Sample	Months	PC	OD280	TT	TA	PA
FR M+ 400L	3	5209.72a	46.43b	334.04a	236.09b	30.10a
FR SR 400L		5431.94a	46.66b	339.274a	223.96a	31.56c
FR M 400L		5029.17a	46.83b	342.181a	233.60b	30.74b
Control		7001.39b	45.18a	461.50b	229.56ab	30.30b
FR M+ 400L	6	7941.67c	45.05b	555.73c	207.47b	32.20b
FR SR 400L		6876.39b	44.91b	572.00c	202.81b	32.41bc
FR M 400L		7895.83c	45.45b	521.60b	206.54b	35.10c
Control		6112.50a	43.13a	398.01a	164.24a	19.76a
FR M+ 400L	9	6277.78a	46.11ab	441.60b	160.35b	40.64b
FR SR 400L		6855.56c	46.73b	493.33c	151.51a	43.53c
FR M 400L		6588.89b	45.99ab	457.60b	155.84ab	44.11d
Control		6038.89a	44.71a	388.00a	166.41b	36.69a
FR M+ 400L	12	5947.22b	46.81c	338.40b	153.51c	43.41b
FR SR 400L		6077.78c	46.51c	394.67c	166.54b	40.91a
FR M 400L		6563.89d	45.70b	300.00a	150.24ab	43.16b
Control		5485.72a	44.59a	336.80b	143.71a	38.31a

TEAC: Trolox Equivalent Antioxidant Capacity (mM); PC: Phenolic Compound (mg/L, gallic acid equivalents); OD280: Total Phenolic Index, TT: Total Tannin (mg/L), TA: Total Anthocyanin, PA: polymeric Anthocyanin (mg/L).

Origin of Oak Wood

The botanical origin of oak also plays an important role in wine aging since the different woods present different morphological and chemical characteristics. Wood from French oak is more porous and a large quantity of oxygen may diffuse into the barrel. This micro-oxygenation may have a stabilising effect on wine colour and polyphenols. Moreover, some studies have shown that French oak provides a greater potential for phenolic compound extraction [58, 59 and 60] and contributes more ellagitannins to wine than American oak [18 and 61]. Ellagitannins present a large number of hydroxyl groups capable of capturing free radicals and therefore present an antioxidant activity [62]. We found similar results since wines aged in French oak showed higher values of OD280 and phenolic compounds as detected by the Folin-Ciocalteau method (Table 5). Together with this high concentration of phenolic compounds, wines aged in French oak wine show a higher AOA (Figure 8).

Table 5. Evolution of chromatic characteristics of Monastrell wines during 12 months of aging in French and American 400 L oak barrels

Sample	months	PC	OD280	TT	TA	PA
US M 400L		6098.61b	46.97b	408.80b	251.95b	1.55c
FR M 400L	3	5029.17a	46.83b	342.18a	233.60a	1.51b
Control		7001.39c	45.18a	461.50c	229.56a	1.49a
US M 400L		7345.83b	45.45b	531.60b	207.57b	31.63b
FR M 400L	6	7895.83c	45.45b	521.60b	206.54b	30.74b
Control		6112.50a	43.13a	398.01a	164.24a	30.30a
US M 400L		6154.17a	45.48ab	453.07b	147.44a	33.97c
FR M 400L	9	6588.89b	45.99b	457.60b	155.84b	35.10b
Control		6038.89a	44.71a	388.00a	166.41c	19.76a
US M 400L		6373.61b	45.10ab	366.00c	142.31a	47.51c
FR M 400L	12	6563.89c	45.70b	300.00a	150.24b	44.11b
Control		5484.72a	44.59a	336.80b	143.71a	38.31a

TEAC: Trolox Equivalent Antioxidant Capacity (mM); PC: Phenolic Compound (mg/L, gallic acid equivalents); OD280: Total Phenolic Index, TT: Total Tannin (mg/L), TA: Total Anthocyanin, PA: polymeric Anthocyanin (mg/L).

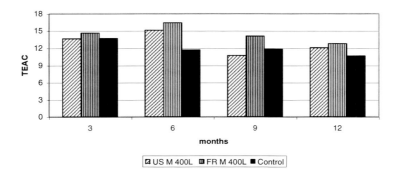

Figure 8. Evolution of TEAC of Monastrell wines during 12 months of aging in French and American oak barrels.

4. CONCLUSION

Our results have shown that the AOA of wines is clearly related with their phenolic content and that aging decreased this capacity, probably as a result of the decrease in total phenolic compounds. This decrease in AOA occurred similarly in wines elaborated with different varieties and therefore with a different phenolic content. It was also found that the decrease in AOA is more pronounced in wines stored in tanks than in oak barrels, probably due to the extraction of phenolic compounds from wood that helped to maintain the AOA of the studied wines. For Monastrell wines, oak aging resulted in positive results after six months of maturation compared with control wines. French oak and medium toasted barrels, since to improve to a largest extent the nutritional characteristics of Monastrell wines. The effect of volume will depend on the duration of the oak aging process. If wines are to be aged, short periods of time and small barrels would lead to more positive results, whereas if aging longer than 6 months, larger barrels would be more appropriate.

REFERENCES

[1] Tang, B.L. Alzheimer's disease: channeling APP to non-amyloidogenic processing. *Biochemical and Biophysical Research Communications*, 2005;331, 358-375.

[2] Villaño, D.; Fernández-Pachón, M.S.; Troncoso, A.M. y García-Parrilla, M.C. Influence of enological practices on the antioxidant activity of wines. *Food Chemistry*, 2006; 95, 394-404.

[3] Lagrue-Lak-Hal, A.H.; Andriantsitohaina, R. Red wine and cardiovascular risks. *Archives des Maladies du Coeur et des Vaisseaux*, 2006, 99, 1230-1235.

[4] Quincozes-Santos, A.; Andreazza, A.C.; Nardin, P.; Funchal, C.; Gonçalves, C.-A.; Gottfried, C. Resveratrol attenuates oxidative-induced DNA damage in C6 Glioma cells. *NeuroToxicology*, 2007, 28, 886-891.

[5] Rajdl, D.; Racek, J.; Trefil, L.; Siala, K. Effect of white wine consumption on oxidative stress markers and homocysteine levels. *Physiological Research*, 2007, 56, 203-212.

[6] Teissedre, P. L.; Frankel, E. N.; Waterhouse, A. L.; Peleg, H.; German, J. B. Inhibition of in vitro human LDL oxidation by phenolic antioxidants from grapes and wines. *Journal of the Science of Food and Agriculture,*1996, 70, 55–61.

[7] Simonetti, P.; Pietta, P.; Testolin, G. Polyphenol content and total antioxidant potential of selected Italian wines. *Journal of Agriculture and Food Chemistry,*1997, 45, 1152–1155.

[8] Rivero-Pérez, M.D.; Muñiz, P.;González-Sanjosé, M.L. Contribution of anthocyanin fraction to the antioxidant properties of wine. *Food and Chemical Toxicology*, 2008, 46, 2815-2822.

[9] De Beer, D; Joubert, E; Gelderblom, C.A.W.; Manley, M. Antioxidant activity of south African red and white cultivar wines: free radical scavenging. *Journal of Agricultural and Food Chemistry*, 2003, 51, 902-909.

[10] Gómez-Cordovés, C.; González-Sanjosé, M. L. Interpretation of color variables during the aging of red wines: Relationship with families of phenolic compounds. *Journal of Agricultural and Food Chemistry*, 1995, 43, 557–561.

[11] Revilla, I.; González-Sanjosé, M. L. Evolution during the storage of red wines with pectolytic enzymes: New anthocyanin pigments formation. *Journal of Wine Research*, 2001, 12, 183–197.

[12] Ortega-Herás, M.; González-Huerta, C.; Herrera, P.; González-Sanjosé, M. L. Changes in wine volatile compounds of varietal wines during ageing in wood barrels. *Analytica Chimica Acta*, 2004, 513, 341–350.

[13] Pérez-Magariño, S.; González-Sanjosé, M. L. Polyphenols and colour variability of red wines made from grapes harvested at different ripeness grade. *Food Chemistry*, 2006, 96, 197–208.

[14] Gómez-Plaza, E.; Miñano, A.; López-Roca, J.M. Comparison of chromatic properties, stability and antioxidant capacity of anthocyanin-based aqueous extracts from grape pomace obtained from different vinification methods. *Food Chemistry*, 2006, 97, 87-94.

[15] Ortega-Regules, A.; Romero-Cascales, I.; Ros-García, J.M.; López-Roca, J.M.; Gómez-Plaza, E. A first approach towards the relationship between grape skin cell wall composition and anthocyanin extractability. *Analytica Chimica Acta*, 2006, 563 (1-2 SPEC. ISS.), 26-32.

[16] Dallas, C.; Ricardo-Da-Silva, J. M.; Laureano, O. Degradation of oligomeric procyanidins and anthocyanins in a Tinta Roriz red wine during maturation. *Vitis*, 1995, 34, 51–56.

[17] Cheynier, V.; Hidalgo, I.; Souquet, J.; Moutounet, M. Estimation of the oxidative changes in phenolic compounds of Carignane during winemaking. *American Journal of Enology and Viticulture*, 1997, 48, 225–228.

[18] Pérez-Prieto, L.J.; López-Roca, J.M.; Martínez-Cutillas, A.; Pardo-Mínguez, F.; Gómez-Plaza, E. Extraction and formation dynamic of oak related volatile compounds from different volume barrels to wine and their behavior during bottle storage. *Journal of Agricultural and Food Chemistry*, 2003, **51**, 5444-5449.

[19] Pérez-Prieto, L. J.; López-Roca, J. M.; Martínez-Cutillas, A.; Pardo-Mínguez, F.; Gómez-Plaza, E. Maturing wines in oak barrels. Effect of oak origin, volume and age of the barrel on the wine volatile composition. *Journal of Agricultural and Food Chemistry*, 2002, 50, 3272-3276.

[20] Larrauri, J.A.; Sanchez-Moreno, C.; Ruperez, P.; Saura-Calixto, F. Free radical capacity in the aging of selected Spanish wines. *Journal of Agricultural and Food Chemistry,* 1999, 47, 1603–1606.

[21] Yamaguchi, F.; Yoshimura, Y.; Nakazawa, H.; Ariga, T. Free Radical Scavenging Activity of Grape Seed Extract and Antioxidants by Electron Spin Resonance Spectrometry in an H_2O_2/NaOH/DMSO System, *Journal of Agricultural and Food Chemistry*, 199, 47, 2544 -2548.

[22] Echeverry, C.; Ferreira, M.; Reyes-Parada, M.; Abin-Carriquiry, J.A.; Blasina, F; González-Neves, G.; Dajas, F. Changes in antioxidant capacity of tannat red wines during early maturation. *Journal of Food Engineering*, 69, 147-154.

[23] Pellegrini, N.; Simonetti, P.; Gardana, C.; Brenna, O.; Brighenti, F.; Pietta, P. Polyphenol content and total antioxidant activity of *Vini NoVelli* (young red wines). *Journal of Agricultural and Food Chemistry,* 2000, 48, 732-735.

[24] Landrault, N.; Poucheret, P.; Ravel, P.; Gasc, F.; Cros, G.; Teissedre, P.-L. Antioxidant capacities and phenolics levels of French wines from different varieties and vintages. *Journal of Agricultural and Food Chemistry,* 2001, 49, 3341-3348.

[25] Roginsky, V; De Beer, D; Harbertson, J.F.; Kilmartin, T.B.; Adams, D.O. The antioxidant activity of Californian red wines does not correlate with wine age. *Journal of the Science of Food and Agriculture,* 2006, 86, 834-840.

[26] Official Methods of Analysis (AOAC) 15th Ed. Association of Official Analytical Chemists. Washington D.C. 1990.

[27] Blouin, J. Tecniques d´analyses des moûtes et des vins. **Ed.** Dujardin-Salleron, Paris, 1992.

[28] Ribéreau-Gayon, P.; Glories, Y.; Maujean, A.; Dubourdieu, D. Traité d´Oenologie.2. Chimie du vin. Stabilisation et traitements. Dunod, Paris. 1998.

[29] Harbertson, J. F.; kennedy, J.A.; Adams, D. O. Tannin in skin and seeds of Cabernet sauvignon, Syrah and Pinot noir berries during ripening. *American Journal of Enology and Viticulture*, 2002, 53, 54-59.

[30] Levengood, J.; Boulton, R. The variation in the color due to copigmentation in young Cabernet Sauvignon wines. In: *Red wine color. Revealing the mysteries.* Waterhouse, A., Kennedy, J. (Eds) American Chemical Society, Washington DC, 35-52. 2004.

[31] Benavente-García,O.; Castillo, J.; Lorente, J.; Ortuño, A. Antioxidant activity of phenolics extracted from Olea europaea L. leaves. *Food Chemistry,* 2000, 68, 457-462.

[32] Pellegrini, N.; Visioli, F.; Buratti, S.; Brighenti, F. Direct Analysis of Total Antioxidant Activity of Olive Oil and Studies on the Influence of Heating. *Journal of Agricultural and Food Chemistry*, 2001, 49, 2532-2538.

[33] Scalfi, L.; Fogliano, V.; Pentangelo, A.; Graziani, G.; Giordano, I.; Ritieni, A. Antioxidant Activity and General Fruit Characteristics in Different Ecotypes of *Corbarini* Small Tomatoes. *Journal of Agricultural and Food Chemistry*, 2000, 48, 1363-1366.

[34] Berg van den, R.; Haenen, G.R.M.M.; Berg van den, H.; Bast, A., 1999. Applicability of an improved Trolox equivalent antioxidant capacity (TEAC) assay for evaluation of antioxidant capacity measurements of mixtures. *Food Chemistry,* 1999, **66,** 511–517.

[35] Arnao, M.B.; Acosta, M.; del Río, J.A.; García-Cánovas, F. Inactivation of peroxidase by hydrogen peroxide and its protection by a reductant agent. *Biochim Biophys Acta*, 1990, 1038, 85–89.

[36] Miller, N.J.; Rice-Evans, C.A.; Davies, M.J.; Gopinathan, V.; Milner, A. A novel method for measuring antioxidant capacity and its application to monitoring the antioxidant status in premature neonates, *Clinical Science,* 1993, 84, 407–412.

[37] Rice-Evans, C.A.; Miller, N.J. Total antioxidant status in plasma and body fluids, *Methods in Enzymology,* 1994, 234, 279–293.

[38] Arnao, M.B.; Cano, A.; Hernández-Ruiz, J.; García-Cánovas, F.; Acosta, M. Inhibition by L-Ascorbic acid and other antioxidants of the 2,2'-azino-bis(3-ethylbenzthiazoline-6-sulfonic acid) oxidation catalyzed by peroxidase: A new approach for determining total antioxidant status of foods. *Analytical Biochemistry,* 1996, 236, 255–261.

[39] Re, R.; Pellegrini, N.; Protegente, A.; Pannala, A.; Yang, M.; Rice-Evans, C. Antioxidant activity applyng an improved ABTS radical cation decolorization assay. *Free Radical Biology and Medicine*, 1999, 26, 1231-1237.

[40] Alonso, A.M.; Domínguez, C.; Guillén, D.A.; Barroso, C.G. Determination of antioxidant power of red and white wines by a new electrochemical method and its correlation with polyphenolic content. *Journal of Agricultural and Food Chemistry,* 2002, 50, 3112-3115.

[41] Villaño, D.; Fernández-Pachón, M.S.; Toncoso, A.M.; García-Parrilla, M.C. The antioxidant activity of wines determined by the ABTS$^{\bullet+}$ method: influence of sample dilution and time. *Talanta,* 2004, 64, 501-509.

[42] Arts, M.J.T.J.; Sebastian-Dallinga, J.; Voss, H.P.; Haenen, G.R.M.M.; Bast, A. A critical appraisal of the use of the antioxidant capacity (TEAC) assay in defining optimal antioxidant structures. *Food Chemistry,* 2003, 80, 409-414.

[43] Li, H.; Wang, X.; Li, Y.; Li, P.; Wang, H. Polyphenolic compounds and antioxidant properties of selected China wines. *Food Chemistry,* 2009, 112, 454-460.

[44] Fernández-Pachón, M.S.; Villaño, D.; García-Parrilla, M.C.; Troncoso, A.M. Antioxidant activity of wines and relation with their polyphenolic composition. *Analytica Chimica Acta,* 2004, 513, 113-118.

[45] Arnous, A.; Makris, D. P.; Kefalas, P. Effect of principal polyphenolic components in relation to antioxidant characteristics of aged red wines. *Journal of Agricultural and Food Chemistry,* 2001, 49, 5736–5742.

[46] Burns, J.; Gardner, P. T.; Matthews, D.; Duthie, G. G.; Lean, M. E. J.; Crozier, A. Extraction of phenolics and changes in antioxidant activity of red wines during vinification. *Journal of Agricultural and Food Chemistry,* 2001, 49, 5797–5808.

[47] Rivero-Pérez, M.D.; González-Sanjosé, M.L.; Muñiz, P.; Pérez-Magariño, S. Antioxidant profile of red-single variety wines microoxygenated before malolactic fermentation. *Food Chemistry,* 2008, 111, 1004–1011.

[48] Rivero-Pérez, M.D.; González-Sanjosé, M.L.; Ortega-Heras, M.; Muñiz, P. Antioxidant potential of single-variety red wines aged in the barrel and in the bottle. *Food Chemistry,* 2008, 111, 957-964.

[49] Cerda, B.; Tomas-Barberán, F.A.; Espín, J.C. Metabolism of antioxidant and chemopreventive ellagitannins from strawberries, raspberries, walnuts, and oak-aged wine in humans: identification of biomarkers and individual variability. *Journal of Agricultural and Food Chemistry,* 2005, 53, 227-235.

[50] Rangkadilok, N.; Sitthimonchai, S.; Worasuttayangkurn, L.; Mahidol, C.; Ruchirawat, M.; Satayavivad, J. Evaluation of free radical scavenging and antityrosinase activities of standardized longan fruit extract. *Food and Chemical Toxicology,* 2007, 45, 328–336.

[51] Kawada, M.; Ohno, Y.; Ri, Y.; Ikoma, T.; Yuugetu, H.; Asai, T.; Watanabe, M.; Yasuda, N.; Akao, S.; Takemura, G.; Minatoguchi, S.; Gotoh, K.; Fujiwara, H.; Fukuda, K. Anti-tumor effect of gallic acid on LL-2 lung cancer cells transplanted in mice. *Anticancer Drugs,* 2001, 12, 847–852.

[52] Yilmaz, Y.; Toledo, R. T. Major flavonoids in grape seeds and skins: antioxidantcapacity of catechin, epicatechin, and gallic acid. *Journal of Agricultural and Food Chemistry,* 2004, 52, 255-260.

[53] Rodríguez-Rodríguez, P; Rabion, P; López-Roca, J.M. y Gómez-Plaza, E. Influencia del envejecimiento en barricas de distinto origen, tostado y volumen en el perfil

aromático de vinos tintos de Monastrell. *Avances en Ciencias y Técnicas Enológicas. Transferencia de Tecnología de la Red GIENOL al Sector Vitivinícola*, 2007, 292-293.

[54] Mosedale, J. R.; Puech, J. L. Wood maturation of distilled beverages. *Food Science and Technology*, 1998, 9, 95-101.

[55] Hale, M. D.; Mccafferty, K.; Larmie, E.; Newton, J.; Swan, J. S. The influence of oak seasoning and toasting parameters on the composition and quality of wine. *American Journal of Enology and Viticulture,* 1999, 50, 495-502.

[56] Giménez-Martínez, R.; López-García de la Serrana, H.; Villalón Mir, M.; Quesada-Granados, J.; López-Martínez, M. C. Influence of wood heat treatment, temperature and maceration time on vanillin, syringaldehyde and gallic acid contents in oak wood and wine spirit mixtures. *American Journal of Enology and Viticulture*, 1996, 47, 441-446.

[57] Moutounet, M.; Rabier, P.; Sarni, F.; Scalbert, A. Les tannins du bois de chene: Les conditions de leur presence dans les vins. Le boit et la qualité des vins et des eaux-de-vie. *Journal International des Sciences de la Vigne et du Vin*, 1992, 26**,** 75-79.

[58] Marco, J.; Artajona, J.; Larrechi, M. S.; Rius, F. X. Relationship between geographical origin and chemical composition of wood for oak barrels. *American Journal of Enology and Viticulture,* 1994, 45, 192-200.

[59] Naudin, R. A. French view of barrel aging. *Wines and Vines*, 1990, 71, 48-55.

[60] Puech, J. L. Characteristics of oak wood and biochemical aspects of Armagnac Aging. . *American Journal of Enology and Viticulture,* 1984, 35; 77-81.

[61] Cadahía, E.; Varea, S.; Muñoz, L.; Fernández de Simón, B.; García-Vallejo, M. Evolution of ellagitannins in Spanish, French, and American oak woods during natural seasoning and toasting. *Journal of Agricultural and Food Chemistry,* 2001, *49,* 3677-3684.

[62] De Beer, D.; Joubert, E.; Marais, J.; Manley, M. Unravelling the total antioxidant capacity of pinotage wines: contribution of phenolic compounds. *Journal of Agricultural and Food Chemistry,* 2006, 54, 2897-2905.

In: Red Wine and Health
Editor: Paul O'Byrne

ISBN: 978-1-60692-718-2
© 2009 Nova Science Publishers, Inc.

Chapter 12

RED WINE AND THE METABOLIC SYNDROME: POSSIBLE CONTRIBUTION OF AN OLD REMEDY FOR AN EMERGENT PROBLEM

Rosário Monteiro[1,2], *Marco Assunção*[3] *and Conceição Calhau*[1]

[1]Department of Biochemistry (U38-FCT), Faculty of Medicine,
University of Porto, Porto, Portugal.
[2]Faculty of Nutrition and Food Sciences, University of Porto, Porto, Portugal.
[3]Department of Anatomy (U121/94-FCT), Faculty of Medicine,
University of Porto, Porto, Portugal.

ABSTRACT

The combination of abdominal obesity with metabolic abnormalities (hyperglycemia, hyperinsulinemia, dyslipidemia, hypertension), collectively termed metabolic syndrome, is increasingly common and largely associated with the risk of developing cardiovascular disease, diabetes and cancer. If traditionally alcoholic beverages were strongly discouraged in the patients presenting these dysfunctions, mounting evidence is now showing that generalization of the deleterious effects of ethanol consumption to all alcoholic beverages is reductive. Since the description of the French paradox, many beneficial effects of red wine have been described, namely those linked to cardiovascular disease protection. Initially, this protective ability was attributed to ethanol. Later on, the relationship has been shown stronger for red wine, and its non-alcoholic components have come into scene, with a special relevance to flavonoids (catechins, procyanidins and anthocyanins) and resveratrol. Conclusive studies revealed that red wine has qualities further than alcohol as de-alcoholized red wine has also been related with health promotion. Considering the central role of visceral obesity and metabolic dysfunction in the metabolic syndrome, we will review the most recent findings regarding the effects of red wine or its components on the adipose tissue. Experimental results on the effects of red wine intake upon body weight and adipose tissue in the rat, from which a new possible red wine mechanism of action is advanced, will also be presented. Often forgotten, and probably making most of the difference for the effects exerted, the amount of beverage consumed as well as the pattern and context of drinking, will also be brought to this discussion.

1. INTRODUCTION

Evidence is being gathered on the health benefits of wine concerning the prevention or improvement of certain disease states. The cardiovascular diseases have received most of the attention concerning the effects of alcoholic beverages, especially red wine, for which improvements in endothelial function, atherosclerotic lesions, plasma lipid profiles and prevention of inflammation, thrombosis and oxidation of low density lipoprotein (LDL) cholesterol particles have been demonstrated [1-3].

It is currently accepted that the metabolic syndrome largely increases the risk for the development of cardiovascular disease, but also type 2 diabetes and cancer [4]. This constellation of disturbances including glucose intolerance, central obesity, dyslipidemia (hypertriglyceridemia, elevated non-esterified fatty acids (NEFA) and decreased high density lipoprotein (HDL) cholesterol) and hypertension can present in several forms, according to the combination of the different components of the syndrome. However, intense debate is ongoing concerning the causes for the onset of the metabolic disturbances that constitute the syndrome. Several explanations have been proposed to explain its origin. While some consider an initial insulin resistant state progressing to the other components, others think that obesity is the main initiator of the syndrome. As a matter of fact, visceral obesity and adipose tissue dysfunction are more and more considered central to the initial metabolic disturbances that lead to disease [5-7]. More recently, the chronic low-grade inflammatory condition as well as the oxidative stress status that accompany visceral obesity have been implicated as major players in both the installation of the metabolic syndrome and of its associated pathophysiological consequences [8, 9].

Considering the vast body of literature related to red wine consumption and the protection of cardiovascular disease, in this review we will focus mainly on the knowledge of red wine or of its components on the adipose tissue, beginning with a revision of the importance of this highly active organ for metabolic homeostasis and the development of the metabolic syndrome.

2. THE ADIPOSE TISSUE IN THE METABOLIC SYNDROME

The primarily known functions of adipose tissue include heat insulation, mechanical cushioning and storage of triglycerides. Furthermore, adipose tissue secretes endocrine, paracrine and autocrine active substances in response to different stimuli [5, 10-12]. Some are specific to adipocytes (the adipokines leptin and adiponectin) and some other may be produced by several cell types in the adipose tissue and include inflammatory cytokines (tumor necrosis factor α (TNFα), interleukin (IL)-6), chemokines (monocyte chemoattractant protein), acute phase reactants, components of the alternative complement system, eicosanoids, as well as molecules with anti-inflammatory properties [13].

The role of the adipose tissue in the pathophysiology of the metabolic syndrome has received much attention in the last few years. Epidemiological evidence linking obesity to the predisposition to develop cardiovascular disease, type 2 diabetes and cancer has encouraged the study of adipose-based mechanisms in the metabolic syndrome. Furthermore, the recognition of the adipose tissue as a true endocrine organ [10-12], rather than a passive storage for energy, with the description of its ability to produce inflammation-active molecules has allowed beginning to understand the links between the adipose tissue and the other pathological manifestations of this syndrome. However, it was not until very recently that a paradigm shift has occurred in the way that we understand the association of the adipose tissue and metabolic disease. Currently, it is not the excess adipose tissue that is considered harmful but the dysfunctional adipose tissue, characterized by visceral fat accumulation and lack of capacity to buffer nutrient excess, mainly carbohydrates and lipids [14]. This justifies also why subcutaneous fat depots are protective and that the lack of adipose tissue, as evident in lipodystrophy, may equally lead to the development of metabolic syndrome [15].

2.1. Adipose Tissue Dysfunction

The most prominent sign of adipose tissue failure is increased circulating concentration of NEFA [5-7]. This reflects the inability of the tissue to buffer the excess nutrient intake and is related to the dyslipidemic state that is typical of the metabolic syndrome. When overload becomes present, the liver increases its production of apo-B containing particles that carry triglycerides to the adipose tissue resulting in LDL formation [4]. When the capacity of adipose tissue is overwhelmed, the conversion of very low density lipoprotein or similar particles is delayed and hypertriglyceridemia originates. Furthermore, neighboring tissues start being used for lipid accumulation (e.g. the liver, muscle, pancreas and heart) [9]. As these organs are not able to store lipids without harm to their functions, lipotoxicity may be the result culminating, in the case of muscle, liver and pancreas, in insulin resistance [9].

2.2. Adipose Tissue Hypertrophy and Inflammation

Another sign of adipose tissue dysfunction is the chronic low grade inflammation that arises with obesity. It has been shown that circulatory inflammatory cytokines (TNFα, IL-6 and C-reactive protein (CRP)) are positively correlated with adipocyte size and, conversely, the plasma concentration of adiponectin is decreased with increasing cell size [16], suggesting that adipocyte hypertrophy is a sign of dysfunction. Adipocyte hypertrophy is also tightly connected to the presence of inflammatory cells in the adipose tissue [17, 18], another feature of dysfunction, but the chemotactic stimulus for their enrolment has not been clearly identified.

We have demonstrated, using the finite element modeling method that adipocyte size determines these cells liability to rupture [19]. Ruptured adipocytes exposing their cellular contents to the extracellular milieu could then constitute the initiation of adipose tissue-originated inflammation. Corroborating this idea is the observation made by Cinti et al. [20] who found that macrophages within the adipose tissue are located in the vicinity of dead adipocytes. Adipocytes enclosed within the visceral cavity may be at the highest risk for rupture as high pressure variations are generated inside the intra-abdominal and the thoracic cavities during physical activities [21, 22], facilitating adipocyte rupture, particularly for larger cells. Macrophage attraction follows, beginning a complex cascade of events that culminates in disease. In good agreement with this hypothesis is the special pathological value of upper body adiposity [23] and the finding that it is associated with a decrease in the number of preadipocytes in the stromal fraction committed to the differentiation program, resulting in a smaller number, although larger, adipose cells [24]. Also important to mention is that bigger adipocytes are also found in insulin resistant patients [25], reinforcing the thought that obesity complications are more associated to adipocyte hypertrophy than hyperplasia.

2.3. Obesity and Insulin Resistance

Both the hypertriglyceridemia that occurs during obesity or adipose tissue dysfunction and overproduction of cytokines by the inflamed tissue contribute to the impairment of insulin signaling. It is known that several kinases phosphorylate the insulin receptor substrate (IRS) in serine residues preventing its activation by the insulin receptor, blunting downstream signaling and facilitating the degradation of IRS protein [9, 26].

There is compelling evidence showing that exposure of adipocytes to several types of stressors (oxidative stress, inflammatory cytokines and elevated concentrations of fatty acids) induces cellular responses mediated by cellular kinases, including mitogen-activated protein kinase (MAPK) (p38MAPK, Jun N-terminal kinase (JNK)), inhibitor of nuclear factor κB kinase (IKK) and various conventional and atypical protein kinases C (PKC) [9, 27-29].

Some of these kinases involved in stress-sensing work in concert to stop the toxic increase of body energy stores, being related to the impairment of insulin action through the stimulation of IRS serine phosphorylation, but also often activate targets related to the inflammatory response. They exert powerful effects on pro-inflammatory gene expression, through activation of activator protein 1 (AP-1) complexes and nuclear factor κB (NFκB) [30]. These transcription factors activate the expression of a wide variety of genes including cytokines, chemokines, adhesion molecules and effector enzymes such as inducible nitric oxide synthase and cycloxygenase-2 [31].

2.4. Adipose Tissue Oxidative Stress in the Metabolic Syndrome

Oxidative stress has been proposed as a potential inducer of an inflammatory status and susceptibility to obesity and related disorders [8, 32-35]. Evidence suggests that it may be involved in the etiology, pathogenesis and development of the metabolic syndrome. It is well known that it occurs more frequently in people with metabolic syndrome than among those without [8, 35-38] although not all studies support this demonstration [39].

Several biomarkers are being suggested as the link between obesity, insulin resistance, cardiovascular disease and metabolic syndrome, and between oxidative stress and metabolic syndrome, such as TNFα, IL-6, IL-18, angiotensinogen, transforming growth factor β, plasminogen activator inhibitor-1 (PAI-1), leptin, resistin, CRP, markers of endothelial dysfunction, adiponectin, isoprostanes, heat shock protein 70 and γ-glutamyltransferase [35, 40-43]. However, the role of many of them concerning inflammatory and oxidative stress processes in humans, as well as the factors involved in their regulation, are currently unclear.

Recent reports on the association of obesity with increased oxidative stress also sustain its implication in pathogenesis. Oxidative stress markers have been shown to be elevated in obese individuals and elevated reactive oxygen species may be implicated in the pathogenesis of atherosclerosis, hypertension and diabetes [44]. However, they also directly affect the adipose tissue. Furukawa et al. [8] showed that oxidative stress suppressed peroxisome proliferator-activated receptor γ (PPARγ) expression in 3T3-L1 preadipocytes and suggested that oxidative stress is an early cause of the metabolic syndrome. In accordance with this, Galinier et al. [45] have recently shown that antioxidant treatment augmented glutathione content and improved its redox status in preadipocytes, this being associated with increased accumulation of triglycerides, an indicator of the differentiated phenotype. These authors also showed that in the absence of metabolic dysfunction and inflammation, adipose tissue levels of antioxidants are high and only when these modifications emerge is there a shift to an oxidative status. Thus, it seems that only when obesity reaches overwhelming proportions, does antioxidant/reactive oxygen species ratio in the adipose tissue decrease. Then, oxidative stress decreases proliferation and differentiation and adipocytes get larger, being more prone to generate reactive oxygen species as the metabolic workload of each individual cell increases [46]. Although no connection with the induction of adipocyte differentiation has been discussed, redox status amelioration has been shown to improve glucose tolerance and insulin sensitivity in *in vivo* models of insulin resistance [47]. The former demonstrations shed light on the meaning of antioxidant ingestion to prevent metabolic diseases and establish new mechanisms through which metabolic improvement may occur.

3. DIETARY INFLUENCES ON THE METABOLIC SYNDROME

The enormous influence of diet and dietary habits in the installation and progression of the metabolic syndrome is currently unarguable. It is without a doubt a disease of excess, where energy surplus is the main instigator leading to systemic overload of nutrients and failure to maintain homeostasis [14]. Although this idea is well accepted, less attention has been paid to the composition of the diet, rather than its energetic value. The scarcity in micronutrients, and relative abundance of sugars, saturated and *trans* fatty acids, are also likely to play important roles in the metabolic deregulation accompanying the syndrome [6].

The implication of oxidative stress and inflammation in the etiology of the metabolic syndrome further supports the paramount importance of food habits to prevent or manage this condition, as it is well known that dietary components may influence antioxidant status and the progression and resolution of inflammatory response within the organism.

3.1. Wine

Wine is produced from different varieties of *Vitis vinifera* grapes, which originate a complex product, given the occurrence of several chemical reactions during the winemaking process [48]. The most important reaction is alcoholic fermentation, due to its impact on wine stability and organoleptic properties. Chemically, wine is composed of a mixture of several hundred different molecules belonging to an extensive array of chemical classes such as alcohols, polyols, polysaccharides, acids, nitrogenous compounds, vitamins, minerals and polyphenols [48, 49].

This later group of compounds has received much attention of the researcher community, since they are widely distributed in nature, and in plant-based foods, and because of a growing list of biological activities they are being endowed with. They constitute an ample group of substances produced during secondary plant metabolism [48-50] that seem to exert defense and signaling actions, such as protection against UV radiation, bacteria and fungi and attraction of polinizing insects [51].

More than 200 polyphenolic compounds have been identified in wine, most of them belonging to the flavonoid group. Among them, the catechins and oligomeric procyanidins, quercetin, kaempferol and the anthocyanin malvidin-3-glucoside are the most abundant. Besides the flavonoids, wine also contains a large amount of phenolic acids, such as gallic acid, and polyphenols from other classes such as the stilbene resveratrol, which can be found in small quantities in red wines [48, 49]. The polyphenols originate in grape seeds and skins and are extracted during fermentation, with the increasing ethanol content of the must [48]. The total amount of polyphenols in red wine may range from 1000-4000 mg/L and approximately 85% are flavonoids [50]. In the present article we will focus mainly on the actions of red wine intake or of its polyphenols and not in white wine for several reasons. The first is that these two beverages greatly differ in their composition, in part due to technological differences in winemaking. This is true not only for the amount, which is much smaller in white wine, but also for the type of polyphenolic compounds [48]. Maybe because of this, most scientific evidence linking wine with health effects deals with red wine.

3.2. Wine and Health

The fist steps given towards the recognition of wine as an important part of the human diet and linking it to heath promoting effects date back to the description that the Mediterranean diet pattern, albeit originally thought to be poor, was associated with low coronary heart disease and cancer prevalence in the population of Crete, in Greece [52]. Already at that time, the consumption of wine, and also olive oil and vinegar, were among the suggested dietary items implicated in this inverse relationship between their consumption and disease.

Later on, the recognition that the French population, despite having a high consumption of saturated fats and displaying elevated blood cholesterol levels, presented an apparently controversial low mortality for coronary heart disease gave birth to the French Paradox [48, 53, 54]. This association was soon explained by their high consumption of wine, particularly red wine [53].

Until then, wine was viewed as just another alcoholic beverage and thought to be mainly toxic as their remaining counterparts. This may have delayed the demonstration of health benefits of wine, as did the thought that their main biological attributes concerned ethanol. Posterior studies demonstrating the wine abundance in polyphenols and other works relating the consumption of a diet rich in such molecules with improved health [55, 56], particularly coronary heart disease, prompted a more detailed study of wine, its distinction from other alcoholic beverages, including from white wine, and the recognition that non-alcoholic components of red wine, played a leading part in its effects.

Even so, this association was not easy to establish and controversial data are still being generated. Some of the reasons for this difficulty are related to red wine content in ethanol. Although this alcohol has been demonstrated to possess benefits underlying the reduced coronary heart disease incidence in red wine drinkers [1-3], effects may largely vary with age, gender and genetic background of the population studied [57]. Furthermore, data on wine consumption generated from food questionnaires may not reflect the drinking pattern or style of drinking. It is understandable that the biological effects of the any alcoholic beverage will vary greatly if a given amount is consumed in the same day (e.g. the binge drinking weekend pattern common in teenagers) or divided by the seven days of the week [58], or even if it drunk as a part of the meal or in between [59]. Any changes in this pattern will have great impact in the time of absorption and metabolism, conditioning the predominance of ethanol (that in high doses is toxic by itself) or of its metabolites (such as acetaldehyde, potentially even more toxic than the precursor) [60].

Thus, for sake of classification and recommendation, it was necessary to define moderate drinking of alcoholic beverages. The definition has been based on the relationship between alcohol consumption and overall mortality. This association has been shown to display a J- or U-shaped pattern, showing that non-consumers or heavy drinkers have higher risk for mortality from all causes, moderate drinkers (1-2 drinks per day) are protected, and that with increasing dose of ethanol the risk for disease rises exponentially [48]. One drink has been defined as the amount of any alcoholic beverage that supplies 15 g of ethanol, and moderate drinking as the consumption of 15 g of ethanol per day for women and 30 g of ethanol per day for men [61].

There has been doubt on whether epidemiological demonstration of the benefits of wine has been confounded by life style patterns associated with wine consumption. Several studies have demonstrated that wine consumption is associated with higher education, better economical status and abundant consumption of fruits and vegetables [57, 62]. This may be true for populations of the north of Europe, where many of these studies were performed and where wine is considered a luxury product due to its expensive price. However, it is not that likely in Mediterranean populations, where wine is a common commodity accessible to almost all social classes.

4. RED WINE, OBESITY AND INSULIN RESISTANCE

Several epidemiological studies have come to the evidence that moderate red wine consumption does not favor obesity or metabolic risk, but may in fact be inversely related to their development [63-65]. A number of investigations have shown that moderate alcohol consumption is associated with enhanced insulin sensitivity (13-17) and that moderate drinkers have a lower risk for type 2 diabetes than non-drinkers or heavy drinkers (18 de Cordain 2000).

Cordain et al. [64] demonstrated that consumption of 190 ml of red wine (13% of ethanol) for 5 days per week during 10 weeks did not affect insulin sensitivity nor body weight and composition, blood lipids and blood pressure. Shedding light and adding to these results, a cross-over design trial study by Beulens et al. [66], also investigated the direct effects of red wine in the adipose tissue. This study involved healthy men with increased waist circumference, drinking 450 ml of red wine (40 g of ethanol) or 450 ml of de-alcoholized red wine daily for 4 weeks. No effect of moderate alcohol consumption was observed in subcutaneous and abdominal fat contents and body weight, but liver fat was slightly higher after consumption of red wine as compared with de-alcoholized red wine. However, the most remarkable finding was that adiponectin, increased 10% after moderate alcohol consumption compared with de-alcoholized red wine. The circulating concentrations of this adipokine have been demonstrated to be inversely correlated with the amount of adipose tissue, having insulin sensitizing effects and inhibiting gluconeogenesis and increasing lipid oxidation [67-69]. Higher circulating concentrations of adiponectin are also related to lower insulin resistance and cardiovascular disease [70]. It has been reported by others that adiponectin is secreted in higher amounts by smaller, adipocytes [16, 71], probably being an index of functionality. It is thus likely that although Beulens et al. did not find changes in body weight nor in adipose tissue distribution there were changes in adipose tissue cellularity, namely in the size or number of differentiated adipocytes.

Djoussé et al. [72] analyzed the association between alcohol consumption and the prevalence odds of metabolic syndrome in 4510 participants of the National Heart, Lung, and Blood Institute Family Heart Study. The results obtained in this study revealed that alcohol consumption was associated with a lower prevalence of metabolic syndrome regardless of the type of beverage consumed. However, in free-living voluntaries (1481 women and 1210 men), a J-shaped relationship was found between total alcohol consumption and waist-to-hip ratio in both sexes and, only in men, between total alcohol consumption and body mass index [73]. The same relationships were observed with wine consumption (less than 100 g ethanol per day) whereas spirits intake was positively associated with body mass index and waist-to-hip ratio in both sexes in a linear fashion and no relationship was found for beer consumption. Also in favor of alcohol ingestion are the results of Dixon et al. [74]. In a cross-sectional study involving severely obese patients, the relationship between alcohol intake and the clinical and serum chemistry features of the metabolic syndrome was determined [74]. Alcohol consumers had lower odds ratio of type 2 diabetes compared with non-consumers. The relationship between the amount and frequency of alcohol consumption and fasting triglyceride, fasting glucose, hemoglobin A1c and insulin resistance showed a U-shaped pattern. For this reason, the authors proposed that light to moderate alcohol consumption should not be discouraged in the severely obese. However no distinction between type of alcoholic beverage was made in this study.

Data on the improvement of inflammation by red wine ingestion is also being gathered. Consumption of red wine for 4 weeks (supplying 30 g of ethanol per day) led to a significant decrease in the serum concentration of CRP and improvement of endothelial function markers in healthy adult men [75]. Lower levels of circulating CRP have also been associated to moderate red wine consumption in cross-sectional studies [76, 77].

In addition to the favorable effects of moderate ethanol intake on metabolic parameters, the abundance of the beverage in polyphenols also contributes to its anti-oxidant, anti-inflammatory, vascular-protective and insulin-sensitizing properties [65]. Experimental data in laboratory animals or cell lines has also contributed to the knowledge of the effect of red wine or its components in the development of obesity insulin resistance and the metabolic syndrome.

It has been shown that grape seed extract and procyanidin treatment of laboratory animals results in reduced weight gain, regulation of energy ingestion having been implicated [78]. More recently, Bargalló et al. [79] reported a decrease in energy intake, decreased epididymal fat mass and whole body weight in lean Zucker rats ingesting a high fat diet and voluntarily drinking red wine, in comparison to high fat diet-fed controls. Weight reduction may be attributed to the effect of procyanidins in fat absorption due to their inhibition of pancreatic lipase [80]. This may also be implicated in the improvement in plasma lipid profile, reduction of triglycerides and fatty acids, decrease in LDL cholesterol and a slight increase in HDL cholesterol observed following an acute dose of grape seed–derived procyanidins [81].

Resveratrol has been shown to have anti-inflammation [82] and anti-platelet properties [83]. A great part of its beneficial effects on atherosclerosis have been related to antioxidative and free radical scavenging activities [84-86]. Some of the mechanisms that explain the biological properties of resveratrol involve down-regulation of the inflammatory response through the inhibition of synthesis and release of pro-inflammatory cytokines, modification of eicosanoid synthesis, inhibition of activated immune cells, or inhibition of indicible nitric oxide synthase and cyclooxygenase-2 via the inhibitory effects on NFκB or AP-1 [87]. The effect on NFκB may explain the suppression of the *ex vivo* production of TNFα, IL-1 and IL-6 by mononuclear blood cells observed after the incubation with resveratrol [88]. These inflammatory actions may determine the impact of this polyphenol in the metabolic syndrome. Indeed, in streptozotocin-induced diabetic rats, resveratrol treatment after 14 days decreased plasma glucose and triglyceride concentration compared to vehicle-treated rats [89]. Furthermore, it resulted in body weight loss and improved diabetes symptoms such as polyphagia, and polydipsia. The same study included results showing that resveratrol stimulated glucose uptake by hepatocytes, adipocytes and skeletal muscle and hepatic glycogen synthesis.

Similar results have been obtained for procyanidins by Pinent et al. [90] who showed that oral administration of procyanidins to streptozotocin-induced diabetic rats had an anti-hyperglycemic effect and was shown to act synergistically with a low dose of insulin. The effect of procyanidins was shown to be abolished by phosphatidylinositol-3-kinase and p38MAPK inhibitors, showing the involvement of these kinases in procyanidin effects.

4.1. Direct Effects of Red Wine on the Adipose Tissue

Many authors now consider adipocyte dysfunction as the instigator of the main metabolic disturbances that constitute the metabolic syndrome and lead to the risk of disease [7]. Despite the growing amount of data linking red wine or alcohol consumption with metabolic syndrome improvement, few studies have been conducted considering the possibility that the protective effects of red wine may be related to its direct effects on the adipose tissue. The need for this kind of study becomes even more emphasized given the fact that adipose tissue dysfunction is considered by many the initiator and central component of the metabolic syndrome.

In an experimental study, Contaldo et al. [91] described that middle-aged men consuming a diet containing 75 g of alcohol as red wine for 2 weeks, adipose tissue lipoprotein lipase activity increased and there was a simultaneous increase in HDL cholesterol, VLDL and serum total triglycerides, despite no change in body weight, fasting blood glucose, serum insulin, total cholesterol and LDL cholesterol were observed. Similarly, resting metabolic rate, postprandial energy expenditure, and postprandial responses of blood glucose, serum insulin, triglyceride, and plasma NEFA also remained unaltered.

The effect of ethanol drinking on some hormonal and metabolic changes and on lipolysis in isolated adipocytes was addressed by Szkudelski et al. [92] in the rats drinking 10% ethanol solution as the only drinking fluid for 2 weeks. They found decreased body weight gain and blood insulin and increased leptin concentration and hepatic triglycerides. In adipocytes isolated from the adipose tissue of these rats it was found that ethanol treatment depressed basal and adrenaline-induced lipolysis and no change was observed in the anti-lipolytic activity of insulin or adenosine. This shows that ethanol in red wine may be responsible for part of the changes in plasma lipid profile and insulin concentration reported after wine ingestion.

The effects of specific polyphenols in have also been investigated in obesity. Tsuda et al. [93] reported that, in male C57BL/6 mice, cyanidin-3-glucoside supplementation (0.2% of the diet) prevented the high fat diet-induced weight gain, adipose tissue weight increase and adipocyte hypertrophy. The mechanisms for these alterations were further explored in human differentiated adipocyte cultures treated for 24 h with cyanidin or cyanidin-3-glucoside. They found by microarray technology and confirmed by real time-PCR increased production of adiponectin and lower transcription of IL-6 and PAI-1 [94, 95]. Another interesting finding by the same group showed that anthocyanins activate cAMP-activated protein kinase through a mechanism that is independent of the AMP/ATP ratio [96].

Procyanidins are also being intensively studied as to their effects in the prevention of obesity and the metabolic syndrome [97]. Concerning effects in adipocytes, studies in 3T3-L1 cells by Ardévol et al. [98] showed that grape seed procyanidin extract induced long-term lipolysis in adipocytes concomitantly with a time-dependent reduction in hormone-sensitive lipase mRNA, suggesting that lipolysis could be mediated by another kind of triglyceride lipase. The same group has also shown that the mechanisms of grape seed procyanidin extract-induced lipolysis involved protein kinase A and PPARγ. This nuclear transcription factor is also down-regulated by long-term treatment with procyanidins [99]. It was suggested that down-regulation of PPARγ by procyanidins could reflect direct binding to PPARγ and consequent reduction of its mRNA concentration. Procyanidins have also been shown to stimulate lipid and glycogen synthesis in 3T3-L1 adipocytes [100] and insulinomimetic effects of these polyphenols were implicated in these actions. Procyanidins also activate glucose uptake by a mechanism that involves glucose transporter-4 translocation to the plasma membrane and requires the activity of the phosphatidylinositol-3-kinase and the p38MAPK, classical mediators of the insulin-signaling pathways but also through complementary pathways [100]. In the same cell line, grape seed procyanidins inhibited differentiation of 3T3-L1 preadipocytes to fully mature adipocytes when added at the onset of differentiation and modulated cell cycle-related genes suggesting that they interfere with the process of preadipocyte proliferation [101].

4.2. Red Wine, Adipocyte Size and Adipose Tissue Aromatase

We also have attempted to address the direct effect of red wine intake in the adipose tissue. We treated three groups of rats for 8 weeks with different beverages: water (control), red wine with 13% ethanol content or 13% ethanol solution. After treatment, we found that subcutaneous adipose tissue expression of aromatase, the enzyme responsible for estrogen synthesis, was increased in red wine- and ethanol-treated rats. In both groups, body weight gain was lower than in controls despite similar energy intake. Another interesting finding was the decrease in adipocyte size in RW-treated rats. These results implied that ethanol could account for part of the effects of red wine in the modulation of aromatase and body weight. Furthermore, there was the suggestion that the increase in aromatase expression could underlie to a certain degree the effects on body weight and adipocyte size (unpublished observations). Indeed, estrogens have recognized effects on body weight that include actions on the central nervous system to regulate food intake and energy expenditure [102, 103] and direct activities on the physiology of the main energy metabolism-regulating organs [104], being usually regarded as opposing excessive body fat accumulation [105]. Red wine components most likely to be responsible for aromatase modulation are ethanol and polyphenols. Several reports exist on the increase of total body aromatization associated with ethanol consumption, which results in increased circulating estrogen concentrations [106]. On the other hand, both others [107-109] and our group [110] have reported the presence of polyphenols in red wine with the capacity to interfere with aromatase activity. Specifically, procyanidin dimers were found to be the most potent aromatase regulators present in grape seed extracts [111]. However, these earlier reports had demonstrated the inhibition of aromatase activity, while we show here that there is an increase in aromatase expression and, therefore, an enhancement in the potential for estrogen synthesis through chronic administration of red wine or ethanol. It is possible that as a result of the continuous effect on estrogen synthesis, aromatase expression may be activated as a counterbalance regulation. Indeed, it has been demonstrated that inhibition of aromatase may result in the increase of aromatase activity in treated cells [112-114]. Furthermore, we have obtained similar effects in aromatase expression in other tissues (i.e. hippocampus) in rats drinking red wine for 2 months [115]

It is known that men and postmenopausal women, whose estrogen levels are low, have increased metabolic risk translated into a higher likelihood to develop cardiovascular diseases, type 2 diabetes and certain forms of cancer. Frequently, several altered metabolic markers are clustered in the same individual justifying its increased risk and visceral obesity is the main component of the metabolic syndrome [4]. The absence of estrogens in animal and human models appears to favor the occurrence of the metabolic syndrome, starting with the facilitation of visceral adipose tissue deposition, which is reverted or prevented by estrogen reposition [116]. Also noteworthy, is that in aromatase knockout mice or in estrogen receptor α knockout mice, obesity and related complications are associated with adipose tissue hypertrophy and hyperplasia [117].

In the adipose tissue, the highest aromatase expression is found in preadipocytes although vascular cells also present aromatase activity [118]. As preadipocytes undergo differentiation, aromatase expression decreases being almost undetectable in fully differentiated adipocytes [119]. The higher aromatase expression in red wine rats in the adipose tissue is thus suggestive of a greater fraction of preadipocytes. Rats treated with red wine had also lower body weight gain and smaller adipocytes. The decrease of adipocyte size can arise from alterations in lipolysis and lipogenesis but could also be due to a negative energy balance. The changes in estrogen production by the adipose tissue are compatible with these observations and the actions of wine components presented above may also be taking part in these effects.

5. CONCLUSION

The results from these investigations showing direct effects of red wine in the adipose tissue, suggest that red wine may favor adipose tissue nutrient buffering capacity, a feature that if exceeded results in metabolic disturbances [120]. Although there is an intense need for further exploration of this subject, the findings here presented open new avenues on possible mechanism of action of red wine in the protection of the metabolic syndrome. In our opinion, adipose tissue remodeling induced by these beverages is of paramount importance in the reduction of metabolic risk associated with obesity. The potential reduction of adipose tissue-originated inflammation may possibly contribute for the proposed protective effects of moderate drinking of red wine for overall health, namely reducing the risk of cardiovascular diseases, type 2 diabetes and cancer.

In a time when people are becoming more health conscious, in part because they recognize that the most prevalent diseases are preventable and also because of the continuous shift of the populations towards a more advanced age, the awareness that food habits, like moderate red wine drinking, may be used to prevent disease is indisputably required.

REFERENCES

[1] Lucas DL, Brown RA, Wassef M & Giles TD. Alcohol and the cardiovascular system research challenges and opportunities. *J Am Coll Cardiol,* 2005, 45, 1916-1924.
[2] Goldberg DM, Hahn SE & Parkes JG. Beyond alcohol: beverage consumption and cardiovascular mortality. *Clin Chim Acta,* 1995, 237, 155-187.
[3] Kannel WB & Ellison RC. Alcohol and coronary heart disease: the evidence for a protective effect. *Clin Chim Acta,* 1996, 246, 59-76.
[4] Eckel RH, Grundy SM & Zimmet PZ. The metabolic syndrome. *Lancet,* 2005, 365, 1415-1428.
[5] Laclaustra M, Corella D & Ordovas JM. Metabolic syndrome pathophysiology: the role of adipose tissue. *Nutr Metab Cardiovasc Dis,* 2007, 17, 125-139.
[6] Mittra S, Bansal VS & Bhatnagar PK. From a glucocentric to a lipocentric approach towards metabolic syndrome. *Drug Discov Today,* 2008, 13, 211-218.
[7] de Ferranti S & Mozaffarian D. The perfect storm: obesity, adipocyte dysfunction, and metabolic consequences. *Clin Chem,* 2008, 54, 945-955.

[8] Furukawa S, Fujita T, Shimabukuro M, Iwaki M, Yamada Y, Nakajima Y, Nakayama O, Makishima M, Matsuda M & Shimomura I. Increased oxidative stress in obesity and its impact on metabolic syndrome. *J Clin Invest,* 2004, 114, 1752-1761.

[9] Hotamisligil GS. Inflammation and metabolic disorders. *Nature,* 2006, 444, 860-867.

[10] Ahima RS & Flier JS. Adipose tissue as an endocrine organ. *Trends Endocrinol Metab,* 2000, 11, 327-332.

[11] Kershaw EE & Flier JS. Adipose tissue as an endocrine organ. *J Clin Endocrinol Metab,* 2004, 89, 2548-2556.

[12] Lafontan M. Fat cells: afferent and efferent messages define new approaches to treat obesity. *Annu Rev Pharmacol Toxicol,* 2005, 45, 119-146.

[13] Bays HE, Gonzalez-Campoy JM, Bray GA, Kitabchi AE, Bergman DA, Schorr AB, Rodbard HW & Henry RR. Pathogenic potential of adipose tissue and metabolic consequences of adipocyte hypertrophy and increased visceral adiposity. *Expert Rev Cardiovasc Ther,* 2008, 6, 343-368.

[14] Sethi JK & Vidal-Puig AJ. Thematic review series: adipocyte biology. Adipose tissue function and plasticity orchestrate nutritional adaptation. *J Lipid Res,* 2007, 48, 1253-1262.

[15] Hegele RA, Joy TR, Al-Attar SA & Rutt BK. Thematic review series: Adipocyte Biology. Lipodystrophies: windows on adipose biology and metabolism. *J Lipid Res,* 2007, 48, 1433-1444.

[16] Bahceci M, Gokalp D, Bahceci S, Tuzcu A, Atmaca S & Arikan S. The correlation between adiposity and adiponectin, tumor necrosis factor alpha, interleukin-6 and high sensitivity C-reactive protein levels. Is adipocyte size associated with inflammation in adults? *J Endocrinol Invest,* 2007, 30, 210-214.

[17] Bouloumié A, Curat CA, Sengenes C, Lolmede K, Miranville A & Busse R. Role of macrophage tissue infiltration in metabolic diseases. *Curr Opin Clin Nutr Metab Care,* 2005, 8, 347-354.

[18] Xu H, Barnes GT, Yang Q, Tan G, Yang D, Chou CJ, Sole J, Nichols A, Ross JS, Tartaglia LA & Chen H. Chronic inflammation in fat plays a crucial role in the development of obesity-related insulin resistance. *J Clin Invest,* 2003, 112, 1821-1830.

[19] Monteiro R, de Castro PM, Calhau C & Azevedo I. Adipocyte size and liability to cell death. *Obes Surg,* 2006, 16, 804-806.

[20] Cinti S, Mitchell G, Barbatelli G, Murano I, Ceresi E, Faloia E, Wang S, Fortier M, Greenberg AS & Obin MS. Adipocyte death defines macrophage localization and function in adipose tissue of obese mice and humans. *J Lipid Res,* 2005, 46, 2347-2355.

[21] Cobb WS, Burns JM, Kercher KW, Matthews BD, Norton JH & Heniford TB. Normal intraabdominal pressure in healthy adults. *J Surg Res,* 2005, 129, 231-235.

[22] Monteiro R, Calhau C & Azevedo I. Obstructive sleep apnoea and adipocyte death. *Eur J Heart Fail,* 2007, 9, 103-104.

[23] Monteiro R, Calhau C & Azevedo I. Comment on: Tchoukalova Y, Koutsari C, Jensen M (2007) Committed subcutaneous preadipocytes are reduced in human obesity. Diabetologia 50:151-157. *Diabetologia,* 2007, 50, 1569.

[24] Tchoukalova Y, Koutsari C & Jensen M. Committed subcutaneous preadipocytes are reduced in human obesity. *Diabetologia,* 2007, 50, 151-157.

[25] Jernås M, Palming J, Sjöholm K, Jennische E, Svensson PA, Gabrielsson BG, Levin M, Sjögren A, Rudemo M, Lystig TC, Carlsson B, Carlsson LM & Lönn M. Separation of

human adipocytes by size: hypertrophic fat cells display distinct gene expression. *FASEB J,* 2006, 20, 1540-1542.

[26] Rudich A, Kanety H & Bashan N. Adipose stress-sensing kinases: linking obesity to malfunction. *Trends Endocrinol Metab,* 2007, 18, 291-299.

[27] Aguirre V, Uchida T, Yenush L, Davis R & White MF. The c-Jun NH(2)-terminal kinase promotes insulin resistance during association with insulin receptor substrate-1 and phosphorylation of Ser(307). *J Biol Chem,* 2000, 275, 9047-9054.

[28] Gao Z, Hwang D, Bataille F, Lefevre M, York D, Quon MJ & Ye J. Serine phosphorylation of insulin receptor substrate 1 by inhibitor kappa B kinase complex. *J Biol Chem,* 2002, 277, 48115-48121.

[29] Griffin ME, Marcucci MJ, Cline GW, Bell K, Barucci N, Lee D, Goodyear LJ, Kraegen EW, White MF & Shulman GI. Free fatty acid-induced insulin resistance is associated with activation of protein kinase C theta and alterations in the insulin signaling cascade. *Diabetes,* 1999, 48, 1270-1274.

[30] Baud V & Karin M. Signal transduction by tumor necrosis factor and its relatives. *Trends Cell Biol,* 2001, 11, 372-377.

[31] Bullo M, Casas-Agustench P, Amigo-Correig P, Aranceta J & Salas-Salvado J. Inflammation, obesity and comorbidities: the role of diet. *Public Health Nutr,* 2007, 10, 1164-1172.

[32] Gregor MF & Hotamisligil GS. Thematic review series: Adipocyte Biology. Adipocyte stress: the endoplasmic reticulum and metabolic disease. *J Lipid Res,* 2007, 48, 1905-1914.

[33] Bastard JP, Maachi M, Lagathu C, Kim MJ, Caron M, Vidal H, Capeau J & Feve B. Recent advances in the relationship between obesity, inflammation, and insulin resistance. *Eur Cytokine Netw,* 2006, 17, 4-12.

[34] Guilherme A, Virbasius JV, Puri V & Czech MP. Adipocyte dysfunctions linking obesity to insulin resistance and type 2 diabetes. *Nat Rev Mol Cell Biol,* 2008, 9, 367-377.

[35] Skalicky J, Muzakova V, Kandar R, Meloun M, Rousar T & Palicka V. Evaluation of oxidative stress and inflammation in obese adults with metabolic syndrome. *Clin Chem Lab Med,* 2008, 46, 499-505.

[36] Hansel B, Giral P, Nobecourt E, Chantepie S, Bruckert E, Chapman MJ & Kontush A. Metabolic syndrome is associated with elevated oxidative stress and dysfunctional dense high-density lipoprotein particles displaying impaired antioxidative activity. *J Clin Endocrinol Metab,* 2004, 89, 4963-4971.

[37] Ford ES. Intake and circulating concentrations of antioxidants in metabolic syndrome. *Curr Atheroscler Rep,* 2006, 8, 448-452.

[38] Cardona F, Tunez I, Tasset I, Montilla P, Collantes E & Tinahones FJ. Fat overload aggravates oxidative stress in patients with the metabolic syndrome. *Eur J Clin Invest,* 2008, 38, 510-515.

[39] Sjogren P, Basu S, Rosell M, Silveira A, de Faire U, Vessby B, Hamsten A, Hellenius ML & Fisher RM. Measures of oxidized low-density lipoprotein and oxidative stress are not related and not elevated in otherwise healthy men with the metabolic syndrome. *Arterioscler Thromb Vasc Biol,* 2005, 25, 2580-2586.

[40] Lee DH, Gross MD & Jacobs DR, Jr. Association of serum carotenoids and tocopherols with gamma-glutamyltransferase: the Cardiovascular Risk Development in Young Adults (CARDIA) Study. *Clin Chem,* 2004, 50, 582-588.

[41] Hozawa A, Jacobs DR, Jr., Steffes MW, Gross MD, Steffen LM & Lee DH. Associations of serum carotenoid concentrations with the development of diabetes and with insulin concentration: interaction with smoking: the Coronary Artery Risk Development in Young Adults (CARDIA) Study. *Am J Epidemiol,* 2006, 163, 929-937.

[42] Vincent HK & Taylor AG. Biomarkers and potential mechanisms of obesity-induced oxidant stress in humans. *Int J Obes (Lond),* 2006, 30, 400-418.

[43] Armutcu F, Ataymen M, Atmaca H & Gurel A. Oxidative stress markers, C-reactive protein and heat shock protein 70 levels in subjects with metabolic syndrome. *Clin Chem Lab Med,* 2008, 46, 785-790.

[44] Reitman A, Friedrich I, Ben-Amotz A & Levy Y. Low plasma antioxidants and normal plasma B vitamins and homocysteine in patients with severe obesity. *Isr Med Assoc J,* 2002, 4, 590-593.

[45] Galinier A, Carriere A, Fernandez Y, Carpene C, Andre M, Caspar-Bauguil S, Thouvenot JP, Periquet B, Penicaud L & Casteilla L. Adipose tissue proadipogenic redox changes in obesity. *J Biol Chem,* 2006, 281, 12682-12687.

[46] Ozcan U, Cao Q, Yilmaz E, Lee AH, Iwakoshi NN, Ozdelen E, Tuncman G, Gorgun C, Glimcher LH & Hotamisligil GS. Endoplasmic reticulum stress links obesity, insulin action, and type 2 diabetes. *Science,* 2004, 306, 457-461.

[47] Houstis N, Rosen ED & Lander ES. Reactive oxygen species have a causal role in multiple forms of insulin resistance. *Nature,* 2006, 440, 944-948.

[48] German JB & Walzem RL. The health benefits of wine. *Annu Rev Nutr,* 2000, 20, 561-593.

[49] Soleas GJ, Diamandis EP & Goldberg DM. Wine as a biological fluid: history, production, and role in disease prevention. *J Clin Lab Anal,* 1997, 11, 287-313.

[50] Bravo L. Polyphenols: chemistry, dietary sources, metabolism, and nutritional significance. *Nutr Rev,* 1998, 56, 317-333.

[51] Santos-Buelga C & Scalbert A. Proanthocyanidins and tannin-like compounds - nature, occurrence, dietary intake and effects on nutrition and health. *J Sci Food Agric,* 2000, 80, 1094-1117.

[52] Simopoulos AP. The Mediterranean diets: What is so special about the diet of Greece? The scientific evidence. *J Nutr,* 2001, 131, 3065S-3073S.

[53] Renaud S & de Lorgeril M. Wine, alcohol, platelets, and the French paradox for coronary heart disease. *Lancet,* 1992, 339, 1523-1526.

[54] St Leger AS, Cochrane AL & Moore F. Factors associated with cardiac mortality in developed countries with particular reference to the consumption of wine. *Lancet,* 1979, 1, 1017-1020.

[55] Hertog MG, Feskens EJ, Hollman PC, Katan MB & Kromhout D. Dietary antioxidant flavonoids and risk of coronary heart disease: the Zutphen Elderly Study. *Lancet,* 1993, 342, 1007-1011.

[56] Keli SO, Hertog MG, Feskens EJ & Kromhout D. Dietary flavonoids, antioxidant vitamins, and incidence of stroke: the Zutphen study. *Arch Intern Med,* 1996, 156, 637-642.

[57] Rosell M, De Faire U & Hellenius ML. Low prevalence of the metabolic syndrome in wine drinkers--is it the alcohol beverage or the lifestyle? *Eur J Clin Nutr,* 2003, 57, 227-234.

[58] Britton A & McKee M. The relation between alcohol and cardiovascular disease in Eastern Europe: explaining the paradox. *J Epidemiol Community Health,* 2000, 54, 328-332.

[59] Van Tol A, Groener JE, Scheek LM, Van Gent T, Veenstra J, Van de Pol H, Hendriks HF & Schaafsma G. Induction of net mass lipid transfer reactions in plasma by wine consumption with dinner. *Eur J Clin Invest,* 1995, 25, 390-395.

[60] Lieber CS. ALCOHOL: its metabolism and interaction with nutrients. *Annu Rev Nutr,* 2000, 20, 395-430.

[61] Gunzerath L, Faden V, Zakhari S & Warren K. National Institute on Alcohol Abuse and Alcoholism report on moderate drinking. *Alcohol Clin Exp Res,* 2004, 28, 829-847.

[62] Panagiotakos DB & Polychronopoulos E. The role of Mediterranean diet in the epidemiology of metabolic syndrome; converting epidemiology to clinical practice. *Lipids Health Dis,* 2005, 4, 7.

[63] Cordain L, Bryan ED, Melby CL & Smith MJ. Influence of moderate daily wine consumption on body weight regulation and metabolism in healthy free-living males. *J Am Coll Nutr,* 1997, 16, 134-139.

[64] Cordain L, Melby CL, Hamamoto AE, O'Neill DS, Cornier MA, Barakat HA, Israel RG & Hill JO. Influence of moderate chronic wine consumption on insulin sensitivity and other correlates of syndrome X in moderately obese women. *Metabolism,* 2000, 49, 1473-1478.

[65] Liu L, Wang Y, Lam KS & Xu A. Moderate wine consumption in the prevention of metabolic syndrome and its related medical complications. *Endocr Metab Immune Disord Drug Targets,* 2008, 8, 89-98.

[66] Beulens JW, van Beers RM, Stolk RP, Schaafsma G & Hendriks HF. The effect of moderate alcohol consumption on fat distribution and adipocytokines. *Obesity (Silver Spring),* 2006, 14, 60-66.

[67] Combs TP, Pajvani UB, Berg AH, Lin Y, Jelicks LA, Laplante M, Nawrocki AR, Rajala MW, Parlow AF, Cheeseboro L, Ding YY, Russell RG, Lindemann D, Hartley A, Baker GR, Obici S, Deshaies Y, Ludgate M, Rossetti L & Scherer PE. A transgenic mouse with a deletion in the collagenous domain of adiponectin displays elevated circulating adiponectin and improved insulin sensitivity. *Endocrinology,* 2004, 145, 367-383.

[68] Fruebis J, Tsao TS, Javorschi S, Ebbets-Reed D, Erickson MR, Yen FT, Bihain BE & Lodish HF. Proteolytic cleavage product of 30-kDa adipocyte complement-related protein increases fatty acid oxidation in muscle and causes weight loss in mice. *Proc Natl Acad Sci U S A,* 2001, 98, 2005-2010.

[69] Yamauchi T, Kamon J, Minokoshi Y, Ito Y, Waki H, Uchida S, Yamashita S, Noda M, Kita S, Ueki K, Eto K, Akanuma Y, Froguel P, Foufelle F, Ferre P, Carling D, Kimura S, Nagai R, Kahn BB & Kadowaki T. Adiponectin stimulates glucose utilization and fatty-acid oxidation by activating AMP-activated protein kinase. *Nat Med,* 2002, 8, 1288-1295.

[70] Fasshauer M, Paschke R & Stumvoll M. Adiponectin, obesity, and cardiovascular disease. *Biochimie,* 2004, 86, 779-784.

[71] Scherer PE, Williams S, Fogliano M, Baldini G & Lodish HF. A novel serum protein similar to C1q, produced exclusively in adipocytes. *J Biol Chem,* 1995, 270, 26746-26749.

[72] Djousse L, Arnett DK, Eckfeldt JH, Province MA, Singer MR & Ellison RC. Alcohol consumption and metabolic syndrome: does the type of beverage matter? *Obes Res,* 2004, 12, 1375-1385.

[73] Lukasiewicz E, Mennen LI, Bertrais S, Arnault N, Preziosi P, Galan P & Hercberg S. Alcohol intake in relation to body mass index and waist-to-hip ratio: the importance of type of alcoholic beverage. *Public Health Nutr,* 2005, 8, 315-320.

[74] Dixon JB, Dixon ME & O'Brien PE. Alcohol consumption in the severely obese: relationship with the metabolic syndrome. *Obes Res,* 2002, 10, 245-252.

[75] Estruch R, Sacanella E, Badia E, Antunez E, Nicolas JM, Fernandez-Sola J, Rotilio D, de Gaetano G, Rubin E & Urbano-Marquez A. Different effects of red wine and gin consumption on inflammatory biomarkers of atherosclerosis: a prospective randomized crossover trial. Effects of wine on inflammatory markers. *Atherosclerosis,* 2004, 175, 117-123.

[76] Albert MA, Glynn RJ & Ridker PM. Alcohol consumption and plasma concentration of C-reactive protein. *Circulation,* 2003, 107, 443-447.

[77] Stewart SH, Mainous AG, 3rd & Gilbert G. Relation between alcohol consumption and C-reactive protein levels in the adult US population. *J Am Board Fam Pract,* 2002, 15, 437-442.

[78] Vogels N, Nijs IM & Westerterp-Plantenga MS. The effect of grape-seed extract on 24 h energy intake in humans. *Eur J Clin Nutr,* 2004, 58, 667-673.

[79] Bargalló MV, Grau AA, Fernández-Larrea Jde D, Anguiano GP, Segarra MC, Rovira MJ, Ferré LA & Olivé MB. Moderate red-wine consumption partially prevents body weight gain in rats fed a hyperlipidic diet. *J Nutr Biochem,* 2006, 17, 139-142.

[80] Moreno DA, Ilic N, Poulev A, Brasaemle DL, Fried SK & Raskin I. Inhibitory effects of grape seed extract on lipases. *Nutrition,* 2003, 19, 876-879.

[81] Del Bas JM, Fernandez-Larrea J, Blay M, Ardevol A, Salvado MJ, Arola L & Blade C. Grape seed procyanidins improve atherosclerotic risk index and induce liver CYP7A1 and SHP expression in healthy rats. *FASEB J,* 2005, 19, 479-481.

[82] Jang DS, Kang BS, Ryu SY, Chang IM, Min KR & Kim Y. Inhibitory effects of resveratrol analogs on unopsonized zymosan-induced oxygen radical production. *Biochem Pharmacol,* 1999, 57, 705-712.

[83] Chung MI, Teng CM, Cheng KL, Ko FN & Lin CN. An antiplatelet principle of Veratrum formosanum. *Planta Med,* 1992, 58, 274-276.

[84] Constant J. Alcohol, ischemic heart disease, and the French paradox. *Coron Artery Dis,* 1997, 8, 645-649.

[85] Frankel EN, Kanner J, German JB, Parks E & Kinsella JE. Inhibition of oxidation of human low-density lipoprotein by phenolic substances in red wine. *Lancet,* 1993, 341, 454-457.

[86] Frankel EN, Waterhouse AL & Kinsella JE. Inhibition of human LDL oxidation by resveratrol. *Lancet,* 1993, 341, 1103-1104.

[87] Rahman I, Biswas SK & Kirkham PA. Regulation of inflammation and redox signaling by dietary polyphenols. *Biochem Pharmacol,* 2006, 72, 1439-1452.

[88] Marier JF, Chen K, Prince P, Scott G, del Castillo JR & Vachon P. Production of ex vivo lipopolysaccharide-induced tumor necrosis factor-alpha, interleukin-1beta, and interleukin-6 is suppressed by trans-resveratrol in a concentration-dependent manner. *Can J Vet Res,* 2005, 69, 151-154.

[89] Su HC, Hung LM & Chen JK. Resveratrol, a red wine antioxidant, possesses an insulin-like effect in streptozotocin-induced diabetic rats. *Am J Physiol Endocrinol Metab,* 2006, 290, E1339-1346.

[90] Pinent M, Blay M, Blade MC, Salvadó MJ, Arola L & Ardévol A. Grape seed-derived procyanidins have an antihyperglycemic effect in streptozotocin-induced diabetic rats and insulinomimetic activity in insulin-sensitive cell lines. *Endocrinology,* 2004, 145, 4985-4990.

[91] Contaldo F, D'Arrigo E, Carandente V, Cortese C, Coltorti A, Mancini M, Taskinen MR & Nikkila EA. Short-term effects of moderate alcohol consumption on lipid metabolism and energy balance in normal men. *Metabolism,* 1989, 38, 166-171.

[92] Szkudelski T, Bialik I & Szkudelska K. Adipocyte lipolysis, hormonal and metabolic changes in ethanol-drinking rats. *J Anim Physiol Anim Nutr (Berl),* 2004, 88, 251-258.

[93] Tsuda T, Horio F, Uchida K, Aoki H & Osawa T. Dietary cyanidin 3-O-beta-D-glucoside-rich purple corn color prevents obesity and ameliorates hyperglycemia in mice. *J Nutr,* 2003, 133, 2125-2130.

[94] Tsuda T, Ueno Y, Kojo H, Yoshikawa T & Osawa T. Gene expression profile of isolated rat adipocytes treated with anthocyanins. *Biochim Biophys Acta,* 2005, 1733, 137-147.

[95] Tsuda T, Ueno Y, Yoshikawa T, Kojo H & Osawa T. Microarray profiling of gene expression in human adipocytes in response to anthocyanins. *Biochem Pharmacol,* 2006, 71, 1184-1197.

[96] Tsuda T, Ueno Y, Aoki H, Koda T, Horio F, Takahashi N, Kawada T & Osawa T. Anthocyanin enhances adipocytokine secretion and adipocyte-specific gene expression in isolated rat adipocytes. *Biochem Biophys Res Commun,* 2004, 316, 149-157.

[97] Pinent M, Blade C, Salvadó MJ, Blay M, Pujadas G, Fernández-Larrea J, Arola L & Ardévol A. Procyanidin effects on adipocyte-related pathologies. *Crit Rev Food Sci Nutr,* 2006, 46, 543-550.

[98] Ardevol A, Blade C, Salvado MJ & Arola L. Changes in lipolysis and hormone-sensitive lipase expression caused by procyanidins in 3T3-L1 adipocytes. *Int J Obes Relat Metab Disord,* 2000, 24, 319-324.

[99] Pinent M, Blade MC, Salvadó MJ, Arola L & Ardévol A. Intracellular mediators of procyanidin-induced lipolysis in 3T3-L1 adipocytes. *J Agric Food Chem,* 2005, 53, 262-266.

[100] Pinent M, Blade MC, Salvadó MJ, Arola L & Ardévol A. Metabolic fate of glucose on 3T3-L1 adipocytes treated with grape seed-derived procyanidin extract (GSPE). Comparison with the effects of insulin. *J Agric Food Chem,* 2005, 53, 5932-5935.

[101] Pinent M, Blade MC, Salvado MJ, Arola L, Hackl H, Quackenbush J, Trajanoski Z & Ardevol A. Grape-seed derived procyanidins interfere with adipogenesis of 3T3-L1 cells at the onset of differentiation. *Int J Obes (Lond),* 2005, 29, 934-941.

[102] Jones ME, Thorburn AW, Britt KL, Hewitt KN, Wreford NG, Proietto J, Oz OK, Leury BJ, Robertson KM, Yao S & Simpson ER. Aromatase-deficient (ArKO) mice have a phenotype of increased adiposity. *Proc Natl Acad Sci U S A,* 2000, 97, 12735-12740.

[103] Geary N, Asarian L, Korach KS, Pfaff DW & Ogawa S. Deficits in E2-dependent control of feeding, weight gain, and cholecystokinin satiation in ER-alpha null mice. *Endocrinology,* 2001, 142, 4751-4757.

[104] Simpson E, Jones M, Misso M, Hewitt K, Hill R, Maffei L, Carani C & Boon WC. Estrogen, a fundamental player in energy homeostasis. *J Steroid Biochem Mol Biol,* 2005, 95, 3-8.

[105] Cooke PS & Naaz A. Role of estrogens in adipocyte development and function. *Exp Biol Med (Maywood),* 2004, 229, 1127-1135.

[106] Ginsburg ES, Mello NK, Mendelson JH, Barbieri RL, Teoh SK, Rothman M, Gao X & Sholar JW. Effects of alcohol ingestion on estrogens in postmenopausal women. *JAMA,* 1996, 276, 1747-1751.

[107] Eng ET, Williams D, Mandava U, Kirma N, Tekmal RR & Chen S. Suppression of aromatase (estrogen synthetase) by red wine phytochemicals. *Breast Cancer Res Treat,* 2001, 67, 133-146.

[108] Eng ET, Williams D, Mandava U, Kirma N, Tekmal RR & Chen S. Anti-aromatase chemicals in red wine. *Ann N Y Acad Sci,* 2002, 963, 239-246.

[109] Wang Y, Lee KW, Chan FL, Chen S & Leung LK. The red wine polyphenol resveratrol displays bilevel inhibition on aromatase in breast cancer cells. *Toxicol Sci,* 2006, 92, 71-77.

[110] Monteiro R, Azevedo I & Calhau C. Modulation of aromatase activity by diet polyphenolic compounds. *J Agric Food Chem,* 2006, 54, 3535-3540.

[111] Eng ET, Ye J, Williams D, Phung S, Moore RE, Young MK, Gruntmanis U, Braunstein G & Chen S. Suppression of estrogen biosynthesis by procyanidin dimers in red wine and grape seeds. *Cancer Res,* 2003, 63, 8516-8522.

[112] Harada N & Hatano O. Inhibitors of aromatase prevent degradation of the enzyme in cultured human tumour cells. *Br J Cancer,* 1998, 77, 567-572.

[113] Kao YC, Okubo T, Sun XZ & Chen S. Induction of aromatase expression by aminoglutethimide, an aromatase inhibitor that is used to treat breast cancer in postmenopausal women. *Anticancer Res,* 1999, 19, 2049-2056.

[114] Yue W & Brodie AM. Mechanisms of the actions of aromatase inhibitors 4-hydroxyandrostenedione, fadrozole, and aminoglutethimide on aromatase in JEG-3 cell culture. *J Steroid Biochem Mol Biol,* 1997, 63, 317-328.

[115] Monteiro R, Faria A, Mateus N, Calhau C & Azevedo I. Red wine interferes with oestrogen signalling in rat hippocampus. *J Steroid Biochem Mol Biol,* 2008, 111, 74-79.

[116] Simpson ER, Misso M, Hewitt KN, Hill RA, Boon WC, Jones ME, Kovacic A, Zhou J & Clyne CD. Estrogen - the good, the bad, and the unexpected. *Endocr Rev,* 2005, 26, 322-330.

[117] Jones ME, Thorburn AW, Britt KL, Hewitt KN, Misso ML, Wreford NG, Proietto J, Oz OK, Leury BJ, Robertson KM, Yao S & Simpson ER. Aromatase-deficient (ArKO) mice accumulate excess adipose tissue. *J Steroid Biochem Mol Biol,* 2001, 79, 3-9.

[118] Rink JD, Simpson ER, Barnard JJ & Bulun SE. Cellular characterization of adipose tissue from various body sites of women. *J Clin Endocrinol Metab,* 1996, 81, 2443-2447.

[119] Simpson ER, Clyne C, Rubin G, Boon WC, Robertson K, Britt K, Speed C & Jones M. Aromatase - a brief overview. *Annu Rev Physiol,* 2002, 64, 93-127.

[120] Smith J, Al-Amri M, Dorairaj P & Sniderman A. The adipocyte life cycle hypothesis. *Clin Sci (Lond),* 2006, 110, 1-9.

In: Red Wine and Health
Editor: Paul O'Byrne

ISBN: 978-1-60692-718-2
© 2009 Nova Science Publishers, Inc.

Chapter 13

RED WINE AND VASCULAR ENDOTHELIUM

Dimitris Tousoulis[*], Nikos Papageorgiou[†], Charalambos Antoniades[‡], Costas Tsioufis[§], Gerasimos Siasos[**] and Christodoulos Stefanadis[††]

ABSTRACT

Light to moderate alcohol consumption may have a beneficial effect on cardiovascular morbidity and mortality. Red wine has been shown to improve endothelial function and decrease oxidative stress. Consumption of red wine induces significant increases in plasma total antioxidant status and significant decreases in plasma malondialdehyde and glutathione in both young and old subjects. Red wine consumption for 2 weeks markedly attenuates insulin-resistance in type 2 diabetic patients, without affecting vascular reactivity and nitric oxide production. In vitro and in animal models, red wine polyphenolics cause substantial falls in blood pressure, mainly by increasing nitric oxide production. Although red wine has beneficial effects on vascular endothelium, more studies are necessary to evaluate these effects on cardiovascular risk.

1. INTRODUCTION

It is well known that light to moderate alcohol consumption may have a beneficial effect on cardiovascular morbidity and mortality [1]. Polyphenols, which are important components of red wine, reduce the risk of coronary artery disease (CAD) by several mechanisms, including reduced low-density lipoprotein (LDL) susceptibility to oxidation [2], reduced platelet aggregation [3,4], increased fibrinolytic activity [5] and increased vasorelaxing activity by increased nitric oxide (NO) production [4,6]. Recent data have demonstrated that consumption of red wine is associated with significant improvement of endothelial function

---

[*] MD PhD
[†] MD
[‡] MD
[§] MD
[**] MD

[7] and several studies, investigating the long-term effects of wine and its constituents on endothelial function, showed that there is a significant improvement of flow-mediated dilatation (FMD), after regular consumption [8]. These data are in accordance with in vitro studies, which showed that in the acute postprandial phase, constituents of red wine such as the polyphenols cause vasorelaxation in aortic rings [9].

Endothelial dysfunction has been proposed to play a pathogenic role in the initiation of vascular disease [10] and there are several studies [9] demonstrating that administration of antioxidants improves endothelial function. These observations suggest that nitric oxide inactivation by oxygen free radicals may contribute to endothelial dysfunction. Polyphenols, which are important components of red wine, have been shown to possess antioxidant properties [8]. This antioxidant capacity of red wine may explain why it has more pronounced cardioprotective effects than other alcoholic beverages. The mechanisms of this association are still unclear, since it is still unknown whether alcohol itself or other substances such as polyphenols included in specific alcoholic beverages like red wine are responsible for this effect [11].

In the present review we will discuss the association between red wine and endothelial function, the relation between alcohol consumption and hypertension, while we will focus on the antioxidant effects of red wine, as these have been highlighted through several studies.

2. OXIDATIVE STRESS HYPOTHESIS AND ATHEROSCLEROSIS

According to the oxidative modification hypothesis, LDL in its native state is not atherogenic. The most biologically relevant modification of LDL is oxidation. Low-density lipoprotein can be easily oxidized by all major cells of the arterial wall [12, 13]. In the early phase, mild oxidation of LDL results in the formation of minimally modified LDL (MMLDL) in the subendothelial space. MM-LDL stimulates production of monocyte chemotactic protein-1 (MCP-1) that promotes monocyte chemotaxis. These molecular events result in monocyte binding to the endothelium and its subsequent migration into the subendothelial space where MM-LDL also stimulates production of monocyte colony stimulating factor (M-CSF). Monocyte colony stimulating factor promotes the differentiation and proliferation of monocytes into macrophages [13].

The initial interest in a role for lipid oxidation in the development of atherosclerotic lesions was in its ability to modify LDL sufficiently to promote its uptake by macrophages. The extensively modified LDL (oxidized LDL, Ox-LDL) is not recognized by the LDL receptor but is taken up avidly by the scavenger receptor pathway in macrophages leading to appreciable cholesterol ester accumulation and foam cell formation [14]. Oxidized LDL has several biological effects [12, 15, 16], as it is pro-inflammatory, it causes inhibition of endothelial nitric oxide synthase (eNOS), it promotes vasoconstriction and adhesion and increases platelet aggregation. Ox-LDL derived products are cytotoxic and can induce apoptosis. Furthermore, it can adversely affect coagulation by stimulating tissue factor and plasminogen activator inhibitor-1 synthesis [17]. Several factors may influence the susceptibility of LDL to oxidation including its site and composition and the presence of endogenous antioxidant compounds. In addition, Ox-LDL stimulates vascular SMCs (smooth

†† MD

muscle cells) proliferation [16]. Thus, intimal thickening further reduces the lumen of blood vessels, leading to further possibility of hypertension and atherosclerosis. As result of the unique localization between circulating blood and the vessel wall, the endothelium has been suggested to play a crucial role in development and progression of atherosclerosis. Therefore, endothelial dysfunction is clearly associated with the disease process. These mechanisms are presented in the **Figure 1**.

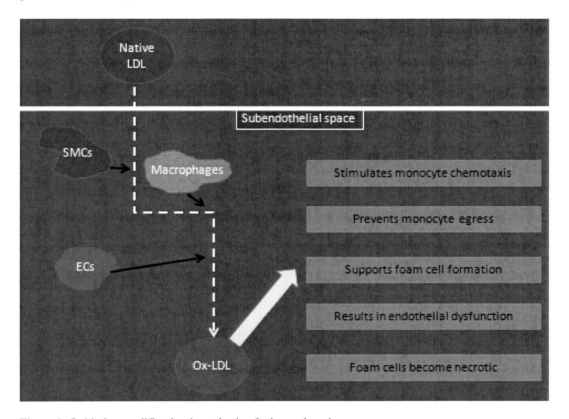

Figure 1. Oxidative modification hypothesis of atherosclerosis

2.1. Reactive Oxygen Species (ROS)

Among factors that result to endothelial dysfunction, reactive oxygen species (ROS) are increasingly recognized as the major responsible for compromising endothelial cell function, **Table 1** [18, 19]. A large amount of evidence implicates reactive oxygen species (ROS), in the development of most cardiovascular diseases. Superoxide ($O_2 \cdot -$) hydroxyl radical ($OH \cdot -$) are two of the most biologically important ROS in the cardiovascular system, and are produced in vascular cells by a number of oxidases, including the NADPH oxidases (Nox) and xanthine oxidase, lipoxygenases, cytochrome p450, uncoupling of the mitochondrial respiratory chain, and uncoupling of eNOS. Production is counterbalanced by antioxidant enzymes such as superoxide dismutases (SOD), catalase, glutathione peroxidase, thioredoxins and peroxiredoxins.

Table 1. Sources of oxidative stress in vascular wall

NANDPH oxidase	
Nitric oxide synthases (eNOS uncoupling, iNOS)	
Xanthine oxidase	**ROS**
Myeloperoxidase	
Lipoxygenase/cyclooxygenase	
Mitochondrial respiratory chain/oxidative phosphorylation	

eNOS: endothelial nitric oxide synthase, iNOS: inducible nitric oxide synthase, ROS: reactive oxygen species

Another important ROS is NO•, produced by eNOS and inducible NOS (iNOS). Superoxide inactivates NO• and counteracts its vasodilatory and anti-inflammatory effects. The interaction of O_2•− and NO• generates peroxynitrite (ONOO•), which has injurious effects on vascular cells. In addition, ONOO• oxidizes tetrahydrobiopterin thereby leading to eNOS uncoupling and diminished NO• production. The importance of ROS in vascular injury lies in the fact that their production is positively regulated by many of the cytokines whose expression is increased after injury, and also by oscillatory shear stress and mechanical disruption [20, 21]. Whereas low levels of ROS are necessary for normal vascular function, excess production or impaired ROS removal, in a pro-inflammatory environment, regulates virtually all of the cellular responses to injury, including monocyte adhesion platelet aggregation, inflammatory gene induction, vascular smooth muscle cell (SMC) apoptosis, proliferation and migration, matrix degradation and impaired endothelium dependent relaxation.

3. THE WINE PARADOX

Renaud et al [22] introduced the term French Paradox to underscore the low mortality rate from ischemic heart disease among people in France despite the highamount of saturated fats in their diet [22-24], which is usually associated with increased mortality from CAD. They attributed this unusual occurrence to red wine consumption based on the findings of the MONICA (MONItoring system for CArdiovascular disease) project, a worldwide program organized by the World Health Organization. Collaborating researchers from 21 countries studied more than 7 million men and women from 37 mostly European populations over a period of 10 years. The investigators observed a lower mortality rate from CAD in France compared with that in the United Kingdom and the United States, despite the high consumption of saturated fats and similar serum cholesterol concentrations. In addition, other risk factors such as blood pressure, body mass index, and cigarette smoking were equivalent in France to what they were in other industrialized countries [25, 26]. Although France and Italy have halved their wine consumption from what it was in the 1960s, and now average 67 and 57 L/capita/year, respectively, these countries still have a much higher intake than the United Kingdom or the United States, where consumption is about 12 and 5 L/capita/year, respectively. Within France, alcohol intake is mostly in the form of red wine. This is particularly true in the south, where CAD is at its lowest, in the north, they consume less wine and more spirits, and have a higher incidence of CAD. Epidemiologic studies suggest that consumption of red wine at a level comparable to that of France can indeed reduce the risk of CAD by preventing arteriosclerosis.

Several reports postulate that this can be attributed to the French consumption of three times more wine [22]. But it is now widely accepted that regular, moderate intake of alcoholic beverages can also decrease the risk of CAD by at least 40% [22, 28, 29]. There are a number of components of red wine that could have an effect on the cardiovascular system, preventing or delaying arteriosclerosis. Alcohol, which is present in up to 15% of the volume of red wine, is one of them. A number of epidemiologic studies have shown an inverse relationship between alcohol consumption and CAD [28, 31]. Even though this beneficial property of ethanol is described for low and moderate intake, high consumption of alcohol leads to increased morbidity and mortality. In this manner, ethanol consumption presents the J-shaped alcohol mortality relation, as shown by a study conducted in a Northern California Health Care Program involving 128,934 adults, with different drinking patterns, followed during a period of 20 years [32]. Red wine also contains a wide variety of polyphenols, most of which derive from grape solids [33, 34].

A number of advantageous properties that help counteract arteriosclerosis have been attributed to polyphenols. Red wine's "polyphenolic aid" inhibits oxidation of human LDL [24,35-38] in vitro and in vivo through several different mechanisms, including scavenging reactive oxygen and nitrogen species, chelating transition metal ions, sparing LDL's associated antioxidants, and increasing or preserving serum paraoxonase activity [36]. Red wine has also been shown to increase high-density lipoprotein (HDL) [39, 40] modulate platelet aggregation [41,42], enhance vasorelaxation, and inhibit smooth muscle cell (SMC) proliferation and vascular hyperplasia [43,44].

4. RED WINE OXIDATIVE STRESS AND ENDOTHELIAL FUNCTION: EVIDENCE FROM CLINICAL STUDIES

Over the last decades a large number of studies has focused on the effects of nutrition on cardiovascular health. Thus, some of them have examined the effects of red wine as a part of nutrition. In addition, studies have shown that red wine has an impact on mechanisms associated to cardiovascular disease such as endothelial dysfunction and oxidative stress **Table 2**.

4.1. Red Wine and Oxidative Stress

The effect of red wine on oxidative stress status has been excessively studied. (red wine os stress) Young and older volunteers were recruited in the study of Micallef et al [45]. Each age group was randomly divided into treatment subjects who consumed 400 mL/day of red wine for two weeks. The results from this study showed that consumption of red wine induced significant increases in plasma total antioxidant status and significant decreases in plasma malondialdehyde and glutathione in both young and old subjects. The results suggested that the consumption of a certain amount of red wine for a specific time period significantly increases antioxidant status and decreases oxidative stress in the circulation.

Another controlled randomized study consisted of healthy volunteers showed similar results [46].

Furthermore, a long-term red wine consumption was examined after a 2 weeks period. Total concentration of phenolics and analysed the individual phenolics in the wine and plasma. The production of conjugated dienes and thiobarbituric acid-reactive substances (TBARS) were measured in oxidized LDL. Plasma total phenolic concentrations increased significantly after 2 weeks of daily red wine consumption and trace levels of metabolites, mainly glucuronides and methyl glucuronides of (+)-catechin and (-)-epicatechin, were detected in the plasma of the red wine group. These flavan-3-ol metabolites were not detected in plasma from the control group. The maximum concentrations of conjugated dienes and TBARS in Cu-oxidized LDL were reduced, while HDL cholesterol concentrations increased following red wine consumption.

The oxidant status was also examined during the study of Ceriello et al [47]. The population of the study consisted of type 2 diabetics. This study examined the acute effects of red wine consumption by patients with increased oxidative status. Red wine consumption during a meal significantly seems to preserve plasma antioxidant defences and reduce LDL oxidation. Moreover, to investigate the effects of moderate red wine consumption in a different population than healthy individuals, patients after an acute coronary syndrome (ACS) were recruited in another study to receive red wine for 2 months [48]. After a 2 months period, while measuring specific blood paparameters associated to oxidative stress, it has been showed that the addition of moderate amounts of red wine did not improve endothelial function beyond conventional therapy, but affected beneficially the parameters of oxidative stress in these patients. Another study regarding to the antioxidant effects of wine on oxidant status compared the impact of red and white wine [49]. Aim of this study was to analyse the relationship between the plasma levels of polyphenols and the antioxidant activity of red and white wine. Healthy subjects were randomly allocated to drink a specific dose of red wine or white in 15 days period. Patients who refrained from any alcohol beverage were used as controls Urinary PGF-2a-III, a marker of oxidative stress and plasma levels of polyphenols were measured. Urinary PGF-2a-III significantly fell in subjects taking wine with a higher percentage decrease in subjects given red wine than in those given white wine. Subjects taking red wine had higher plasma polyphenols than those taking white wine.

4.2. Red Wine and Endothelial Function

It has been shown that apart from the antioxidant effects of red wine, the latter seems to affect positively endothelial function. Endothelial nitric oxide synthase (eNOS) exerts vasoprotective effects and moderate consumption of red wine seems to offer more benefits in endothelia function than any other type of drink. However, the molecular basis of this protective effect is unclear. Thus human endothelial cells were treated with red wine from different countries [50]. The results of the study showed an important effect of red wine coming from a specific country such as France while other types red wine from other countries had a less or no effect. Incubation of endothelial cells with red wines from France upregulated eNOS mRNA and protein expression. Endothelial cells treated with French red wines produced up to three times more bioactive NO than did control cells. In addition, the eNOS mRNA stability was also increased by red wine. Recently we were also able to highlight the effects of red wine on endothelial function.

We [51] compared the acute effects of several alcoholic beverages on endothelial function in young adults. In this randomized intervention trial, healthy young individuals with no risk factor for atherosclerosis were randomized into 5 equally sized groups and received an equal amount of alcohol, as red wine, white wine, beer, whisky or water. Endothelial function was estimated by using strain-gauge plethysmography. The results of the study showed that reactive hyperemia was significantly increased 1 h after red wine (same with beer consumption) consumption, while it returned at baseline at 4 h but remained unchanged in all the other groups. The levels of vonWillebrand Factor were decreased in the red wine as well as the beer group only. This study also suggested that red wine may be even more beneficial from other alcohol beverages.

In another study of Whelan et al [52] the effects of acute ingestion of white wine were compared with those of red wine on endothelial function in subjects with coronary artery disease (CAD). Flow-mediated dilatation (FMD) of the brachial artery was used to evaluate endothelial function, At baseline, FMD was similar for the two types of wine. At 360 min after ingestion of wine there was no difference in FMD, which improved nearly threefold after both wines and there was no detectable change in plasma polyphenol levels after either wine. In controversy to Pignatelli et al [49] who showed that red wine is more antioxidant than white wine, Whelan et al showed that the 2 types of wine seem to share the same beneficial effects on endothelial function. Whether alcohol has an impact on endothelial function was the aim of another study of Agewall et al [53]. The study consisted of healthy subjects who were randomized to drink a single dose of red wine with or without alcohol. Endothelial function was evaluated with the use of FMD and the subjects were studied a second time within a week of the first study in across-over design. After the red wine with alcohol, the resting brachial artery diameter, resting blood flow, heart rate and plasma–ethanol increased significantly. After the *de-alcoholized red wine* these parameters were unchanged. Flow-mediated dilatation of the brachial artery was significantly higher after drinking *de-alcoholized red wine* than after drinking red wine with alcohol and before drinking. After ingestion of red wine with alcohol the brachial artery dilated and the blood flow increased. These changes were not observed following the de-alcoholized red wine and were thus attributable to ethanol. These haemodynamic changes may have concealed an effect on flow-mediated brachial artery dilatation which did not increase after drinking red wine with alcohol. Flow-mediated dilatation of the brachial artery increased significantly after *de-alcoholized red wine* and this finding may support the hypothesis that antioxidant qualities of red wine, rather than ethanol in itself, may protect against cardiovascular disease. Similarly to Agewall et al, Karatzi et al [54] showed that acute ingestion of red wine without alcohol led to higher FMD than ingestion of regular red wine in CAD patients.

The acute effect of red wine on endothelial function may be different than its long-term effect and it could be attributed to its constituents other than alcohol. Finally, to determine whether red wine improves insulin resistance in diabetic patients and to explore the relation between insulin sensitivity and endothelial function, Napoli et al [55] studied vascular reactivity and insulin-mediated glucose uptake in 9 type 2 diabetic patients before and after 2 weeks of red wine consumption. Vascular reactivity was evaluated by plethysmography during intraarterial infusion of vasoactive agents. The basal forearm blood flow and the response to vasoactive agents such as acetylocholine were unchanged both in the wine-treated and in the control diabetics. In contrast, insulin mediated whole body glucose disposal improved by after red wine consumption but did not change in the control group. Thus, it seems that red wine consumption for 2 weeks markedly attenuates insulin-resistance in type 2 diabetic patients, without affecting vascular reactivity and nitric oxide production.

5. THE EFFECTS OF RED WINE IN HYPERTENSIVES

During the last years, several studies have examined the association of acohol consumption and hypertension. The origins of the scientific interest on the link between alcohol and hypertension go back to a French report published in 1915 [56], but it was almost a half a century later that further research was performed on this subject [57-59]. Nowadays, it is well-established that alcohol consumption increases both blood pressure (BP) levels and the incidence of hypertension, whereas exerts significant favorable effects on atherosclerotic cardiovascular disease morbidity and mortality even in the setting of hypertension [57, 58]. Thus, there is a growing emphasis on reassessing the clinical implications of alcohol-related hypertension in the light of recent epidemiological and interventional data that led to this ongoing debate as to the relative risks and benefits of alcohol use in hypertensive patients [57-59].

In vitro and in animal models, red wine polyphenolics cause substantial falls in BP, mainly by increasing nitric oxide production [60]. Although, some studies showed that wine drinking is associated with weaker effects on BP than beer and spirits [57, 59, 61, 62], recent reports exhibited no link between the type of drink and BP response [63,64]. On the contrary, liquor drinkers had significantly higher odds ratio for isolated systolic hypertension, while the incidence of systolic-diastolic and isolated diastolic hypertension was not related to the type of alcohol in another cross-sectional study [57, 65, 66]. Therefore, based on the available data so far it is the amount and not the type of alcohol beverage consumed that is the most important determinant of the link between blood pressure status and alcohol.

The stimulation of the sympathetic nervous system is the most probable pathophysiological mechanism responsible for the association of alcohol with BP. It is established that when heavy drinkers withdraw from alcohol a significant sympathetic responsiveness is produced [59, 67]. Additionally, the fact that wine and beer consumption is accompanied by augmented excretion of 24-hour endothelin-1, a powerful vasocontrictor, provides another mechanistic link of alcohol with pressure responses [64]. Finally, one could not rule out the impact of adverse large vessel structure and function taking into account the J-shaped relation between alcohol intake and measures of stiffness in middle-aged and older subjects of both sexes [68-70].

Table 2. Red wine studies: effects on endothelial function and oxidative stress

Study	Population (number)	Dose	Type of wine	Duration	Associated to	Comments
Wallerath et al [50]	HECs	unknown	Different types of red wine	unknown	Endothelial function	Increased expression of eNOS especially after French red wine
Tousoulis et al [51]	Healthy subjects (83)	264ml	Red vs other alcohol beverages	Acute consumption	Endothelial function	Increased reactive hyperemia and decreased vWF levels after red wine consumption
Agewall et al [53]	Healthy subjects (12)	250ml	Red (alcohol vs dealcohol)	Acute consumption	Endothelial function	Flow-mediated dilatation of the brachial artery increased significantly after de-alcoholized red wine
Karatzi et al [54]	CAD (15)	250ml	Red (alcohol vs dealcohol)	Acute consumption	Endothelial function	Acute ingestion of red wine without alcohol led to higher FMD than ingestion of regular red wine in CAD patients.
Whelan et al [52]	CAD (14)	4ml/kg	Red vs White	Acute consumption	Endothelial function	Wine acutely improves endothelial function in patients with CAD
Napoli et al [55]	Diabetes type II (17)	360ml/day	Red vs controls	2 weeks	Endothelial function	Red wine consumption for 2 weeks markedly attenuates insulin-resistance in type 2 diabetic patients, without affecting vascular reactivity and nitric oxide production
Micallef et al [45]	Healthy subjects (40)	400ml/day	Red	2 weeks	Oxidative stress	Red wine provides general oxidative protection and to lipid systems in circulation via the increase in antioxidant status
Tsang et al [46]	Healthy subjects (20)	375ml/day	Red vs controls	2 weeks	Oxidative stress	Evidence for potential protective effects of moderate consumption of red wine in healthy volunteers
Pignatelli et al [49]	Healthy subjects (20)	300ml/day	Red vs white vs controls	15 days	Oxidative stress	Red wine is more antioxidant than white wine in virtue of its higher content of polyphenols, an effect that may be dependent upon a synergism among polyphenols
Guarda et al [48]	ACS (20)	250ml/day	Red vs controls	2 months	Oxidative stress	The addition of moderate amounts of red wine did not improve endothelial function beyond conventional therapy, whereas it showed benefits in parameters of oxidative stress in these patients
Ceriello et al [47]	Diabetes type II (20)	300ml	Red vs controls	Acute consumption	Oxidative stress	Red wine significantly preserves plasma antioxidant defences and reduces LDL oxidation

HECs: human endothelial cells, CAD: coronary artery disease, FMD: flow-mediated dilatation, ACS: acute coronary syndromes, LDL: low-density lipoprotein

6. CONCLUSIONS

Evidence suggests that light to moderate alcohol consumption may have a beneficial effect on cardiovascular morbidity and mortality. Red wine has been shown to improve endothelial function and decrease oxidative stress, which are associated to cardiovascular disease. Consumption of red wine induces significant increases in plasma total antioxidant status and significant decreases in plasma malondialdehyde and glutathione in both young and old subjects. Moreover, red wine consumption for 2 weeks markedly attenuates insulin-resistance in type 2 diabetic patients, without affecting vascular reactivity and nitric oxide production. In vitro and in animal models, red wine polyphenolics cause substantial falls in blood pressure, mainly by increasing nitric oxide production. Although red wine has beneficial effects on vascular endothelium, more studies are necessary to evaluate these effects on cardiovascular risk.

REFERENCES

[1] Rimm EB, Klatsky A, Grobbee D, Stampfer MJ. Review of moderate alcohol consumption and reduced risk of coronary heart disease; is the effect due to beer, wine or spirits? *BMJ* 1996;312:731e6.

[2] Frankel E, Kanner J, German J, Parks E, Kinsella JE. Inhibition of oxidation of human low – density lipoprotein by phenolic substances in red wine. *Lancet* 1993; 341:454–457.

[3] Keevil G, Osman H, Reed J, Folts JD. Grape juice, but not orange juice or grapefruit juice inhibits human platelet aggregation. *J Nutr 2000*; 130:53–56.

[4] Freedman J, Parker C, Li L et al. Select flavonoids and whole juice from purple grapes inhibit platelet function and enhance nitric oxide release. *Circulation 2001*; 103:2792–2798.

[5] Pendurthi U, Williams T, Vijaya M. Resveratrol, a polyphenolic compound found in wine, inhibits tissue factor expression in vascular cells. *Arterioscler Thromb Vasc Biol 1999*; 19:419–426.

[6] Wollny T, Aiello L, di Tommaso D et al. Modulation of haemostatic function and prevention of experimental thrombosis by red wine in rats: a role for increased nitric oxide production. *Br J Pharmacol 1999*; 127:747–755.

[7] Hashimoto M, Kim S, Eto M, et al. Effect of acute intake of red wine on flow mediated vasodilation of the brachial artery. *Am J Cardiol 2001*;88(12):1457e60.

[8] Teissedre PL, Frankel EN, Waterhouse AL, Peleg H, German JB. Inhibition of in vitro human LDL oxidation by phenolic antioxidants from grapes and wines. *J Sci Food Agric 1996*; 70: 55–61.

[9] Kugiyama K, Ohgushi M, Motoyama T et al. Intracoronary infusion of reduced glutathione improves endothelial vasomotor response to acetylcholine in human coronary circulation. *Circulation 1998*; 97: 2299–301.

[10] Cohen R. The role of nitric oxide and other endotheliumderived vasoactive substances in vascular disease. *Prog Cardiovasc Dis 1995*; 38: 105–28.

[11] Frankel EN, Kanner J, German JB, Parks E, Kinsella JE. Inhibition of oxidation of human low density lipoprotein by phenolic substances in red wine. Lancet 1993;341:454e7.

[12] Keaney J.F. Oxidative stress and the vascular wall: NADPH oxidases take center stage, *Circulation2005*; 112: 2585–2858.

[13] Singh U, Devaraj S, Jialal I. Vitamin E, oxidative stress and inflammation, *Annu. Rev. Nutr. 2005*;25:151–174.

[14] Witzum J, Steinberg D. Role of oxidized low-density lipoprotein in atherogenesis, *J. Clin. Invest. 1991*;88:1785–1792.

[15] Madamanchi N.R, Vendrov A, Runge M.S, Oxidative stress and vascular disease, *Arterioscler. Thromb. Vasc. Biol. 2005*;25: 29–38.

[16] Stocker R, Keaney J.F. Role of oxidative modifications in atherosclerosis, *Physiol. Rev. 2001*;84:1381–1478.

[17] Jialal I. Evolving lipoprotein risk factors: lipoprotein(a) and oxidized low-density lipoprotein, *Clin. Chem. 1998*;44:1827–1832.

[18] U. Rueckschloss, N. Duerrschmidt, H. Morawietz, NADPH oxidase in endothelial cells: impact on atherosclerosis, *Antioxid. Redox Signal 2003*;5: 171–180.

[19] U. Rueckschloss, M.T. Quinn, J. Holtz, H. Morawietz, Dosedependent regulation of NAD(P)H oxidase expression by angiotensin II in human endothelial cells: protective effect of angiotensin II type 1 receptor blockade in patients with coronary artery disease, *Arterioscler. Thromb. Vasc. Biol. 2002*;22: 1845–1851.

[20] Papaharalambus C, Griendling K. Basic mechanisms of oxidative stress and reactive oxygen species in cardiovascular injury. *Trends Cardiovasc Med. 2007*; 17(2): 48–54.

[21] Singh U, Ishwarlal Jialal I. Oxidative stress and atherosclerosis. *Pathophysiology* 2006;13: 129–142

[22] Renaud S, de Lorgeril M. Wine, alcohol, platelets, and the French paradox for coronary heart disease. *Lancet* 1992;339: 1523–1526.

[23] Teissedre PL,Waterhouse AL. Inhibition of oxidation of human low density lipoproteins by phenolic substances in different essential oils varieties. *J Agric Food Chem* 2000;48:3801–3805.

[24] Howard A, Chopra M, Thurnham D, et al. Red wine consumption and inhibition of LDL oxidation: what are the important components? *Med Hypotheses* 2002;59:101–104.

[25] Tunstall-Pedoe H, Kuulasmaa K, Mahonen M, et al. Contribution of trends in survival and coronary-event rates to changes in coronary heart disease mortality: 10-year results from 37WHO MONICA Project populations. *Lancet* 1999;353:1547–1557.

[26] Kuulasmaa K,Tunstall-Pedoe H, Dobson A, et al. Estimation of contribution of changes in classic risk factors to trends in coronary-event rates across the MONICA Project populations. *Lancet* 2000;355:675–687.

[27] Yarnell JW. The Mediterranean diet revisited-toward resolving the (French) paradox. *Q J Med* 2000;93:783–785.

[28] Kozararevic D, McGeeD,Vojvodic N et al. Frequency of alcohol consumption and morbidity and mortality. *Lancet* 1980;1:613–616.

[29] Marmot MG, Rose G, Shipley MJ, Thomas BJ. Alcohol and mortality: explaining the U-shaped curve. *Lancet* 1981;1:580– 583.

[30] Sumpio BE, Pradhan S. Artherosclerosis. Biological and surgical considerations. In: Ascher E, Hollier L, Strandness DE, eds. *Haimovici's vascular surgery. 5th ed. Malden, MA: Blackwell Science, Inc*; 2004:137–163.

[31] Shaper AG, Wattamethee G, Walker M. Alcohol and mortality in British men: explaining the U-shaped curve. *Lancet* 1988;1: 1267–273.

[32] Klatsky AL, Friedman GD, Armstrong MA, Kipp H. Wine, liquor, beer, and mortality. *AmJ Epidemiol 2003*;158:585–595.

[33] Cordova A, Jackson L, Berke-Schlessel D, Sumpio B,. The Cardiovascular Protective Effect of Red Wine. *J Am Coll Surg*. 2005;200(3):428-439.

[34] Wollin S, Jones P. Alcohol, Red Wine and Cardiovascular Disease. *J. Nutr.* 2001;131: 1401–1404.

[35] Fuhrman B, Volkova N, Suraski A, Aviram M. White wine with red wine-like properties: increased extraction of grape skin polyphenols improve the antioxidant capacity of the derived white wine. *J Agric Food Chem* 2001;49:3164–3168.

[36] Fuhrman B, Aviram M. Flavonoids protect LDL from oxidation and attenuate atherosclerosis. *Curr Opin Lipidol* 2001;12:41–48.

[37] Nigdikar SV, Williams NR, Griffin BA, Howard AN. Consumption of red wine polyphenols reduces the susceptibility of low-density lipoproteins to oxidation in vivo. *Am J Clin Nutr* 1998;68:258–265.

[38] Waterhouse AL. Wine phenolics. *Ann NY Acad Sci* 2002;957: 21–36.

[39] Perret B, Ruidavets JB, Vieu C, et al. Alcohol consumption is associated with enrichment of high-density lipoprotein particles in polyunsaturated lipids and increased cholesterol esterification rate. *Alcohol Clin Exp Res* 2002;26:1134–1140.

[40] Araya J, Rodrigo R, Orellana M, Rivera G. Red wine raises plasma HDL and preserves long-chain polyunsaturated fatty acids in rat kidney and erythrocytes. *Br J Nutr* 2001;86:189–195.

[41] Pace-Asciak CR, Rounova O, Hahn SE, et al. Wines and grape juices as modulators of platelet aggregation in healthy human subjects. *Clin Chim Acta* 1996;246:163–182.

[42] Pace-Asciak CR, Hahn S, Diamandis EP, et al. The red wine phenolics trans-resveratrol and quercitin block human platelet aggregation and eicosanoid synthesis: implications for protection against coronary heart disease. *Clin Chim Acta* 1995;236: 207–219.

[43] Rivard A, Andres V. Vascular smooth muscle cell proliferation in the pathogenesis of atherosclerotic cardiovascular diseases. *Histol Histopathol* 2000;15:557–571.

[44] Zou J, Huang Y, Cao K, et al. Effect of resveratrol on intimal hyperplasia after endothelial denudation in an experimental rabbit model. *Life Sci* 2000;68:153–163.

[45] Micallef M, Lexis L, Lewandowski P. Red wine consumption increases antioxidant status and decreases oxidative stress in the circulation of both young and old humans. *Nutrition Journal 2007*;6:27 1-8

[46] Tsang C, Higgins S, Duthie G et al. The influence of moderate red wine consumption on antioxidant status and indices of oxidative stress associated with CHD in healthy volunteers. *Br J Nutr* 2005;93:233–240.

[47] Ceriello A, Bortolotti N, Motz E et al. Red wine protects diabetic patients from meal-induced oxidative stress and thrombosis activation : a pleasant approach to the prevention of cardiovascular disease in diabetes. *Eur J Clin Invest.* 2001;31(4):322-328.

[48] Guarda E, Godoy I, Foncea R, Pérez DD, Romero C, Venegas R, Leighton F. Red wine reduces oxidative stress in patients with acute coronary syndrome. *Int J Cardiol.* 2005;104(1):35-8.

[49] Pignatelli P, Ghiselli A, Buchetti B et al. Polyphenols synergistically inhibit oxidative stress in subjects given red and white wine. *Atherosclerosis.* 2006;188(1):77-83.

[50] Wallerath T, Poleo D, Li H, Förstermann U. Red wine increases the expression of human endothelial nitric oxide synthase: a mechanism that may contribute to its beneficial cardiovascular effects. *J Am Coll Cardiol.* 2003;41(3):471-8.

[51] Tousoulis D, Ntarladimas I, Antoniades C et al. Acute effects of different alcoholic beverages on vascular endothelium, inflammatory markers and thrombosis fibrinolysis system. *Clin Nutr.* 2008 Feb 22. [Epub ahead of print]

[52] Whelan AP, Sutherland WH, McCormick MP, Yeoman DJ, de Jong SA, Williams MJ. Effects of white and red wine on endothelial function in subjects with coronary artery disease. *Intern Med J.* 2004;34(5):224-8.

[53] Agewall S, Wright S, Doughty RN, Whalley GA, Duxbury M, Sharpe N. Does a glass of red wine improve endothelial function? *Eur Heart J.* 2000;21(1):74-8.

[54] Karatzi K, Papamichael C, Aznaouridis K et al. Constituents of red wine other than alcohol improve endothelial function in patients with coronary artery disease. *Coron Artery Dis.* 2004;15(8):485-90.

[55] Napoli R, Cozzolino D, Guardasole V et al. Red wine consumption improves insulin resistance but not endothelial function in type 2 diabetic patients. *Metabolism.* 2005;54(3):306-13.

[56] Lian C. L' alcoolisme cause d'hypertension arterielle. *Bull Acad Med* 1915;74: 525-528.

[57] Puddey IB, Lawrence JB. Alcohol is bad for blood pressure. *Clin Exp Phramacol Physiol* 2006; 33:868-871.

[58] Kodavali L, Townsend RR. Alcohol and its relationship to blood pressure. *Curr Hypertens Rep* 2006; 8:338-344

[59] Klatsky AL. Alcohol, cardiovascular diseases and diabetes mellitus. *Pharmacol Res* 2007; 55: 237-247.

[60] Diebolt M, Bucher B, Andriantsitohaina R. Wine polyphenols decrease blood pressure, improve NO vasodilation and induce gene expression. *Hypertension* 2001; 38: 159-165.

[61] Criqui MH, Wallace RB, Mishkel M, Barret-Connor E, Heiss G. Lacohol comsumption and blood pressure. The Lipid research clinis Prevalence Study. *Hypertension* 1981; 3: 557-565.

[62] Marques-Vidal P, Montaye M, Haas B, et al. Relationships between alcoholic beverages and cardiovascular risk factor levels in middle-aged men, the PRIME study. *Atheroscleorosis* 2001; 157: 431-440.

[63] Stranges S, Wu T, Dorn JM et al. Relationship of alcohol drinking pattern to risk of hypertension: A population-based study. *Hypertension* 2004; 44: 813-819.

[64] Zilkens RR, Burke V, Hodgson JM, et al. Red wine and beer elevate blood pressure in normotensive men. *Hypertension* 2005; 45: 874-879.

[65] Wildman RP, Gu DF, Muntner P et al. Alcohol intake and hypertension subtypes in Chinese men. *J Hypertens* 2005; 23: 737-743.

[66] Okamura T, Tanaka T, Yoshita K et al. Specific alcoholic beergae and blood pressure in a middle-aged Japanese population: The High-risk and Population Strategy for Occupational Health Promotion (HIPOP-OHP) Study. *J Hum Hypertens* 2004; 8: 9-16.
[67] Randin D, Vollenweider P, Tappy L, Jequier E, Nicod P, Sherrer U. Suppression of alcohol-induced hypertension by dexamethasone. *N Engl J Med* 1995; 332: 1733-1777.
[68] Beilin LJ, Puddey IB. Alcohol and hypertension. An update. *Hypertension* 2996; 47: 1035-1048.
[69] Van den Elzen AP, Sierkma A, Oren A et al. Alcohol intake and aortic stiffness in young men and women. *J Hypertens* 2005; 23: 731-735.
[70] Nakanishi N, Kawashimo H, Nakamura K et al. Association of alcohol consumption with increase in aortic stiffness: a 9-year longitudinal study in middle-aged Japanese men. *Ind Health* 2001; 39: 24-28.

In: Red Wine and Health
Editor: Paul O'Byrne

ISBN 978-1-60692-718-2
© 2009 Nova Science Publishers, Inc.

Chapter 14

A Prooxidant Mechanism of Red Wine Polyphenols in Chemoprevention of Cancer

S.M. Hadi[1,*], M.F. Ullah[1], Uzma Shamim[1], Sarmad Hanif[1], Asfar S. Azmi[2] and Showket H. Bhat[3,†]

[1]Department of Biochemistry, Faculty of Life Sciences,
AMU, Aligarh-202002 (U.P.) India
[2] Department of Pathology, Karmanos Cancer Institute,
Wayne State University School of Medicine, Detroit, Michigan, USA
[3]Center for Cancer Pharmacology, University of Pennsylvania
School of Medicine, Philadelphia, PA

Abstract

Moderate consumption of red wine is considered to have a preventive effect against cardiovascular disease and cancer. The effect is attributed to the presence of polyphenols in red wine such as resveratrol, delphinidin, quercetin and gallic acid. Plant derived polyphenols are recognized as naturally occurring antioxidants but also act as prooxidants catalyzing DNA degradation in the presence of transition metal ions such as copper. The mechanism of pharmacological action of polyphenols present in red wine has been the subject of considerable interest as the identification of such mechanisms may lead to the development of novel anticancer and other drugs. Of particular interest is the observation that several polyphenols in red wine such as resveratrol and gallic acid have been found to induce internucleosomal DNA fragmentation in cancer cell lines but not in normal human cells. Some data in the literature suggests that the antioxidant properties of polyphenols may not fully account for their chemopreventive effect against cancer. Studies in our laboratory have shown that quercetin, resveratrol and delphinidin are able to bind Cu(II) leading to its reduction to Cu(I), whose reoxidation in the presence of molecular oxygen leads to the generation of a variety of reactive oxygen species (ROS).

---

* To whom correspondence may be addressed, E-mail: smhadi@vsnl.com, Tel: +91-571-2700741 , Mobile: +919837266761
† Address: Center for Cancer Pharmacology, 841-850 Biomedical Research Building II/III, University of Pennsylvania School of Medicine, 421 Curie Boulevard, Philadelphia, PA 19104-616

Copper is an important metal ion present in chromatin and is closely associated with DNA bases particularly guanine. Based on our own studies and those of others we have proposed that the prooxidant action (i.e. generation of ROS) may be an important mechanism of anticancer properties of plant polyphenols. We have shown that resveratrol, delphinidin, quercetin and gallic acid in the presence of copper ions are capable of causing DNA degradation in cells such as lymphocytes. We have further shown that these polyphenols alone are also capable of causing DNA breakage in cells. Neocuproine (a Cu(I) specific sequestering agent) inhibits such DNA degradation. Bathocuproine, which is unable to permeate through the cell membrane, did not cause such inhibition. We have also shown that delphinidin and resveratrol are able to degrade DNA in cell nuclei and that such DNA degradation is also inhibited by neocuproine, suggesting that nuclear copper is mobilized in this reaction. Neocuproine was also shown to inhibit the oxidative stress generated in lymphocytes indicating that the cellular DNA breakage involves the formation of ROS. These results indicate that the generation of ROS occurs through mobilization of endogenous copper ions. It is well established that tissue, cellular and serum copper levels are considerably elevated in various malignancies. Therefore, cancer cells may be more subject to electron transfer between copper ions and polyphenols to generate ROS. Thus, our results are in support of our hypothesis that anticancer mechanism of plant polyphenols involves mobilization of endogenous copper possibly chromatin bound copper and the consequent prooxidant action.

1. INTRODUCTION

In recent years evidence has emerged to suggest that moderate consumption of beverages such as red wine and green tea has a preventive effect against a number of diseases including cardiovascular disease and cancer. Red wine is a rich source of polyphenolic compounds that include flavonols (quercetin), stilbenes (resveratrol), anthocyanidins (delphinidin) and hydroxybenzoic acid (gallic acid). These phytochemicals are known to possess a wide range of pharmacological properties the mechanisms of which have been the subject of considerable interest. They are recognized as naturally occurring antioxidants and have been implicated as antiviral and antitumor compounds [1, 2]. In recent years, a number of reports have appeared which have shown that red wine extracts as well as isolated poyphenolic constituents of red wine are able to induce apoptosis in various cancer cell lines [3,4]. Resveratrol has been shown to inhibit the initiation and promotion of hydrocarbon induced skin cancer as well as the progression of breast cancer in mice models [5]. The consumption of green tea is also considered to reduce the risk of various cancers such as that of bladder, prostate, esophagus and stomach [6]. The chemopreventive efficacy of red wine polyphenols has been observed to be comparable to those of green tea polyphenolic constituents. Of particular interest is the observation that the green tea polyohenol epigallocatechin-3-gallate (EGCG) was found to induce internucleosomal DNA fragmentation in cancer cell lines such as human epidermoid carcinoma cells, human carcinoma keratinocytes, human prostate carcinoma cells, mouse lymphoma cells but not in normal human epidermal keratinocytes [4]. Similarly resveratrol, a major polyphenol in red wine, was also shown to induce apoptotic cell death in HL60 human leukemia cell lines but not in normal peripheral blood lymphocytes [4]. Gallic acid, another constituent of red wine showed cytotoxicity for a number of tumor cell lines but primary cultured rat hepatocytes and macrophages were found to be refractory to the cytotoxic effect

[7]. The hallmark of apoptosis is internucleosomal DNA fragmentation, which distinguishes it from necrosis. Other changes such as shrinkage of cells, membrane blebbing and the dissociation of the nucleus into chromatoid bodies also occur. It is to be noted that most clinically used anticancer drugs can activate late events of apoptosis (DNA degradation and morphological changes) and there are differences in essential signaling pathways between pharmacological cell death and physiological induction of programmed cell death [8]. Based on our own observations and those of others we have proposed a mechanism of DNA fragmentation in cancer cells by plant polyphenolics that involves mobilization of intracellular copper. Studies on chemopreventive and therapeutic plant-derived phytonutrients assume significance in view of the fact that such compounds exhibit negligible or low toxicity even at relatively high concentrations. Further they may also act as lead compounds for the synthesis and development of novel anticancer drugs. Table 1 gives the concentrations of some polyphenols present in red wines. However, it must be emphasized that such concentrations exhibit considerable variation depending on the vintage and the region where the wine is produced. Figure 1 provides the chemical structures of four polyphenols in red wine studied in our laboratory for their mechanism of action.

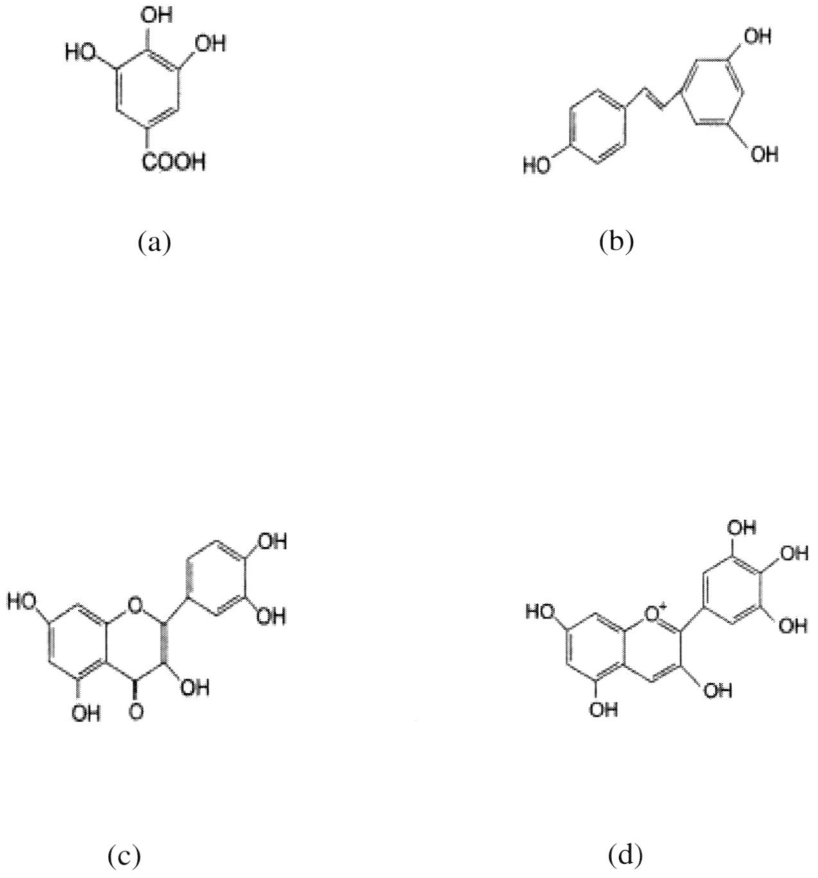

Figure 1. Chemical structures of (a) gallic acid, (b) resveratrol, (c) quercetin, (d) delphinidin

Table 1. Concentrations of some polyphenols present in popular red wines

Representative red wine	Polyphenolic constituent	Concentration (mg/L)	Reference
Burgundy	Catechin	136.0	[9]
Burgundy	Epicatechin	50.2	[9]
Chateauneuf	*trans*-resveratrol	4.7	[9]
Australian Shiraz	Quercetin	9.7	[9]
Muscadine	Ellagic acid	8.5	[10]
Muscadine	Gallic acid	73.0	[10]
Teroldego Rotaliano	Delphinidin	22.5	[11]
Teroldego Rotaliano	Malvidin	197.7	[11]

2. OXIDATIVE DNA BREAKAGE BY RED WINE POLYPHENOLS *IN VITRO* IN THE PRESENCE OF COPPER IONS

Studies in our laboratory have shown that a number of red wine polyphenols including gallic acid [12], quercetin [13,14], resveratrol [15] and delphinidin [16] cause oxidative strand breakage in DNA either alone or in the presence of transition metal ions such as copper. Such DNA degradation action appears to be a common property of all plant derived polyphenolic compounds. Recent studies by Liu and co-workers [17] demonstrated that resveratrol as well as its certain synthetic analogs namely 3,4,4-trihydroxy-*trans*-stilbene, 3,4-dihydroxy-*trans*stilbene, 3,4,5-trihydroxy-*trans*-stilbene, which are generally effective antioxidants, can switch to prooxidants in the presence of Cu(II) to induce DNA damage. Copper is an important metal ion present in chromatin and is closely associated with DNA bases particularly guanine [18,19]. It is also one of the most redox active of the various metal ions present in cells. We have also shown that the polyphenol quercetin is capable of binding to DNA and copper [14]. Evidence deduced in our laboratory has shown that polyphenols such as the flavonoid quercetin and the stilbene resveratrol can not only bind copper ions but also catalyze their redox cycling [15]. In the case of quercetin a mechanism was proposed which involves the formation of a ternary complex of DNA–quercetin–Cu(II) [14,20]. A redox reaction of the compound and Cu(II) in the ternary complex may occur leading to the reduction of Cu(II) to Cu(I), whose reoxidation generates a variety of ROS (Fig. 2). Most of the pharmacological properties of plant polyphenols are considered to reflect their ability to scavenge endogenously generated oxygen radicals or those free radicals formed by various xenobiotics, radiation etc. However, some data in the literature suggests that the antioxidant properties of the polyphenolic compounds may not fully account for their chemopreventive effects [21,22]. Most plant polyphenols possess both antioxidant as well as prooxidant properties [7,13] and we have proposed that the prooxidant action of plant polyphenolics may be an important mechanism of their anticancer and apoptosis inducing properties [22]. Such a mechanism for the cytotoxic action of these compounds against cancer cells would involve mobilization of endogenous copper ions and the consequent prooxidant action.

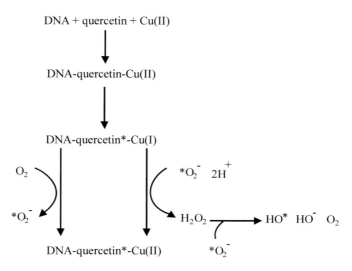

Figure 2. Involvement of a ternary complex of quercetin, DNA and Cu(II)/Cu(I) in the generation of active oxygen species. The oxidized forms of quercetin (represented as quercetin*) are not necessarily identical.

3. CU(II) MEDIATED DNA BREAKAGE INDUCED BY RED WINE POLYPHENOLS IN HUMAN PERIPHERAL LYMPHOCYTES

Using a cellular system of lymphocytes isolated from human peripheral blood and alkaline single cell gel electrophoresis (comet assay), we have confirmed that the plant polyphenol–Cu(II) system is indeed capable of causing DNA degradation in cells such as lymphocytes [23]. Further, the DNA degradation of lymphocytes is inhibited by scavengers of ROS and neocuproine, a Cu(I) specific sequestering agent. Also, similar to the *in vitro* results, *trans*-stilbene which does not have any hydroxyl group is inactive in the lymphocyte system. These findings demonstrate that the polyphenol–Cu(II) system for DNA breakage is physiologically feasible and could be of biological significance.

4. EVIDENCE FOR THE PROOXIDANT ACTION OF POLYPHENOLS AS AN IMPORTANT MECHANISM FOR THEIR ANTICANCER PROPERTIES

We give below several lines of indirect evidence in literature, which strongly suggest that the prooxidant action of plant derived polyphenolics rather than their antioxidant activity may be an important mechanism for their anticancer and apoptosis inducing properties:

1) Apoptotic DNA fragmentation properties of several anticancer drugs [24,25] and γ-radiation [26] are considered to be mediated by ROS. It may also be mentioned that doxorubicin induced apoptosis in human osteocarcinoma Saos-2 cells is mediated by

ROS and is independent of p-53 [27]. Interestingly, certain properties of polyphenolic compounds, such as binding and cleavage of DNA and the generation of ROS in the presence of transition metal ions [14] are similar to those of certain known anticancer drugs [28].

2) Structure activity studies carried out in our laboratory with gallic acid (a structural constituent of tannic acid) indicate that if two of the three hydroxyl groups are methylated (syringic acid), the DNA degrading capacity decreases sharply [12]. The results correlate with those of Inoue et al. [7] who showed that modification of hydroxyl groups, such as that resulting in the formation of syringic acid, abolishes the apoptotic activity of gallic acid.

3) Evidence suggests that the antioxidant properties of polyphenolics may not fully account for their chemopreventive effects. For example, it was shown that although ellagic acid is an antioxidant ten times more potent than tannic acid, the latter was more effective in inhibiting skin tumor promotion by 12-O-tetradecanoyl phorbol-13 acetate (TPA) than the former [21]. It was suggested that the antioxidant effects of these polyphenols might be essential but not sufficient for their antitumor promotion. In any case ROS scavenging properties of plant polyphenols may account for their chemopreventive effects but not for any therapeutic action against cancer cells [25]. Expression of the *bcl*-2 proto-oncogene, which blocks apoptosis, decreases cellular production of ROS [29], whereas the coadministration of antioxidant enzymes such as superoxide dismutase (SOD) and catalase prevents curcumin mediated apoptosis in human leukemia cells [30]. Further it has been shown that the programmed cell death induced by curcumin in human leukemic T-lymphocytes is independent of the involvement of mitochondria and caspases suggesting the existence of pathways other than the 'classical' ones [31]. Caspases are essential for both Fas and mitochondria mediated apoptosis. However, inhibition of caspases or the use of cells with defective apoptosis machinery has demonstrated that alternative types of programmed cell death could occur as well and such alternative death mechanisms are divided into "apoptosis-like" and "necrosis-like" [32].

4) Fe^{3+} and Cu^{2+} are the most redox-active of the metal ions in living cells. Wolfe et al. [33] have proposed that a copper mediated Fenton reaction, generating site-specific hydroxyl radicals, is capable of inducing apoptosis in thymocytes. In a study with thiol-containing compounds, apoptosis was induced in different cell lines when either free copper or ceruloplasmin (a copper binding protein) was added; however such activity was not observed when either free iron or the iron-containing serum protein transferrin was added [34]. Most of the copper present in human plasma is associated with ceruloplasmin, which has six tightly held copper atoms and a seventh, easily mobilized one [35]. In another study supporting these observations, copper was found to enhance the apoptosis-inducing activity of polyphenolic antioxidants, whereas iron was inhibitory [36]. Although iron is considerably more abundant in biological systems, the major ions in the nucleus are copper and zinc [19]. Further, although in general, tumors are considered to contain less total iron and have less iron saturation in ferritin than do normal cells that is not always the case [37]. As already mentioned copper ions occur naturally in chromatin and can be mobilized by metal chelating agents. Burkitt et al. [38] suggested that the internucleosomal DNA fragmentation might be caused not only by endonuclease but

also by metal-chelating agents such as 1,10-phenanthroline (OP), which promotes the redox activity of endogenous copper ions and the resulting production of hydroxyl radicals. Thus, the internucleosomal DNA "laddering" often used as an indicator of apoptosis may also reflect DNA fragmentation by non-enzymatic processes. Several reports indicate that serum [39,40], tissue [41] and intracellular copper levels in cancer cells [42] are significantly increased in various malignancies. Indeed, such levels have been described as a sensitive index of disease activity of several hematologic and non-hematologic malignancies [43].

5) A comparison of the properties of complexes formed between plant polyphenolics and Cu2+ and Fe3+ should indicate which of these two metal ions could lead to DNA fragmentation in the nucleus when complexed. Not much is known about the properties of such complexes. However, considerable information is available about OP chelation of copper and iron ions. Burkitt et al. [38] cited several reasons why Cu2+ rather than Fe3+ may be responsible for OP-stimulated internucleosomal DNA fragmentation in isolated nuclei. For example, the cumulative affinity constants ($\beta 3$ in 0.1M salt) for chelation of various metal ions by OP are in the order $Cu^{2+} \approx Fe^{2+} > Zn^{2+} > Fe^{3+}$. The complex formed between OP and Cu2+ has a redox potential ($E°$ for Cu^{2+}/Cu^{+} = 0.17 V) that favors redox cycling, whereas that for Fe^{3+}/Fe^{2+} is 1.1V, presumably because of stabilization in the ferrous state. Copper is also shown to be present in chromosomes as Cu+ ions because of stabilization in the presence of DNA. This overcomes the need for the reduction of Cu^{2+} to Cu^{+} and can directly generate the hydroxyl radicals. Finally, copper and zinc are major metal ions present naturally in chromosomes [19]. Because most polyphenolics are also polycyclic compounds similar in size to OP, conceivably their metal binding properties are also similar.

6) Mechanistic studies have indicated that the apoptosis induction by delphinidin may involve an oxidation/JNK mediated caspase pathway. Delphinidin treatment increased the levels of intracellular ROS, which may be a sensor to activate JNK. Concomitant with the apoptosis, JNK pathway activation such as JNK phosphorylation, *c-jun* gene expression and caspase 3 activation was observed in delphinidin treated cells. Antioxidants such as N-acetyl-L-cysteine (NAC) and catalase effectively blocked delphinidin induced JNK phosphorylation, caspase 3 activation and DNA fragmentation [44].

7) It has been shown that the polyphenol curcumin mediated apoptosis of HL60 cells is closely related to an increase in the concentrations of ROS possibly generated through the reduction of transition metals in cells [45].

5. OXIDATIVE DNA BREAKAGE BY RED WINE POLYPHENOLS IN HUMAN PERIPHERAL LYMPHOCYTES AND LYMPHOCYTE NUCLEI

Using the comet assay our laboratory has shown that red wine polyphenols cause DNA breakage in isolated human peripheral lymphocytes [46]. Photographs of comets seen on treatment with different concentrations of resveratrol are shown in Fig. 3. At 50 and 100 µM concentrations resveratrol did not damage the lymphocyte DNA to any significant extent whereas at 200 μM concentration a comet with a tail indicative of DNA breakage was observed. The results demonstrate that resveratrol alone is capable of DNA breakage in lymphocytes. We have further reported that several other polyphenols such as gallic acid and delphinidin are also able to catalyze DNA breakage in lymphocytes [16].

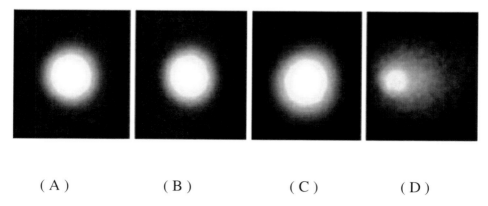

(A)   (B)   (C)   (D)

Figure 3. Alkaline single cell gel electrophoresis (comet assay) of human peripheral lymphocytes showing comets (100×) after treatment with different concentrations of resveratrol: (A) untreated, (B) 50 μM, (C) 100 μM and (D) 200 μM.

Further studies in this laboratory using a lysed version of comet assay have shown that delphinidin is able to cause considerably greater DNA breakage in lymphocyte nuclei as compared to intact lymphocytes [Fig 4].

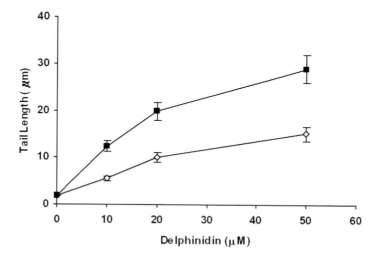

Figure 4. A comparison of DNA breakage in intact lymphocytes (◊) and lymphocyte nuclei (■) using increasing concentrations of delphinidin. Values reported are ± S.E.M. of three independent experiments.

This is explained by the elimination of cell membrane and cytoplasmic barrier in the lysed version of comet assay. Thus, delphinidin is able to directly interact with cell nuclei leading to an enhanced DNA breakage[16] Table 2 gives the results of an experiment where three scavengers of ROS have been tested namely, SOD and catalase, which remove superoxide and H_2O_2, respectively and thiourea, which is a scavenger of several ROS. All three cause significant inhibition of DNA breakage induced by delphinidin in lymphocytes as evidenced by decreased tail lengths. We conclude that superoxide anion and H_2O_2 are essential components in the pathway that leads to the formation of hydroxyl radical and other species which would be the proximal DNA cleaving agents.

Table 2. Effect of scavengers of reactive oxygen species on Delphinidin induced DNA breakage in lymphocytes

Treatment	Tail length (µm)	% inhibition
Untreated	1.5 ± 0.15	-
Delphinidin (100 µM)	25.0 ± 2[a]	0
+ thiourea (1mM)	10.36 ± 1.03*	58.5
+ SOD (100 µg/ml)	8.5 ± 0.85*	66
+ catalase (100µg/ml)	10.3 ± 1*	58.8

All values represent S.E.M of three independent experiments.
* p values < 0.05 when compared to control[a].

6. PUTATIVE MOBILIZATION OF NUCLEAR COPPER BY RED WINE POLYPHENOLS

In a previous study [23] we have shown that the resveratrol–Cu(II) mediated degradation of cellular DNA is inhibited by neocuproine which is a Cu(I) specific chelating agent and is membrane permeable [47]. In the experiment shown in Fig. 5, we have also used bathocuproine disulphonate, the water soluble membrane impermeable analog of neocuproine to show that whereas neocuproine inhibits resveratrol induced DNA breakage in intact lymphocytes, bathocuproine as expected is ineffective in causing such inhibition (Fig. 5a). However, when these two copper specific chelators (both of which are able to permeate the nuclear pore complex), were tested for DNA breakage inhibition in lymphocyte nuclei, both were found to inhibit DNA breakage in a dose dependent manner (Fig. 5b) [48]. From the results we conclude that the DNA breakage by the polyphenols involves nuclear copper and that Cu (I) is an essential intermediate that leads to DNA breakage.

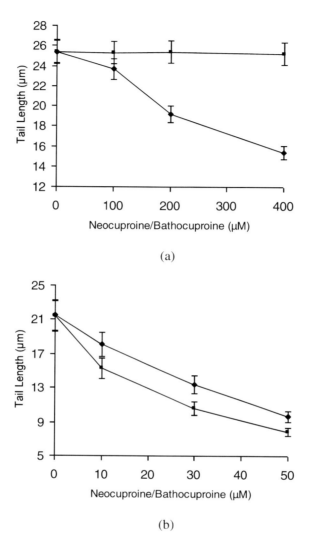

Figure 5. Effect of increasing concentrations of bathocuproine (■)/ neocuproine (♦) on resveratrol induced DNA breakage in lymphocytes (a) and lymphocyte nuclei (b). Concentration of resveratrol was 200μM and 50μM in lymphocyte and lymphocyte nuclei respectively. Values reported are ±S.E.M. of three independent experiments.

7. OXIDATIVE DNA BREAKAGE BY RED WINE POLYPHENOLS IS MEDIATED BY INTRACELLULAR PRODUCTION OF REACTIVE OXYGEN SPECIES

It is well known that polyphenols autooxidize in cell culture media to generate H_2O_2 that can enter cells/nuclei causing damage to various macromolecules [49].We have therefore determined the resveratrol induced formation of H_2O_2 in the incubation medium of nuclei (0.4N phosphate buffer) and also compared it with a known generator of H_2O_2 namely tannic acid [50]. The results showed that the rate of H_2O_2 formation by resveratrol is almost negligible but that of tannic acid is quite significant. However, the DNA breakage efficiencies of the two polyphenols follow a reverse trend where resveratrol was found to be considerably more effective than tannic acid [48]. .It is therefore indicated that the nuclear DNA breakage observed in our studies is not the result of extraneous generation of ROS. We thus presume that the lymphocyte DNA breakage is the result of the generation of hydroxyl radicals and other ROS *in situ*. Oxygen radical damage to deoxyribose or DNA is considered to give rise to thiobarbituric acid reactive substance (TBARS) [51,52]. We therefore determined the formation of TBARS in lymphocytes as a measure of oxidative stress with increasing concentrations of resveratrol. The effect of preincubating the cells with neocuproine and thiourea was also studied. Results given in Fig. 6 show that there is a dose dependent increase in the formation of TBARS in lymphocytes. However, when the cells were preincubated with neocuproine and thiourea there was a considerable decrease in the rate of formation of TBARS by resveratrol. These results indicate that both DNA breakage and oxidative stress in cells is inhibited by Cu(I) chelation and scavenging of ROS. Thus, it can be concluded that the formation of ROS by polyphenols in lymphocytes involves their interaction with intracellular copper as well as its reduction to Cu(I).

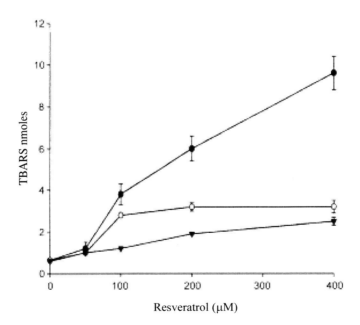

Figure 6. Effect of preincubation of lymphocytes with neocuproine and thiourea on TBARS generated by increasing concentrations of resveratrol. Resveratrol alone (●); resveratrol + neocuproine (1mM) (O); resveratrol + thiourea (1mM) (▼). The isolated cells (1×10^5) suspended in RPMI 1640 were preincubated with the indicated concentrations of neocuproine and thiourea for 30 min at 37 °C. After pelleting the cells were washed twice with PBS (Ca2+ and Mg2+ free) before resuspension in RPMI and further incubation for 1 h in the presence of increasing resveratrol concentrations. Viability of lymphocytes after preincubation with neocuproine and thiourea was more than 90%. Values reported are ±S.E.M. of three independent experiments.

8. CONCLUSIONS

The above studies lead to the conclusion that red wine polyphenols are able to cause (i) cellular DNA degradation in mammalian cells (ii), such DNA breakage is caused by the generation of reactive oxygen species (ROS) and (iii) involves the mobilization of nuclear copper. In view of the findings in our laboratory [53] and those of others we suggest that the red wine polyphenols possessing anticancer and apoptosis inducing activities are able to mobilize nuclear copper leading to the formation of ROS such as the hydroxyl radical close to the proximity of the site of DNA cleavage. Essentially this would be an alternative, non-enzymatic and copper-dependent pathway for the cytotoxic action of polyphenols in red wine that are capable of mobilizing and reducing endogenous copper. As such this would be independent of Fas and mitochondria mediated programmed cell death. It is conceivable that such a mechanism may also lead to internucleosomal DNA breakage (a hallmark of apoptosis) as internucleosomal spacer DNA would be relatively more susceptible to cleavage by ROS. Indeed such a common mechanism better explains the anticancer effects of polyphenols with diverse chemical structures as also the preferential cytotoxicity towards cancer cells. The generation of ROS in normal cells is under tight homeostatic control [54]. However, increased generation of ROS resulting in oxidative stress can be induced by a large number of factors including metals, drugs and prooxidants such as H_2O_2 resulting in the induction of apoptosis. Since in various malignancies, copper levels are known to be elevated, presumably the oxidative stress is further enhanced in cancer cells. Most cancer cells have an imbalance in antioxidant enzymes compared with normal cells [55]. In cancer cells, ROS levels can overwhelm the cells' antioxidant capacity, leading to irreversible damage and apoptosis [56]. The generation of hydroxyl radicals in the proximity of DNA is well established as a cause of strand scission. It is generally recognized that such reaction with DNA is preceded by the association of a ligand with DNA followed by the formation of hydroxyl radicals at that site. Among oxygen radicals the hydroxyl radical is most electrophilic with high reactivity and therefore possesses a small diffusion radius. Thus, in order to cleave DNA it must be produced in the vicinity of DNA [57]. The location of the redox-active metal is of utmost importance because the hydroxyl radical, due to its extreme reactivity, interacts exclusively in the vicinity of the bound metal [58]. As already mentioned cancer cells are known to contain elevated levels of copper [39–42] and therefore may be more subject to electron transfer with antioxidants to generate ROS [17]. Thus, because of higher intracellular copper levels in cancer cells it may be predicted that the cytotoxic concentrations of polyphenols required would be lower in these cells as compared to normal cells. Indeed, some plant polyphenols have shown such a differential effect for certain cancer cell lines [59].

ACKNOWLEDGMENT

The authors acknowledge the financial assistance provided by University Grants Commission, New Delhi, under the DRS Program.

REFERENCES

[1] Hanasaki Y, Ogawa S, Fukui S. The correlation between active oxygen scavenging and antioxidative effects of flavonoids. *Free Radic Biol Med* 1994;16:845–50.

[2] Mukhtar H, Das M, Khan WA, Wang ZY, Bik DP, Bickers DR. Exceptional activity of tannic acid among naturally occurring plant phenols in protecting against 7,12-dimethyl benz(a)anthracene-, benzo(a)pyrene-, 3-methyl cholanthrene- and N-methyl-N nitrosourea-induced skin tumorigenesis in mice. *Cancer Res* 1988;48:2361–5.

[3] Susanne UM, Susan SP, Stephen TT. Extracts from red muscadine and cabernet sauvignon wines induce cell death in MOLT-4 human leukemia cells. *Food Chemistry* 2008;108:824-832.

[4] Clement MV, Hirpara JL, Chawdhury SH, Pervaiz S. Chemopreventive agent resveratrol, a natural product derived from grapes, triggers CD95 signalling-dependent apoptosis in human tumor cells. *Blood* 1998;92:996–1002.

[5] Jang M, Cai L, Udeani GO, Slowing KV, Thomas CF, Beecher CW, Fong HH, Farnsworth NR, Kinghorn AD, Mehta RG, Moon RC, Pezzuto JM. Cancer chemoprevention activity of resveratrol, a natural product derived from grapes. *Science* 1997; 275:218-220

[6] Ahmad N, Feyes DK, Nieminen AL, Agarwal R, Mukhtar H. Green tea constituent epigallocatechin-3-gallate, and induction of cell cycle arrest in human carcinoma cells. *J Natl Cancer Inst* 1997;89:1881–6.

[7] Inoue M, Suzuki R, Koide T, Sakaguchi N, Ogihara Y, Yabu Y. Antioxidant, gallic acid, induces apoptosis in HL60RG cells. *Biochem Biophys Res Commun* 1994;204:898–904.

[8] Smets LA. Programmed cell death (apoptosis) and response to anticancer drugs. *Anticancer Drugs* 1994;5:3–9.

[9] Goldberg GM, Tsang E, Karumanchiri A, Diamandis EP, Soleas G, Ng E. Methods to assay the concentrations of phenolic constituents of biological interest in wines. *Anal Chem* 1996;68: 1688-1694

[10] Talcott SUM, Percival SS, Talcott ST. Extracts from red muscadine and cabernet sauvignon wines induce cell death in MOLT-4 human leukemia cells. *Food chem* 2008;108: 824-832

[11] Canali R, Ambra R, Stelitano C, Mattivi F, Scaccini C, Virgili F. A novel model to study the biological effects of red wine at the molecular level. *British J Nutr* 2007;97:1053-1058

[12] Khan NS, Hadi SM. Structural features of tannic acid important for DNA degradation in the presence of Cu(II). *Mutagenesis* 1998;13:271–4.

[13] Ahmad MS, Fazal F, Rahman A, Hadi SM, Parish JH. Activities of flavonoids for the cleavage of DNA in the presence of Cu(II): correlation with the generation of active oxygen species. *Carcinogenesis* 1992;13:605–8.

[14] Rahman A, Shahabuddin A, Hadi SM, Parish JH. Complexes involving quercetin, DNA and Cu(II). *Carcinogenesis* 1990;11:2001–3.

[15] Ahmad A, Asad SF, Singh S, Hadi SM. DNA breakage by resveratrol and Cu(II): reaction mechanism and bacteriophage inactivation. *Cancer Lett* 2000;154:29–37.

[16] Hanif S, Shamim U, Ullah MF, Azmi AS, Bhat SH, Hadi SM. The anthocyanidin delphinidin mobilizes endogenous copper ions from human lymphocytes leading to oxidative degradation of cellular DNA. *Toxicology* 2008;249:19-25

[17] Zheng LF,Wei QY, Cai YJ, Fang JG, Zhou B, Yang L, et al. DNA damage induced by resveratrol and its synthetic analogues in the presence of Cu(II) ions: mechanism and structure-activity relationship. *Free Radic Biol Med* 2006;41:1807–16.

[18] Kagawa TF, Geierstanger BH, Wang AH, Ho PS. Covalent modification of guanine bases in double-stranded DNA: the 1:2-AZ-DNA structure of d(CGCGCG) in the presence of CuCl2. *J Biol Chem* 1994;266:20175–84.

[19] Bryan SE. Metal ions in biological systems. New York: *Marcel Dekker*; 1979.

[20] Rahman A, Shahabuddin A, Hadi SM, Parish JH, Ainley K. Strand scission in DNA induced by quercetin and Cu(II): role of Cu(I) and oxygen free radicals. *Carcinogenesis* 1989;10:1833–9.

[21] Gali HU, Perchellet EM, Klish DS, Johnson JM, Perchellet JP. Hydrolyzable tannins: potent inhibitors of hydroperoxide production and tumor promotion in mouse skin treated with 12-O-tetradecanoyl phorbol-13- acetate in vivo. *Int J Cancer 1992*;51:425–32.

[22] Hadi SM, Asad SF, Singh S, Ahmad A. Putative mechanism for anticancer and apoptosis inducing properties of plant-derived polyphenolic compounds. *IUBMB Life* 2000;50:1–5.

[23] Azmi AS, Bhat SH, Hadi SM. Resveratrol–Cu(II) induced DNA breakage in human peripheral lymphocytes: implications for anticancer properties. *FEBS Lett* 2005;579:3131–5.

[24] Kaufmann SH. Induction of endonucleolytic DNA cleavage in human acute myelogenous leukemia cells by etoposide, camptothecin, and other cytotoxic anticancer drugs: a cautionary note. *Cancer Res* 1989;49:5870–8.

[25] Radin NS. Designing anticancer drugs via the achilles heel: ceramide, allylic ketones, and mitochondria. *Bioorg Med Chem* 2003;11:2123–42.

[26] Sellins KS, Cohen JJ. Gene induction by n-irradiation leads to DNA fragmentation in lymphocytes. *J Immunol* 1987;139:3199–206.

[27] Tsang WP, Chau SPY, Kong SK, Fung KP, Kwok TT. Reactive oxygen species mediated doxorubicin induced p53-independent apoptosis. *Life Sci* 2003;73:2047–58.

[28] Ehrenfeld GM, Shipley JB, Heimbrook DC, Sugiyama H, Long EC, van Boom JH, et al. Copper dependent cleavage of DNA by bleomycin. *Biochemistry* 1987;26:931–42.

[29] Kane DJ, Sarafian TA, Anton R, Hahn H, Gralla EB, Selverstone VJ, et al. Bcl-2 inhibition of neural death: decreased generation of reactive oxygen species. *Science* 1993;262:1274–7.

[30] Kuo ML, Huang TS, Lin JK. Curcumin, an antioxidant and antitumor promoter, induces apoptosis in human leukemia cells. *Biochem Biophys Acta* 1996;1317:95–100.

[31] Piwocka K, Zablocki K, Wieckowski MR, Skierski J, Feiga I, Szopa J, et al. A novel apoptosis-like pathway, independent of mitochondria and caspases, induced by curcumin in human lymphoblastoid T (Jurkat) cells. *Exp Cell Res* 1999;249:299–307.

[32] Leist M, Jaattela M. Four deaths and a funeral: from caspases to alternative mechanisms. *Nat Rev Mol Cell Biol* 2001;2:589–98.

[33] Wolfe JT, Ross D, Cohen GM. A role for metals and free radicals in the induction of apoptosis in thymocytes. *FEBS Lett* 1994;352:59–6

[34] Held KD, Sylvester FC, Hopcia KL, Biaglow JE. Role of Fenton chemistry thiol-induced toxicity and apoptosis. *Radiat Res* 1996;145:542–53.
[35] Swain J, Gutteridge JMC. Prooxidant iron and copper, with ferroxidase and xanthine oxidase activities in human atherosclerotic material. *FEBS Lett* 1995;368:513–5.
[36] Satoh K, Kodofuku T, Sakagami H. Copper, but not iron, enhances apoptosis inducing activity of antioxidants. *Anticancer Res* 1997;17:2487–90.
[37] Halliwell B, Gutteridge JMC. Oxygen toxicity, oxygen radicals, transition metals and disease. *Biochem J* 1984;219:1–14.
[38] Burkitt MJ, Milne L, Nicotera P, Orrenius S. 1,10-Phenanthroline stimulates internucleosomal DNA fragmentation in isolated rat liver nuclei by promoting redox activity of endogenous copper ions. *Biochem J* 1996;313:163–9.
[39] Ebadi M, Swanson S. The status of zinc, copper and metallothionein in cancer patients. *Prog Clin Biol Res* 1988;259:161–75.
[40] Margalioth EJ, Udassin R, Cohen C, Maor J, Anteby SO, Schenker JG. Serum copper level in gynecologic malignancies. *Am J Obstet Gynecol* 1987;157:93–6.
[41] Yoshida D, Ikeda Y, Nakazawa S. Quantitative analysis of copper, zinc and copper/zinc ratio in selective human brain tumors. *J Neurooncol* 1993;16:109–15.
[42] Ebara M, Fukuda H, Hatano R, Saisho H, NagatoY, Suzuki J, et al. Relationship between copper, zinc and metalothionein in hepatocellular carcinoma and its surrounding liver parenchyma. *J Hepatol* 2000;33:415–22.
[43] Pizzolo G, Savarin T, Molino AM, Ambrosette A, Todeschini G, Vettore L. The diagnostic value of serum copper levels and other hematochemical parameters in malignancies. *Tumorigenesis* 1978:;64:55–61.
[44] Hou DX, Ose T, Lin S, et al. Anthocyanidins induce apoptosis in human promyelocytic leukemia cells: structure-activity relationship and mechanisms involved. *Int J Oncol* 2003;23:705–712.
[45] Yoshino M, Haneda M, Naruse M, Htay HH, Tsuboushi R, Qiao SL, et al. Prooxidant activity of curcumin: copper-dependent formation of 8-hydroxy-2-deoxyguanosine in DNA and induction of apoptotic cell death. *Toxicol In Vitro* 2004;18:783–9.
[46] Azmi AS, Bhat SH, Hanif S, Hadi SM. Plant polyphenols mobilize endogenous copper in human peripheral lymphocytes leading to oxidative DNA breakage: a putative mechanism for anticancer properties. *FEBS Lett* 2006;580:533–8.
[47] Barbouti A, Doulias PE, Zhu BZ, Feri B, Galaris D. Intracellular iron, but not copper plays a critical role in hydrogen peroxide-induced DNAdamage. *Free Radic Biol Med* 2001;31:490–8.
[48] Shamim U, Hanif S, Ullah MF, Asfar S. Azmi, Showket H. Bhat, S.M. Hadi .Plant polyphenols mobilize nuclear copper in human peripheral lymphocytes leading to oxidatively generated DNA breakage: Implications for an anticancer mechanism. *Free Rad Res* 2008 (In press)
[49] Long LH, Clement MV, Halliwell B. Artifacts in cell culture: rapid generation of hydrogen peroxide on addition of (−)-epigallocatechin, (−)- epigallocatechin gallate, (+)-catechin and quercetin to commonly used cell culture media. *Biochem Biophys Res Commun* 2000; 273:50–3.
[50] Bhat R, Hadi SM. DNA breakage by tannic acid −Cu(II): sequence specificity of the reaction and involvement of Cu(II). *Mutat Res* 1994; 313:39-48

[51] Quinlan GJ, Gutteridge JMC. Oxygen radical damage to DNA by rifamycin SV and copper ions. *Biochem Pharmacol* 1987;36:3629–33.
[52] Smith C, Halliwell B, Arouma OI. Protection by albumin against prooxidant action of phenolic dietary components. *Food Chem Toxicol* 1992;30: 483–9.
[53] Hadi SM, Azmi AS, Bhat SH, Hanif S, Shamim U, Ullah MF. Oxidative breakage of cellular DNA by plant polyphenols: A putative mechanism for anticancer properties.*Semin Cancer Biol* 2007;17: 370–376
[54] Klein JA, Ackerman SL. Oxidative stress, cell cycle and neurodegenartion. *J Clin Invest* 2003; 111: 785-793
[55] Oberly TD, Oberly LW. Antioxidant enzyme levels in cancer. *Histol Histopathol* 1997; 12: 525-535
[56] Kong Q, Beel JA, lilleihei KO. A threshold concept for cancer therapy. *Med Hypothesis* 2000; 55: 29-35
[57] Pryor WA. Why is hydroxyl radical the only radical that commonly adds to DNA? Hypothesis: it has rare combination of high electrophilicity, thermochemical reactivity and a mode of production near DNA. *Free Radic Biol Med* 1988;4:219–33.
[58] Chevion M. Site-specific mechanism for free radical induced biological damage. The essential role of redox-active transition metals. *Free Radic Biol Med* 1988;5:27–37.
[59] Chen ZP, Schell JB, Ho CT, Chen KY. Green tea epigallocatechin gallate shows a pronounced growth inhibitory effect on cancerous cells but not on their normal counterparts. *Cancer Lett* 1998;129:173–9.

In: Red Wine and Health
Editor: Paul O'Byrne

ISBN 978-1-60692-718-2
© 2009 Nova Science Publishers, Inc.

Chapter 15

HOW DO WE DEMONSTRATE THAT THERE IS A POTENTIAL THERAPEUTIC ROLE FOR MODERATE WINE CONSUMPTION?

Creina S. Stockley
The Australian Wine Research Institute Australia

ABSTRACT

The light to moderate consumption of alcoholic beverages has been observed to reduce the risk of, and death from, cardiovascular disease (CVD) by potentially 20-50% compared to abstention and excessive consumption. The main component considered responsible for the reduced risk is ethanol. One of the alcoholic beverages, wine, additionally contains phenolic compounds, that are also observed in fruits and vegetables, the consumption of which is associated with a similar reduced risk of CVD. It has thus been proposed that consumers of wine have a greater reduction in the risk of CVD than do consumers of beer and spirits, but potential confounders include the drinking pattern and associated diet and lifestyle of consumers.

What is perplexing scientists, however, is the amount of phenolic compound that is necessary to elicit a cardioprotective effect e.g. on platelet aggregation or coagulation. In *in vitro* studies effects are generally elicited with a 10- or 100-fold greater concentration of phenolic compounds than is present in blood and at cellular sites of action following moderate consumption. This suggests that the metabolites of phenolic compounds may also be bioactive.

This paper reviews the data generated to date on the amount of phenolic compounds necessary to elicit certain cardioprotective effects, and whether isolated individual phenolic compounds are as effective as those administered in a wine medium. The data suggests that although the phenolic compounds are absorbed into the blood stream in measurable amounts, the metabolite is more likely to be the biologically active compound *in vitro*. Furthermore, when seed-derived phenolic compounds are together with the skin and flesh-derived phenolic compounds in wine, they exhibit greater cardioprotective effects than when present individually in a non-wine medium and are potentially equipotent to certain conventional pharmaceutical products at reducing the risk of CVD.

This data may have implications for national alcohol and dietary guidelines, for medical practitioners who 'prescribe' daily moderate wine consumption, as well as for the wine industry per se redeveloping healthier wine styles and types.

INTRODUCTION

From earliest times wine has been used as a therapeutic agent. For example, the physician Hippocartes of Cos (c 460–370 BC) prescribed it as a wound dressing, as a nourishing dietary beverage, as a cooling agent for fevers, as a purgative and as a diuretic (Lucia 1963: 63). Similarly, Claudius Galenus (Galen) (c AD 130–201) recommended that wine be used for the dressing of wounds, for fevers and for debility, therapies that became widely adopted throughout medieval Europe. Wine remained a therapeutic agent into the middle-ages through the *Liber de Vinis*, which was written by Arnaldus de Villanova (c AD 1235–1311), who again recommended wine as an antiseptic, a restorative, and for the preparation of poultices. Wines then fell from favour as a therapeutic agent, which is attributed to the Puritan religious movement led by Oliver Cromwell (c AD 1599 –1658) that spread to the New World when the Pilgrim Fathers settled the east coast of North America in 1620. Wine only found favour again as a therapeutic agent in the last decades of the twentieth century, although, in the first decades, the first population-based study observed that there was a linear relationship between the prevalence of hypertension and cardiovascular disease (CVD) and the amount of wine consumed by French Troops on the western front during World War I (Lian 1915).

A J-shaped relationship between amount of wine consumed and risk of cardiovascular diseases such as hypertension was, however, first observed in 1974 by Klatsky et al. and independently by St Leger et al. in 1979. It only came to public prominence in 1992 (Renaud and de Lorgeril 1992) when French wine drinkers were observed to have a reduced risk of cardiovascular disease (CVD) compared to other population groups which had similar high risk factors for CVD, such as in the USA. Interestingly, in contrast to beer and spirits drinkers in the USA, US wine drinkers are observed to have a similar reduced rate to that of French wine drinkers (Klatsky and Armstrong 1993).

Why is This Observation Important?

CVD accounts for 25 to 50% of all deaths in developed countries and its incidence is increasing in developing countries (Tunstall-Pedoe et al. 1994). According to World Health Organization (WHO) estimates, in 2005, 17.5 million people died of CVD. This is 30% of all deaths globally, while at least 20 million people survived heart attacks and strokes, many require continuing costly clinical care (WHO 2006). The main factors responsible for these alarming figures are represented by the unacceptably high rates of patients with uncontrolled hypertension and dyslipidaemia, and the epidemic of obesity and type 2 diabetes, which tend to appear together as the metabolic syndrome (MS) (Dunstan et al. 2002, Zimmet et al. 2005).

The WHO estimates that there are currently 1.1 billion people who are overweight and expect this total to rise to over 1.5 billion by 2015 (WHO 2006); overweight is defined as a BMI ≥ 25 kg/m^2 (WHO 2002). It is estimated globally that the prevalence of diabetes mellitus is 5.1% of the adult population where type 2 diabetes mellitus is now found in almost every population (International Diabetes Federation 2006). Approximately 75–80% of diabetics die of CVD. In the Hoorn Study, a 10-year population-based cohort study, the metabolic syndrome, however defined, was associated with an approximate two-fold increased risk of incident CVD morbidity and mortality in a European population (Dekker et al. 2005).

Factors Modifying the Risk of CVD

Notably, CVD incidence varies 10-fold across different countries. Sources of the variation include impact of different risk factors for CVD such as body mass index (BMI), diet and exercise, diabetes, genetic predisposition, blood pressure, serum cholesterol concentration, cigarette smoking and socioeconomic status, as well as differences in the amount, pattern and even type of alcoholic beverage consumed, such as beer, wine or spirits (Wietlisbach et al.1997).

Dietary Factors Modifying the Risk of CVD

Diet is also a significant source of variation in CVD risk. For example, in a 30-year follow-up study in seven countries, the risk of CVD was at least two- to three-fold lower in countries consuming a Mediterranean-style diet compared to that in northern Europe and USA where the diet was generally higher in fat (de Lorgeril et al. 1999). The core components of a Mediterranean-style diet include the high consumption of cereals, fruits, legumes and vegetables, which typically contain a high concentration of phenolic compounds, and have previously been associated with a reduced risk of CVD (Trichopoulou and Lagiou 1997). Diet is a risk factor that can be readily modified to reduce the risk of CVD and the impact of other important cardiovascular risk factors. For example, subjects placed on a Mediterranean-style diet for 46 months had a 50–70% lower risk of recurrent CVD, compared to control subjects on a higher fat diet, (Kris-Etherton et al. 2001). Furthermore, 55% of patients with MS who followed a Mediterranean diet for two years were symptom-less and had a reduced risk of CVD at follow-up compared with only 14% of patients in the control group (Esposito et al. 2004).

Influence of Wine on the Risk of CVD

Wine is a major component of a Mediterranean-style diet (Kris-Etherton et al. 2001). Epidemiological studies have indicated that consumers of wine have a reduced risk of CVD, similar but additive to that for consumers of a traditional Mediterranean diet. This is exemplified in an epidemiological study assessing the geographical distribution of CVD in Spain, one of the 18 Mediterranean countries. A higher rate of CVD was observed in those Spanish regions with the lowest per capita wine consumption, despite having, overall, a Mediterranean-style diet. The rate of CVD was, however, still less than that of countries consuming a higher fat and lower phenolic compound diet (Rodriguez et al. 1996). The amount of wine associated with a reduced risk of CVD is generally considered as two to four glasses of wine per day consumed with food, which would attenuate a high blood alcohol concentration associated with cellular and tissue damage, prolong any acute and short-term anti-atherosclerotic, blood pressure and haemostatic effects, and prevent any rebound effects of the ethanol components of the beverage (Rodriguez et al. 1996, Klatsky 2003).

CVD involves a complex interplay between multiple altered cellular and molecular functions in heart muscle (such as cardiomyocytes), blood vessels (such as endothelial cells), vascular smooth muscle cells, blood cells (such as platelets and monocytes) and plasma components (such as lipoproteins, and blood clotting and blood flow factors) as well as gene function (Booyse et al. 2007).

The mechanisms involved in the CVD risk reduction provided by a Mediterranean-style diet are equally multifactorial, and include anti-inflammatory effects and enhanced endothelial function, thus providing a protective effect during the early phases of atherosclerosis (Esposito et al. 2004, Lopez-Garcia et al. 2004, Ross 1999). The endothelium plays a crucial role in regulating peripheral blood flow and oxygen supply to organs and tissues through the production of nitric oxide (NO) (Ignarro et al. 2002). NO tonically regulates arterial and arteriolar tone and exerts significant anti-inflammatory and anti-atherosclerotic effects (Ignarro et al. 2002). Endothelial dysfunction has been shown to be an independent predictor of CVD even after adjusting for traditional risk factors (Lerman and Zeiher 2005), such as hypertension and hypercholesterolaemia, which are characterized by an impairment of endothelium-dependent vasodilatation. Therefore, improving endothelial function by means of pharmacological and non-pharmacological strategies such as moderate wine consumption with food might represent an important therapeutic target (Lerman and Zeiher 2005, Kawashima et al. 2001)).

WINE-DERIVED PHENOLIC COMPOUNDS

The components of wine that might confer a reduced risk of CVD, by enhancing endothelial function and exerting anti-inflammatory and anti-atherosclerotic effects, are represented by the phenolic compounds. These compounds, also present in the fruit and vegetable components of a Mediterranean-style diet, have been associated with a reduced risk of CVD (Kris-Etherton et al. 2001; Genkinger et al. 2004).

Catechin, quercetin and resveratrol represent some of the primary phenolic compounds in wine (Carando et al. 1999). For example, *in vitro* and animal studies have demonstrated that catechin, quercetin, and resveratrol, administered either acutely or chronically, exert significant beneficial or positive effects on established markers of CVD risk such as endothelial function (Benito et al. 2002, Chen and Pace-Asciak 1996, Cishek et al. 1997, Wallerath et al. 2002; Wallerath et al. 2005; Sanchez et al. 2006) and blood pressure (Negishi et al. 2004, Garcia-Saura et al. 2005, Duarte et al. 2002, Liu et al. 2005). In both red and white wines, catechin is the most abundant and resveratrol is the least (Cabanis et al. 1999).

Catechin

The flavanol catechin, a simple monomeric compound, is found in both the seed and the skin of the grape berry as well as in the leaves and stems. The average concentration of catechin in red wine is 191.3 mg/L and is 34.9 mg/L in white wine (Soleas et al. 1997). A dose of 35 mg catechin in red wine yields a plasma total catechin concentration of *ca.* 91 nmol/L (Donovan et al. 1999). Free catechin and its free primary metabolite 3'-O-methylcatechin, was detected in plasma at 1 h post consumption but was not detected at 3-4 h. This implies that, immediately after absorption, catechin is metabolised to polar conjugates (glucuronate or sulfate) either in the epithelial cells or in the liver, before systemic circulation (Donovan et al. 1999). The presence or absence of alcohol does not influence the absorption or metabolism of catechin (Bell et al. 2000).

It has been shown that as atherosclerosis develops, vascular smooth muscle cells are released by platelets and endothelial cells, which proliferate and accumulate within the intima of the blood vessel wall, to further develop the atherosclerotic lesion or plaque. The primary mitogenic and chemotactic compound for the release of the vascular smooth muscle cells is platelet-derived growth factor, which exerts its effects via activation of two subtypes of trans-membrane receptor tyrosine kinases, α and β platelet-derived growth factor receptors (Tanizawa et al. 1996, Schwartz 1997, Heldin and Westermmark 1999, Rosenkranz and Kazlauskas 1999). Recent *in vitro* research suggests that catechin, for example, may inhibit the activation of the β platelet-derived growth factor receptors, and hence platelet-derived growth factor and the subsequent proliferation and migration of vascular smooth muscle cells (Kerry and Abbey 1997).

Endothelial cells synthesise proteins such as tissue-type plasminogen activator (t-PA) and urokinase-type PA (u-PA) which activate fibrinolysis and plasminogen activator inhibitor type-1 (PAI-1) which activates thrombosis. Catechin has been observed to promote fibrinolysis by up-regulating both t-PA and u-PA gene transcription (Abou-Agag et al. 2001, Booyse et al. 2007) as well as by suppressing that of PAI-1 gene transcription (Pasten et al. 2007) in the human coronary artery, by activating the mitogen-activated protein kinases ERK and JNK signalling pathways at the transcription level.

Normal endothelial function depends on a controlled balance between the production of endothelium-derived relaxing factors such as nitric oxide and prostacyclin, and the release of constricting factors such as prostaglandins and thromboxane A2. An imbalance towards an increased release of constricting factors is associated with endothelial dysfunction. Catechin has also been observed to induce endothelium dependent vasorelaxation in the rat aorta (Benito et al. 2002) and mouse renal artery (Gendron and Thorin 2007) by promoting NO production by promoting endothelial nitric oxide synthase (eNOS) mRNA expression and by preventing the release of the vasoconstrictor, thromboxane A2; NO also inhibits lipid peroxidation in LDL and is hence anti-atherogenic (Hogg et al. 1993, 1998).

Quercetin

The simple flavonol quercetin is produced and found in the skin of the grape berry and in grape rachis and leaves. The average concentration of quercetin in red wine is 7.7 mg/L but can range from 2.0–29 mg/L (Soleas et al. 1997, McDonald et al. 1998), and is generally not found in white wine. There have been no human pharmacokinetic studies on quercetin following red wine consumption. Generally, however, quercetin is not found in plasma as the free form or as the parent glycoside but exclusively as methyl, sulfate or glucuronic acid conjugates (Day et al. 2001). Lower doses of quercetin are more methylated than higher doses, potentially yielding compounds such as tamarixetin and isorhamnetin, which may exert certain cardioprotective effects (Dragoni et al. 2006). As quercetin has a relatively long half-life compared with catechin, a 50 mg dose of quercetin would yield a plasma concentration of *ca.* 0.75–1.5 µmol/L (Scalbert and Williamson 2000, Manach et al. 2005), and its metabolites may accumulate in plasma if it is consumed regularly.

Platelet function is pivotal in the formation and progression of atherosclerotic plaques and a diet high in fruits and vegetables has been observed to reduce the risk of thrombus formation. Quercetin has been observed to influence platelet function by inhibiting, for example, collagen-induced platelet aggregation through inhibition of GPVI-mediated signalling, as well as both thrombin-induced and ADP-induced platelet aggregation (Pace-Asciak et al. 1995, Hubbard et al. 2003). Quercetin has also been observed to inhibit the tyrosine phosphorylation and/or kinase activity of a number of critical components of the GPVI signalling pathway, such as the non-receptor tyrosine kinase Syk, phospholipase Cγ2 and PI3-K (Hubbard et al. 2003, 2004). All inhibitions were dose-dependent.

Endothelial cells also release metabolites of arachidonic acid, most notably prostacyclin but also hydroxyeicosatetraenoic acids (HETEs), which influence platelet aggregation and quercetin has also been observed to inhibit 12-HETE synthesis from arachidonate by platelets (Pace-Asciak et al. 2005); in particular, 12-HETE impairs endothelial function. In addition, quercetin has been observed to promote fibrinolysis by up-regulating both tissue- and urokinase-type plasminogen activator gene transcription (Abou-Agag et al. 2001, Booyse et al. 2007, Pan et al. 2008). Furthermore quercetin, as well as catechin, increases the expression and activity of eNOS (Wallerath et al. 2005), while decreasing NADPH oxidase-mediated superoxide anion (O_2^-) generation (Pignatelli et al. 2006); the excessive generation of O_2^- is involved in the degradation of NO associated with endothelial dysfunction in clinical and experimental hypertension.

Resveratrol

The non-flavonoid stilbene phenolic compound, resveratrol, exists in both *cis* and *trans* forms in wine, but *trans*-resveratrol predominates in grapes. The average concentration of resveratrol in red wine is 7 mg/L, 2 mg/L in rosé and 0.5 mg/L in white wine (Waterhouse 2002). Recent research has demonstrated that while approximately 70% of resveratrol was relatively rapidly absorbed following oral administration to healthy humans, only trace amounts (<5 ng/mL) of un-metabolized resveratrol could be detected in the systemic circulation following a 25 mg dose (Walle et al. 2004). Sulfate and glucuronic acid conjugates were, however, measured in plasma and urine. The latter study utilized ^{14}C-labelled resveratrol administered both orally and intravenously. The maximum plasma concentration of both the parent compound and metabolites was, however, *ca.* 490 ng/mL or 2.146 µmol/L. Boocock et al (2007) recently observed that a 5 g single oral dose of resveratrol provided a plasma resveratrol concentration of 2.4 µmol/L, while the concentration of the sulfate and glucuronide metabolites was observed to be 3- and 8-fold higher. No adverse effects were observed at such an inflated dose. These human data appear to be consistent with those observed in animals, although the doses of resveratrol were significantly higher in animal studies (Meng et al. 2004). Both animal and human studies suggest that resveratrol has sufficient bioavailability to reach cellular target sites (Jannin et al. 2004). The chemopreventative effects of resveratrol *in vitro* require a concentration of at least 5 µmol/L.

Purified or synthetic resveratrol enhances endothelial function, and inhibits inflammation. The endothelial effects of resveratrol, in addition to the potentiating effects on NO synthesis and release (Wallerath et al.2002, Wallerath et al. 2005, Ekshyyan et al. 2007), can also be ascribed to its inhibitory effects on the most potent vasoconstrictor hormone in humans, that is, endothelin-1 (ET-1). ET-1 overproduction is another risk factor for the development and progression of atherosclerosis and is observed to increase in rabbits fed a high fat diet. Indeed, resveratrol has been observed *in vitro* to inhibit the synthesis of ET-1 by suppressing transcription of the prepro-ET-1 gene and by changing the morphology of the endothelial cell to modify tyrosine-kinase signalling and hence tyrosine phosphorylation (Zou et al. 2003). This inhibitory effect is dose-dependent, emphasizing the need for controlled studies aimed at assessing different concentrations of resveratrol on vascular and platelet function. Concerning the upregulation of NO, of the phenolic compounds, resveratrol has been observed to be the most efficacious stimulator of human eNOS expression and transcription, but this compound alone does not explain the total stimulatory effect of red wine on eNOS (Wallerath et al. 2005), such that the effects of the individual phenolic compounds appear to be additive and complementary.

The anti-inflammatory properties of resveratrol are secondary to the inhibition of the expression of the monocyte and endothelial adhesion molecules, vascular cell adhesion molecule-1 (VCAM-1) and intercellular adhesion molecule-1 (ICAM-1), and the attachment of monocytes to endothelial cells, as well as inhibiting the lipopolysaccharide (LPS)-induced synthesis of the pro-inflammatory cytokine, tumor necrosis factor-α (TNF-α), and interleukin-1-β, and the release of interleukin 6 from monocytes, partly via a modulatory effect on the nuclear factor kappa B (NF-kappaB) and other signaling pathways (Carluccio et al. 2003).

Furthermore, resveratrol has independently been observed to interfere with the multiple protein kinase pathways and vascular smooth muscle cell protein synthesis activated by angiotensin II, the angiotensin-converting enzyme, which converts angiotensin I to angiotensin II, and thus may also decrease the plasma concentration of angiotensin II and thereby inhibit the vascular smooth muscle cell hypertrophy (Hernandez-Ledesma et al. 2003).

Bioavailability of Wine-Derived Phenolic Compounds

At the same time as the phenolic compounds are observed to enhance endothelial function and reduce blood pressure, they appear, however, to undergo extensive first-pass phase II metabolism in the small intestine and in the liver (Manach and Donovan 2004). Metabolites conjugated with methyl, glucuronate, and sulfate groups are the predominant forms present in plasma, but these are usually not measured in human intervention studies (Kroon et al. 2004). Accordingly, it is thus suggested that these metabolites may actually exert the biological effects *in vivo*, although has yet to be confirmed. For example, metabolites of catechin, quercetin and resveratrol have been shown to exert endothelial, anti-inflammatory and anti-thrombotic effects *in vitro* (Day et al. 2000, Koga and Meydani 2001, Williamson et al. 2005).

CONCLUSION

Phenolic compounds are absorbed into the blood stream in measurable amounts following moderate wine consumption but are relatively rapidly and extensively metabolised such that their metabolites may actually exert the beneficial or positive biological effects on CVD in addition to or instead of the parent compound.

When the seed-derived phenolic compounds such as catechin are together in wine with the skin and flesh-derived phenolic compounds such as quercetin and resveratrol, they exhibit greater endothelial, anti-inflammatory, and anti-thrombotic cardioprotective effects than when present individually in a non-wine medium. The vast majority of the available data, however, have been obtained from *in vitro* studies using concentrations of the phenolic compounds that are not necessarily consistent with those observed in wine. Indeed, attempts to extend *in vitro* and animal findings to human studies have resulted in few studies in which effectiveness was shown at moderate oral 'doses' of wine and correspondingly, wine-derived catechin, quercetin and resveratrol. It is unknown as to whether these phenolic compounds *in vivo* reach the multiple proposed sites of action beyond the gastrointestinal tract, and although recent studies have been undertaken to determine their bioavailability, there is still limited information on their pharmacokinetics in humans. Therefore, the paucity of human data on the pharmacokinetics and pharmacodynamics of catechin, quercetin and resveratrol and their metabolites warrants more research, using escalating doses in accurately controlled human *in vivo* studies in conjunction with reliable and established markers of endothelial function, thombogenic activity and inflammation.

REFERENCES

Abou-Agag, L.H.; Aikens, M.L.; Tabengwa, E.M.; Benza, R.L.; Shows, S.R., Grenett, H.E., and Booyse, F.M. Polyphenolics increase t-PA and u-PA gene transcription in cultured human endothelial cells. *Alcohol. Clin. Exp. Res.* 2001; 25(2):155–62 .

Bell, J.R.; Donovan, J.L.; Wong, R.; Waterhouse, A.L.; German, J.B.; Walzem, R.L.; Kasim-Karakas, S.E. (+)-Catechin in human plasma after ingestion of a single serving of reconstituted red wine. *Am J Clin Nutr.* 2000;71(1):103-8.

Benito, S.; Lopez, D.; Saiz, M.P. et al. A flavonoid-rich diet increases nitric oxide production in rat aorta. *Br.J.Pharmacol.* 2002; 135:910-916.

Boocock, D.J.; Faust, G.E.; Patel, K.R.; Schinas, A.M.; Brown, V.A. et al. Phase I dose escalation pharmacokinetic study in healthy volunteers of resveratrol, a potential cancer chemopreventive agent.*Cancer Epidemiol Biomarkers Prev.* 2007; 16(6):1246-52.

Booyse, F.M.; Pan, W.; Grenett, H.E.; Parks, D.A.; Darley-Usmar, V.M.; Bradley, K.M.; Tabengwa, E.M. Mechanism by which alcohol and wine polyphenols affect coronary heart disease risk. *Ann Epidemiol.* 2007; 17(5 Suppl):S24-31.

Carluccio, M.A. et al. Olive oil and red wine antioxidant polyphenols inhibit endothelial activation: antiatherogenic properties of Mediterranean diet phytochemicals. *Arterioscler. Thromb. Vasc. Biol.* 2003; 23: 622-9.

Carando, S.; Teissedre, P.L.; Pascual-Martinez, L.; Cabanis, J.C. Levels of flavan-3-ols in French wines. *J.Agric.Food Chem.* 1999; 47:4161-4166.

Chen, C.K.; Pace-Asciak, C.R. Vasorelaxing activity of resveratrol and quercetin in isolated rat aorta. *Gen.Pharmacol.* 1996; 27:363-366.

Cishek, M.B.; Galloway, M.T.; Karim, M.; German, J.B.; Kappagoda, C.T. Effect of red wine on endothelium-dependent relaxation in rabbits. *Clin.Sci.*(Lond) 1997; 93:507-511.

Day, A.J.; Mellon, F.; Barron, D.; Sarrazin, G.; Morgan, M.R.; Williamson, G. Human metabolism of dietary flavonoids: identification of plasma metabolites of quercetin. *Free Radic.Res.* 2001; 35:941-952.

Dekker, J.M.; Girman, C.; Rhodes, T.; Nijpels, G.; Stehouwer, C.D.; Bouter, L.M.; Heine, R.J. Metabolic syndrome and 10-year cardiovascular disease risk in the Hoorn Study. *Circulation.* 2005;112(5):666-73

Donovan, J.L.; Bell, J.R.; Kasim-Karakas, S. et al. Catechin is present as metabolites in human plasma after consumption of red wine. *J.Nutr.* 1999; 129:1662-1668.

Dragoni, S.; Gee, J.; Bennett, R.; Valoti, M.; Sgaragli, G. Red wine alcohol promotes quercetin absorption and directs its metabolism towards isorhamnetin and tamarixetin in rat intestine in vitro. *Br.J.Pharmacol.* 2006; 147:765-771.

Dunstan, D.W.; Zimmet, P.Z.; Welborn, T.A. et al. The rising prevalence of diabetes and impaired glucose tolerance: the Australian Diabetes, Obesity and Lifestyle Study. *Diabetes Care* 2002; 25:829-834.

Duarte, J..; Jimenez, R.; O'Valle, F. et al. Protective effects of the flavonoid quercetin in chronic nitric oxide deficient rats. *J.Hypertens.* 2002; 20:1843-1854.

Ekshyyan, V.P.; Hebert, V.Y.; Khandelwal, A.; Dugas, T.R. Resveratrol inhibits rat aortic vascular smooth muscle cell proliferation via estrogen receptor dependent nitric oxide production. *J Cardiovasc Pharmacol.* 2007;50(1):83-93.

Esposito, K.; Marfella, R.; Ciotola, M. et al. Effect of a mediterranean-style diet on endothelial dysfunction and markers of vascular inflammation in the metabolic syndrome: a randomized trial. *JAMA* 2004; 292:1440-1446.

Garcia-Saura, M.F.; Galisteo, M.; Villar, I.C. et al. Effects of chronic quercetin treatment in experimental renovascular hypertension. *Mol.Cell Biochem.* 2005; 270:147-155.

Gendron, M.E.; Thorin, E. A change in the redox environment and thromboxane A2 production precede endothelial dysfunction in mice. *Am J Physiol Heart Circ Physiol.* 2007;293(4):H2508-15.

Genkinger, J.M.; Platz, E.A.; Hoffman, S.C.; Comstock, G.W.; Helzlsouer, K.J. Fruit, vegetable, and antioxidant intake and all-cause, cancer, and cardiovascular disease mortality in a community-dwelling population in Washington County, Maryland. *Am J Epidemiol.* 2004; 160:1223-1233.

Heldin, C.H.; Westermark, B. Mechanism of action and in vivo role of platelet-derived growth factor. *Physiol. Rev.* 1999; 79(4):1283–316.

Hernandez-Ledesma, B.; Martin-Alvarez, P.J.; Pueyo, E. Assessment of the spectrophotometric method for determination of angiotensin-converting-enzyme activity: influence of the inhibition type. *J Agric. Food Chem.* 2003; 51: 4175-9.

Higashi, Y.; Yoshizumi, M. New methods to evaluate endothelial function: method for assessing endothelial function in humans using a strain-gauge plethysmography: nitric oxide-dependent and -independent vasodilation. *J. Pharmacol. Sci.* 2003; 93:399-404.

Hogg, N.; Kalyanaraman, B.; Joseph, J.; Struck, A.; Parthasarathy, S. Inhibition of low-density lipoprotein oxidation by nitric oxide. Potential role in atherogenesis. *FEBS Lett.* 1993; 334(2):170-4.

Hogg, N.; Kalyanaraman, B. Nitric oxide and low-density lipoprotein oxidation. *Free Radic Res.* 1998; 28(6):593-600.

Hubbard, G.P.; Wolffram, S.; Lovegrove, J.A,; Gibbins, J.M. Ingestion of quercetin inhibits platelet aggregation and essential components of the collagen-stimulated platelet activation pathway in humans. *J Thromb Haemost.* 2004; 2(12):2138-45.

Hubbard, G.P.; Stevens, J.M.; Cicmil, M.; Sage, T.; Jordan, P.A.; Williams, C.M.; Lovegrove, J.A.; Gibbins, J.M. Quercetin inhibits collagen-stimulated platelet activation through inhibition of multiple components of the glycoprotein VI signaling pathway. *J Thromb Haemost.* 2003; 1(5):1079-88.

Ignarro, L.J.; Napoli, C.; Loscalzo, J. Nitric oxide donors and cardiovascular agents modulating the bioactivity of nitric oxide: an overview. Circ Res. 2002; ;90(1):21-8.International Diabetes Federation. *Diabetes Atlas. 3rd edn.* Brussels:. *International Diabetes Federation,* 2006.

Jannin, B.; Menzel, M.; Berlot, J.P.; Delmas, D.; Lancon, A.; Latruffe, N. Transport of resveratrol, a cancer chemopreventive agent, to cellular targets: plasmatic protein binding and cell uptake. *Biochem Pharmacol.* 2004; 68(6):1113-8.

Kawashima, S. et al. Endothelial NO synthase overexpression inhibits lesion formation in mouse model of vascular remodeling. *Arterioscler. Thromb. Vasc. Biol.* 2001; 21:201-7.

Kerry, N.L.; Abbey, M. Red wine and fractionated phenolic compounds prepared from red wine inhibit low density lipoprotein oxidation in vitro. *Atherosclerosis* 1997; 135:93–102.

Koga, T.; Meydani, M. Effect of plasma metabolites of (+)-catechin and quercetin on monocyte adhesion to human aortic endothelial cells. *Am J Clin Nutr.* 2001;73(5):941-8.

Klatsky, AL. Drink to your health? Sci. Am. 2003; 288(2):74–81.Klatsky, A.L.; Armstrong, M.A. Alcoholic beverage choice and risk of coronary artery disease mortality: do red wine drinkers fare best? *Am. J. Cardiol.* 1993; 71(5):467–9.

Klatsky, A.L.; Friedman, G.D.; Siegelaub, A.B. Alcohol consumption before myocardial infarction. Results from the Kaiser-Permanente epidemiologic study of myocardial infarction. *Ann. Intern. Med* . 1974; 81(3):294–301.

Kris-Etherton, P.; Eckel, R.H.; Howard, B.V.; St Jeor, S.; Bazzarre, T.L. AHA Science Advisory: Lyon Diet Heart Study. Benefits of a Mediterranean-style, National Cholesterol Education Program/American Heart Association Step I Dietary Pattern on Cardiovascular Disease. *Circulation* 2001; 103:1823-1825.

Kroon, P.A.; Clifford, M.N.; Crozier, A. et al. How should we assess the effects of exposure to dietary polyphenols in vitro? *Am.J.Clin.Nutr.* 2004; 80:15-21.

Lerman, A.; Zeiher, A.M. Endothelial function: cardiac events. *Circulation* 2005; 111:363-368.

Lian, C. L'alcoolisme, cause d'hypertension arterielle. Bull. Acad. Med. 1915; 74:525–8.

Liu, Z. ; Song, Y. ; Zhang, X. et al. Effects of trans-resveratrol on hypertension-induced cardiac hypertrophy using the partially nephrectomized rat model. *Clin. Exp. Pharmacol. Physiol* 2005; 32:1049-1054.

Lopez-Garcia, E.; Schulze, M.B.; Fung, T.T. et al. Major dietary patterns are related to plasma concentrations of markers of inflammation and endothelial dysfunction. *Am J Clin Nutr.* 2004; 80:1029-1035.

de Lorgeril, M.; Salen, P.; Martin, J.L.; Monjaud, I.; Delaye, J.; Mamelle, N. Mediterranean diet, traditional risk factors, and the rate of cardiovascular complications after myocardial infarction: final report of the Lyon Diet Heart Study. *Circulation* 1999; 99:779-785.

McDonald, M.S.; Hughes, M.; Burns, J.; Lean, M.E.; Matthews, D.; Crozier, A. Survey of the free and conjugated myricetin and quercetin content of red wines of different geographical origins. *J Agric Food Chem.* 1998; 46(2):368–75.

Manach, C.; Donovan, J.L. Pharmacokinetics and metabolism of dietary flavonoids in humans. *Free Radic.Res.* 2004; 38:771-785.

Manach, C.; Williamson, G; Morand, C; Scalbert, A; Remesy, C. Bioavailability and bioefficacy of polyphenols in humans. I. Review of 97 bioavailability studies. *Am J Clin Nutr.* 2005; 81(1 Suppl):230S-242S.

Meng, X.; Maliakal, P.; Lu, H.; Lee, M.J.; Yang, C.S. Urinary and plasma levels of resveratrol and quercetin in humans, mice, and rats after ingestion of pure compounds and grape juice. *J Agric Food Chem.* 2004; 52(4):935-42.

Negishi, H.; Xu, J.W.; Ikeda, K.; Njelekela, M.; Nara, Y.; Yamori, Y. Black and green tea polyphenols attenuate blood pressure increases in stroke-prone spontaneously hypertensive rats. *J. Nutr.* 2004; 134:38-42.

Pan, W.; Chang, M.J.; Booyse, F.M.; Grenett, H.E.; Bradley, K.M.; Wolkowicz, P.E.; Shang, Q.; Tabengwa, E.M. Quercetin induced tissue-type plasminogen activator expression is mediated through Sp1 and p38 mitogen-activated protein kinase in human endothelial cells. *J Thromb Haemost.* 2008; 6(6):976-85.

Pasten, C.; Olave, N.C.; Zhou, L.; Tabengwa, E.M.; Wolkowicz, P.E.; Grenett, H.E. Polyphenols downregulate PAI-1 gene expression in cultured human coronary artery endothelial cells: molecular contributor to cardiovascular protection. *Thromb Res.* 2007; 121(1):59-65.

Pace-Asciak, C.R.; Rounova, O.; Hahn, S.E.; Diamandis, E.P.; Goldberg, D.M. Wines and grape juices as modulators of platelet aggregation in healthy human subjects. *Clin. Chim. Acta* 1996; 246(1–2):163–82.

Pace-Asciak, C.R., Hahn, S., Diamandis, E.P., Soleas, D and Goldberg, D.M. The red wine phenolics trans-resveratrol and quercetin block human platelet aggregation and eicosanoid synthesis: implications for protection against coronary heart disease. *Clin. Chim. Acta* 1996; 235:207–19.

Pignatelli, P.; Di Santo, S.; Buchetti, B.; Sanguigni, V.; Brunelli, A.; Violi, F. Polyphenols enhance platelet nitric oxide by inhibiting protein kinase C-dependent NADPH oxidase activation: effect on platelet recruitment. *FASEB J.* 2006; 20(8):1082-9.

Renuad, S.; de Lorgeril, M. The French Paradox: dietary factors for coronary heart disease. *Lancet* 1992; 339:1523–6.

Rodriguez, A.F.; Banegas, J.R.; Garcia, C.C.; del Rey, C.J. Lower consumption of wine and fish as a possible explanation for higher ischaemic heart disease mortality in Spain's Mediterranean region. *Int J Epidemiol*. 1996; 25:1196-1201.

Rosenkranz, S.; Kazlauskas, A. Evidence for distinct signaling properties and biological responses induced by the PDGF receptor alpha and beta subtypes. *Growth Factors* 1999; 16(3):201–16.

Ross, R. Atherosclerosis--an inflammatory disease. *N. Engl. J Med*. 1999; 340:115-126.

Ignarro, L.J. Wei Lun Visiting Professorial Lecture: Nitric oxide in the regulation of vascular function: an historical overview. *J. Card Surg*. 2002; 17:301-306.

Sanchez, M.; Galisteo, M.; Vera, R.; Villar, I.C.; Zarzuelo, A.; Tamargo, J.; Perez-Vizcaino, F.; Duarte, J. J Hypertens. 2006; 24(1):75-84. Comment in: *J Hypertens*. 2006; 24(2):259-61. Quercetin down regulates NADPH oxidase, increases eNOS activity and prevents endothelial dysfunction in spontaneously hypertensive rats.

Scalbert A.; Williamson G. Dietary intake and bioavailability of polyphenols. *J Nutr*. 2000; 130(8S Suppl):2073S-85S.

Schwartz, S.M. Smooth muscle migration in atherosclerosis and restenosis. *J. Clin. Invest.*, 1997; 100(11 Suppl):S87–9

Soleas, G.J.; Diamandis, E.P.; Goldberg, D.M. Wine as a biological fluid: history, production, and role in disease prevention. *J. Clin. Lab. Anal*. 1997; 11(5):287–313.

St Leger, A.S.; Cochrane, A.L.; Moore, F. Factors associated with cardiac mortality in developed countries with particular reference to the consumption of wine. *Lancet* 1979; 1 1017–20.

Tanizawa, S.; Ueda, M.; van der Loos, C.M.; van der Wal, A.C.; Becker, A.E. Expression of platelet derived growth factor B chain and beta receptor in human coronary arteries after percutaneous transluminal coronary angioplasty: an immunohistochemical study. *Heart* 1996; 75(6):549–56

Trichopoulou, A.; Lagiou, P. Healthy traditional Mediterranean diet: an expression of culture, history, and lifestyle. *Nutr.Rev*. 1997; 55:383-389.

In: Red Wine and Health
Editor: Paul O'Byrne

ISBN 978-1-60692-718-2
© 2009 Nova Science Publishers, Inc.

Chapter 16

KIDNEY PROTECTION BY WINE THROUGH AN ENHANCEMENT OF THE ANTIOXIDANT DEFENSE SYSTEM

Ramon Rodrigo and Joaquin Toro*

Laboratory of Renal Pathophysiology, Molecular and Clinical Pharmacology Program, Institute of Biomedical Sciences, Faculty of Medicine, University of Chile

INTRODUCTION

Over the last decade the favorable consequence of moderate alcohol beverages consumption, especially wine, has been widely studied in rodents and humans. As opposed to what we might think at first sight, the results of those experiences have supported the view that moderate wine intake could play a protective role in several systems, including cardiovascular, digestive and neuroendocrine ones. Moreover, wine might be helpful for the prevention of pandemical diseases and its complications. The latter is remarkable, considering the fact that chronic pathologies increase every year because of the worldwide lifespan rise and non healthy lifestyle.

The effects on cardiac and circulatory systems are probably the most revised. Strong evidence shows that common diseases such as arterial hypertension, heart stroke and atherosclerosis, among others, are prevented or even more, have decreased death risk between patients who include wine as a part of their diet [Da Luz & Coimbra 2004; Mukamal & Ascherio 2005; Renaud & de Lorgeril 1992, Tsang et al. 2005]. Also, there is an inverse association between moderate red wine intake and risk of type II diabetes, which is considered as a cardiovascular "equivalent"[Hodge & English 2006].

Recently, in digestive system, it has been reported that wine plays a protective role against the development and progression of different cancer forms [Gledovic & Grgurevic 2007; Kuo & Hsu 2008, Kim & Kim 2006]. The diminished risk of uncontrolled cell growth

---

* Corresponding author: Dr. Ramon Rodrigo, Molecular and Clinical Pharmacology Program, Institute of Biomedical Sciences, Faculty of Medicine, University of Chile, Adress: Independencia #1027, casilla 70058, Santiago , Chile., Email: rrodrigo@med.uchile.cl, Fax: 56-2-7372783, Phone: 56-2-9786126

is also applicable for lung cancer [Chao 2007] which, according to Mayo Clinic, is the most common cause of cancer-related death in men and women in USA.

Other less understood conditions, like nonalcoholic fatty liver disease, metabolic syndrome and Alzheimer disease are seemingly less prevalent in moderate wine drinkers [Dunn & Xu 2008; Baik & Shin 2008; Marambaud & Zhao 2005].

On the other hand, the understanding of wine effects on the human kidney is still very limited. Also, most part of these studies has been performed in rodents. Nevertheless, it is expected that if beneficial wine effects are due to a positive interference in commonly pathological ways, particularly oxidative stress, herein it should be also useful for renal diseases. In fact, several investigations agree that moderate wine intake has a renoprotective effect in humans.

Moreover, the impact of these results in the outcome of patients, and the improvement on the knowledge of the mechanism causing oxidative injury have opened a new potential therapeutic door in humans, thereby stimulating more researches including other patophysiological models such as chronic renal failure, nephrosclerosis, glomerulonephritis, myoglobinuric acute renal failure and other renal syndromes.

The aim of this chapter is to examine the pathophysiological basis for the prevention of renal damage through the beneficial effects of wine, based on functional, biochemical and ultrastructural evidence.

1. OXIDATIVE STRESS: A GENERAL PATHWAY FOR SEEMINGLY UNRELATED DISEASES

According to the theory of reduction/oxidation in cellular functioning, the oxidation and reduction reactions in biological systems (redox reactions) represent the basis for numerous biochemical mechanisms of methabolic changes [Valko&Rhodes 2006]. In biological terms, instead of using words reductant and oxidant, it is more appropriate to use the terms antioxidant and pro-oxidant, respectively [Nyska&Kohen 2002]. A reducing agent, or antioxidant, is a substance which donates electrons, whereas an oxidant, or pro-oxidant agent, is a substance that accepts electrons.

Cells are constantly exposed to oxidants from both physiological processes, such as mitochondrial respiration [Chance&Schoener 1979] and pathophysiological conditions such as inflammation, foreign compound metabolism, and radiation among others [Ames&Tanaka 1995].

Oxidative stress constitutes a unifying mechanism of injury of many types of disease processes. It occur when there is an imbalance between the production of reactive oxygen species (ROS) and the biological system's ability to readily detoxify these reactive intermediates or easily repair the resulting damage.

ROS are a family of highly reactive species that can be beneficial, as they are used by the immune system as a way to attack and kill pathogens, or might cause cell damage either directly or through behaving as intermediates in diverse signaling pathways. Some of the most important ROS are described on table N°1.

1.1. Generation of ROS

In mammalian cells ROS might be formed through different pathways, either enzymatically or non-enzymatically. For instance, the generation of superoxide radical anion (O2•−), as well as other ROS, requires cell activation involving alteration of the cell membrane structure what in turn activates the generation of lipid peroxidation product molecules. In the context of this chapter, relevant pathways will be described below.

1.1.1. Fenton Reaction

The enzymes contain metal ions. If the concentration of their substrates increases, these enzymes are decomposed and metal ions (mainly iron ions) are liberated. Then, iron ions react with H_2O_2, generating •OH

$$(Fe(II) + H_2O_2 \rightarrow Fe(III) + \bullet OH + {}^-OH) \text{ [Stohs \& Bagchi 1995]}.$$

1.1.2. Haber-Weiss Reaction

The superoxide radical participates in the Haber-Weiss reaction (O2•− + $H_2O_2 \rightarrow O_2$ + •OH+OH−), which combines a Fenton reaction and the reduction of Fe(III) by superoxide, yielding Fe(II) and oxygen (Fe(III) + $O_2^{\bullet-} \rightarrow$ Fe(II) + O_2) [Liochev & Fridovich 2002]

1.1.3. Mitochondrial Generation

The generation of water from oxygen in mitochondria is an enzymatic process in physiological cellular metabolism. The oxygen molecule itself is reduced to water after forming, as successive intermediates, superoxide, hydrogen peroxide (H_2O_2) and hydroxyl radical. Intermediates do not leave the complex before the process is finished, but in some pathophysiological conditions ROS can leave the respiratory burst.

1.1.4. Xanthine Axidase

The enzyme xanthine oxidase (XO), catalyzes the oxidation of hypoxanthine to xanthine and can further catalyze the oxidation of xanthine to uric acid, generating superoxide anion on the first reaction.

1.1.5. NADPH Oxidase

The enzyme NADPH oxidase (NOX), catalyzes one electron reduction of molecular Oxygen to generate $O_2^{\bullet-}$, using NADPH as the source of electrons. $O_2^{\bullet-}$ is known as a central and initial ROS molecule that may convert to more active and toxic ROS, such as those mentioned previously.

1.1.6. Nitric Oxide Synthase

Uncoupling of the nitric oxide synthase enzyme (NOS) results in $O_2^{\bullet-}$ formation instead of nitric oxide (NO).

1.1.5. Generation by Mieloperoxidase

The mieloperoxidase enzyme (MPO) produces hypochlorous acid (HOCl) from H_2O_2 and chloride anion (Cl-) during the neutrophil's respiratory burst. It requires heme as a cofactor. In addition, it oxidizes tyrosine to tyrosyl radical using hydrogen peroxide as oxidizing agent [Heinecke & Li 1993]. HOCl and tyrosyl radical, both cytotoxic, are used by the neutrophil to kill bacteria and other pathogens.

1.1.6. Generation by Cytochrome-P450

The membrane-bound microsomal monooxygenase is a multienzyme system that generally summarizes as cytochrome p450 (C-p450), as the terminal oxidase and an FAD/FMN-containing NADPH-cytochrome p450 reductase (CPR). The most common reaction catalyzed by the C-p450 is a monooxygenase reaction. This might be, for example, the insertion of one atom of oxygen into an organic substrate (RH) while the other oxygen atom is reduced to water (RH + O_2 + 2H+ + 2e– → ROH + H_2O).

One ROS-generating way is given by ferric p450. Once bounded to the substrate, ferric P450 reduces CPR by accepting its first electron, thereby being reduced. Then, this new ferrous hemoprotein binds an oxygen molecule to form oxycomplex, which is further reduced to give peroxycomplex. The input of protons to this intermediate can result in the heterolytic cleavage of the O–O bond, producing H_2O and the 'oxenoid' complex, the latter of which then inserts the heme-bound activated oxygen atom into the substrate molecule. The decomposition of this final one-electron-reduced ternary complex results in $O_2^{\bullet-}$ release. The second ROS-producing branch is the protonation of the peroxycytochrome P450 with the formation of H_2O_2 [Davydov 2001].

1.2. Pathophysiological Conditions

In pathophysiological conditions, sources of ROS include the mitochondrial respiratory electron transport chain, xanthine oxidase activation through ischemia–reperfusion, the respiratory burst associated with neutrophil activation, and arachidonic acid (AA) metabolism.

Activated neutrophils produce O2•– as a cytotoxic agent as part of the respiratory burst via the action of membrane-bound NADPH oxidase on molecular oxygen. Neutrophils also produce NO that can react with superoxide to produce peroxynitrite, a powerful oxidant, which may decompose to form hydroxyl radical.

Additionally, in ischemia-reperfusion xanthine oxidase (XO) catalyzes the formation of uric acid with the co-production of superoxide. Superoxide release results in the recruitment and activation of neutrophils and their adherence to endothelial cells, which in turn stimulates the formation of xanthine oxidase in the endothelium, with further superoxide production, as a positive feedback model pathway. Accordingly, allopurinol, a xanthine oxidase inhibitor, has been demonstrated that blocks the superoxide production in ischemia–reperfusion settings involving organs such as heart [Tan&Yokoyama 1993], liver [Granger 1988], kidney [Terada&Dormish 1992], and small intestine [Grisham&Hernandez 1986].

1.3. ROS-Mediated Cell Damage

ROS have physiological essential roles in mitochondrial respiration, prostaglandin production pathways and host defense [Webster&Nunn 1988].

However, ROS have well known involvement in common-shared pathophysiological models causing cell damage, either directly or through behaving as intermediates in diverse signaling pathways, including DNA damage, protein oxidation and lipid peroxidation resulting in membrane damage, among others [Zimmerman 1995]

1.3.1. DNA Damage

Oxidative DNA modifications are frequent in mammalian and have been suggested as important contributory factors to the mechanism in carcinogenesis, diabetes and natural aging.

DNA damages are considered as the most serious ROS-induced cellular modifications as DNA is not synthesized de novo but copied, perpetuating by means of this way those modifications and hence inducing mutations and genetic instability.

The main responsible ROS of DNA damage is •OH, which reacts with all components of the DNA molecule, damaging both purine and pyrimidine bases and the deoxyribose backbone. This is explained by the diffusion-limited hydroxyl radical ability to add to double bonds of DNA bases, abstracting a hydrogen atom from the methyl group of thymine and each of the five carbon atoms of 2¢ deoxyribose [Dizdaroglu&Jaruga 2002]. Further reactions of base and sugar radicals generate a variety of modified bases and sugars, base-free sites, strand breaks and DNA-protein cross-links.

In addition, reactive nitrogen species such as peroxynitrite and nitrogen oxides have also been implicated in DNA damage [Brown & Borutaite 2001]

1.3.2. Lipid Peroxidation

It is known that ROS attacks cellular components involving polyunsaturated fatty acid (PUFA) residues of phospholipids, which are extremely sensitive to oxidation [Esterbauer&Schaur 1991; Marnett 1999]. The overall process of lipid peroxidation consists of three stages: initiation, propagation, and termination [Pinchuk & Schnitzer 1998; Nyska & Kohen 2002]. Once formed, peroxyl radicals can be rearranged via a cyclization reaction to endoperoxides, being malondialdehyde (MDA) as the final product [Marnett 1999]. MDA is a minor lipid peroxidation product generated by heating of endoperoxides derived from AA. The main PUFA in tissue is linoleic acid, five times more abundant than AA. Linoleic acid generates only traces of MDA [Pryor & Stanley 1976], but is transformed as easily as AA to peroxyl radicals. F2-isoprostanes are useful to demonstrate the occurrence of non-enzymatic lipid peroxidation processes, nevertheless they are only trace products formed through free radicals catalyzed attack on esterified arachidonate, providing a reliable tool to identify population with enhanced rates of lipid peroxidation [Patrignani & Tacconelli 2005].

Lipid peroxidation involves low-density lipoprotein (LDL) oxidation as well as high-density lipoprotein (HDL). It is well known that the LDL oxidation is a key process in the pathogenesis of atherosclerosis [Spiteller 2003]. The oxidized cholesterol esters are directly incorporated into lipoproteins and transferred to endothelial cells via the LDL where they induce damage and start the sequence of events leading to atherosclerosis.

1.3.3. Protein Oxidation

The side chains of all amino acid residues of proteins are susceptible to oxidation by the action of ROS [Stadtman 2004]. The protein carbonyl group is generated by ROS through many different mechanisms and its concentration is a good measure of protein oxidation via oxidative stress. NO reacts rapidly with superoxide radical to form the highly toxic peroxynitrite anion that is able to nitrosate the cysteine sulfhydryl groups of proteins, to nitrate tyrosine and tryptophan residues of proteins and to oxidize methionine residues to methionine sulfoxide [Valko&Rhodes 2006]. Oxidation of proteins is associated with a number of age-related diseases and aging [Stadtman 2001; Levine & Stadtman 2001].

1.3.4. Others

Oxidative damage to the mitochondrial membrane can also occur, resulting in membrane depolarization and the uncoupling of oxidative phosphorylation, with altered cellular respiration [Nathan & Singer 1999]. This can ultimately lead to mitochondrial damage, with release of cytochrome c, activation of caspases and apoptosis [Macdonald & Galley 2003].

2. ANTIOXIDANT DEFENSE SYSTEM

All forms of life maintain a reducing environment within their cells. The maintenance of this status is achieved possibly through the antioxidant defense system, which is in action to protect cellular homeostasis against harmful ROS produced during normal cellular metabolism as well as in the pathophysiological states. The antioxidant system is preserved by antioxidant substances that maintain the reduced state by a constant input of metabolic energy.

Antioxidant substances are molecules that can scavenge free radicals by accepting or donating an electron to eliminate the unpaired condition. Typically, this means that the antioxidant molecule becomes a free radical in the process of scavenging a ROS to a more stable and less reactive molecule. In most cases the scavenger molecule provides hydrogen radical that combines with the free radical. Consequently, it is generated a new radical that has an enhanced lifetime compared with the starting one, for instance, due to a conjugated system [Spiteller 2003].

The extended lifetime of this radical enables it to react with a second radical by formation of a new molecule and thus one scavenger molecule can eliminate two radicals.

Antioxidant molecules can be produced endogenously or provided exogenously through diet or antioxidant supplements. The main endogenous antioxidant enzymes are superoxide dismutase (SOD), catalase (CAT), and glutathione peroxidase (GSH-Px). They are described on table N°2.

Exogenous antioxidants, such as vitamins E and C, exist at a number of locations namely on the cell membrane, intracellularly and extracellularly. They react with ROS to either remove or inhibit them. The hydrophobic lipid interior of membranes requires a different spectrum of antioxidants. Fat-soluble vitamin E is the most important antioxidant in this environment, which protects against the loss of membrane integrity.

Fat-soluble antioxidants are important in preventing membrane PUFA from undergoing lipid peroxidation. Glutathione removes already generated radical, if no radicals are present, the PUFA cannot be attacked. Therefore, they shield the membrane rich in PUFA against ROS [Spiteller 2002]. In addition, water-soluble antioxidants including vitamin C play a key role in scavenging ROS in the hydrophilic phase.

Other small antioxidant molecules are also naturally present in the plasma, such as uric acid and bilirubin. Recently, it was found that fish, fish oils, and vegetables contain furan fatty acids that are radical scavengers, responsible for the beneficial efficiency of a fish diet [Spiteller 2005]

3. OXIDATIVE STRESS: ROS AS PROVED FACTORS FOR DISEASES DEVELOPMENT AND WINE EFFECTS

In physiological conditions, both enzymatic and non-enzymatic systems preserve the oxidant/antioxidant status. However, these systems are overwhelmed during oxidative stress, which is a metabolic derangement due to an imbalance caused either by an excessive generation of ROS or by a diminished capacity of the antioxidant defense system.

As a simplified way, it could be certainly mentioned that diseases are the result of cell functioning disorders that might lead or not into systemic alterations as a chain reaction. Impairment of cell function might be caused by several factors, typically more than one acting at the same time, enhancing the same pathophysiological pathway or other. In the other hand, we have exposed the most important conditions involving ROS either as direct cellular damage agents or their behavior as mediators implicated in pathophysiological pathways [Freeman & Crapo 1982; Mantle & Preedy 1999].

Then, it should be expected that the interaction between oxidant and antioxidant agents, and thus ROS generation, is somehow implicated in different kinds of diseases development, as well as in its prevention by means of enhancing the antioxidant system.

3.1. Antioxidant Compounds of Wine

Grapes contain a wide variety of polyphenols including resveratrol, catechins, flavonoids and its derivatives, flavons, flavonols, and anthocyanins.

Several studies are in agreement that, among other alcoholic beverages, particularly wine shows healthy properties [Di Castelnuovo et al 2002; Böhm et al 2004; Rimm & Stampfer 2002]. A likely explanation can be its peculiar composition due to the methods employed to obtain it. Maturation in oak barrels distinguishes wine from beer, thereby enriching the polyphenol content in wine.

Polyphenolic compounds could play a major role in enhancing the antioxidant system, since they behave as ROS scavengers, metal chelators and enzyme modulators [Pietta et al. 1998]. In general, more than two thirds of the polyphenols consumed in the diet are flavonoids.

Red wine flavonoids have generated a great interest especially due to their *in vivo* and *in vitro* antioxidant capabilities. Indeed, these compounds are particularly abundant in red wine and possess a number of biological effects that might participate in vascular protection, including anti-aggregatory, antioxidant and free radical scavenging properties.

Quercetin and resveratrol are probably the most investigated wine polyphenols. The first is a bioflavonoid that is present not only in grape but also in tea and many fruits and vegetables (onion and apple). Resveratrol is a notable polpolyphenolic phytoalexin compound, more specifically a stilbenoid. It has recently attracted great attention due to its role in mimicking calorie restriction and lifespan extension in rats [Barger et al 2008], or even more, its property on the inhibition of migration and invasion of human breast-cancer cells. [Tang et al 2008]

3.2. Wine Protective Effect Against ROS Mediated Diseases

ROS are thought to contribute to the pathogenesis of a number of seemingly unrelated disorders, including tissue inflammation, cancer, heart failure, hypertension, preeclampsia and atherosclerosis. All of these have been extensively studied over the past few years and, in-between them, deleterious effect of ROS seems to be a constant

In order to explain this, some examples of widely known syndromes and wine effects will be described as follow:

3.2.1. Metabolic Syndrome

The metabolic syndrome (MS) include a variety of cardio-metabolic abnormalities associated with a high risk of developing type 2 diabetes and cardiovascular disease (CVD), first cause of death among elder population. Recent studies have demonstrated multiple beneficial effects of moderate wine consumption in the protection against development of the MS and its related medical complications.

Polyphenols, possess multiple benefits on the MS beyond alcohol through their anti-oxidant, anti-inflammatory, vascular-protective and insulin-sensitizing properties.

For instance, resveratrol can act as a potent activator of the NAD+-dependent deacetylases to expand the life span and to prevent the deleterious effects of excess eating on insulin resistance and metabolic derangement. Also, resveratrol has multiple protective effects against the MS thereby stimulating cAMP-activated protein kinase and promoting mitochondria biogenesis [Liu L et al. 2008]

3.2.2. Cardiovascular diseases

Many epidemiological studies have shown that regular intake of natural polyphenols in grape juice, red wine and in some other beverages is associated with reduced risk of cardiovascular diseases [Fuster et al. 1992, Middleton et al. 2000]. Also, the Mediterranean diet, rich in fruits, vegetables and red wine was suggested to protect against the development of cardiovascular diseases [Hertog et al.1995, De Lorgeril et al. 1996].

The association of moderate wine consumption with lower incidence of atherosclerotic heart disease has been repeatedly documented in numerous epidemiological studies on diverse ethnic groups. For instance, flavonoids might interfere with atherosclerotic plaque development and stability, vascular thrombosis and occlusion, explaining by means of this way their vascular protective properties [Zenebe & Pecháňová 2002; Curin & Andriantsitohaina 2005; Andriantsitohaina et al. 2005; Brito et al. 2006]. In fact, resveratrol is able to regulate the expression of genes involved in lipid uptake and efflux strongly suggesting that polyphenols could limit cholesterol accumulation in human macrophages, thus delaying the onset of atheromatous lesions [Sevov et al. 2006]. Moreover, resveratrol protects human umbilical vein endothelial cells against oxidized LDL-induced cytotoxicity, apoptosis, generation of ROS, and intracellular calcium accumulation [Ou et al 2006].

On the other hand, flavonoids may interact with the generation of NO from vascular endothelium, which leads not only to vasodilation, but also to the expression of genes that protect the cardiovascular system [Middleton et al. 2000; Zenebe & Pecháňová 2002; Curin & Andriantsitohaina 2005]. Flavonoids might also protect different tissues against ischemic damage on stroke disease, as they reduce oxidative and nitrosative stress responsible for cellular death.

Finally, other polyphenols may also contribute to the preservation of the integrity of cells belonging to the vascular wall, mainly those in the endothelium, by acting on the signaling cascades implicated in endothelial apoptosis [Corder et al. 2006].

3.3.3. Hypertension

In rats, long-term ethanol ingestion significantly increases both diastolic and systolic blood pressures, by means of down-regulating the eNOS and the vascular endothelial growth factor, leading to depletion of aortic NO levels. In addition, the aortic NADPH oxidase activity is significantly enhanced, thereby increasing lipid peroxidation and depressing the reduced to oxidized ratio of gluthathione. Thus, ethanol finally leads into impaired vasorelaxation and hypertension in rats [Husain 2007].

However, several authors have reported that extracts from grape and wine induce endothelium-dependent relaxation *via* enhanced generation and/or increased biological activity of NO which leads to the elevation of cGMP level [Fitzpatrick *et al.* 1993; Andriambeloson *et al.* 1997]. The increase in the intracellular Ca^{2+} level proceeds *via* a redox-sensitive pathway to the activation of NO synthase, the production of NO and thus endothelium-dependent vasodilation in different types of arteries from various species [Andriambeloson *et al.* 1999, Zenebe *et al.* 2003, Duarte *et al.* 2004]. The latter is also applicable in short-term oral administration of red wine polyphenolic compounds, which decreases blood pressure in normotensive rats [Diebolt et al. 2001].

Because the action of red wine polyphenolic compounds has been associated with the improvement of endothelium-dependent relaxation and elevation of NO synthase activity and/or expression in several *in vitro* and *in vivo* experiments [Andriambeloson *et al.* 1998, Pecháňová *et al.* 2004], it may be assumed about a possible therapeutic effect of polyphenols in diseases associated with reduced NO bioavailability such as endothelial dysfunction or atherosclerosis

4. KIDNEY, ROS AND BENEFICIAL WINE EFFECTS

There exists very limited data concerning the relationship between wine consumption and kidney disease. However, considerable experimental evidence supports the view that ROS could play a key role in the pathophysiological processes of seemingly unrelated renal diseases [Rodrigo&Rivera 2002].

The abundance of PUFA makes the kidney an organ particularly vulnerable to ROS attack [Kubo el at. 1997]. The involvement of ROS in the mechanism of renal damage is supported by two lines of experimental evidence: (i) detection of products of oxidant injury in renal tissue or urine, and (ii) experimental demonstration of a protective effect of metabolic inhibitors of ROS [Ishikawa et al. 1994].

4.1. ROS-Related Renal Diseases

Oxidative stress upregulates the expression of adhesion molecules, chemoattractant compounds and cytokines [Klahr 2001], mediating a wide range of renal impairments like chronic renal failure, hemodialysis, rhabdomyolysis, renal fibrosis, glomerulosclerosis, kidney stones, and hyperlipidemia, among others, leading to glomerular damage.

4.1.1. Chronic Renal Failure And Hemodialysis:

In chronic renal failure (CRF), ROS causes glomerular and tubulointerstitial damage by activating and maintaining vicious cycles through cytokine release, leukocyte infiltration, fibrosis, and mesangial and endothelial cell apoptoses. Also, endothelial dysfunction is present in subjects with CRF and is inter-related to oxidative stress [Annuk et al 2003]. An increased synthesis of $O_2\bullet^-$ reduces NO bioavailability by inactivation, leading to peroxynitrite formation. Following peroxynitrite protonation it will break off with liberating the highly peroxidant OH•. Endothelium is affected by this reaction in two different ways: 1) NO scavenging impairs its vasodilating activity and 2) OH• causes cell damage [Galle&Wanner 1997].

In the progression of renal diseases a key role is played by cytokines, particularly by transforming growth factor beta (TGF-β). This molecule has several biological effects, including an increase of glomerular permeability to proteins [Sharma et al. 2000] and stimulation of extracellular matrix synthesis. It has been demonstrated that oxidative stress is interrelated with both increased TGF-β production and upregulation of its expression [Sharma et al. 2000; Klahr&Morrissey 2000].

There exist basically two kinds of treatments for terminal CRF: kidney transplant or hemodialysis.

On transplanted patients, the isquemia/reperfusion cycle is inevitable, and it is widely known that this mechanism is one of the most important source of ROS generation on tissues, including of course kidney, thereby generating renal damage immediately after surgery. In the other hand, oxidative stress contributes to morbidity in hemodializyed patients. In order of importance, three possible sources of ROS have been suggested to contribute to the development of oxidative stress: the uremic state, the dialyzer membrane, and bacterial contaminants from the dialysate [Ward & McLeish 2003].

4.1.2. Renal Fibrosis

In renal fibrosis (RF), a major role is played by Plasminogen Activator Inhibitor-1 (PAI-1), which promotes the accumulation of the extracellular matrix through the inhibition of plasmin-dependent extracellular matrix degradation [Kimura 2005].

Local production of TGF-β, by intrinsic renal cells or by macrophages invading the kidney, is also a key mediator of renal fibrosis. Activation of TGF-beta stimulates endothelin production which, in turn, is a potent stimulus for fibrogenesis [Klahr 2001].

Additionally, transcription factors such as nuclear factor-κB (NF-κB), which is a regulator of many genes involved in the control of immune and inflammatory responses, has a leading role in RF along with diabetes and atherosclerosis development. The activation of these transcriptional factors is directly influenced by ROS and inflammatory signals, such as tumor necrosis factor-alpha (TNF-α) [Baldwin 2001]. Moreover, •O_2- and peroxynitrite are involved in the apoptosis of mesangial cells produced by TNF-α and this effect is mediated by tyrosine kinase [Kitamura & Ishikawa 1999]. However, it was recently shown that, in human mesangial cells, intracellular calcium, but not ROS, mediates proinflammatory cytokine-induced NF-κB activation [Chang 2006].

4.1.3. Glomerulonephritis

ROS are increasingly believed to be important intracellular signaling molecules in mitogenic pathways involved in the pathogenesis of glomerulonephritis (GN). In rats treated with anti-Thy1, as nephritis induced model, an increased expression of glomerular TGF-β and mRNA nephritis was found. ROS production was increased by four or five times. This was significantly attenuated and mesangial cell transformation into myofibroblasts was completely prevented by treatment with alpha-lipoic acid. The effects of alpha-lipoic acid were at least partially due to inhibition of oxidative stress [Budisavljevic et al. 2003]. In mesangioproliferative GN, the increase of ROS is thought to be produced by a pronounced dysregulation of pro-oxidative and antioxidative enzymes leading to a net increase in glomerular ROS levels [Gaertner et. al 2002].

4.1.4. Glomerulosclerosis: Hyperlipidemia and Hyperlipoproteinemia

Either both of these conditions can aggravate glomerulosclerosis (GE) or renal tubulointerstitial damage in kidneys without primary immunologic disease. Enhanced generation of ROS is demonstrated by a rise in oxidant enzymes activity, and generation of hypochlorite-modified proteins in renal tissue and urine, thereby contributing to the deleterious effects of hyperlipidemia on the renal damage [Scheuer et al., 2000].

The glomerulus is considerably more sensitive to oxidative injuries than other nephron segments. Oxidative stress may alter the structure and function of the glomerulus because of the effects of ROS on mesangial and endothelial cells [Klahr, 1997].

Lipoprotein glomerulopathy has been characterized by a relatively rapid progression to renal impairment and the development of GE [Sakatsume et al., 2001]. The glomerular oxidative damage leading to GE is mediated by oxidized forms of LDL (LDL-ox), which increase in oxidative stress status. In CRF, LDL frequently undergoes glycation, oxidation, and carbonylation [Galle & Wagner 1999]. Oxidation of LDL is induced by infiltrating leukocytes resulting in increased glomerular damage. LDL-ox induces a dual effect in cultured human endothelial cells: they promote cell proliferation at low concentrations but stimulate apoptosis at higher concentrations and both actions are related to oxidative stress [Galle et. al 2001]. LDL-ox may stimulate the genic expression of fibronectin through the autocrine secretion of TGF-β in cultured human glomerular epithelial cells [Ding et al., 1997].

On the other hand, native LDL has shown a dose-dependent stimulation of proliferation of cultured mesangial cells [Nishida et al., 1999], a response attributed to an enhancement of expression of c-jun and c-fos genes, involved in the cellular proliferation and DNA synthesis in mesangial cells during LDL exposure [Gröne et al., 1996]. Antioxidant enzymes, such as CAT and SOD, but not GSH-Px, may partially inhibit the effect of LDL on DNA synthesis [Greiber et al., 1996]. Native LDL was also found to induce the generation of ROS in rat glomerular cells [Wanner et al., 1997], although other studies found no effect of LDL in the production of $O_2^{\cdot-}$ anion by mesangial and endothelial cells in vitro [Galle et al., 1999]. In addition, native LDL can also stimulate fibronectin secretion by mesangial cells.

Atherogenic lipoproteins induce formation of ROS not only in arteries, but also in glomeruli and juxtaglomerular cells, causing an inhibition of NO-mediated vasodilation, stimulation of renin release, and modulation of mesangial cell growth and proliferation. The damaging effect of the lipoproteins can be prevented by antioxidant enzymes and HDL [Wanner et al. 1997]. Also, low concentrations of lipoprotein(a) (Lp(a)) stimulated growth of mesangial cells, whereas higher concentrations had antiproliferative or toxic effects. The stimulation on mesangial cell proliferation, as well as the cytotoxic effects caused by Lp(a) are both likely to have a negative impact on the course of renal disease. Indeed, serum levels of the Lp(a) are elevated in patients with nephrotic syndrome and Lp(a) deposits have been identified in diseased glomeruli [Greiber et. al 1996].

These data support a role of oxidative stress and dyslipoproteinemia in the pathogenesis of glomerulosclerosis associated with renal diseases. Although the presence of an excessive amount of LDL is recognized as a factor of glomerular damage, its role in the production of oxidative stress has yet to be fully elucidated.

4.1.5. Myoglobinuria, Rhabdomyolysis And Acute Renal Failure

Myoglobinuria plays a key role in the pathophysiology of both acute renal failure in clinical settings that are characterized by muscle tissue injury [Vanholder et al. 2000], and in a widely used animal model of glycerol-induced rhabdomyolysis.

The term rhabdomyolysis refers to disintegration of striated muscle, which results in the release of muscular cell constituents into the extracellular fluid and the circulation. One of the key compounds released is myoglobin, an 18,800-Dalton oxygen carrier. It resembles hemoglobin, but contains only one heme moiety.

Normally, myoglobin is loosely bound to plasma globulins and only small amounts reach the urine. However, when massive amounts of myoglobin are released, the binding capacity of the plasma protein is exceeded. Myoglobin is then filtered by the glomeruli and reaches the tubules, where it may cause obstruction and renal dysfunction [Zager 1996]. The intratubular degradation of myoglobin results in a massive generation of ROS that overwhelms the scavenging capacity of the antioxidant system, thereby generating renal damage. In fact, myoglobin induces proximal tubular cell death through the generation of H_2O_2 [Zager 1997]. Also, during rhabdomyolysis potentially toxic myocyte contents are released into the systemic circulation, and the renal consequences of this disturbance have been attributed to both intense vasoconstriction and renal tubular necrosis.

4.1.6. Angiotensin II Increase And Kidney Stones

Numerous pharmacologic interventions that ameliorate the increased expansion of the interstitial volume, decrease the expression of TGF-β, and down-regulate the production of extracellular matrix and the infiltration of the interstitium by macrophages have been described, attempting to inhibit the activity of Angiotensin II enzyme (AT-II). One of the most widely known kinds of those drugs are angiotensin converting enzyme inhibitors.

It is also known that ROS play a mayor role in renal vasoconstrictor responses to acute and chronic stimulation by AT-II and norepinephrine, as well as in long-term effects of endothelin-1 (ET-1) [Just et al. 2008]. AT-II plays a pivotal role in the progression of renal diseases, including obstructive nephropathy. The increased levels of AT-II in obstructive nephropathy upregulate the expression of several factors, including TGF-β, TNF-α and NF-κB, among others [Klahr 2001], and the activation of membrane-bound NADPH-ox, thereby generating •O_2- which, in turn, leads to hypertrophy of renal tubular cells [Hannken 1998]. NF-κB is also implicated in the setting of ureteral obstruction, leading to sustained obstructive nephropathy and apoptosis of tubular epithelial cells.

Renal damage resulting from unilateral ureteral obstruction (UUO) may be aggravated by ROS. It is known that obstructive nephropathy and sodium wasting or depletion leads to progressive renal tubular atrophy and interstitial fibrosis. In rats, it was found that sodium depletion without UUO increased several renal antioxidant enzymes, what is consistent with a stress response to increased ROS production. Furthermore, UUO not only reduced antioxidant enzyme activities but also inhibited increases seen with sodium depletion [Kinter et al. 1999]. Then, it could be concluded that that suppression of renal antioxidant enzyme activities by UUO contributes to the progression of renal injury in obstructive nephropathy, which indeed is exacerbated by sodium depletion.

4.1.7. Diabetic Nephropathy

Oxidative stress has been known to play an important role in the development and progression of diabetic nephropathy. High glucose induces intracellular ROS either directly via glucose metabolism and auto-oxidation or indirectly through the formation of advanced glycation end products and their receptor binding. ROS mimic the stimulatory effects of elevated glycemia and upregulate TGF-β, PAI-1, and other extracellular matrix proteins by glomerular mesangial cells, thus leading to mesangial expansion and subsequent renal damage [Ha & Lee 2001]

4.2. Red Wine Effects on the Kidney

Before explaining the positive consequences of moderate wine intake, we must distinguish the actions effected by alcohol *per se* on the kidney and those from the non-alcoholic wine components, mainly polyphenols. Some observations deriving from experimental studies and human diseases indicate a negative effect of high doses of ethanol on kidney function, but moderate doses could have some beneficial effects. In turn, wine polyphenols seem to be protective through different mechanisms: they act as antioxidants, protect the endothelium, and interfere with apoptotic mechanisms. These effects will be separately analyzed in the following sections.

4.2.1. Alcohol Effects on the Kidney

In rats, despite the evidence supporting that acute ethanol administration causes a dose-dependent impairment of the antioxidant system [Scott et. al 2000], or glomerular damage [Cecchin & De Marchi, 1996], a protection against oxidative injury may also be postulated on the basis of data found in experimental models of ethanol consumption. In fact, several studies confirm that long-term consumption increases the activity of antioxidant enzymes such as catalase [Orellana et al. 1998], superoxide dismutase [Dreosti et al. 1982], and glutathione peroxidase [Rodrigo et al 2002].

To test the hypothesis that ethanol might be able to inhibit tissue fibrosis and therefore progression of renal diseases, some investigators used a rat model of glomerulonephritis induced by injection of anti-thy1 antibodies [Peters et al. 2003]. The acute form of renal damage (ARF) was a reversible mesangioproliferative glomerulonephritis; whereas the chronic one (CRF) was an irreversible and progressive glomerulosclerosis with tubulointerstitial fibrosis. However, in both forms the daily administration of 40 mL of beer (the equivalent of 2 mL ethanol intake) did not influence TGF-β level or renal matrix protein production and accumulation. Then, prevailing long-term effect is difficult to predict, even in this animal organ.

In humans, it was demonstrated in autopsy studies that long-term alcohol abuse is associated with renal alterations, including tubular dysfunction, acute tubular necrosis, and immunoglobulin A (IgA) nephropathy. Also, structural and functional renal abnormalities have been observed in the fetal alcohol syndrome, which occurs in children prenatally exposed to ethanol [Cecchin & De Marchi 1996].

Alcohol consumption could interact with other risk factors [McCann et al. 2003]. For instance, alcohol intake and smoking are often related to each other, and cigarette smoking has been positively associated to the number of drinks consumed [Volpato 2004]. Recent studies confirmed that long-term intake of ethanol and nicotine may produce similar and, in some occasions, additive tissue injuries based on increased oxidative stress [Husain et al. 2001].

4.2.2. Non-Alcoholic Wine Compounds Effects on the Kidney: Polyphenols

After long-term exposure to polyphenol-rich red wine, an enhancement of antioxidant defenses was demonstrated in rat plasma and kidney [Rodrigo et al 2002]. In addition, in autoradiographic studies, 3 hours after oral administration, labeled *trans*-resveratrol was found in different mouse tissues, occurring kidney as the second most labeled organ [Vitrac 2003]. Thus, it is reasonable to hypothesize that long-term wine consumption allows the obtaining of effective resveratrol concentration in human kidney. Cis-resveratrol, another resveratrol isomer, is critically involved in regulating the expression of the genes involved in NF-κB signaling [Leiro 2005] whose leading role in renal damage was previously described.

Recently, it was demonstrated that resveratrol, suppresses the proteinuria, hypoalbuminemia and hyperlipidemia induced by anti-rat kidney serum in a glomerulonephritis rat model [Nihei et al 2001]. Resveratrol is also a powerful inhibitor of human c-p450 [Chun et al 1999], whose activity is enhanced by long-term ethanol ingestion. In rat kidney red wine administration attenuated c-p450 activity, suggesting an inhibition by non-alcoholic wine components [Orellana et al. 2002]. Additionally, pretreatment with resveratrol in rat kidney had antioxidant and anti-inflammatory effects [Bertelli et al. 2002], resulting in prevention of leukocyte recruitment and less endothelial barrier damage [Shigematsu et al. 2003].

In rats, resveratrol [Giovannini et al. 2001] and quercetin [Kahraman et al. 2003] exerted protective effects in renal ROS scavenging challenges like, for example, models of renal ischemia/reperfusion injury. Quercetin administration reduced oxidative stress and improved renal function [Anjaneyulu et al. 2004].

In the experimental model of ARF through myoglobinuric renal damage caused by glycerol, the administration of quercetin provide a protective effect due to its radical-scavenging and iron-chelating activities [Rodrigo et al. 2002; Chander&Chopra 2005]. This is explained on the basis of its ability to inhibit apoptosis of mesangial cells by blocking tyrosine phosphorylation [Li et al. 2005]], as was confirmed *in vitro* and *in vivo* [Ishikawa & Kitamura 2000]. Although these studies have been performed in rodents, it was suggested that this protection may be useful to prevent or treat myoglobinuric acute renal failure in humans [Stefanovic at al. 2000], two species having a great similarity on the mechanism of renal injury in this setting.

Quercitin also protects the rat kidney against oxidative stress-related damage caused by cyclosporine [Satyanarayana et al. 2001]. In this field, provinol administration showed a similar renoprotective effect. [Buffoli et al. 2005]

In the mouse kidney tannic acid, another plant polyphenol, has been demonstrated to reduce ROS production by modulating enzymes involved in oxidative metabolism [Krajka-Kuzniak & Baer-Dubowska 2003]. Alpha-G-rutin, another wine polyphenol, served to prevent oxidative renal damage in mice treated with Fe-NTA [Shimoi et al., 1997].

4.2.3. Beneficial Red Wine Effects on the Kidney

Accordingly to the evidence here presented, it could be hypothesized that interventions aimed to favor the scavenging and/or depuration of ROS, like those involving long-term exposure to red wine polyphenols through moderate wine intake, should attenuate or prevent the new onset oxidative stress. This effect should protect the kidney against the subsequent oxidative damage. Since the kidney is a highly perfused organ, it is reasonable to asume that favorable wine effects could be enhanced in comparison to others tissues.

It is remarkable the fact that the antioxidant protection by wine is possible through the combined effects of ethanol and nonalcoholic wine components with antioxidant and chelating properties. Indeed, although dietary supplements containing polyphenols have been used in humans, a safety assessment of the applied dose has been recommended due to the possibility of some adverse effect of this mode of consumption [Mennen et al., 2005]. For instance, in mice, it was demonstrated that the renoprotective effect against rhabdomyolysis following glycerol injection was significantly higher in chronic red wine intake, rather than alcohol-free red wine or ethanol (Fig. 1). The morphological consequences of this experience are illustrated in figures 2, 3 and 4 [Rodrigo et. al 2004].

A recent meta-analysis has underlined that ethanol consumption is directly related to the relative risk of arterial hypertension [Corrao et al. 2004]. However, hypertensive subjects who are moderate wine drinkers seem to have a lower hypertension-related mortality compared with hypertensive subjects who are not drinkers [Renaud et al. 2004]. In fact, in rat kidney, it was found that long-term exposure to ethanol increased sodium-potassium-activated adenosine triphosphatase activity [(Na + K)-ATPase], with a consequent antinatriuretic effect [Rodrigo & Thielemann 1997].

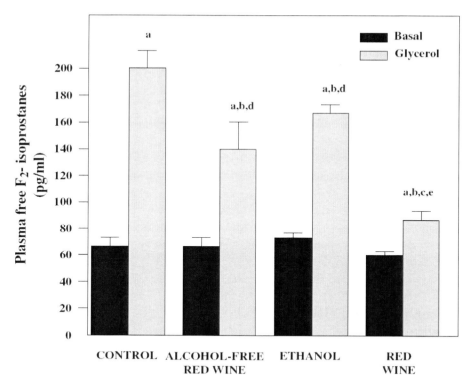

Figure 1. Effects of rhabdomyolysis on plasma levels of free F2- isoprostanes in control, ethanol, red wine and alcohol-free red wine groups. Values are means±SE (n¼20). Statistically significant differences, at $P<0.05$, are indicated by superscript letters: avs basal, bvs control-glycerol, cvs ethanol-glycerol, dvs red wineglycerol and evs alcohol-free red wine-glycerol.

However, when red wine or alcohol-free red wine was used, (Na + K)-ATPase activity was not influenced [Rodrigo & Rivera 2002]. Also, the influence of polyphenols on NO-dependent vasodilation, described previously, might be particularly beneficial in CRF which is accompanied by an impairment of NO-signaling mechanisms in peripheral arterioles [Bagi et al. 2003]. Thus, in subjects with CRF who are frequently hypertensive, wine consumption might reduce the hypertension-related organ injury. In fact, recently the possible advantage of a moderate wine consumption in patients with chronic renal failure was hypothesized [Caimi et al., 2004].

Atherosclerosis development is accelerated in CRF and constitutes the major cause of death in this clinical setting. Both increased oxidative stress and endothelial dysfunction are relevant aspects of atherogenesis in CRF patients and should be targets for antioxidant treatment, such as red wine polyphenols [Caimi et al. 2004].

Strong evidence shows that there is an inverse association between moderate alcohol intake, especially red wine, and the risk of renal cell cancer. The lower risk did not change even among population with high risk factors of cancer development [Greving et al. 2007; Lee et al. 2007].

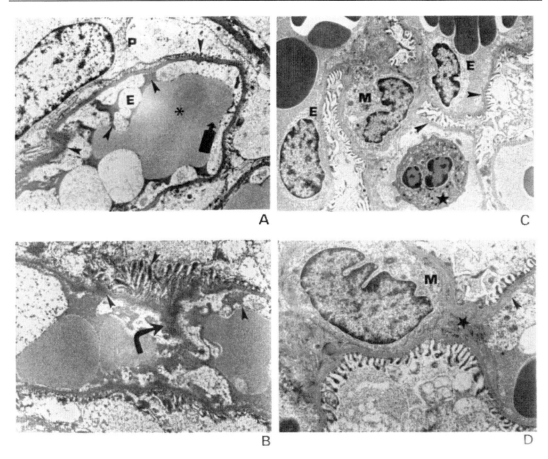

Figure 2. Electron micrographs of the kidneys of rats from the control (A and B) and red wine (C and D) groups showing the ultrastructural characteristics of the glomerulus of a nephron, after 6 h of glycerol injection. (A) The swelling of the endothelium (E), electron-dense deposits within the endothelial cells, the foot processes and the Glomerular basement membrane (GBM) (arrow heads) and glomerular capillary lumen (thick arrow) with dark plasma (*) (original_25 000) are shown. (B) The electron-dense deposits causing the GBM to protrude into the capillary lumen (arrow). The same deposits were present in the cytoskeleton of the foot processes, the endothelial cells, and the GBM (arrow heads). The foot processes were all intact and detachments from the GBM were not seen (originalx35 000). (C) The normal endothelium (E), mesangium (M) and filtration barrier (arrow heads). Presence of a neutrophil in the capillary lumen (star) (originalx35 000). (D) A normal mesangium (M) and filtration barrier (arrow heads) and mesangial matrix (star) are shown. Electron-dense deposits were not seen (originalx38 500).

In diabetic patients the administration of moderate amounts of red wine and a carbohydrate-restricted, low-iron available and polyphenol-enriched diet was significantly more effective than a standard diet in slowing the progression of diabetic nephropathy [Facchini & Saylor 2003]. It is also notable that moderate prandial wine consumption has no adverse effects on the glycemic control on these patients [Gin et al. 1992], and it did not improve or impair insulin sensitivity in overweight women or change any of the known correlates of insulin sensitivity, including body weight and composition, blood lipid profile, and blood pressure [Cordain et al. 2000].

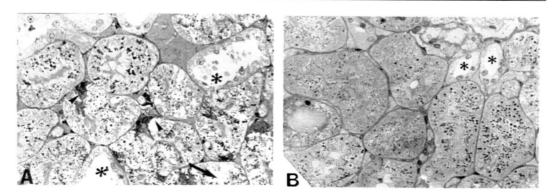

Figure 3. Micrographs of the kidneys of rats from the control (A) and red wine (B) groups showing the histological characteristics of the tubular epithelium at 6 h after glycerol injection. (A) The proximal convoluted tubules displaying tubular necrosis with vacuolar and hydropic cell degeneration (arrow) and tubulorhexis (arrow heads) are shown. The distal convoluted tubules showed exfoliated cells (*) (originalx400). In contrast, kidneys from the red wine group (B) showed normal distal convoluted tubules (*) and proximal convoluted tubules without tubular necrosis (originalx400).

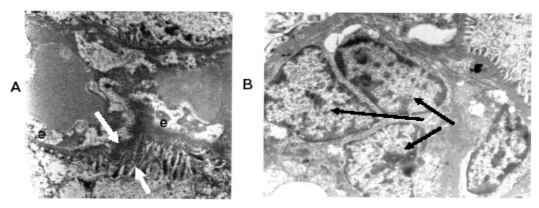

Figure 4. Electron micrographs of the kidney of rats from the control (A) and red wine (B) groups, showing in (A) the endothelium with obliteration of the pores and electron-dense deposits in the foot processes and the (GBM). (B) shows only the expansion of the mesangial cells.

Studies in rats demonstrated that long-term wine exposure reduced LDL-cholesterol through its nonalcoholic components, thereby protecting the kidney against the deleterious effects of LDL and their oxidized derivatives on the glomerulus [Cascon et al., 2001]. This effect could be reinforced by a preservation of polyunsaturated fatty acids of kidney phospholipids, also attributed to polyphenols [Araya et al., 2001].

Another possible *in vivo* beneficial action of red wine beverages in kidney was induced by decreasing the activity of ATII, in a short-term administration model in rats [Honsho et al. 2005].

5. CONCLUSION

Oxidative stress plays a mayor role in cellular damage, and it is involved in several mechanisms leading to a variety of unrelated diseases, including of course renal injury.

Chronic red wine intake should ameliorate the renal damage caused by oxidative stress. The renoprotective effects of red wine have been attributed to the synergistic effects of both alcohol and polyphenolic compounds, although the effects of the latter seem to dominate in this matter. However, the relative contributions of polyphenols and ethanol remain to be fully elucidated, especially in humans. Further investigations, like controlled clinical trials, are needed to confirm the possible efficacy of a new therapeutic door based on the beneficial effects of red wine compounds, especially polyphenols.

Table 1.

Oxidant	Chemical Name	Description	Process
$\cdot O_2^-$,	Superoxide radical anion	One-electron reduction state of O_2, formed in many auto-oxidation reactions and by the electron transport chain	Rather unreactive but can release Fe^{2+} from iron-sulfur proteins and ferritin
H_2O_2,	Hydrogen peroxide	Two-electron reduction state, formed by dismutation of $\cdot O_2^-$ or by direct reduction of O_2	Lipid soluble and thus able to diffuse across membranes
$\cdot OH$,	Hydroxyl radical	Three-electron reduction state, formed by Fenton reaction and decomposition of peroxynitrite.	Extremely reactive, will attack most cellular components
$^1O_2$	Singlet oxygen	It is the lowest electronically excited singlet state of molecular oxygen	Not a free radical but highly reactive; its oxidation induces citotoxic damage.

From [Sies 1985; Docampo 1995; Rice-Evans&Gopinathan 1995]

Table 2.

Antioxidant enzyme	Chemical Name	Scavenged Oxidant agent	General characteristics
GSH-Px	Glutathione peroxidase	H_2O_2	It is the major endogenous antioxidant molecule. It catalyzes the conversion of H2O2 and organic peroxides into water or alcohols, respectively.
SOD	superoxide dismutase	$\cdot O_2^-$,	It catalyzes the conversion of O2•− to O2 and to less-reactive species like H2O2. Necessary for the release of biologically active NO. It protects NO from inactivation.
CAT	Catalase	H_2O_2,	It catalyzes the break down of H2O2 to water and molecular oxygen.

From [Valko&Rhodes 2006].

REFERENCES

[1] Ames J.B., Tanaka T., Ikura M., Stryer L. Nuclear magnetic resonance evidence for Ca(2+)-induced extrusion of the myristoyl group of recoverin. *J. Biol. Chem.* (1995) 270: 30909–30913.

[2] Andriambeloson E, Kleschyov AL, Muller B, Beretz A, Stoclet JC, Andriantsitohaina R. Nitric oxide production and endothelium-dependent vasorelaxation induced by wine polyphenols in rat thoracic aorta. *Br J Pharmacol* (1997) 120: 1053-1058.

[3] Andriambeloson E, Magnier C, Haan-Archipoff G, Lobstein A, Anton R, Beretz A, Stoclet JC, Andriantsitohaina R: Natural dietary polyphenolic compounds caused endothelium-dependent vasorelaxation in rat thoracic aorta. *J Nutr* (1998) 128: 2324-2333,.

[4] Andriambeloson E, Stoclet JC, Andriantsitohaina R: Mechanism of endothelial nitric oxidedependent vasorelaxation induced by wine polyphenols in rat thoracic aorta. *J Cardiovasc Pharmacol* (1999) 33: 248-254.

[5] Andriantsitohaina R, Curin Y, Ritz MF, Gerald R, Alves A, Mendelowitsch A, Elbaz M. Polyphenols: protection of neurovascular unit in stroke and inhibition of in-stent-neointimal growth. *Physiol Res* (2005) 54: 51P.

[6] Anjaneyulu M, Chopra K. Quercetin, an anti-oxidant bioflavonoid, attenuates diabetic nephropathy in rats. *Clin Exp Pharmacol Physiol* (2004) 21: 244–8.

[7] Annuk M, Zilmer M, Fellstrom B. Endothelium-dependent vasodilation and oxidative stress in chronic renal failure: impact on cardiovascular disease. *Kidney Int* (2003) 63:S50 –3.

[8] Araya J, Rodrigo R, Orellana M, Rivera G. Red wine raises plasma HDL and preserves long-chain polyunsaturated fatty acids in rat kidney and erythrocytes. *Br J Nutr.* (2001) 86:189-95.

[9] Bagi Z, Hamar P, Antus B, Rosivall L, Koller A. Chronic renal failure leads to reduced flow-dependent dilation in isolated rat skeletal muscle arterioles due to lack of NO mediation. *Kidney Blood Press Res* (2003) 26:19 –26.

[10] Baik I, Shin C. Prospective study of alcohol consumption and metabolic syndrome. Am *J Clin Nutr.* (2008) 87:1455-63.

[11] Baldwin AS Jr. Series introduction: the transcription factor NF-kappaB and human disease. *Clin Invest.* (2001) 107:3-6.

[12] Baldwin AS Jr. The transcription factor NF-kB and human disease. *J Clin Invest* (2001) 107:3– 6.

[13] Barger JL, Kayo T, Vann JM, Arias EB, Wang J, Hacker TA, Wang Y, Raederstorff D, Morrow JD, Leeuwenburgh C, Allison DB, Saupe KW, Cartee GD, Weindruch R, Prolla TA.1 A low dose of dietary resveratrol partially mimics caloric restriction and retards aging parameters in mice. *PLoS ONE.* (2008) 3:2264.

[14] Bertelli AA, Migliori M, Panichi V, et al. Resveratrol, a component of wine and grapes, in the prevention of kidney disease. *Ann N Y Acad Sci* (2002) 957:230–8.

[15] Böhm M, Rosenkranz S, Laufs U. Alcohol and red wine: impact on cardiovascular risk. *Nephrol Dial Transplant* (2004) 19:11– 6.

[16] Brito PM, Mariano A, Almeida LM, Dinis TCP. Resveratrol affords protection against peroxynitrite-mediated endothelial cell death: a role for intracellular glutathione. *Chem Biol Interact* (2006) 164:157–66.

[17] Brown GC, Borutaite V. Nitric oxide, mitochondria, and cell death. *IUBMB Life*. (2001) 52:189-95.

[18] Budisavljevic MN, Hodge L, Barber K, Fulmer JR, Durazo-Arvizu RA, Self SE, Kuhlmann M, Raymond JR, Greene EL. Oxidative stress in the pathogenesis of experimental mesangial proliferative glomerulonephritis. *Am J Physiol Renal Physiol*. (2003) 285:F1138-48.

[19] Buffoli B, Pechanovà O, Kojsovà S, Andriantsitohaina R, Giugno L, Bianchi R, Rezzani R. Provinol prevents CsA-induced nephrotoxicity by reducing reactive oxygen species, iNOS, and NF-kB expression. *J Histochem Cytochem* (2005) 53:1459–68.

[20] Caimi, G., Carollo, C., Lo Presti, R.,. Chronic renal failure: oxidative stress, endothelial dysfunction and wine. *Clin. Nephrol* (2004) 62: 331–335.

[21] Cecchin E, De Marchi S. Alcohol misuse and renal damage. *Addict Biol* (1996) 1:7–17.

[22] Cecchin E, De Marchi S. Alcohol misuse and renal damage. *Addiction Biology* (1996) 1:7–17.

[23] Chance B., Schoener B., Oshino R., Itshak F., Nakase Y. Oxidation-reduction ratio studies of mitochondria in freezetrapped samples. NADH and flavoprotein fluorescence signals. *J. Biol. Chem.* (1979) 254: 4764–4771.

[24] Chander V, Chopra K. Role of nitric oxide in resveratrol-induced renal protective effects of ischemic preconditioning. *J Vasc Surg* (2005) 42:1198 –205.

[25] Chang JW, Kim CS, Kim SB, Park SK, Park JS, Lee SK. Proinflammatory cytokine-induced NF-kappaB activation in human mesangial cells is mediated through intracellular calcium but not ROS: effects of silymarin. *Nephron Exp Nephrol* (2006) 103:156 –165.

[26] Chao C. Associations between beer, wine, and liquor consumption and lung cancer risk: a meta-analysis. *Cancer Epidemiol Biomarkers*. (2007) 16:2436-47.

[27] Chun YJ, Kim MY, Guengerich FP. Resveratrol is a selective human cytochrome P450 1A1 inhibitor. *Biochem Biophys Res Commun* (1999) 262:20–4.

[28] Cordain, L.; Melby, C. L.; Hamamoto, A. E.; O'Neill, D. S.; Cornier, M. A.; Barakat, H. A.; Israel, R. G.; Hill, J. O. Influence of moderate chronic wine consumption on insulin sensitivity and other correlates of syndrome X in moderately obese women. *Metabolism* (2000) 49:1473–1478.

[29] Corder R, Mullen W, Khan NH, Marks SC, Wood EG, Carrier MJ, Crozier A. Oenology: red wine procyanidins and vascular health. *Nature* (2006) 444: 566.

[30] Corrao G, Bagnardi V, Zambon A, La Vecchia C. A meta-analysis of alcohol consumption and the risk of 15 diseases. Prev Med (2004) 38:613–9.

[31] Curin Y, Andriantsitohaina R: Polyphenols as potential therapeutic agents against cardiovascular diseases. *Pharmacol Rep* (2005) 57: 97-107.

[32] Da Luz PL, Coimbra SR. Wine, Alcohol and atherosclerosis: clinical evidences and mechanism. *Braz J Med Biol Res*. (2004) 37:1275-95.

[33] Davydov DR. Microsomal monooxygenase in apoptosis: another target for cytochrome c signaling?. *Trends Biochem Sci*. (2001) 26:155-60.

[34] De Lorgeril M, Salen P, Martin JL, Mamelle N, Monjaud I, Touboul P, Delaye J. Effect of a Mediterranean type of diet on the rate of cardiovascular complications in patients

with coronary artery disease. Insights into the protective effect of certain nutrients. *J Am Coll Cardiol* (1996) 28: 1103-1108.
[35] Di Castelnuovo A, Rotondo S, Iacoviello L, Donati MB, De Gaetano G. Meta-analysis of wine and beer consumption in relation to vascular risk. *Circulation* (2002) 105:2836–44.
[36] Diebolt M, Bucher B, Andriantsitohaina R. Wine polyphenols decrease blood pressure, improve NO vasodilatation, and induce gene expression. *Hypertension.* (2001) 38:159-65.
[37] Ding G, van Goor H, Ricardo SD, Orlowski JM, Diamond JR. Oxidized LDL stimulates the expression of TGF-beta and fibronectin in human glomerular epithelial cells. *Kidney Int.* (1997) 51:147-54.
[38] Dizdaroglu M., Jaruga P., Birincioglu M., Rodriguez H. Free radical-induced damage to DNA: mechanisms and measurement. *Free Radic. Biol. Med.* (2002) 32: 1102–1115.
[39] Docampo, R.. "Antioxidant mechanisms", in J. Marr and M. Müller, (Eds.): *Biochemistry and Molecular Biology of Parasites.* London: Academic Press, (1995)147-160.
[40] Dreosti IE, Manuel SJ, Buckley RA. Superoxide dismutase (EC1.15.1.1), manganese and the effect of ethanol in adult and foetal rats. *Br J Nutr* (1982) 48:205–10.
[41] Duarte J, Andriambeloson E, Diebolt M, Andriantsitohaina R: Wine polyphenols stimulate superoxide anion production to promote calcium signaling and endothelial-dependent vasodilatation. *Physiol Res* (2004) 53: 595-602.
[42] Dunn W, Xu R, Schwimmer JB. Modest wine drinking and decreased prevalence of suspected nonalcoholic fatty liver disease. *Hepatology* (2008) 47: 1947-54.
[43] Esterbauer H., Schaur R.J., Zollner H. Chemistry and biochemistry of 4-hydroxynonenal, malonaldehyde and related aldehydes. *Free Radic. Biol. Med.* (1991) 11: 81–128.
[44] Facchini FS, Saylor KL. A low-iron-available, polyphenol-enriched, carbohydrate-restricted diet to slow progression of diabetic nephropathy. *Diabetes* (2003) 52:1204 –9.
[45] Fitzpatrick D, Hirschfield SL, Coffey RG: Endothelium-dependent relaxing activity of wine and other grape products. *Am J Physiol* (1993) 265: H774-H778,
[46] Freeman BA, Crapo JD. Biology of disease: free radicals and tissue injury. *Lab Invest.* (1982) 47: 412-26.
[47] Fuster V, Badimon JJ, Chesebro JH: The patogenesis of coronary artery disease and the acute coronary syndromes. *New Engl J Med* (1992) 326: 242-250,.
[48] Gaertner SA, Janssen U, Ostendorf T, Koch KM, Floege J, Gwinner W. Glomerular oxidative and antioxidative systems in experimental mesangioproliferative glomerulonephritis. *J Am Soc Nephrol.* (2002) 13:2930-7.
[49] Galle J, Heinloth A, Wanner C, Heermeier K. Dual effect of oxidized LDL on cell cycle in human endothelial cells through oxidative stress. *Kidney Int* (2001) 78:S120 –3.
[50] Galle J, Wanner C. Modification of lipoproteins in uremia: oxidation, glycation and carbamoylation. *Miner Electrolyte Metab* (1999) 25: 263–8.
[51] Galle J, Wanner C. Oxidative stress and vascular injury-relevant for atherogenesis in uraemic patients? *Nephrol Dial Transplant* (1997)12: 2480–3.
[52] Gin, H.; Morlat, P.; Ragnaud, J. M.; Aubertin, J. Short-term effect of red wine (consumed during meals) on insulin requirement and glucose tolerance in diabetic patients. *Diabetes Care* (1992) 15:546–548.

[53] Giovannini L, Migliori M, Longoni BM, et al. Resveratrol, a polyphenol found in wine, reduces ischemia reperfusion injury in rat kidneys. *J Cardiovasc Pharmacol* (2001) 37:262–70.

[54] Gledovic Z, Grgurevic A, Pekmezovic T et al. Risk factors for esophageal cancer in Serbia. *Indian J Gastroenterol*. (2007) 6:265-8.

[55] Granger D.N. Role of xanthine oxidase and granulocytes in ischemia-reperfusion injury. *Am. J. Physiol*. (1988) 255: 1269–1275.

[56] Greiber, S.; Kramer-Guth, A.; Pavenstadt, H.; Gutenskunt, M.; Schollmeyer, P.; Wanner, C. Effects of lipoprotein(a) on mesangial cell proliferation and viability. *Nephrol. Dial. Transplant.* (1996) 11:778–785.

[57] Greving JP, Lee JE, Wolk A, Lukkien C. Lindblad P, Bergstro A. Alcoholic beverages and risk of renal cell cancer. *British Journal of Cancer* (2007) 97: 429-433.

[58] Grisham M.B., Hernandez L.A., Granger D.N. Xanthine oxidase and neutrophil infiltration in intestinal ischemia. *Am. J. Physiol*. (1986) 251: G567–G574.

[59] Gröne HJ, Hohbach J, Gröne EF. Modulation of glomerular sclerosis and interstitial fibrosis by native and modified lipoproteins. *Kidney Int Suppl*. (1996) 54: S18-22.

[60] Ha H, Lee HB. Oxidative stress in diabetic nephropathy: basic and clinical information. *Curr Diab Rep*. (2001) 1: 282-7.

[61] Hannken T, Schroeder R, Stahl RAK, Wolf G: Angiotensin IImediated expression of p27 Kip1 and induction of cellular hypertrophy in renal tubular cells depend on the generation of oxygen radicals. *Kidney Int* (1998) 54: 1923–1933.

[62] Heinecke JW, Li W, Francis GA, Goldstein JA. Tyrosyl radical generated by myeloperoxidase catalyzes the oxidative cross-linking of proteins. *J Clin Invest* (1993) 91:2866-72.

[63] Hertog MGL, Kromhout D, Aravanis C, Blackburn H, Buzina R, Fidanza F, Giampaolis S, Jansen A, Menotti A, Nedeljkovic S. Flavonoid intake and long term risk of cardiovascular disease in the Seven Countries Study. *Arch Intern Med* (1995) 155: 381-386.

[64] Hodge AM, English DR, O'Dea K, Giles GG. Alcohol intake, consumption pattern and beverage type, and the risk of Type 2 diabetes. *Diabet Med*. (2006) 23:690-7.

[65] Honsho S, Sugiyama A, Takahara A, Satoh Y, Nakamura Y, Hashimoto K. A red wine vinegar beverage can inhibit the renin-angiotensin system: experimental evidence in vivo. *Biol Pharm Bull* (2005) 28:1208-10.

[66] Husain K, Scott BR, Reddy SK, Somani SM. Chronic ethanol and nicotine interaction on rat tissue antioxidant defense system. *Alcohol* (2001) 25:89-97.

[67] Husain K. Vascular endothelial oxidative stress in alcohol-induced hypertension. *Cell Mol Biol* (2007) 53:70-77.

[68] Ishikawa Y, Kitamura M. Bioflavonoid quercetin inhibits mitosis and apoptosis of glomerular cells in vitro and in vivo. *Biochem Biophys Res Commun* (2000) 279:629 – 34.

[69] Ishikawa, I.; Kiyama, S.; Yoshioka, T. Renal antioxidant enzymes: their regulation and function. *Kidney Int*. (1994) 45:1–9.

[70] Just A, Whitten CL, Arendshorst WJ. Reactive oxygen species participate in acute renal vasoconstrictor responses induced by ETA and ETB receptors. *Am J Physiol Renal Physiol*. (2008) 294:719-28.

[71] Kahraman A, Erkasap N, Serteser M, Koken T. Protective effect of quercetin on renal ischemia/reperfusion injury in rats. *J Nephrol* (2003) 16:219 –24.

[72] Kim MJ, Kim YJ, Park HJ et al. Apoptotic effect of red wine polyphenols on human colon cancer SNU-C4 cells. *Food Chem Toxicol.* (2006) 44:898-902.

[73] Kimura H. Increased expression of plasminogen activator inhibitor-1 in hypoxic renal injury and its pathological significance in progression of advanced renal disease. *Rinsho Byori* (2005) 53:749 –58.

[74] Kinter, M.; Wolstenholme, J. T.; Thornhill, B. A.; Newton, E. A.; McCormick, M. L.; Chevalier, R. L. Unilateral ureteral obstruction impairs renal antioxidant enzyme activation during sodium depletion. *Kidney Int.* (1999) 55:1327–1334.

[75] Kitamura M, Ishikawa Y. Oxidant-induced apoptosis of glomerular cells: intracellular signaling and its intervention by bioflavonoid. *Kidney Int* (1999) 56:1223–9.

[76] Klahr S, Morrissey JJ. The role of vasoactive compounds, growth factors and cytokines in the progression of renal disease. *Kidney Int* (2000) 75:S7–14.

[77] Klahr S. Oxygen radicals and renal diseases. *Miner Electrolyte Metab.* (1997) 23:140-3.

[78] Klahr, S. Urinary tract obstruction. *Semin. Nephrol.* (2001) 21:133-145.

[79] Krajka-Kuźniak V, Baer-Dubowska W. The effects of tannic acid on cytochrome P450 and phase II enzymes in mouse liver and kidney. *Toxicol Lett.* (2003) 143: 209-16.

[80] Kubo, K.; Saito, M.; Tadocoro, T.; Maekawa, A. Changes in susceptibility of tissues to lipid peroxidation after ingestion of various levels of docosahexanoic acid and vitamin E. *Br. J. Nutr.* (1997) 78:655–669

[81] Kuo PL, Hsu YL. The grape and wine constituent piceatannol inhibits proliferation of human bladder cancer cells via blocking cell cycle progression and inducing Fas/membrane bound Fas ligand-mediated apoptotic pathway. *Mol Nutr Food Res.* (2008) 52:408-18.

[82] Lee JE, Hunter DJ, Spiegelman D, Adami HO, Albanes D, Bernstein L, van den Brandt PA, Buring JE, Cho E, Folsom AR, Freudenheim JL, Giovannucci E, Graham S, Horn-Ross PL, Leitzmann MF, McCullough ML, Miller AB, Parker AS, Rodriguez C, Rohan TE, Schatzkin A, Schouten LJ, Virtanen M, Willett WC, Wolk A, Zhang SM, Smith-Warner SA. Alcohol intake and renal cell cancer in a pooled analysis of 12 prospective studies. *J Natl Cancer Inst.* (2007) 99:801-10.

[83] Leiro J, Arranza JA, Fraiz N, Sanmartin ML, Quezada E, Orallo F. Effect of cis-resveratrol on genes involved in nuclear factor kappa B signaling. *Int Immunopharmacol* (2005) 5:393– 406.

[84] Levine R.L., Stadtman E.R. Oxidative modification of proteins during aging. *Exp. Gerontol.* (2001) 36: 1495–1502.

[85] Li X, Kimura H, Hirota K, Kasuno K, Torii K, Okada T, et al. Synergistic effect of hypoxia and TNF-alpha on production of PAI-1 in human proximal renal tubular cells. *Kidney Int* (2005) 68:569–83.

[86] Liochev S.I,. Fridovich I, The Haber-Weiss cycle - 70 years later: an alternative view, *Redox report* (2002) 7 55–57.

[87] Liu L, Wang Y, Lam KS, Xu A. Moderate wine consumption in the prevention of metabolic syndrome and its related medical complications. *Endocr Metab Immune Disord Drug Targets.* (2008) 8:89-98.

[88] Macdonald J., Galley H.F., Webster N.R. Oxidative stress and gene expression in sepsis. *Br. J. Anaesth.* (2003) 90: 221–232.

[89] Mantle D, Preedy VR. Free radicals as mediators of alcohol toxicity. *Adverse Drug React Toxicol Rev.* (1999) 18: 235-52.

[90] Marambaud P, Zhao H, Davies P. Resveratrol promotes clearance of Alzheimer's disease amyloid-beta peptides. *J Biol Chem.* (2005) 280:37377-82.

[91] Marnett L.J. Lipid peroxidation – DNA damage by malondialdehyde. *Mut. Res. Fund. Mol. Mech. Mutagen* (1999) 424: 83–95.

[92] McCann SE, Sempos C, Freudenheim JL, et al. Alcoholic beverage preference and characteristics of drinkers and nondrinkers in western New York (United States). *Nutr Metab Cardiovasc Dis* (2003) 13:2–11.

[93] Mennen, L.I., Walker, R., Bennetau-Pelissero, C., Scalbert, A. Risks and safety of polyphenol consumption. *Am. J. Clin. Nutr.* (2005) 81: 326S–329S.

[94] Middleton EJR, Kandaswami C, Theoharides TC: The effect of plant flavonoids on mammalian cells: implications for inflammation, heart disease and cancer. *Pharmacol Rev* (2000) 52: 673-751.

[95] Mukamal KJ, Ascherio A, Mittleman MA Alcohol and risk for ischemic stroke in men: the role of drinking patterns and usual beverage. *Ann Intern Med.* (2005) 142:11-9.

[96] Nathan A.T., Singer M. The oxygen trail: tissue oxygenation. *Br. Med. Bull.* (1999) 55: 96–108.

[97] Nihei T, Miura Y, Yagasaki K. Inhibitory effect of resveratrol on proteinuria, hypoalbuminemia and hyperlipidemia in nephritic rats. *Life Sci* (2001) 68:2845–52.

[98] Nishida Y, Oda H, Yorioka N. Effect of lipoproteins on mesangial cell proliferation. *Kidney Int Suppl.* (1999) 71:S51-3.

[99] Nyska A., Kohen R, Oxidation of biological systems: oxidative stress phenomena, antioxidants, redox reactions, and methods for their quantification, *Toxicol. Pathol.* (2002) 30:620–650.

[100] Nyska A., Kohen R. Oxidation of biological systems: oxidative stress phenomena, antioxidants, redox reactions, and methods for their quantification. *Toxicol. Pathol.* (2002) 30: 620–650.

[101] Orellana M, Araya J, Guajardo V, Rodrigo R. Modulation of cytochrome P450 activity in the kidney of rats following long-term red wine exposure. *Comp Biochem Physiol C* (2002) 132:399–405.

[102] Orellana M, Valdes E, Fernandez J, Rodrigo R. Effects of chronic ethanol consumption on extramitochondrial fatty acid oxidation and ethanol metabolism by rat kidney. *Gen Pharmacol* (1998) 30:719 –23.

[103] Orellana M, Valdés E, Fernández J, Rodrigo R. Effects of chronic ethanol consumption on extramitochondrial fatty acid oxidation and ethanol metabolism by rat kidney. *General Pharmacology* (1998) 30:719–23.

[104] Ou HC, Chou FP, Sheen HM, Lin TM, Yang CH, Sheu WHH. Resveratrol, a polyphenolic compound in red wine, protects against oxidized LDL-induced cytotoxicity in endothelial cells. *Clin Chim Acta* (2006) 364:196 –204.

[105] Patrignani P., Tacconelli S. Isoprostanes and other markers of peroxidation in atherosclerosis. *Biomarkers* (2005) 10: S24–S29.

[106] Pechanová O, Bertanová I, Babál P, Martinez MC, Kyselá S, Štvrtina S, Andriantsitohaina R. Red wine polyphenols prevent cardiovascular alterations in L-Name-induced hypertension. *J Hypertens* (2004) 22: 1551-1559.

[107] Peters H, Martini S, Woydt R, et al. Moderate alcohol intake has no impact on acute and chronic progressive anti-thy1 glomerulonephritis. *Am J Physiol Renal Physiol* (2003) 284:F1105–14.

[108] Pietta, P., Simonetti, P., Gordana, C., Brusamolino, A., Morazzoni, P., Bombardelli, E. Relationship between rate and extent of cathechin absorption and plasma antioxidant status. *Biochem. Mol. Biol. Int.* (1998) 46: 895–903.

[109] Pinchuk I., Schnitzer E., Lichtenberg D. Kinetic analysis of copper-induced peroxidation of LDL. *Biochim. Biophys. Acta* (1998) 1389: 155–172.

[110] Pryor W.A., Stanley J.P., Blair E. Autoxidation of polyunsaturated fatty acids: II. A suggested mechanism for the formation of TBA-reactive materials from prostaglandin-like endoperoxides. *Lipids* (1976) 11: 370–379.

[111] Renaud S, de Lorgeril M. Wine, alcohol, platelets, and the French paradox for coronary heart disease. Renaud S, de Lorgeril M. *Lancet.* (1992) 339:1523-6.

[112] Renaud SC, Gueguen R, Conard P, Lanzmann-Petithory D, Orgogozo JM, Henry O. Moderate wine drinkers have lower hypertensionrelated mortality: a prospective cohort study in French men. *Am J Clin Nutr* (2004) 80:621–5.

[113] Rice-Evans CA, Gopinathan V. "Oxygen toxicity, free radicals and antioxidants in human disease: biochemical implications in atherosclerosis and the problems of premature neonates". *Essays Biochem.* (1995) 29: 39–63.

[114] Rimm EB, Stampfer MJ. Wine, beer and spirits: are they really horses of a different color? *Circulation* (2002) 105:2806 –7.

[115] Rodrigo R, Bosco C, Herrera P, Rivera G. Amelioration of myoglobinuric renal damage in rats by chronic exposure to flavonol-rich red wine. *Nephrol Dial Transplant* (2004) 19: 2237–2244.

[116] Rodrigo R, Rivera G, Orellana M, Araya J, Bosco C. Rat kidney antioxidant response to long-term exposure to flavonol rich red wine. *Life Sci* (2002) 71:2881–95.

[117] Rodrigo R, Rivera G. Renal damage mediated by oxidative stress: A hypothesis of protective effects of red wine. *Free Radical Biology and Medicine* (2002) 33:409–22.

[118] Rodrigo R, Thielemann L. Effects of chronic and acute ethanol exposure on renal (Na⁺ K)-ATPase in the rat. *Gen Pharmacol* (1997) 29:719 –23.

[119] Sakatsume M, Kadomura M, Sakata I, Imai N, Kondo D, Osawa Y, Shimada H, Ueno M, Miida T, Nishi S, Arakawa M, Gejyo F. Novel glomerular lipoprotein deposits associated with apolipoprotein E2 homozygosity. *Kidney Int.* (2001) 59:1911-8.

[120] Satyanarayana PS, Singh D, Chopra K. Quercetin, a bioflavonoid, protects against oxidative stress-related renal dysfunction by cyclosporine in rats. *Methods Find Exp Clin Pharmacol* (2001) 23:175– 81.

[121] Scheuer, H.; Gwinner, W.; Hohbach, J.; Grone, E. F.; Brandes R. P.; Malle, E.; Olbricht, C. J.; Walli, A. K.; Grone, H. J. Oxidant stress in hyperlipidemia-induced renal damage. *Am. J. Physiol.* (2000) 278:F63–F74.

[122] Scott RB, Reddy HS, Husain K, Schlorff EC, Rybak RP, Somani SM. Dose response of ethanol on antioxidant defense system of liver, lung, and kidney in the rat. *Pathophysiology* (2000) 7:25–32.

[123] Scott RB, Reddy KS, Husain K, Schlorff EC, Rybak LP, Somani SM. Dose response of ethanol on antioxidant defense system of liver, lung, and kidney in rat. *Pathophysiology* (2000) 7:25–32.

[124] Sevov M, Elfineh L, Cavelier LB. Resveratrol regulates the expression of LXR- in human macrophages. *Biochem Biophys Res Commun* (2006) 348:1047–54.

[125] Sharma R, Khanna A, Sharma M, Savin VJ. Transforming growth factor-beta1 increases albumin permeability of isolated rat glomeruli via hydroxyl radicals. *Kidney Int* (2000) 58:131– 6.

[126] Shigematsu S, Ishida S, Hara M, et al. Resveratrol, a red wine constituent polyphenol, prevents superoxide-dependent inflammatory responses induced by ischemia/reperfusion, platelet-activating factor, or oxidants. *Free Radic Biol Med* (2003) 34:810 –7.

[127] Shimoi K, Shen B, Toyokuni S, Mochizuki R, Furugori M, Kinae N. Protection by alpha G-rutin, a water-soluble antioxidant flavonoid, against renal damage in mice treated with ferric nitrilotriacetate. *Jpn J Cancer Res.* (1997) 88: 453-60

[128] Sies, H.. "Oxidative stress: introductory remarks", in H. Sies, (Ed.): *Oxidative Stress*. Academic Press, (1985)1-7.

[129] Spiteller G. Are changes of the cell membrane structure causally involved in the aging process? Ann. N. Y. *Acad. Sci.* (2002) 959: 30–44.

[130] Spiteller G. Are lipid peroxidation processes induced by changes in the cell wall structure and how are these processes connected with diseases? *Med. Hypotheses* (2003) 60: 69–83.

[131] Spiteller G. The relation of lipid peroxidation processes with atherogenesis: a new theory on atherogenesis. *Mol. Nutr. Food Res.* (2005) 49: 999–1013.

[132] Stadtman E.R. Protein oxidation in aging and age-related diseases. Ann. N. Y. *Acad. Sci.* (2001) 928: 22–38.

[133] Stadtman E.R. Role of oxidant species in aging. *Curr. Med. Chem.* (2004) 11: 1105–1112.

[134] Stefanovic, V., Savic, V., Vlahovic, P., Cvetkovic, T., Najman, S., Mitic- Zlatkovic, M.,. Reversal of experimental myoglobinuric acute renal failure with bioflavonoids from seeds of grape. (2000) *Ren. Fail.* 22: 255–266

[135] Stohs S.J,. Bagchi D, Oxidative mechanisms in the toxicity of metal-ions, *Free Rad. Biol. Med.* (1995) 18: 321–336.

[136] Tan S., Yokoyama Y., Dickens E., Cash T.G., Freeman B.A., Parks D.A. Xanthine-oxidase activity in the circulation of rats following hemorrhagic shock. *Free Radic. Biol. Med.* (1993) 15: 407–414.

[137] Tang FY, Su YC, Chen NC, Hsieh HS, Chen KS. Resveratrol inhibits migration and invasion of human breast-cancer cells. *Mol Nutr Food Res.* (2008) 52: 683-91

[138] Terada L.S., Dormish J.J., Shanley P.F., Leff J.A., Anderson B.O., Repine J.E. Circulating xanthine oxidase mediates lung neutrophil sequestration after intestinal ischemia-reperfusion. *Am. J. Physiol.* (1992) 263: L394–L401.

[139] Tsang C, Higgins S, Duthie GG, Duthie SJ, Howie M, Mullen W, et al. The influence of moderate red wine consumption on antioxidant status and indices of oxidative stress associated with CHD in healthy volunteers. *Br J Nutr* (2005) 93:233-40.

[140] Valko M., Rhodes C.J., Moncol J., Izakovic M., Mazur M. Free radicals, metals and antioxidants in oxidative stress-induced cancer. *Chem. Biol. Interact.* (2006) 160: 1–40.

[141] Vanholder R, Sever MS, Erek E, Lamiere N. Rhabdomyolysis. *J Am Soc Nephrol* (2000) 11: 1553–1561

[142] Vitrac X, Desmouliere A, Brouillaud B, et al. Distribution of [14C]-trans-resveratrol, a cancer chemopreventive polyphenol, in mouse tissues after oral administration. *Life Sci* (2003) 72:2219 –33.

[143] Volpato S, Pahor M, Ferrucci L, et al. Relationship of alcohol intake with inflammatory markers and plasminogen activator inhibitor-1 in well-functioning older adults. *Circulation* (2004) 109:607–12.

[144] Wanner, C.; Greiber, S.; Kramer-Guth, A.; Heinloth, A.; Galle, J. Lipids and progression of renal disease: role of modified low density lipoprotein and lipoprotein(a). *Kidney Int.* (1997) 52:S102–S106

[145] Ward RA, McLeish KR. Oxidant stress in hemodialysis patients: what are the determining factors? *Artif Organs.* (2003) 27:230-6.

[146] Webster N.R., Nunn J.F. Molecular structure of free radicals and their importance in biological reactions. *Br. J. Anaesth.* (1988) 60: 98–108.

[147] Zager RA: Rhabdomyolysis and myohemoglobinuric acute renal failure. *Kidney Int* (1996) 49:314 -326.

[148] Zager, R. A.; Burkhart, K. Myoglobin in proximal human kidney cells: roles of Fe, Ca^{2+}, H_2O_2, a mitochondrial electron transport. *Kidney Int.* (1997) 51:728–738.

[149] Zenebe W, Pechanová O, Andriantsitohaina R: Red wine polyphenols induce vasorelaxation by increased nitric oxide bioactivity. *Physiol Res* (2003) 52: 425-432,.

[150] Zenebe W, Pechanová O. Effects of red wine polyphenolic compounds on the cardiovascular system. *Bratisl Lek Listy* (2002) 103: 159-165.

[151] Zimmerman J.J. Defining the role of oxyradicals in the pathogenesis of sepsis. *Crit. Care Med.* (1995) 23: 616–617.

In: Red Wine and Health
Editor: Paul O'Byrne

ISBN 978-1-60692-718-2
© 2009 Nova Science Publishers, Inc.

Chapter 17

KEEPING THE TRACK OF QUALITY: AUTHENTICATION AND TRACEABILITY STUDIES ON WINE

Maurizio Aceto*, Massimo Baldizzone and Matteo Oddone
Department of Environmental and Life Sciences,
University of Eastern Piedmont, via Bellini, 25/G – 15100 Alessandria

ABSTRACT

The quality of a wine is one of the most valuable features in the consumer's view. This is a consequence of a higher level of knowledge and culinary education among consumers: most people are now definitely ready to spend some more money to yield a higher quality product. At present, though, this feature seems not to be a matter of strict control from governments. In so many times laws have been violated that it is impossible not to see how inefficiently the present regulations on wine are working. The number of sophistication procedures is increasing constantly and becoming sophisticated and hard to recognize. More strict analytical controls should be developed and routinely used. An important concept in this field is *traceability*. In commodity economics this concept means "monitoring of goods fluxes from raw materials to the consumers' table" but this process is only based on production of documentation, easily subjected to falsification. Here traceability is expressed in a different way than before: in the chemical sense, *traceability* means to individuate chemical markers to find a link among the geographical zone where a wine is made and the final product of winemaking process, i.e. wine itself. It is mandatory that analytical techniques should be used to fulfill this task. The condition for this to happen is that wines grown on different zones should carry with them a fingerprint from soil to the bottle to be expressed in chemical terms, be it isotope ratios or elemental distributions. As long as this fingerprint is not altered along the whole winemaking process, its recognition could allow one to check whether a wine had been effectively produced in a certain area.

Another key feature in wine research is *authentication*, a concept expressing the possibility to identify and discriminate true samples from false samples. This concept, though not being a synonym of traceability, points to the same direction, i.e. quality.

---

* Corresponding author, email maurizio.aceto@unipmn.it, tel. +39 0131 360265, fax +39 0131 360250

Among the different techniques available for wine analysis and control, two seem to be highly promising for fingerprint recognition and authentication: isotope ratio – MS for determination of light and heavy elements and ICP-MS for determination of trace and ultra-trace concentrations of elements acting as markers, with particular focus devoted to lanthanides. An increasing amount of publications is being devoted in the last years to the application of these techniques to wine authentication and traceability, a review of state-of-the-art of which is the task of the present work.

1. INTRODUCTION

It is possibly a consequence of the human condition the fact that fraud has accompanied transactions since ancient ages. There have always been dishonest wine dealers who used to maximize profits by diluting their product with water, i.e. with a cheaper ingredient. Ancient Romans said *caveat emptor*, i.e. who is going to purchase must be well aware. Today, though laws and rules had been imposed on every kind of foodstuff, the number of frauds is amazingly high, with particular reference to higher quality – and therefore higher price – foodstuffs. Products such as truffles, cheese, olive oil are subjected to adulteration or falsification all over the world, at the expense of those working with earnestness in the agriculture field and, finally, of consumers who, faced with this problem, cannot do much about it.

Wine is by no means an exception in this view. Though legislation on wine is among the most complete in the food sector and wine therefore among the most controlled foodstuffs, diffusion of fraud is so high that is virtually impossible to quantify it. Several kinds of frauds are committed every year on the wine market, an example of which can be the following:

- Adulteration
  - with water
- Sophistication
  - with sugars and/or alcohols obtained by species different from *Vitis vinifera*
  - with not allowed additives, flavors and dyestuffs
  - with addition of wines obtained by eating grapes
- Counterfeiting
  - wines totally obtained by musts and/or eating grapes commercialized as products grown out of wine grapes
  - wines commercialized with protected denominations (DOC and/or DOCG) without having chemical, physical, organoleptic and documentary requisites prescribed by laws

Authentication of wine is strictly bound to its labeling. A wine labeled as "table wine" will be obtained with grapes of whatever origin, while a DOC wine will be obtained only from grapes of a certain area. Behind labels there are always rules imposing given features from the technical point of view. Nowadays there is an increasing interest about foodstuffs provenance, due to the request of consumers of additional warranties of quality, authenticity, and typicality. The *Controlled Denomination of Origin* (*Appellation d'Origine Controlee* or AOC in French, *Denominazione di Origine Controllata* or DOC in Italian) of wines represents an unambiguous reference to the geographical origin and is an important indicator of quality.

Problems arise, though, where rules change from country to country. Some countries pursue more strict rules in the commercialization of foodstuffs, others are less strict, requesting to respect analytical parameters more or less restrictive. A clear example is the addition of sugar in wine processing, a practice allowed in France but not in Italy.

Moreover, it is virtually impossible to define a wine in terms of a single scientific description. Nearly 1000 different chemical compounds are known to be present in it, among which not less than 400-500 are active in terms of taste and flavor, though being at concentrations of µg/l or less. The same wine can show slight but significant differences according to its geographic provenance, year of harvest, wine processing, etc. To be able to define an "authentic" wine product, a database might be available with all possible variants of major, minor and trace ingredients, continuously updated taking into account new agricultural and process technologies and, most important, collected by a *super partes* organism.

In this context there is a concept that is acquiring a wide importance: *traceability* or *chain traceability*. In the food-agricultural sector this word has become in the last years the subject of particular attention among entrepreneurs and consumers as a consequence of its connection with problems concerning safety and origin of products. The concept of traceability expresses the possibility to trace, through the different passages in the production chain, up to the provenance of raw materials with which a product is made. This can be done by a procedure of self certification or, in a more expensive but scientifically more accurate way, through determination of some chemical or physical parameters that we can guess as unaltered along the path that brings from raw materials to the final product reaching our table.

1.1. Traceability in Commodity Sense

Usually when one speaks about chain traceability he means *commodity traceability*. It consists in monitoring of material fluxes from production of raw materials up to final selling. That means it could be possible, in principle, to identify every single parcel of grapes used during winemaking and, on another side, to tell where a wine bottle come from; it is the most basic way to control processes. Moreover, it is also an assumption of responsibility towards consumers which cannot help appreciating an effort to guarantee quality. The new European regulation 178/2002 (applicable on January 1st, 2005), imposing the requirements for the traceability of food [1], seems to reinforce this concept. The weak point of commodity traceability, though, is that it has documental bases only, in some cases involving self-certification.

1.2. Traceability in Chemical Sense

Chemical analysis of materials is never considered a crucial point in traceability as expressed in commodity sense. In few occasions there are procedures in which chemical tests are scheduled to be performed along the chain. Indeed, chemical traceability should be regarded as the only *true* traceability: it is only by individuating one o more chemical markers that the link among raw materials and the final product can be revealed. More than this, chemical traceability can sometimes reveal the link among the final product and soil, i.e. the geographic zone from which a product comes from.

Analytical chemistry has therefore an important role in the safeguard of food quality. Apart from commodity aspects, that is to satisfy need of control on chain, several analytical techniques are used to recognize frauds that are committed at detriment of quality foods. In the last years scientific studies have shown that powerful and sophisticated techniques such as mass spectrometry and NMR are able to recognize foodstuffs coming from different countries or regions, in reason of chemical parameters linked to soil or to the production cycle used. Real possibilities do exist to develop routine procedures in order to apply these techniques to food analysis.

1.3. Traceability and Authentication

It is noteworthy at this stage to point out the difference among *traceability* and *authentication*. While traceability aims at finding out the link among a product and its raw materials, the concept of authentication implies the possibility to verify the features declared by a product label. Therefore traceability will be addressed to identify chemical parameters useful to keep the chain tracks in its different stages, while authentication will be more addressed to individuate chemical variables allowing to discriminate *authentic* products from *non authentic* products. A common scheme of authentication can involve using one or more groups of chemical compounds or parameter, whose distribution is evaluated with reference to geographic provenance, botanic or animal variety, age or production technologies of samples of a particular food. These variables are employed to individuate groups or classes of samples with homogeneous chemical features, evaluating differences among groups and comparing identified structures with reference samples and with unassigned samples. Such procedure is termed *classification*. To carry out these studies, multivariate mathematical analysis is needed and in particular the procedures used by *chemometrics*.

If a wine can be traced it will be certainly authentic; on the contrary, if a wine is authentic, that is, if it satisfies all parameters requested by law, not necessarily it might be considered as traceable. These two concepts are therefore not synonyms. It is apparent, though, that they are strictly bound one to each other. An analytical technique able to authenticate a wine product will support a traceability study on that product. These concepts point in the same direction, which is to guarantee the quality of foodstuffs to the consumers' advantage.

Authentication and traceability studies on foodstuffs are usually done by individuation of physico-chemical variables that must present well-defined values or ranges. It is more than obvious that these values are identified starting from reference samples, i.e. samples whose authenticity, in terms of composition, geographic provenance, processing, etc., could be documented above every doubt.

Several physico-chemical parameters can be used to authenticate or trace a wine. They can be classified into three groups:

- elements and isotopes: these parameters, with particular reference to trace and ultratrace elements, can be linked to soil, so that they can be considered eligible for traceability; they are useful also for authentication

- compounds: a wide range of organic and inorganic compounds can be exploited analytically to classify and therefore authenticate wines; usually the same is not true for traceability
- spectral parameters: it is possible to use some spectral features, i.e. absorbance values at determinate wavelengths, as variables for classification of wines; again, this is more useful to authentication than to traceability

For what concerns data treatment, multivariate analysis techniques are needed to yield information useful for classification. This is usually done through application of *chemometrics*, with particular reference to *pattern recognition* techniques. Unsupervised techniques, such as Principal Components Analysis (PCA) or Cluster analysis (CA), and supervised techniques, such as Discriminant Analysis (DA) or Soft Independent Modeling of Class Analogy (SIMCA) are widely used in this field. Discussion on application of chemometrics to wine classification can be found in Forina *et al.* [2,3,4]. Applications were reviewed by Arvanitoyannis *et al.* [5].

2. ANALYTICAL TECHNIQUES FOR AUTHENTICATION AND TRACEABILITY OF WINES

2.1. Introduction

To determine the physico-chemical parameters cited before, a wide range of analytical techniques are available. In the past it was nearly impossible to identify an adulterated wine, the only way being tasting by highly-trained oenologists. Today highly sophisticated instrumentations coupled with advanced mathematical methods allow authentication and traceability studies to be performed in order to identify frauds.

The most useful analytical techniques are the following:

- Stable Isotope Analysis (SIA) is unquestionably the most powerful technique for authentication and traceability of wine and food in general. High resolution mass spectrometry or NMR spectrometry can be used to evidence isotopic distribution that are characteristic of samples of different origin, be it geographical, varietal or technological;
- Elemental analysis techniques (GF-AAS, ICP-AES, ICP-MS) are able to determine nearly all elements in the periodic table down to trace and ultratrace level concentrations. Of particular interest for traceability is the determination of lanthanides or rare earths (REE);
- Chromatographic techniques can be used in the classification of wine, due to the great number of organic compounds present in its composition.

2.2. Stable Isotope Analysis

Isotope techniques were developed in the early '80s in France (University of Nantes) and rapidly found great interest in all sector of scientific research. Quantification of the ratio of two isotopes of the same element is highly powerful in verifying whether two chemically analogous objects differ in provenance with relation to the respective raw materials. Phenomena of various kind, either biological, geological or anthropogenic, can influence isotopic distribution of elements in raw materials, determining differences in the final products that can be revealed by isotope analysis techniques. Of particular interest are *stable isotopes*, i.e. non artificial. All techniques quantifying isotope ratios can be resumed under the name Stable Isotope Ratio Analysis (SIRA or SIA) but from the technological point of view only High Resolution Mass Spectrometry and NMR Spectrometry can be used.

SIA finds many applications in food authentication. On the basis of different isotope ratios, it is possible to discriminate among molecules, present in one food, having the same chemical structure but coming from different raw materials or produced as a consequence of different processes, for example by biological or industrial synthesis. Examples of applications are the following:

- discrimination among natural and artificial flavors (es. vanillin)
- discrimination among acetic acid coming from acetic fermentation and from industrial synthesis
- discrimination among wild and farming salmons, on the basis of a typical lipid compound
- addition of sugars different from the ones naturally present in a food
- addition of water to milk, wine, orange juices, etc.
- identification of geographic provenance of foodstuffs

To fully describe the theoretical and technological aspects of SIA some textbooks can be suggested [6]. It is important here to evidence the basis on which SIA can be used in authentication and traceability of food and wine in particular. The possibility to discriminate among samples according to isotope ratios of some elements is linked to *fractionation* phenomena, that is deviation from a starting natural isotope distribution, occurring in raw materials as a consequence of biogeochemical phenomena, either natural and artificial [7,8]. According to the composition of wine, two groups of nuclides and the corresponding ratios must be considered:

- light elements such as hydrogen ($^2H/^1H$), carbon ($^{13}C/^{12}C$), nitrogen ($^{15}N/^{14}N$), oxygen ($^{18}O/^{16}O$, $^{18}O/^{17}O$, $^{17}O/^{16}O$) and sulphur ($^{34}S/^{32}S$, $^{34}S/^{33}S$, $^{36}S/^{34}S$)
- heavy elements such as strontium ($^{87}S/^{86}S$) and lead ($^{206}Pb/^{207}Pb$, $^{208}Pb/^{206}Pb$, $^{208}Pb/^{207}Pb$, $^{206}Pb/^{204}Pb$)

2.2.1. Analysis of Light Elements

Light elements are of major interest in biosynthetic processes and their isotopes are consequently subjected to wide fractionation. Hydrogen, carbon and oxygen form two fundamental molecules in the life of plants: water and carbon dioxide. According to several phenomena such as climate conditions (cold or hot weather, dry or wet, latitude, altitude, etc.), water cycle, transpiration and many other processes which are typical of every vegetal species, plants will have at their disposal water with a particular isotopic signature, to be used in photosynthesis. The same holds for carbon dioxide but with lower changes.

Photosynthesis, with production of glucose, causes one more isotope change for what concerns D/H ratio but more than this it is highly selective for what concerns fixation of CO_2 and, therefore, value of $^{13}C/^{12}C$ ratio. It is, indeed, its main variation source. Plants incorporate CO_2 according to three biosynthetic mechanisms:

- the *Calvin* or *C3 cycle* (typical of, for example, vine and sugar beet)
- the *Hatch-Slack* or *C4 cycle* (typical of sugar cane and maize)
- the *Crassulean Acid Metabolism* or *CAM cycle*, less common

Glucose and ethanol synthesized from plants of different metabolic pathway can be clearly discriminated, as can be seen from Figure 1.

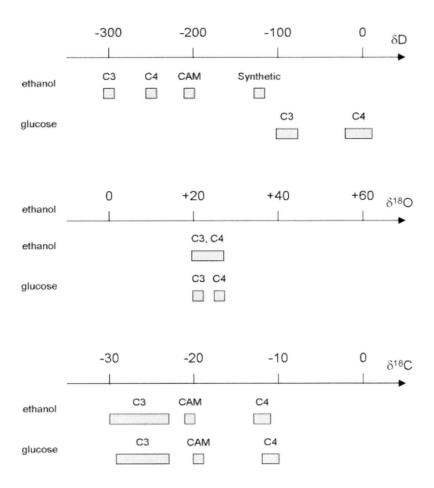

Figure 1. Isotope ratio ranges for plants of C3, C4 and CAM type

At the end of the biosynthetic cycle, glucose molecules are produced with an isotope signature correlated with those of water and CO_2 involved, as well as of the photosynthesis cycle followed. The subsequent alcoholic fermentation occurring in wine modifies only slightly the isotope ratios consolidated up to this stage (except for D/H ratio) so that they can be found almost unaltered in wine. Finally, according to the above mentioned processes it is clear that water and ethanol, the two predominant molecules in wine, will have their isotopic signatures determined by all these phenomena.

SIA of light elements has many applications in wine authentication, with particular reference of identification of fraudulent practices. To clarify the importance of the introduction of SIA methods, it must be considered that, before their development, no method was efficient enough to identify fraudulent practices. The most important information provided by SIA of light elements is reported in Table 1.

Table 1. Information provided by SIA of light elements.

Isotope ratio	Fractionation source	Information provided
$^{13}C/^{12}C$, D/H	Metabolism (C3, C4, CAM)	Illicit addition of cane or beet sugar
$^{18}O/^{16}O$, D/H	Water source	Dilution with water
$^{13}C/^{12}C$, D/H	Chemical synthesis	Addition of synthetic compounds
$^{18}O/^{16}O$, D/H, $^{15}N/^{14}N$, $^{13}C/^{12}C$	Geographic provenance	Characterization of DOC and DOCG wines

Two main aspects can be singled out:

1. sophistication of wine by addition of sugars obtained by plants others than vine (sugar beet, sugar cane or maize)
2. adulteration of wine by addition of water

Saccarose fraudulently added to musts hydrolyzes rapidly to fructose and glucose (Figure 2), which are already present in wines and are therefore indistinguishable from the molecules added.

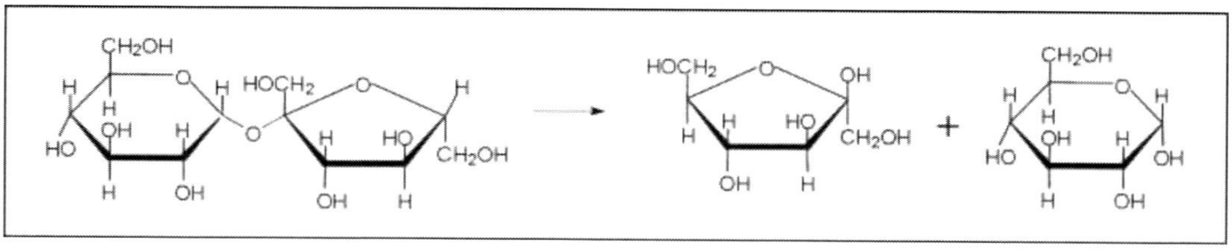

Figure 2. Hydrolysis of saccarose to fructose + glucose

Fructose and glucose molecules added retain still a track of their origin which is hidden in the isotope distribution of their elements: carbon, hydrogen and oxygen. These distributions are definitely different from the natural, according to the vegetal origin of saccarose or to processes used to obtain it. Addition of sugars from other plants is relatively easy to find out, according to D/H ratio: the value of vine sugar is in the range 98-102 ppm, higher values suggest addition of cane or maize sugars, while lower values stand for addition of beet sugar. Determination of D/H ratio is usually performed by NMR. A more subtle fraudulent practice, that is the addition of a well-balanced mixture of cane and beet sugars, will not modify D/H ratio but can be still evidenced by change in typical values of $^{13}C/^{12}C$ ratio.

For what concerns dilution of wine, this fraud can be revealed through measurement of $^{18}O/^{16}O$ value: added water, in fact, usually has a lower content of ^{18}O isotope and will therefore diminish accordingly the expected value. Determination of $^{18}O/^{16}O$ ratio is usually performed by high resolution MS.

Potentiality of SIA of light elements is such that in the last years these methods have been adopted as official by European Union (EU) and by the International Organization of Vine and Wine (OIV) for the analysis of wines. EU regulation 2676/90 [9], determining Community methods for the analysis of wines, provides for identification of raising of alcoholic grade of musts and wines through fraudulent addition of saccarose through NMR analysis of D/H ratio. EU Regulation 822/97 [10] provides for determination of $^{18}O/^{16}O$ in water of wines to identify possible fraudulent dilution of a sample. Finally EU regulation 440/2003 [11] adds determination of $^{13}C/^{12}C$ ratio to identify enrichment with mixtures of sugars of various origins and acidification of wines using malic acid.

For what concerns determination of geographic provenance of a wine, light elements are at present less effective in providing useful information. This is due, almost paradoxically, to the extreme ease of isotope distribution of light elements to vary as a consequence of various phenomena, as described before. The Δm/m parameter, linked to mass difference, shows very high values for these elements so that mass fractionation effects will influence heavily the final values of ratios in food samples. All reactions depending on mass, in fact, will cause fractionation. Examples of Δm/m values are reported in Table 2.

Table 2. Values of Δm/m for light elements

Element	Ratio	Δm/m	value
Hydrogen	D/H	(2-1)/2	0.5
Carbon	$^{13}C/^{12}C$	(13-12)/13	0.0769
	$^{13}CO_2/^{12}CO_2$	(45-44)/45	0.0222
Oxygen	$^{18}O/^{16}O$	(18-16)/18	0.111
	$H_2^{18}O/H_2^{16}O$	(20-18)/20	0.1

Ease of fractionation, due to significative mass difference among isotopes of the same element, is at the same time strong point and limitation of SIA applied to light elements: from the point of view of fraud control this behavior greatly helps recognition of fraudulent practices but from the point of view of determination of geographic provenance it is apparent that the natural variability of data renders hard to have precise references to classify samples of wines. As an example we can consider a vintage series of similar wines: Rossmann [12] analyzed white wines from Franken (Germany) in the series 1991-1999 and showed that $δ^{18}O$ values changed substantially according to different vintages. For these reasons SIA of light elements is still at an experimental stage in determining geographic provenance of wines.

Wide data collection is needed, to be able to take into account all possible sources of variability, either seasonal and climatic and the effect of artificial variations, i.e. those induced by wine chain in the form of addition of compounds with different isotope distribution. To illustrate the state-of-the-art in determination of the geographic provenance of wines through SIA of light elements, some studies can be cited [13,14,15]. Results from these studies show that good geographic discrimination can be obtained if more parameters are taken into account, i.e. both hydrogen, carbon and oxygen isotope ratios. As an example, in fact, according to values of $\delta^{18}O$ for wines from countries with different climate, differences are only slightly significative among samples from countries with mild climate (Spain, Portugal), from temperate countries (France, Italy) and from countries with continental climate (Germany, Austria).

To improve geographic classification, at present some national authorities are working to collect as more as possible data on wine, grapes and musts. In Italy a Data Bank was founded in 1987 who every year collects and analyzes not less than 500 samples of grapes from all Italian regions, together with information about vineyards, production and climate; these grapes are then processed in order to obtain wine samples to be analyzed. Italian Data Bank is validated through a UE Commission in accordance with the Joint Research Centre at Ispra. In Europe, according to UE regulation 2676/90 a wine database exists from 1990, gathering data from certified European wines. D/H ratio, $\delta^{13}C$ of ethanol and $\delta^{18}O$ of water are routinarily determined on these samples; wines from extra European countries are also analyzed, in order to take into account the possibility of adulteration with rectified musts, sugars or various products from these countries.

Recently a study by Coetzee *et al.* [16] proposed use of boron isotopes in provenance determination. Authors showed that $^{11}B/^{10}B$ ratio can be used to characterize wines from different geographical origins.

Finally, for what concerns traceability, light elements are simply not efficient at all. To find a connection between raw materials and wine as the final product, it would be necessary to investigate along wine chain in order to find a link with soil. Determination of light elements isotope ratios is hard to perform on soil, due to its unhomogeneity: many compounds are present formed by light elements, unlike wine in which ethanol and water are absolutely prevailing and can be used to determine C, H and O isotope ratios. SIA of soil has therefore no practical application.

2.2.2. Analysis of Heavy Elements

Heavy elements are of major interest in geochemical processes. The main source of their isotope fractionation is formation of daughter radiogenic nuclides starting from mother radioactive nuclides, as a consequence of nuclear transmutations continuously occurring (if we refer to a geological scale). The amount of mother nuclides varies from mineral to mineral so that rocks of different origin will contain proportionally different amounts of daughter nuclides, from site to site. In Table 3 some of the most important radioactive mother and radiogenic daughter nuclides are reported; they are considered as petrogenetic tracers and, as such, useful to determine age of rocks.

Table 3. Mother and daughter nuclides of heavy elements

Mother nuclides	Decay type	$T_{1/2}$	Daughter nuclides	Reference isotope
^{40}K	E.C.	$1.193 \cdot 10^{10}$	^{40}Ar	^{36}Ar
^{87}Rb	β^-	$4.88 \cdot 10^{10}$	^{87}Sr	^{86}Sr
^{147}Sm	α	$1.06 \cdot 10^{11}$	^{143}Nd	^{144}Nd
^{187}Re	β^-	$4.23 \cdot 10^{10}$	^{187}Os	^{186}Os
^{232}Th	$6\alpha + 4\beta^-$	$1.40 \cdot 10^{10}$	^{208}Pb	^{204}Pb
^{235}U	$7\alpha + 4\beta^-$	$7.04 \cdot 10^{8}$	^{207}Pb	^{204}Pb
^{238}U	$8\alpha + 6\beta^-$	$4.47 \cdot 10^{9}$	^{206}Pb	^{204}Pb

It is apparent that isotopes of heavy elements are subjected to wide fractionation at a preliminary stage, that is when rocks are formed. Moreover, most of heavy elements are considered as nonessential for life or at least with a minor role with respect of light elements and this limits the possibility of isotope fractionation by biological processes. During uptake of mineral substances by plants from soil there is no significant isotope fractionation of these nuclides in such a way that their isotope ratios could act as good provenance markers. According to these features, the link among food and soil can be studied with SIA of heavy elements, whose isotope signatures are different from soil to soil and can act as geographic fingerprints.

Heavy elements usually occur in food as trace or ultratrace elements. Their origin can be a sum of factor, including geographic provenance. In wine two heavy elements show interesting features: strontium and lead, occurring at concentration of mg/l or below. To illustrate the possibility of using SIA on these elements to recognize geographic provenance, let us consider the difference among absolute concentration and isotope ratio. The concentration of Sr in wine varies in the range 60 ppb - 7 ppm according to origin; it is therefore a trace element in wine. Along wine chain, Sr concentration tends to increase from grape to must up to wine, possibly as a consequence of release of Sr^{2+} ions contained in seeds and skins. Moreover artificial contributions can be due to fertilizers or to winemaking practices such as clarification with bentonite, deacidification with $CaCO_3$ or other Ca compounds that can contain Sr impurities (Sr^{2+} ion is vicariant of Ca^{2+} ion). Total Sr concentration is therefore not useful to trace a wine chain. A different behavior can be expected from isotope ratios, in particular from the $^{87}Sr/^{86}Sr$ ratio. ^{87}Sr is radiogenic, being formed from radioactive decay of ^{87}Rb, so that its concentration gradually increases with time in minerals and rocks (unlike other Sr isotopes), and so does the $^{87}Sr/^{86}Sr$ ratio. This is the basis for a commonly used dating method in geochemistry: the system Rb/Sr is a true radioactive clock for dating minerals and it is used to date ancient terrestrial igneous and metamorphic rocks and samples of moon rocks. For example, in granite rocks, more ancient geologically, the value of $^{87}Sr/^{86}Sr$ is typically 0.710, while in basaltic, younger rocks, the value is in the range 0.702 - 0.705. Moreover, the value of $\Delta m/m$ for $^{87}Sr/^{86}Sr$ is low with respect of light elements, being around 0.0115. According to this value it can be esteemed that mass effects have low influence on Sr fractionation.

From the point of view of wine traceability, it is important to note that $^{87}Sr/^{86}Sr$ varies according to geologic age of soil. Older soils will show higher values while younger soils will have lower values. As a consequence, Sr isotope ratio can play as provenance markers. Use of

Sr isotopes as wine markers was indeed introduced in 1993 by German researchers [17] and later discussed by other authors [18]. Naturally it is necessary to verify whether isotope distribution of Sr keep unaltered in transfer of nutrients from soil to plants and in the various passages of wine chain. If this would be the case, isotope distribution in wine should reflect that of soil. This was brilliantly demonstrated by Almeida and Vasconcelos [19] in a study on red wines coming from Duero (Northeastern Portugal). Two wines were obtained from grapes cultivated on two different vineyards, one ancient and one young but grown on the same type of soil, with two different winemaking techniques. Authors determined $^{87}Sr/^{86}Sr$ with ICP-MS in samples of soil, musts, fined and aged wines for both chains and results showed clearly that neither winemaking nor ageing were effective in changing Sr isotope ratio, which resulted to be determined only to soil age.

Another heavy element with great potential for traceability is lead (Pb). This element is an effective tracker of anthropogenic activity, being a witness of the impact mankind has on environmental cycles. From the start of Industrial Age and in particular from the introduction of lead tetraethyl in gasoline as antiknocking agent, an increase has been recorded in the lead pollution in environment, due to the fact that this metal was vehiculated in all atmospheric compartments and found even at unexpected latitudes. Strong correlations among Pb emissions and Pb content in soils and plants was demonstrated. This trend was inverted in '70s thanks to the reduction of Pb addition to gasoline and the introduction of *green* fuel; Pb pollution in vegetables is accordingly lowering.

Apart from being an interesting, though sinister, marker for environmental change, Pb can be used as geographic provenance marker of wine. Four stable isotopes exist: ^{204}Pb, ^{206}Pb, ^{207}Pb and ^{208}Pb. The last three are radiogenic as they derive from radioactive decay of, respectively, ^{238}U, ^{235}U and ^{232}Th. whereas ^{204}Pb is non radiogenic. Abundance of radiogenic isotopes tends therefore to increase in time. In a similar way to Sr, relative ratios of Pb isotopes change as a function of rocks genesis, as these different rocks will contain different amounts of U and Th. According to the geologic age of rocks and their geographic position, corresponding soils will have different Pb isotope ratios and this is an even more favorable situation with respect to Sr, as more fractionation schemes are possible. One more profitable point is that the variations of Pb isotope distributions in rocks from the average distribution are naturally high, in a different way from variations for light elements. As an example, consider that the difference in Pb isotope distribution for the two most important lead mines in the world, that is Joplin in Missouri and Broken Hill in Australia, is near 30‰, an enormous value. That causes wines from USA and from Australia to be readily distinguished on the basis of $^{208}Pb/^{208}Pb$ or $^{206}Pb/^{207}Pb$ ratio values, accordingly to the use of local lead minerals as raw materials for antiknocking agents.

The value of $\Delta m/m$ for Pb ratio is very low, being around 0.0096. Isotope fractionation induced by biological or artificial phenomena is irrelevant with respect of geochemical processes, so that Pb isotope ratios will reflect only geochemical differences already existing in nature. This feature can be exploited in wine authentication and traceability. It is interesting to compare again, as already done with Sr, total Pb concentration with Pb isotope ratios in wines with similar features. Rosman *et al.* [20] analyzed vintages of a French wine from 1950 to 1991, coming from the same vineyard; authors reported the results shown in Table 4.

Table 4. Isotopic composition and Pb concentration in vintages of wine coming from the same vineyard

Year	^{206}Pb/^{207}Pb	^{208}Pb/^{207}Pb	^{206}Pb/^{204}Pb	Total Pb concentration (µg/l)
1950	1.1607	2.4456	18.153	128
1962	1.1689	2.4551	18.274	78
1966	1.1606	2.4452	18.132	164
1967	1.1597	2.4460	18.127	126
1970	1.1690	2.4555	18.274	174
1971	1.1642	2.4485	18.220	125
1974	1.1567	2.4374	18.054	119
1976	1.1519	2.4360	18.004	113
1978	1.1734	2.4534	18.326	179
1980	1.1726	2.4560	18.351	227
1981	1.1568	2.4368	18.064	96
1984	1.1525	2.4328	17.982	67
1985	1.1567	2.4373	18.057	57
1986	1.1590	2.4395	18.112	92
1987	1.1586	2.4395	18.110	60
1988	1.1570	2.4364	18.070	62
1989	1.1569	2.4371	18.090	55
1990	1.1550	2.4337	18.067	40
1991	1.1617	2.4415	18.165	54

It can be noted that isotope ratios have little variations, in contrast with Pb total concentration that changes in a fivefold range. Apparently Pb concentration can change in time according to different effects, mostly anthropogenic, while Pb isotope ratios do not.

As a consequence of suitability of Pb as markers, some studies have recently demonstrated the advantageous application of SIA of Pb isotope ratios to determine the geographic provenance of wines [21,22]. In certain cases [23] problems were reported with traceability: Pb ratios were found to be different from soil to wine, possibly due to the fact that interception of airborne Pb by plants was greater than its uptake by the root system. This phenomenon was found to occur in polluted and industrial areas.

2.3. Elemental Analysis

Atomic spectroscopy is the technique of choice in the field of element determination at trace and ultra-trace level, with particular reference to Graphite Furnace Atomic Absorption Spectrometry (GF-AAS), Inductively Coupled Plasma – Atomic Emission Spectrometry (ICP-AES) and, above all, Inductively Coupled Plasma – Mass Spectrometry (ICP-MS). Application of these techniques in wine analysis can be considered as straightforward [24,25, 26,27,28], both in control procedures and in authentication and traceability studies. Sometimes trace and ultratrace elements act as markers, providing information on the origin of raw materials with which a food or a wine was prepared. Several studies are present in the literature on the classification of wine samples according to their elemental content, as will be shown later.

2.4. Chromatographic Techniques

Chromatography has been fully applied to wine characterization, either to determine volatile compounds with gas chromatography and to determine nonvolatile compounds with HPLC and ion chromatography. Nearly all analytes present in wine can be separated and identified with chromatographic methods and several thousands of publications could be cited for separation of flavors, carboxylic acids, polyphenols, aldehydes, cations, inorganic anions, amines, aminoacids, sugars etc. As a consequence, many chromatographic methods have been developed for authentication of wines on the basis of distribution of one or more classes of compounds. Hyphenation of chromatography to more specific and powerful detection systems has increased even more the possibility to apply it to classification schemes [29,30].

2.5. Molecular Spectroscopic Techniques

The methods of control and classification of wine cited up to this point were based on qualitative and quantitative determinations of analytes, be them elements, isotopes or compounds. A different approach can be considered, consisting in determination of spectroscopic parameters such as absorbance at fixed wavelength, due to the presence in samples of molecules able to absorb light. These parameters can be used as variables for classification, without need to make reference to the molecules responsible for absorption. In this way a complete absorbance spectrum can yield several tens or hundreds of variables, according to the desired resolution or discrimination power. Again, mathematical multivariate methods are needed to handle the great amount of information deriving. The spectral ranges utilized can be typically in the UV-visible, NIR or IR field [31,32]. Spectra can be recorded on untreated wines or, with better results, on methanolic extracts after solid-phase extraction on a C18 column, in order to avoid contribution from major components, i.e. water, ethanol, sugars and carboxylic acids. The advantage of applying such a procedure lies in the fact that to record an UV-visible, NIR or FTIR spectrum is usually simpler and faster than to perform a chromatographic run or an elemental analysis.

3. THE WINE CHAIN

When developing analytical methods for wine, a perfect comprehension of its production chain, i.e. of all transformation passages occurring from soil to the final product (the bottled wine) is mandatory to study traceability, since all passages can influence more or less deeply the possibility to control material flux by chemical analysis. This is less mandatory in authentication, when one wants to distinguish a true product from one which is fake, but it must be considered that knowledge of different passages in chain could allow to individuate more efficiently the analytical tests to be performed.

For this reason it is appropriate to investigate inside the production chain of wine (Figure 3).

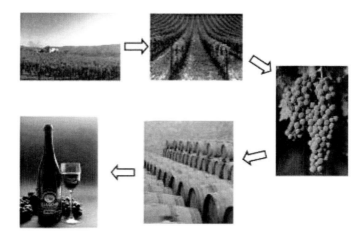

Figure 3. The wine production chain

The different passages of production chain imply modifications in the raw materials in reason of chemical and physical treatments and of addition of various compounds. Links among various passages are regulated by natural and artificial phenomena. Natural phenomena can be the following:

1. biological:
   A. assumption of mineral substances from soil by vine
   B. ferment reactions (alcoholic, acetic, malolactic)
2. geological:
   C. differentiation among soil and soil

Artificial phenomena comprehend all variations imposed by human processing:

- use of pesticides on field
- addition of concentrated musts, yeasts, microbic starters, ferment activators
- addition of clarification, filtration, stabilization and antioxidizing agents
- storage (in casks, in steel)
- bottling

Differences set by process are added to those set by nature and all these phenomena are reflected on the composition of the product that goes from raw materials gradually to bottled and marketed wine. This sometimes can be used to discriminate among wines but more frequently overlap of natural and artificial contributions brings the situation to be complicate.

When taking into consideration the role of metals we can imagine that wine chain works as shown in Table 5.

Table 5. Change in metal distribution according to wine chain.

Primary raw materials	Secondary raw materials	Action on metals
vineyard soil		
⇓	pesticides	addition of Cu and Zn compounds
grapes (one or more vines)		
⇓		
must		
⇓	concentrated musts, fermenting yeast strains, microbic starters, ferment activators	addition of K, Ca, P compounds; depletion of metals by precipitation as sulphides
unfined wine		
⇓	clarification, filtration agents, stabilization and antioxidizing agents	metal precipitation or increase
fined wine		
⇓	storage materials	release of Cr, Fe, Ni ions
wine kept in containers		
⇓	packaging materials	
finished product		

Since many classes of organic compounds, typical of determinate passages of wine chain, can be used in wine classification, it is useful to have a look to the role of other analytes as shown in Table 6.

Table 6. Change in metal distribution according to wine chain

Primary raw materials	Species useful for classification
vineyard soil	
	primary flavors (terpenes)
⇓	anthocyans
	other polyphenols
grapes (one or more vines)	
⇓	secondary flavors (prefermentative)
must	
⇓	secondary flavors (fermentative)
unfined wine	
⇓	
fined wine	
⇓	tertiary flavors
wine kept in containers	
⇓	
finished product	

In some particular wines, procedures are undertaken introducing variability that must be taken into account. Some examples are the following:

1. the so-called *fortified wines* (*Marsala*, *Sherry*, *Porto*, *Madeira*) are those wines for which addition of alcohol is permitted, not just to increase ethanol level but to modify perception of aromatic compounds and therefore the overall taste. Unfortunately added alcohol will have most probably an isotopic fingerprint, in terms of $^2H/^1H$, $^{13}C/^{12}C$ and $^{18}O/^{16}O$ ratios, different from the natural fingerprint formed according to alcoholic fermentation. In the final product these two contributions will be indistinguishable and the bottled wine will have a mixed isotopic fingerprint, probably not correlated anymore to origin;

2. in *sparkling wines* two fermentation stages are planned, the first one being alcoholic fermentation to produce ethanol, the second one induced to produce further carbon dioxide. Usually the second fermentation is obtained with addition of small amounts of sugar, accordingly to current regulations in the different countries. Again, carbon in CO_2 generated in the second fermentation will add its isotopic fingerprint to natural CO_2.

According to features of the wine chain, it seems to be reasonable to resume as follows:

- trace metals and isotopes can be more useful for traceability but also for authentication
- organic compounds can be useful for authentication

These concepts will be illustrated by the examples in the next paragraph.

4. Classification of Wines

A great number of studies on classification of wines have been published in the last years as a consequence of the improving interest in certification of wine quality by consumers. Methods of classification and analysis of wine were recently reviewed by Kelly *et al.* [33] and by Reid *et al.* [34] inside works dealing with food authenticity.

4.1. Meaning of Classification

Classification studies on wine can be thought of as based on three main schemes:

- according to *geographic provenance*, that is discriminating wines coming from different regions or produced with raw materials coming from different regions
- according to *variety*, that is discriminating wines produced from different vines
- according to the *technological processes* used in winemaking

Condition to develop a powerful classification study, allowing to authenticate or trace a wine, is the availability of certified samples, that is wines of known geographic provenance, vine or technological process used. It must be noted that both authentic and false samples are requested in order to achieve affordable results.

The use of chemical variables in the classification of wines dates back to the end of 70s: first studies, in fact, are those of Kwan e Kowalski [35] who were able to distinguish among European and American *Pinot Noir* samples on the basis of relative ratios of some organic compounds. Sometimes it is possible to individuate in wine chemical compounds typical of vine or somehow linked to soil and therefore typical of a territory, but more frequently a single element or compound is not enough to obtain a good discrimination. In most cases several analytes must be taken into consideration, which implies the need for suitable analytical techniques (multiresidues techniques) and mathematical multivariate analysis.

Classes of analytes suitable for classifying wines can be the following:

1. trace elements
2. isotopes
3. volatile compounds
4. polyphenolic compounds
5. other organic compounds
6. spectroscopic parameters, .i.e. absorbance values at fixed □ in the UV-visible, NIR or IR range

Usually volatile compounds are more fit in the varietal classification, while trace elements and isotopes, being more linked to soil, are more useful for geographic classification. Other compounds, such as polyphenols, are less specific in their classification power. In several cases it is appropriate to use different classes of analytes, raising in this way the possibility of discrimination.

4.2. Geographic Classification

The relation among a wine and its territory can be determined either by authentication and by traceability. At present the most of geographic provenance studies on food are devoted to wine, due to its economical importance. Besides this, wine chemistry is known enough to allow individuation of chemical markers that are effective in classification. Classification of wine according to geographic provenance is extraordinarily important from the economical point of view, as long as we think about the difference in price among a wine coming from Langhe (Southern Piedmont, one of the most important wine-producing regions in the world) and a product coming from a less renowned region. Local and typical products, such as wines obtained from narrow areas if not single vineyards, should be acknowledged of added value determined by being referred to a localized and recognizable geographic zone, as well as by the relative hardness in obtaining such limited productions. Moreover, it must be considered that the trade supremacy of regions with historically consolidated oenological vocation (Italy, France) is at present challenged by emergent countries such as California, Chile, Argentina, Australia or New Zealand, producing wines at definitely competitive prices. To contrast phenomena bound to globalization it is mandatory to direct efforts on quality and on acknowledgement of local typicality, features that can be thwarted if non authentic products get into the market. The need to link a wine to its area of origin or production is therefore pressing. For this reason traditional countries such as France, Spain or Germany (but also California or Australia) invest resources in the field of oenological research, trying to satisfy the need to authenticate wines from the geographic point of view.

Before describing examples of scientific studies on geographic provenance of wines, it is important to underline the difference among the *provenance* area of raw materials with which a wine is produced and the production area of a wine. From the regulatory point of view there can be sometimes no difference. DOC and DOCG specifications can refer to well delimited areas of origin of raw materials AND/OR areas of production, i.e. where raw materials are transformed to obtain the final product. These areas are not always identical and sometimes regulations are permissive enough to allow wine growers to exploit to their advantage this ambiguity, producing in their areas wines starting from raw materials, i.e. grapes or musts, coming from other areas, even achievable at cheaper prices. The following examples will clarify this concept.

Example A: the Barolo
Barolo wine was acknowledged of DOCG specification in 1980. It is usually called "the King of wines and the wine of the Kings". DOCG specification imposes that production of *Barolo* must observe, among others, three typical rules:

- only *Nebbiolo* grapes (actually only three clones of that vine, that is *Lampia*, *Michet* and *Rosé*) can be used for winemaking
- grapes must come from whole or partial territory of 11 municipal districts in the province of Cuneo (Southern Piedmont): Barolo, Castiglione Falletto, Serralunga d'Alba, Monforte d'Alba, Novello, La Morra, Verduno, Grinzane Cavour, Diano d'Alba, Cherasco and Roddi (Figure 4)
- winemaking and ageing procedures must be done inside the area delimited by the above cited 11 municipal districts.

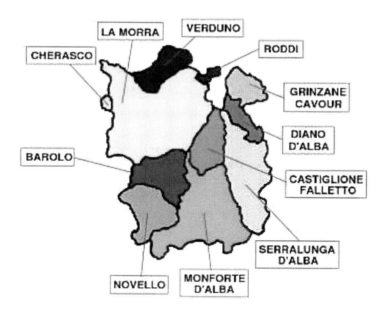

Figure 4. Territory of production of DOCG *Barolo* wine

It is apparent that specifications are quite restrictive: *both* raw materials *and* production chain are linked to the area delimited by DOCG. In this case we have as a consequence that specifications would simplify the possibility to trace or authenticate the final product.

Example B: the Langhe Nebbiolo
The Langhe specification was acknowledged in 1994 to wines produced inside the whole province of Cuneo. Despite being produced from the same vine as Barolo (the Nebbiolo

vine), Langhe is quite less esteemed. This is due to the fact that the production area is much wider and therefore less selected than the area from which Barolo is produced.

As shown, production specifications impose precise rules for what concerns both origin of grapes and winemaking location. The possibility to discriminate wines coming from different regions is therefore connected, at first instance, to soil features and secondarily to winemaking procedures. It is apparent that trace elements and isotopes, being more linked to soil, be considered the most useful variables for geographic classification.

Let us now consider the role of elements as discrimination variables. Among different factors influencing element content in wine we can consider, making reference to Table 5:

- contribution from soil on which vines grow;
- efficiency of vines to take up mineral substances from soil;
- contribution from various passages of the production chain, from grape to bottled wine (preliminary treatments, fermentation reactions, addition of compounds, storage, ageing, bottling);

The final distribution results from a sum of factors, some of which typical of a territory soil, some other out of control or with no discrimination power. On the basis of previous considerations and according to some literature sources [36,37,38,39,40,41] we can divide elements in three groups according to their discrimination power as chemical variables.

1. *elements with only natural contributions*: these are elements whose concentration in wine is not influenced by the production chain, but is determined by mineral contribution from soil and by efficiency of vines to assume this contribution for its metabolism.
    a. Al, B, Ba, Li, Mn, Mo, Rb, Si, Sr and Ti behave this way (occasionally some of these elements can receive artificial contributions if illicit treatments are used in winemaking);
    b. trace and ultratrace elements such as lanthanides and II and III series transition metals too show this behavior
2. *elements with natural and artificial contributions*: these are elements whose concentration is a sum of different factors, some natural, some artificial; among these we can cite
    a. Ca and Mg are natural constituents of grapes and musts but their concentration in wine is increased by corresponding carbonates used for deacidification;
    b. Cu and Zn are withdrawn naturally from soil or from fungicidal treatments (Bordeaux mixture, Zn thiocarbamates) or from winemaking equipment;
    c. Fe comes partly from natural contributions (assumption from soil, residual soil particles in must), partly from artificial contributions (winemaking equipment, steel containers for storage);
    d. K is the main cation in grape and consequently in wine but it is also added to wine as metabisulfite or carbonate during winemaking;
    e. Na comes from soil or from illicit salting addition as chloride

  f. P is naturally present as organic or inorganic phosphates but also added as Ca or ammonium salt
3. *elements with only artificial contributions*: these are elements whose concentration in wine is almost exclusively derived from artificial source.
  a. Pb comes mainly from fungicidal treatments, tinned containers or environmental pollution, with a minimal natural contribution from soil. Examples of exceptions can be wines from Sardinia, whose vineyards are often located in proximity or lead mines
  b. Co, Cr, Ni and V, present in wine at low concentrations, come mostly from interaction of wine and must with metallic containers for storage

  From the point of view of traceability, most promising variables are the elements of chiefly natural origin (group 1) in that these can reflect distinctiveness of soil or vine. From the point of view of authentication, indeed, even elements belonging to the group 2 can yield discrimination power as they can reflect distinctiveness of winemaking besides of soil.

  It is important to stress out the need to have several variables at disposal as a key to obtain good discrimination. Particularly suitable are therefore multielemental techniques such as ICP-MS or ICP-AES.

4.2.1. Authentication

  The starting point in authentication studies on wines is finding one or few analytes allowing discrimination in groups of the wine samples analyzed. If this is not possible in a simple way, as is usually the case, data need to be elaborated with chemometric methods, either unsupervised (PCA and CA) or supervised (DA). In the selection of chemical variables for geographic authentication, it must be considered that every classification scheme accounts for itself, in the sense that variables fit for a good classification in one case can result unfit in other cases. Studies in which metal ions were exploited as variables recommend in some cases use of alkali (Li, Na, Rb) and alkali-earth metals (Ca, Mg, Sr, Ba), in other cases use of transition metals (Mn, Ni) or of lanthanides. This is due to the great complexity and heterogeneity of wine, a chemical matrix that can reflect typical features of soils, vines and winemaking processes different from area to area. For this reason it is quite hard or impossible to single out variables useful for every classification scheme.

  Nevertheless, elemental analysis has been and still is often used in provenance studies of wines. Application of the SIA technique, with reference to Sr and Pb isotope ratios, has been already discussed in paragraph 2.2.2 and is at present potentially the most efficient method for geographic provenance of wines. In addition to studies cited in paragraph 2.2.2, some more studies are noteworthy. Ogrinc *et al.* [42] investigated the authenticity and geographical origin of Slovenian wines using a combination of IRMS and SNIF-NMR to determine isotopic ratios of H, C and O. Results allowed authors to discriminate between coastal and continental wine regions. Christoph *et al.* [43] discussed the relationship between meteorological data and isotopic composition of wines with reference to German wines produced in the regions of Franconia and Lake Constance between 1992 and 2001. In another study of these authors, discussion was extended to Hungarian and Croatian wines produced between 1997 and 2001 [44].

  Besides isotope analysis, it is relatively recent the indication that trace elements also could be helpful in the geographic discrimination. A pioneering study on German wines was done by Siegmund and Bächmann in 1977 [45] who determined 15 elements in 70 wines using Neutron Activation Analysis and Cluster analysis. Among first studies is noteworthy one by McCurdy and Medina [46] who in 1992 determined with ICP-MS lanthanides and other trace and ultratrace elements in wines coming from different countries, verifying differences in the distribution; the number of samples analyzed was scarcely significative, though. A simple classification was obtained by Latorre *et al.* [47] in which 42 white wines from Galicia (Northwestern Spain) were analyzed with AAS for their content of Li, Rb, Na, K, Mn, Fe and Ca, in order to discriminate wines of *Rias Baixas* Certified Brand of Origin, considered to be more valuable, from other wines often used as possible substrates for falsification. Authors showed that discrimination could be obtained from just two variables, in this case Li and Rb, but this must be seen as an extremely fortuitous case. A study by Baxter *et al.* [48] was among the first in which ICP-MS was used to obtain variables; authors classified 55 wines from Spain and 57 from England through determination of not less than 48 trace elements and data treatment with discriminant analysis. Among the set of samples red, white and roseé wines were present, showing that geographic provenance was stronger than variety in determining elemental content in wine. On a smaller scale, in another study [49] 88 samples of German white wines were analyzed. Samples were from four typical wine regions (Dienheim and Ingelheim from of the Rheinhessen area, Bad Dürkheim and Landau from Pfalz) and from three varieties (*Riesling*, *Silvaner* and *Weißburgunder*). Among 33 elements determined with ICP-MS, highly significative for discrimination resulted to be As, Be, Cs, Li, Sn, Sr, Ti, W and Y at trace level and B, Mg, Pb, Si as minor elements. A study by Castiñeira Gomez *et al.* [50] proposed different chemometric approaches to treatment of data obtained with ICP-MS; authors reviewed also the state-of-the-art of geographic classification of wines with elemental analysis. On a slightly different side, Taylor *et al.* [51] analyzed 95 samples of *Riesling*, *Pinot Blanc*, *Chardonnay* and *Gewürztraminer* wines from Okanagan Valley (British Columbia) and Niagara Peninsula (Ontario), two important wine regions in Canada who are quite different from a geochemical point of view. Authors verified differences of composition in soil sampled from vineyards of the two regions, in particular for Sr content, which reflected well in wines, allowing discrimination of the two groups on the basis of elemental content. Rb and Sr, but also Al, Co, Mn, Mo, Sb, U, V and Zn were the best variables for classification using Discriminant Analysis.

As seen before, in many cases elements are efficient variables for classification. In many other cases, though, this is not true, in particular when wines coming from nearby regions are considered. In such cases it is highly possible that differences induced by soil be negligible or anyway less significant than those induced by winemaking processes or vine varieties. When this happens it is suitable to support elemental analysis with determination of other parameters, such as organic compounds, routine parameters (i.e. density, alcohol content, acidity, dry extract etc.) or spectroscopic parameters; in this way datasets can be generated with higher probability of classification success. Among the several studies that can be cited concerning this subject, Etievant *et al.* [52] combined inorganic and organic parameters to classify French red wines. Martin *et al.* [53,54,55] were among the first to combine isotope ratio analysis and metal determination to improve geographic classification. Brescia *et al.* [56] analyzed several wines from Apulia (Southern Italy) determining routine and NMR parameters, metals, inorganic anions, carboxylic acids and classifying samples according to geographic provenance into three groups: Central, Northern and Southern Apulia.

4.2.2. Traceability

Traceability of wine could be studied through determination of elements in the various section of wine chain. The main concept underpinning this kind of study is the following: if concentration of an element is not altered by artificial factors, it should be possible to find it in wine in amount proportional to its concentration in soil. It is necessary to point out, though, that in a typical food chain the concentration of most elements tends to change inside wide ranges from soil to the final product. Most soluble ions (or most *bioavailable* ions) will be uptaken best by plants and their concentration will be consequently higher in food. Therefore, since a single element can hardly be significant for discrimination of foodstuffs of different geographic provenance, it is more suitable to concentrate on the *distribution* of several elements. The meaning of distribution is to take into consideration globally the concentrations of a range of elements instead of one element only, so that this concept is linked to relative ratios among these elements. This concept will be explained in depth when speaking about lanthanides.

The link of a wine with soil could therefore be put into evidence through determination of distribution of selected elements in the different chain sections. Vine soaks up from soil all mineral substances needed for its metabolism. Some studies [57,58] suggest that element distribution (or at least a part of it) in soil, could be found unaltered in plants feeding from that soil, constituting in this way a sort of fingerprint propagating to plants and finally to fruits, up to final products such as wine [59].

Among trace elements, lanthanides or Rare Earths Elements (REE) seem to be powerful markers for traceability of plants [60,61,62,63,64,65] and wine [66] in reason of their similar chemical behavior. REE are 14 elements with atomic number ranging from 57 and 71. They occur mainly as trivalent ions Me^{3+}, with exceptions concerning Ce^{4+} and Eu^{2+}, and can be divided into two subgroups: from La to Gd with a more basic behavior and higher solubility, from Tb to Lu with a more acid behavior and lower solubility. Their electronic configuration is $(Xe)4f^x6s^2$, i.e. they have 4f orbitals partially to completely filled, according to atomic number, but external 6s orbitals are always filled. In reason of this configuration, all REE show similar chemical behavior. Moreover, REE seem not to have a definite role in plant physiology, so that plants tend to treat their ions without distinction. It is assumed that trivalent ions could compete with calcium in same instances but no discrimination is reported among different REE. According to these features, it is highly probable that REE distribution in soil could remain unaltered in grapes, in must and eventually in wine. This is because elements showing similar chemical behavior should answer consequently to the various physico-chemical processes occurring along the wine chain such as precipitation, complexation or plant uptake. There should not be, therefore, any *fractionation* of distribution, that is, depletion or enrichment of some REE. These characteristics make REE an ideal group of elements for tracing food and, in particular, wine.

To better evaluate the meaning of distribution, let us first consider metal content in soil-plants-fruits chains. To fix ideas, we can state, according to what is shown in Table 7, that for lanthanides an average lowering of nearly 100.000 times occurs from soil to fruits and finally to wine. Concentrations of REE in plants are very low compared to those in soils and rocks because these elements are largely insoluble.

Table 7. Average ranges of some lanthanides in soil, plants and wine

Section of chain	La	Ce	Pr	Nd	Sm	Eu	Gd
Rocks	1-200 mg/Kg	1-250 mg/Kg	1-30 mg/Kg	1-80 mg/Kg	1-20 mg/Kg	0.01-4 mg/Kg	1-20 mg/Kg
Plants	1-15000 µg/Kg	2-16.00 µg/Kg	1-600 µg/Kg	10-3000 µg/Kg	0.2-800 µg/Kg	0.04-170 µg/Kg	2-500 µg/Kg
Wine	30-1200 ng/l	70-2000 ng/l	10-250 ng/l	10-1000 ng/l	20-200 ng/l	10-70 ng/l	10-200 ng/l

For what concerns wine, variation of concentration of trace elements from soil to grapes, must and wine is very high. In Figure 5 the concentration of lanthanum and cerium in a sample wine chain is shown.

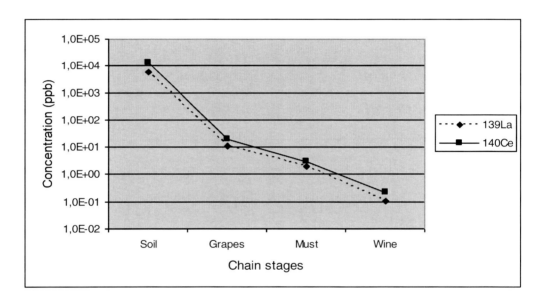

Figure 5. Lanthanum and cerium concentration along a sample wine chain (log scale)

This is the reason why we must not evaluate traceability according to absolute concentration data but to relative data, that is *distribution* data. Compare as an example ratios of lanthanum concentration vs. other metals concentrations in different section of a sample wine chain as shown in Table 8.

Table 8. Ratios of lanthanum vs. other metals in wine chain

Section of chain	La	Ce	Nd	Fe	Cu
Soil	100 µg/Kg	200 µg/Kg	10 µg/Kg	1000 mg/Kg	100 mg/Kg
Grapes	10 µg/Kg	20 µg/Kg	1 µg/Kg	10 mg/Kg	5 mg/Kg
Wine	1 µg/l	2 µg/l	0.1 µg/l	10 mg/l	1 mg/l
ratio La/Me	1	0.5	10	various	various

It is apparent that, while the absolute concentrations of the analytes reported is lowering from soil to wine, the distribution of lanthanides Ce and Nd, here expressed as ratios with lanthanum, is constant. Note that Fe and Cu do not behave the same way: their initial concentration is changed by several factors, either natural and anthropogenic.

In view of these initial results, it appears that REE could be suitable for wine traceability. Several studies in the scientific literature discussed this possibility in the last 20 years. Starting from the cited work by McCurdy and Medina in 1992, there have been some notable contributions. There is general agreement on the fact that the whole winemaking cycle had to be considered: some authors were in fact skeptical about suitability of REE as fingerprint for the provenance of wines [67,68,69], due to possible contamination from bentonites usually applied for purification during wine fining; other authors [70,71,72,73,74,75] reported that different types of bentonites behave in a different way, some altering distribution, some not. According to this studies, it can be hypothesized that a proper choice of fining agents could allow to perform traceability studies. More data are needed on this subject and effects of winemaking must be taken carefully into consideration.

Oddone *et al.* [76] evaluated the role of REE in four chains of wines from Piedmont (Italy). Data were obtained by ICP-MS analysis of soil, grapes, must and wine of *Gavi* (a white wine), *Barbera*, *Brachetto d'Acqui* and *Freisa* (red wines). Results reported by authors showed that REE distribution was clearly maintained from soil to must, while some fractionation occurred in wines as an effect of winemaking. As an example, results from a *Gavi* chain are shown in Figure 6

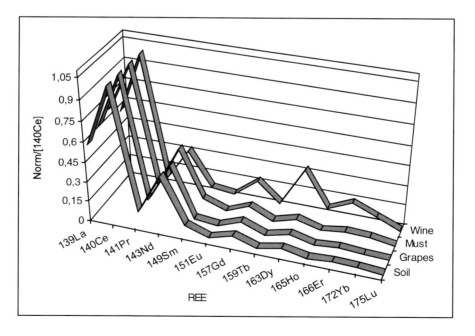

Figure 6. Distribution of REE in various stages of a chain of *Gavi*

In order to better compare data from the different stages of this sample chain, in every stage (soil, grapes, must and wine) concentration data are normalized to Ce so that [Ce] is always equal to 1. It is apparent that REE behave like group 1 elements as described before. Similar results were reported by Bertoldi *et al.* [77]. Authors found a good correlation among REE content in grapes and in soil after extraction with aqua regia.

For what concerns distribution of REE in the last chain stage, i.e. wine, results from Oddone *et al.* showed that some fractionation occurred on heavier analytes (Gd-Lu) when passing from must to wine as an effect of winemaking processes, while lighter analytes (La-Eu) seem to maintain a constant distribution. It must be considered also that concentrations of heavy REE in wines are usually lower than 50 ppt, as can be seen in Table 9, so that corresponding analytical data as determined with ICP-MS must be considered less robust.

Table 9. REE Concentrations in a sample of *Gavi*

Element	Concentration	Element	Concentration
Lanthanum	0,064	Terbium	0,01
Cerium	0,16	Dysprosium	0,029
Praseodymium	0,002	Holmium	0,021
Neodymium	0,098	Erbium	0,042
Samarium	0,026	Thulium	0,022
Europium	0,014	Ytterbium	0,05
Gadolinium	0,025	Lutetium	0,011

Finally, the powerful and unique role of REE in traceability is well demonstrated in comparing Figure 6 with Figure 7, where distribution of some transition metals determined in the same chain is reported: in this case distribution is not maintained constant, as a consequence of winemaking processes, so that transition metals behave apparently like groups 2 or 3 and are not therefore suitable as markers.

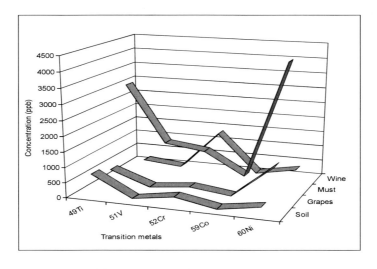

Figure 7. Distribution of some transition metals in various stages of a chain of *Gavi*

4.3. Varietal Classification

Another common classification scheme of wines is on the basis of variety. This aspect is important from the commodity point of view since specifications, as said before, provide for precise rules on the use of raw materials, indicating which varieties and to what maximum percentages can be used. In more restrictive specifications (such as *Barolo* DOCG) not only the vine variety is specified but also the cultivars. It is apparent that the possibility to recognize grape varieties in a wine is therefore important. In V.Q.P.R.D wines from EU countries, all varieties classified belong to species *Vitis vinifera* or come from a crossing among this species and other species of the *Vitis* genus [78].

Variables allowing to discriminate and recognize vine varieties are mainly organic compounds, among which of particular relevance are the following:

- volatile compounds, accounting for wine aroma;
- polyphenolic compounds, among which anthocyanins are the most important;

Such as in geographic classification one element only cannot guarantee efficient discrimination, in varietal classification one compound only is not enough to distinguish different varieties. In few cases a specific compound can be associated with a vine variety [79], such as some monoterpenes which are responsible for floral aroma in *Muscat*, *Gewürztraminer* and *Riesling* or cis-Rose oxide which is a key aroma constituent of *Gewürztraminer*. As a rule, compounds formed biosynthetically in food are similar in every variety of that food; the same holds for compounds formed as a consequence of technological processes. What is changing from variety to variety is, again, the distribution of these compounds.

It must be considered that the equivalence a vine ⇔ a wine is not a common rule in winemaking, in reason of the fact that the interest of wine producers is to obtain a valuable wine, not to work for the analytical chemist! A common problem in varietal classification is therefore when a wine is produced starting from two or more vine varieties. In some cases this is not allowed (example: *Barolo* made from other vines than *Nebbiolo*) and it is relatively simple to find out frauds; in some other cases, that is, when mixing is allowed according to specifications, it is quite difficult or impossible to check for possible frauds. For example *Chianti*, a valuable DOCG wine from Tuscany, can be produced using not less than four different vines, as can be seen in Table 10.

Table 10. Composition of *Chianti*

Vines	Percentage allowed
Sangiovese	75.0% - 100.0%
Canaiolo Nero	0.0% - 10.0%
Malvasia Bianca Lunga	0.0% - 10.0%
Trebbiano Toscano	0.0% - 10.0%
Other red grape vines	0.0% - 15.0% according to zone and type

This is quite an hindrance from the authentication point of view, as the distribution of some vine markers such as anthocyans will result in a mixture of different contributions.

4.3.1. Volatile Compounds

Volatile compounds are responsible for wine flavor. They belong to the groups of terpenes, alcohols, aldehydes, ketons, acids, esters and other minor groups. These compounds can be divided in three classes:

1. *primary* or *grape-derived* compounds, mostly terpenes, also called *varietal flavors* because they are typical of different varieties of *Vitis vinifera*;
2. *secondary* or *fermentation-derived* compounds are given off during winemaking processes, in particular during pressing (*prefermentative flavors*) and during fermentations (*fermentative flavors*);
3. *tertiary* or *ageing-derived* compounds are generated during maturity and ageing, in relation to conservation conditions that can be either oxidizing (with air contact) or reducing (without air)

Volatile compounds are very important from the point of view of wine classification. Primary flavors can be used in varietal classification, being specific for every vine variety. Secondary flavors are generated by fermentations, without meaningful differences among varieties. Tertiary flavors, finally, can assume typical features according to vine or conservation method. After all, flavors can be considered as promising variables in classification studies, with particular reference to terpenic profile.

For what concerns varietal classification of wines, several studies can be cited on the use of volatile compounds as discriminating variables, most of them using GC-MS coupled with extraction methods such as SPE or SPME. Best studies are those devoted to classification of aromatic wines which are rich in terpenes. Weber *et al.* [80] classified 90 samples of white wines from Germany belonging to three valuable varieties: *Mueller-Thurgau*, *Silvaner* and *Riesling* varieties. A good classification was obtained using as variables terpenes such as linalool oxide (trans), α-terpineol, 2,6-dimethyl-3,7-octadien-2,6-diol and β-citronellol and other compounds such as benzyl alcohol, phenyl ethyl alcohol and hexanoic acid. In a similar study Danzer *et al.* [81] classified wines of *Müller-Thurgau*, *Riesling*, *Silvaner*, *Scheurebe*, *Weißer Burgunder* and *Gewürztraminer* varieties by using a combination of terpenes and some vintage-dependent components such as 1-hexanol, 2-furancarboxaldehyde, diethyl succinate, phenyl ethyl alcohol, benzyl alcohol, and hexanoic acid. Falqué *et al.* [82] classified samples of *Loureira*, *Treixadura* and *Dona Branca* wines, produced from autochthonous varieties typical of Galicia and Northern Portugal. Other studies were those of Pozo-Bayo *et al.* [83] on Spanish wines and of Pet'ka *et al.* [84] on Slovak white wines.

4.3.2. Polyphenolic Compounds

Among polyphenolic compounds, anthocyanins are the most important from the varietal point of view. In the *Vitis vinifera* grape, used to produce wines all over Europe, only five different anthocyanins are present as 3-O-monoglucosides: delphinidin, cyanidin, petunidin, peonidin and malvidin (Figure 8).

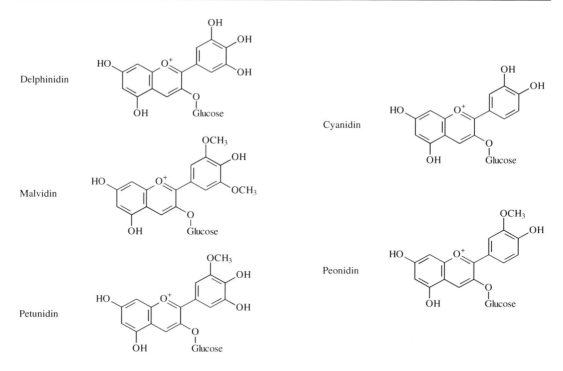

Figure 8. The five anthocyanins of *Vitis vinifera*

In non-*Vitis vinifera* grapes, such as *Vitis labrusca*, 3,5-O-diglucosides are present; since in some countries the production and commercialization of wines from non-*Vitis vinifera* grape is prohibited, hybrid grapes may be identified by their anthocyanin profile, because of their 3,5-O-diglucoside anthocyanin contents which are practically absent in the *Vitis vinifera* grapes [85]. Moreover, extracts from other botanical varieties (elderberry, strawberry, blackcurrant, cherry, etc.) are sometimes illicitly added to improve wine color but this fraud can be easily revealed as the corresponding anthocyanins are different, containing different sugar residues. The study of anthocyanic composition is therefore a useful tool to characterize grapes and wines, all the more it is one of the parameters used in taxonomic classification of grapes.

Some studies demonstrate the possibility to exploit anthocyanin profile in the varietal classification of red and roseé wines, provided that samples be produced in purity, i.e. using a single grape variety. Anthocyanins are usually determined by HPLC. It must be considered that the anthocyanin content of these wines depends on variety, vintage and technology and decreases with time; as in the case of metals for geographic classification, the determination of absolute anthocyanin concentrations can give scarce information regarding variety because the effects of technology and age are greater. However, the anthocyanin distribution, that is, the ratio of anthocyanins to each other, is determined by the variety and shows more stability in time. In a study by Zeppa *et al.* [86] the anthocyanin composition was determined in four autochthonous vines from Piedmont: *Avanà, Becouet, Grisa nera* and *Grisa roussa*. The four vine varieties showed completely different anthocyanin distributions, in particular *Grisa roussa* was found to be composed nearly exclusively by cyanidin. Carreño *et al.* [87] discriminated 32 varieties of grapes cultivated in the Murcia region (Southeastern Spain) according to their anthocyanin profile. For what concerns wines, Berente *et al.* [88] analyzed 52 German wines of 7 different varieties and were able to obtain a good varietal classification with PCA analysis. Similar results were proposed by Arozarena *et al.* [89] in a study on Spanish wines. Some authors [90] pointed out the fact that anthocyanin patterns could be different in skin extracts and wines of the same cultivar, as a consequence of winemaking, suggesting the need of extensive databases of varietal wines from different geographical and oenological origins.

4.3.3. IR analysis

While previous classification examples were based on identification of well-defined analytes, another possibility of varietal classification is given by spectroscopic analysis of wine samples, with particular interest to IR analysis. The IR spectrum of a wine can be used to extract variables, i.e. absorbances at different wavelengths, useful to obtain a classification without any reference to the compounds responsible for absorption in the IR spectrum. Edelmann *et al.* [32] were able to obtain an efficient varietal classification of red Austrian wines of Cabernet Sauvignon, Merlot, Pinot Noir, Blaufränkisch, St. Laurent and Zweigelt varieties; in order to improve classification power, spectra were recorded on dried extracts after passing samples on SPE RP-C18 columns, so that polyphenolic compounds could be evidenced. In the spectra the main absorption bands are similar for all samples but little, significant shifts in absolute position are present from sample to sample, in such a way that IR spectrum can be considered a fingerprint of the polyphenolic profile of a wine variety. Even better classification results were obtained by the authors when first derivative spectra of the samples were used.

4.4. Technological Classification

The third classification scheme is based on technology of production. It aims to distinguish among wines produced with different winemaking technologies or ageing. The main aspect with technological classification is again the economical one. Wines produced with more onerous processes, such as ageing or rigid selection of grapes, should see this charge acknowledged by a higher price. Wines from organic agriculture, for example, should be sold at a higher price than wines from industrial production, as well as an aged wine is expected to be more expensive than a young one. It is also important, of course, to be able to discriminate among *regular* and *illicit* winemaking practices. To summarize, the following aspects can be pointed out in technological classification:

1. distinction among young and aged wines: differences exist that can be detected already by tasting but are more apparent upon chemical analysis and can be exploited for classification if chemistry of the involved reactions is well understood;
2. distinction among different vintages in a wine series: it is well-known that some vintages, as a consequence of favorable climatic conditions, can reach extra-quality and therefore higher prices. As an example, *Barolo* vintages 1958, 1961, 1964, 1971, 1978, 1979, 1982, 1985, 1989, 1990, 1993 and 1995 are considered highly valuable or *five stars* vintages;

3. distinction among wines produced with organic or industrial agriculture practices: residues of industrial processes can be identified
4. distinction among type of ageing (i.e. oxidizing or reducing conditions): different flavors can develop in either cases
5. distinction among type of containers (wood, barrique, steel, cement etc.): same as previous case

In all cases it is important to be able to identify compounds acting as markers of the technological processes involved. Sometimes these compounds can be present in wine at trace or ultratrace concentration levels, though being already active from the organoleptic point of view if their concentration is beyond perception threshold. Flavors developing in ageing, for example, are still partly unknown and are at present the object of scientific research [79]. Some of them are formed in oxidant or reducing conditions starting from compounds already present in wine, while others are released by cask wood. Their identification could greatly support authentication of aged wines; moreover, casks assembled with wood coming from different geographic areas could generate different flavor profiles in aged wines. Among these flavors, some can be considered as effective markers for ageing:

1. *furans* such as 5.6-dihydro-4-methyl-2H-pyran-2-one, imparting to wine a *candy floss* aroma;
2. *lactones* such as β-methyl-γ-octalactone 15, commonly known as *oak* or *whiskey lactone*, imparting a woody, oaky, coconut-like aroma;
3. *aldehydes* such as 4-hydroxy-3-methoxybenzaldehyde or vanillin, imparting the typical vanilla aroma;
4. *phenols* such as 4-vinylguaiacol, responsible for unpleasant *burnt* aroma

As for geographic and varietal classification, many studies are present in the literature dealing with technological classification of wines. In this case it is harder to identify well-defined classes of compounds useful as variables; volatile compounds are perhaps the most powerful.

For what concerns discrimination among young and aged wines, it is noteworthy a study by Marengo *et al.* [91] who discriminated 68 samples of wines from Piedmont produced with vine *Nebbiolo* but differing for ageing. Samples belonged to 5 different specifications:

1. *Barolo*, the most valuable among *Nebbiolos*, with 3 years of ageing
2. *Barbaresco*, almost as valuable as *Barolo*, with 2 years of ageing
3. *Nebbiolo d'Alba*, with 1 years of ageing
4. *Roero*, with 8 months of ageing
5. *Langhe Nebbiolo*, the youngest and less valuable, with 6 months of ageing

The possibility to discriminate among *Nebbiolos* is very important, as the difference in price can be as high as 20 times among aged and younger types. This classification is interesting also from the varietal point of view, since selected clones of *Nebbiolo* are used for the most valuable specifications, and from the geographic point of view since areas delimited by specifications are different (this is the subject of another study by Marengo and Aceto [92]) as shown in Figure 9.

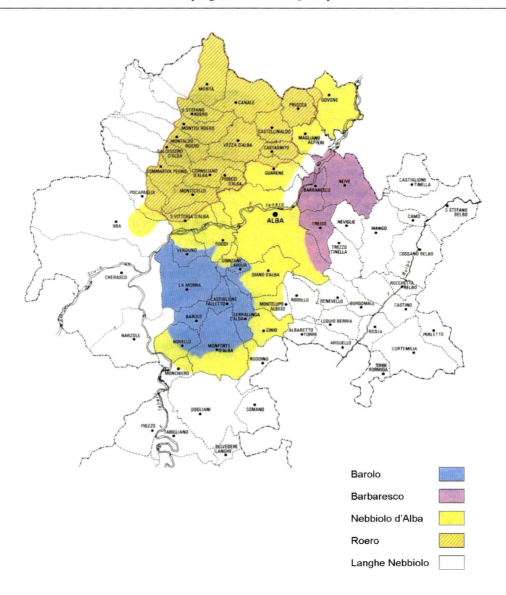

Figure 9. Areas of production of the 5 Nebbiolos

Varietal discrimination was obtained by authors on the basis of volatile compounds distribution as determined with SPME-GC-MS. 35 compounds, mostly alcohols, esters and terpenes, were selected as variables. PCA analysis allowed to discriminate well the 5 specifications and it is interesting to note that the first PC was found to be anticorrelated with ageing time. The most discriminating variables were found among esters: ethyl 2-methylpropanoate, 3-methylbutyl hexanoate, ethyl decanoate, diethyl succinate, ethyl 3-methylbutanoate and ethyl octanoate. This can be explained by having a look inside chemistry of wine ageing:

- esters formed by reaction of ethanol with carboxylic acids (tartaric, malic, lactic, succinic) tend to increase their concentration with ageing, though esterification rates be very low, with lactate and succinate more reactive and tartrate less reactive;
- esters formed during fermentation processes or *neutral esters* (non ethylic esters, ethyl hexanoate, ethyl octanoate, ethyl decanoate) tend to hydrolyze and so decrease their concentration because in young wines they are produced at concentration higher that allowed in equilibrium conditions

For what concerns technology of ageing, it is interesting to make reference to *Sherry*. This typical Spanish wine is obtained following a hard production cycle. Several different types of *Sherry* are produced, according to different winemaking processes used including ageing. Categories *Fino, Oloroso* and *Amontillado* are produced in different conditions during ageing: in *Fino* reducing processes, due to *flor* yeasts, are prevailing, in *Oloroso* oxidative processes are prevailing while in *Amontillado* both conditions are present who globally give rise to a more complex organoleptic profile. As a consequence, *Amontillado* is considered to be the more valuable category of *Sherry*. The three cited categories can be discriminated according to chemical parameters such as volatile compounds and polyphenols distributions:

- aromatic profiles of the three categories, determined with SPME-GC-MS, can be resumed as follows: *Fino* is characterized by fruity and floral aroma due to compounds such as farnesol, β-citronellol and β-ionone, by rancid taste due to butanoic acid and by stinging aroma due to acetaldehyde; *Oloroso* shows smoky and ethereal aromas due respectively to ethyl guaiacol and ethyl acetate; *Amontillado* shows an intermediate, more complex profile
- polyphenols distribution, determined with HPLC, can be described as follows: in *Fino* polyphenols derived from cynnamic and benzoic acids are prevalent; in *Oloroso* the polyphenolic content is higher and more variegated; *Amontillado* shows again an intermediate profile

In a work by Garcia Moreno and Barroso [93] the three categories were well discriminated according to the variables described before, that is aromatic profile and polyphenolic profile. In the first classification scheme the compound 5-(hydroxymethyl)-2-furaldehyde was found to be highly discriminant; PCA analysis revealed that that the first component explained the degree of oxidation of the samples while the second component explained the effect of the process of biological aging. In the second classification scheme, discrimination was obtained on the basis of low molecular weight polyphenols; discrimination was already apparent at the beginning of ageing process.

For what concerns discrimination among vintages, one of the first studies was proposed by Seeber *et al.* [94] who were able to discriminate among different vintage years (1986, 1987,1988) of Chardonnay musts and wines from Trentino (Northern Italy). Several parameters, either organic and inorganic, were determined by authors. In a study based on determination of similar parameters, Giaccio and Del Signore [95] analyzed 156 samples of *Montepulciano d'Abruzzo* of three different vintages, 1994, 1995 and 1996; samples were produced in different zones of Abruzzo (Central Italy) with slightly different winemaking procedures. Classification according to vintage year, connected with climatic conditions, was found to be the more efficient, allowing to identify single vintages.

5. CONCLUSIONS

As can be seen, scientific research is greatly supporting the search for quality in wine production. As soon as more sophisticated and powerful analytical techniques are available, authentication and traceability studies of wine are becoming more and more popular among scientists; in the meantime, consumers can take advantage of these results. Contextually, illicit processes become more and more difficult to be discovered.

After all, to be able to follow the wine chain is a hard task to perform; authentication of wine samples is slightly simpler but sometimes puzzling. Human intervention, be it allowed or illicit, contributes heavily to the final product. On the other hand, it must be remembered that, while the task of the analytical chemist is to distinguish among authentic and false wine samples or to find the link among soil and wine, the main aim of wine producers is quality of their products, not traceability nor authentication.

REFERENCES

[1]   European Commission Regulation No 178/2002. *Off. J. Eur. Comm.* 2002, L31/1.
[2]   Forina, M.; Lanteri, S. In Chemometrics, Mathematics and Statistics in Chemistry; Kowalski, B.; Ed.; Riedel: Dordrecht, *The Netherlands*, 1984; pp 305-350.
[3]   Forina, M.; Armanino, C.; Castino, M.; Ubigli, M. *Vitis*, 1986, 5, 189-201.
[4]   Forina, M.; Drava, G. *Analusis*, 1997, 25, M38-M42.
[5]   Arvanitoyannis, I. S.; Katsota, M. N.; Psarra, E. P.; Soufleros, E. H.; Kallithraka, S. *Trends Food Sci. Technol.* 1999, 10, 321-336.
[6]   De Groot, P. A. Handbook of stable isotope analytical techniques; Elsevier: Amsterdam, *The Netherlands*, 2004, Vol. 1, pp 1258.
[7]   Martin, G. J. Rev. Fr. *Oenol.* 1988, 28, 53-60.
[8]   Martin, G. J.; Guillou, C.; Martin, M. L.; Cabanis, M. T.; Tep, Y.; Aerny, J. J. *Agric. Food Chem.* 1988, 36, 316-322.
[9]   European Commission Regulation No 2676/90. *Off. J. Eur. Comm.* 1990, L272/64.
[10] European Commission Regulation No 822/97. *Off. J. Eur. Comm.* 1997, L117/10.
[11] European Commission Regulation No 440/2003, *Annex II. Off. J. Eur. Comm.* 2003, L66/17.
[12] Rossmann, A. *Food Rev. Int.* 2001, 17, 347-381.
[13] Rossmann, A.; Schmidt, H. L.; Reniero, F.; Versini, G.; Moussa, I.; Merle, M. H. Z. Lebensm. *Unters. Forsch.* 1996, 203, 293-301.
[14] Versini, G.; Monetti, A.; Reniero, F. In Wine - Nutritional and Therapeutic Benefits; Watkins, T. R.; Ed.; ACS Symposium Series 661; *American Chemical Society*: Washington, DC, 1997; pp 113-130.
[15] Rossmann, A.; Reniero, F.; Moussa, I.; Schmidt, H. L.; Versini, G.; Merle, M. H. Lebensm. *Unters. Forsch.* 1999, 208, 400-407.

[16] Coetzee, P. P.; Vanhaecke, F. *Anal. Bioanal. Chem.* 2005, 383, 977-984.
[17] Horn, P.; Schaaf, P.; Holbach, B.; Holzl, S.; Eschnauer, H. Z. Lebensm. *Unters. Forsch.* 1993, 196, 407-409.
[18] Barbaste, M.; Robinson, K.; Guilfoyle, S.; Medina, B.; Lobinski, R. *J. Anal. At. Spectrom.* 2002, 17, 135-137.
[19] Almeida, C. M. R.; Vasconcelos, M. T. S. D. *Food Chem.* 2004, 85, 7–12.
[20] Rosman, K. J. R.; Chisholm, W.; Jimi, S.; Candelone, J. P.; Boutron, C. P.; Teissedre, P. L.; Adams, F. C. *Environ. Res.* 1998, 78, 161-167.
[21] Larcher, R.; Nicolini, G.; Pangrazzi, P. *J. Agric. Food Chem.* 2003, 51, 5956-5961.
[22] Medina, B.; Augagneur, S.; Barbaste, M.; Grouset, F. E.; Buat-Meard, P. *Food Addit. Contam.* 2000, 17 435-445.
[23] Mihaljevic, M.; Ettler, V.; Sebek, O.; Strnad, L.; Chrastny, V. *J. Geochem. Explor.* 2006, 88, 130-133.
[24] Gonzalvez, A.; Armenta, S.; Pastor, A.; de la Guardia, M. *J. Agric. Food Chem.* 2008, 56, 4943-4954.
[25] Dessuy, M. B.; Vale, M. G. R.; Souza, A. S.; Ferreira, S. L. C.; Welz, B.; Katskov, D. A. *Talanta* 2008, 74, 1321-1329.
[26] Catarino, S.; Curvelo-Garcia, A. S.; de Sousa, R. B. *Talanta* 2006, 70, 1073-1080.
[27] Aceto, M.; Abollino, O.; Bruzzoniti, M.C.; Malandrino, M.; Mentasti, E.; Sarzanini, C. *Food Addit. Contam.* 2002, 19, 126-133.
[28] Pyrzynska, K. *Crit. Rev. Anal. Chem.* 2004, 34, 69-83.
[29] Flamini, R. *Mass Spectrom. Rev.* 2003, 22, 218-250.
[30] Flamini, R.; Panighel, A. *Mass Spectrom. Rev.* 2006, 25, 741-774.
[31] Liu, L.; Cozzolino, D.; Cynkar, W. U.; Dambergs, R. G.; Janik, L.; O'Neill, B. K.; Colb, C. B.; Gishen, M. *Food Chem.* 2008, 106, 781-786.
[32] Edelmann, A.; Diewok, J.; Schuster, K. C.; Lendl, B. *J. Agric. Food Chem.* 2001, 49, 1139-1145.
[33] Kelly, S.; Heaton, H.; Hoogewerff, J. *Trends Food Sci. Technol.* 2005, 16, 555-567.
[34] Reid, L. M.; O'Donnell, C. P.; Downey, G. *Trends Food Sci. Technol.* 2006, 17, 344-353.
[35] Kwan, W.; Kowalski, B. *J. Food Sci.* 1978, 43, 1320-1323.
[36] Zoecklein, B. W.; Fugelsang, K. C.; Gump, B. H.; Nury, F. S. Wine analysis and production; *Chapman & Hall*: New York, NY, 1995.
[37] Aceto, M. In Reviews in food and nutrition toxicity; Preedy, V. R.; Watson, R. R.; Eds.; *Taylor & Francis*: London, UK, 2003; *Vol. 1*, pp 169-203.
[38] Kment, P.; Mihaljevic, M.; Ettler, V.; Sebek, O.; Strnad, L.; Rohlova, L. *Food Chem.* 2005, 91, 157-165
[39] Greenough, J. D.; Mallory-Greenough, L. M.; Fryer, B. J. *Geosci. Can.* 2005, 32, 129-137.
[40] Greenough, J. D.; Mallory-Greenough, L. M.; Fryer, B. J. *Geochim. Cosmochim. Acta* 2006, 70, A215-A215.
[41] Pohl, P. *Trends Anal. Chem.* 2007, 26, 941-949.
[42] Ogrinc, N.; Košir, I. J.; Kocjančič, M.; Kidrič, J. *J. Agric. Food Chem.* 2001, 49, 1432-1440.
[43] Christoph, N.; Rossmann, A.; Voerkelius, S. Mitt. *Klosterneuburg* 2003, 53, 23-40.

[44] Christoph, N.; Baratossy, G.; Kubanovic, V.; Kozina, B.; Rossmann, A.; Schlicht, C.; Voerkelius, S. Mitt. *Klosterneuburg* 2004, 54, 155-169.
[45] Siegmund, H.; Bächmann, K. Z. *Lebensm. Unters. Forsch.* 1977, 164, 1-7.
[46] McCurdy, E., Potter, D., Medina, B. *Lab. News* 1992, 9, 10-11.
[47] Latorre, M. J.; Garcia-Jares, C.; Medina, B.; Herrero, C. J. *Agric. Food Chem.* 1994, 42, 1451-1455.
[48] Baxter, M. J.; Crews, H. M.; Dennis, M. J.; Goodall, I.; Anderson, D. *Food Chem.* 1997, 60, 443-450.
[49] Thiel, G.; Geisler, G.; Blechschmidt, I.; Danzer, K. *Anal. Bioanal. Chem.* 2004, 378, 1630-1636.
[50] Castiñeira Gomez, M. D. M.; Feldmann, I.; Jakubowski, N.; Andersson, J. T. J. *Agric. Food Chem.* 2004, 52, 2962-2974.
[51] Taylor, V. F.; Longerich, H. P.; Greenough, J. D. J. *Agric. Food Chem.* 2003, 51, 856-860
[52] Etievant, P.; Schlich, P.; Bouvier, J. C.; Symonds, P.; Bertrand, A. J. *Sci. Food Agric.* 1988, 45, 25-41.
[53] Martin, G. J.; Mazure, M.; Jouitteau, C.; Martin, Y. L.; Aguile, L.; Allain, P. Am. J. *Enol. Vitic.* 1999, 50, 409-417.
[54] Day, M. P.; Zhang, B.; Martin, G. J. Am. J. Enol. *Vitic.* 1994, 45, 79-85.
[55] Day, M. P.; Zhang, B.; Martin, G. J. J. Sci. *Food Agric.* 1995, 67, 113-123.
[56] Brescia, M. A.; Caldarola, V.; De Giglio, A.; Benedetti, D.; Fanizzi, F. P.; Sacco, A. Anal. *Chim. Acta* 2002, 458, 177-186.
[57] AA.VV. Trace and Ultratrace Elements in Plants and Soil; Shtangeeva, I.; Ed.; *Advances in Ecological Sciences, Vol 20*; WIT Press: Southampton, UK, 2004, pp 364.
[58] Kabata-Pendias, A.; Pendias, H. Trace elements in soils and plants; *3ed.*; CRC: Boca Raton, USA, 2001, pp 413.
[59] Taylor, V. F.; Longerich, H. P.; Greenough, J. D. *Geosci. Can.* 2002, 29, 110-120.
[60] Brown, P. H.; Rathjen, A. H.; Graham, R. D.; Tribe, D. E. In Handbook on the Physics and Chemistry of Rare Earths; Gschneider, K. A.; Eyring, L.; Eds.; *Elsevier: Amsterdam, The Netherlands*, 1990, Vol. 13, pp 423-450.
[61] Wyttenbach, A.; Schleppi, P.; Bucher, J.; Furrer, V.; Tobler, L. *Biol. Trace Elem. Res.* 1994, 41, 13-29.
[62] Wyttenbach, A.; Furrer, V.; Schleppi, P.; Tobler, L. *Plant Soil*, 1998, 199, 267–273.
[63] Zhang, Z. Y.; Wang, Y. Q.; Li, F. L.; Xiao, H. Q.; Chai, Z. F. J. *Radioanal. Nucl. Chem.*, 2002, 252, 461-465.
[64] Tyler, G. *Plant Soil* 2004, 267, 191-206.
[65] Liang, T.; Ding, S. M.; Song, W. C.; Chong, Z. Y.; Zhang, C. S.; Li, H. T. J. *Rare Earths 2008*, 26, 7-15.
[66] Augagneur, S.; Medina, B.; Szpunar, J.; Lobinski, R. J. *Anal. At. Spectrom.* 1996, 11, 713-721.
[67] Jakubowski, N.; Brandt, R.; Stuewer, D.; Eschnauer, H. R.; Gortges, S. Fresenius J. *Anal. Chem.* 1999, 364, 424-428.
[68] Rossano, E.C.; Szilagyi, Z.; Malorni, A.; Pocsfalvi, G. J. *Agric. Food Chem.* 2007, 55, 311-317.
[69] Catarino, S.; Madeira. M.; Monteiro, F.; Rocha, F.; Curvelo-Garcia, A. S.; de Sousa, R. B. J. *Agric. Food Chem.* 2008, 56, 158-165.

[70] Castiñeira Gomez, M. D. M.; Brandt, R.; Jakubowski, N.; Andersson, J. T. *J. Agric. Food Chem.* 2004, 52, 2953-2961.

[71] Tatar, E.; Mihucz, V. G.; Virag, I.; Racz, L.; Zaray, G. *Microchem. J.* 2007, 85, 132-135.

[72] Almeida, C. M. R.; Vasconcelos, M. T. S. D. *J. Agric. Food Chem.* 2003, 51, 4788-4798.

[73] Mihucz, V. G. ; Done, C. J.; Tatar, E.; Virag, I.; Zaray, G.; Baiulescu, E. G. *Talanta*, 2006, 70, 984-990

[74] Larcher, R., Nicolini, G. In Hyphenated Techniques in Grape and Wine Chemistry; Flamini, R.; Ed.; *J. Wiley & Sons:* New York, NY, 2008, pp 423-450.

[75] Larcher, R., Nicolini, G., Bertoldi, D., Bontempo, L., Camin, F. In *TRACE - 4th Annual meeting and conference*, Torremolinos, 23rd-25th April 2008, pp 50-51.

[76] Oddone, M.; Robotti, E.; Marengo, E.; Baldizzone, M.; Aceto, M. In *Proceedings of VI Italian Congress "Chimica degli Alimenti";* Coisson, J. D.; Arlorio, M.; Martelli, A.; Eds.; Taro: Alessandria, IT, 2007; pp 573-577.

[77] Bertoldi, D., Larcher, R., Nicolini, G., Bontempo, L., Bertamini, M., Concheri, G. In *TRACE - 4th Annual meeting and conference, Torremolinos, 23rd-25th April 2008*, pp 51-52.

[78] European Commission Regulation No 1493/99. Off. *J. Eur. Comm.* 1999, L 179/15.

[79] Ebeler, S. E. *Food Rev. Int.* 2001, 17, 45-56.

[80] Weber, J.; Beeg, M.; Bartzsch, C.; Feller, K. H.; De la Calle Garcia, D.; Reichenbächer, M.; Danzer, K. J. High Resol. *Chromatogr.* 1999, 22, 322-326.

[81] Danzer, K.; De la Calle Garcia, D.; Thiel, G.; Reichenbächer, M. *Am. Lab.* 1999, 26-34.

[82] Falqué, E.; Fernandez, E.; Dubourdieu, D. J. Agric. *Food Chem.* 2002, 50, 538-543.

[83] Pozo-Bayo, M. A.; Pueyo, E.; Martın-Alvarez, P.J.; Polo, M. C. J. *Chromatog*r. A 2001, 922, 267-275.

[84] Petka, J.; Mocak, J.; Farkaš, P.; Balla, B.; Kovač, M. J. Sci. *Food Agric.* 2001, 81, 1533-1539.

[85] Flamini, R. J. *Mass Spectrom.* 2005, 40, 705-713.

[86] Zeppa, G.; Rolle, L.; Gerbi, V.; Guidoni, S. Ital. J. *Food Sci.* 2001, 13, 405-412.

[87] Carreño, J.; Almela, L.; Martınez, A.; Fernandez-Lopez, J. A. *Lebensm.-Wiss. Technol.* 1997, 30, 259-265.

[88] Berente, B.; De la Calle Garcıa, D.; Reichenbächer, M.; Danzer, K. J. *Chromatog*r. A 2000, 871, 95-103.

[89] Arozarena, I.; Casp, A.; Marín, R.; Navarro, M. *Eur. Food Res. Technol.* 2000, 212, 108-112.

[90] Garcia-Beneytez, E.; Cabello, F.; Revilla, E. J. Agric. *Food Chem.* 2003, 51, 5622-5629.

[91] Marengo, E.; Aceto, M.; Maurino, V. *J. Chromatogr.* 2001, 943, 123-137.

[92] Marengo, E.; *Aceto, M. Food Chem.* 2003, 81, 621-630.

[93] Garcia Moreno, M. V.; Barroso, C. G. J. *Agric. Food Chem.* 2002, 50, 7556-7563.

[94] Seeber, R.; Sferlazzo, G.; Leardi, R.; Dalla Serra, A.; Versini, G. J. *Agric. Food Chem.* 1991, 39, 1764-1769.

[95] Giaccio, M.; Del Signore, A. J. *Sci. Food Agric.* 2004, 84, 164-172.

In: Red Wine and Health
Editors: Paul O'Byrne

ISBN: 978-1-60692-718-2
© 2009 Nova Science Publishers, Inc.

Chapter 18

HUMAN HEALTH BENEFITS, ANTIMICROBIAL PROPERTIES AND THE FUTURE OF PHENOLIC COMPOUNDS AS PRESERVATIVES IN THE FOOD INDUSTRY

María Cristina Manca de Nadra[*]
and María José Rodríguez Vaquero

Facultad de Bioquímica, Química y Farmacia – Universidad Nacional de Tucumán, and Centro de referencias de lactobacillus (Cerela) – CONICET, Tucumán. Argentina

ABSTRACT

Phenolic compounds are found in fruit, vegetables, nuts, seeds, stems and flowers as well as tea, wine, propolis and honey, and represent a common constituent of the human diet. Dietary flavonoids have attracted interest because they have a variety of beneficial biological properties, which may play an important role in the maintenance of human health. Flavonoids are potent antioxidants, free radical scavengers and metal chelators; they inhibit lipid peroxidation and exhibit various physiological activities including anti-inflammatory, antiallergic, anticarcinogenic, antihypertensive, antiarthritic and antimicrobial activities. Consumption of phenol-rich beverages, fruit and vegetables has commonly been associated to a reduction of the risk of cardiovascular diseases in epidemiological studies and the regular consumption, during several weeks or months, was shown to reduce cholesterolemia, and oxidative stress. The total polyphenols amounts determined from the same plant and their corresponding antioxidant and antimicrobial activities may vary widely, depending on extraction conditions applied.

Food contamination and spoilage by microorganisms are a serious problem because they have not yet been brought under adequate control despite the news preservation techniques available. Food-borne illness resulting from consumption of food contaminated with pathogenic bacteria has been of vital concern to public health.

---

[*] Correspondence to: Facultad de Bioquímica, Química y Farmacia – Universidad Nacional de Tucumán, ayacucho 471 and Centro de referencias de lactobacillus (Cerela) – CONICET, Chacabuco 145. Tucumán. Argentina. E-mail: mcmanca@fbqf.unt.edu.ar

Unfortunately there is a dramatic increase throughout the world in the number of reported cases of food-borne illness. To reduce the incidence of food poisoning and spoilage by pathogenic microorganisms many synthetic chemicals were utilized. The exploration of natural antimicrobials for food preservation receives increased attention due to consumer awareness of natural food products and a growing concern of microbial resistance towards conventional preservatives. The use of phenolic compounds as antimicrobial agents would provide an additional benefits, including dual-function effects of both preservation and delivery health benefits. Knowing the antimicrobial effect of the phenolic compounds from vegetables on the principal pathogenic microorganisms from the different foods, it is possible to search strategies to combine the synergic antimicrobial effects of phenolic compounds with their natural biological properties. The results will permit to formulate new products to be used as food preservatives or to be included in the human diet.

INTRODUCTION

Phenolic compounds are secondary metabolites which are synthesized by plants and play important structural roles in the cell wall, act as a defense against UV light, protect against pathogen ingress and are involved in repair of injury. Many foods and beverages contain high levels of phenolic compounds, which often provide colour, taste, astringency and other sensory characteristics (Williamson *et al.*, 2000).

Derived from the basic structure of phenol (hydroxybenzene), the term "phenolic" refers to any compound with a phenol-type structure.

Basical chemical structure of phenolic compounds

There are three classes of phenolics compounds in terms of chemical structures:

1. Non-flavonoids

Phenols with only one aromatic ring, derivatives of hydroxycinnamic acid (caffeic, ferulic acids) or of hydroxybenzoic acid (gallic, protocatechuic, vanillic acids). Some of them that are present in red wines are:

Hydroxybenzoic Acid Derivatives

Gallic acid *Protocatechuic acid* *Vanillic acid*

Hydroxycinnamic Acid Derivates

Caffeic acid *Ferulic acid*

2. Flavonoids

Flavonoids are one of the better-known groups of polyphenols. They are most common in edible plant products, particularly fruits and vegetables (excluding algae and mushrooms) (Bravo, 1998). Food products abundant in flavonoid compounds are green leafed, yellow and red vegetables (e.g., onion, cabbage, broccoli, cauliflower, Brussels sprouts, pulse seeds, tomatoes, and peppers), fruit (e.g., grapefruits, oranges, berries, red and black currants, dark grapes and apples) (Bengoechea et al.,1997; Buren et al.,1976; Lu & Foo, 1997; Oleszek et al., 1988), but also tea (especially green tea) (Hojden, 2000; Perucka, 2001) and red wine (Pelegrinin, et al., 2000; Vinson & Hontz, 1995).

They have a common core, the flavane nucleus, consisting of two benzene rings (A and B) linked by an oxygen-containing pyrane ring (Van de Wiel et al., 2001). They are classified according to substitutions and differ in the arrangements of hydroxyl, methoxy, and glycosidic side groups, and in the conjugation between the A- and B- rings (Heim et al., 2002).

Based on the saturation and oxidation of heterocyclic C-ring, flavonoids are subdivided in flavan, flavanone, flavone, flavonol, dihydroflavonol, flavan-3-ol, flavan-4-ol, and flavan-3, 4-diol (Marais et al., 2006). The well-known flavonoids, belonging to the flavan-3-ol class, include catechin (*trans*) and epicatechin (*cis*), which differ from each other on the configuration of carbons 2 and 3, which are linked to a catechol ring and to a hydroxyl group, respectively. (de Souza et al., 2008)

Basical chemical structure of flavonoids compounds

Flavonols

Rutin

Quercetin

Miricetina

Kaempferol

Flavanols

(+)-Catechin

3. Tannins

Tannins could be divided into hydrolysable and condensed tannins and these are classified by structure and susceptibility to acid hydrolysis. Hydrolysable tannins are comprised of a polyol carbohydrate core (usually D-glucose) esterified to phenolic acids such as gallic or ellagic acids, forming gallotannins and ellagitannins, respectively. Mild acid hydrolysis of these tannins yields carbohydrates and phenolics. Tannic acid is a gallotannin consisting of esters of gallic acid and glucose, containing galloyl groups esterified directly to the glucose molecule (Rodríguez *et al*, 2008).

Other flavonoids structurally related to (epi)catechin included gallocatechin/epigallocatechin and afzelechin/epiafzelechin. These compounds can be linked to a gallic acid residue, giving rise to gallate derivatives, or forming oligomers among themselves, giving rise to proanthocyanidins, known as condensed tannins. Condensed tannins have also been found, consisting of di-, tri-, tetra-, and penta-, hexa, and heptamers (de Souza *et al*, 2008).

BENEFICIAL EFFECTS OF PHENOLIC COMPOUNDS

Interest in phenolic compounds has increased in recent years because of their potential beneficial effects on human health. Phenolic compounds are well documented for their biological effects, which led to the belief that diet rich in fruit and vegetables contributes to good health (Williamson *et al*, 2000).

The total polyphenols amounts determined from the same plant and their corresponding antioxidant and antimicrobial activities may vary widely, depending on extraction conditions applied (Wach *et al.*, 2007).

Flavonoids (mg/kg or mg/l)	Major sources
< 10	Cabbage, spinach, carrots, peas, peaches, berries, orange juice, coffee, white wine.
< 50	Lettuce, beans, red pepper, tomatoes, apples, grapes, tea, cherries, red wine.
> 50	Broccoli, endive, celery, onion, cranberry.

Apple pulp contains catechin, procyanidin, caffeic and chlorogenic acids among other components. The skin contains all the afore mentioned substances as well as flavonoids, not present in pulp, such as quercetin glycosides and cyanidin glycosides (Escarpa & Gonzalez, 1998; Van der Sluis *et al.*, 2001). Apples are fruits consumed worldwide in different forms fresh, juices and cider. Their beneficial properties to human health are related to the high content of phenol compounds.

In *Granny Smith* and *Royal Gala* apple varieties, the phenolic compounds concentration depend on extraction conditions applied. Extractions were carried out twice for 8 h at 60°C (Jayaprakasha *et al*, 2003) with 400 ml of the following solvents: A, acetone:water:acetic acid; B, ethyl acetate:methanol:water and C, ethanol:water. The most effective extraction method for polyphenols from apples was with acetone:water:acetic acid. By this method the *Granny Smith* variety contained 49% more total polyphenols than *Royal Gala*.

Grapes and wines contain a large array of phenolic compounds. The specific amounts and types of phenolics present in grapes and wine depend on a number of factors, including variety of grape, maturity, seasonal conditions, storage, and processing practices (Amerine & Ough, 1980): phenol carboxylic acids, 100-200 mg/l, catechin, 10-400 mg/l, quercetin, 5-20 mg/l (Cheynier & Teissedre, 1998). The total concentration polyphenols in red Argentinean wines from a same winemaking depend of the grape variety. Cabernet Sauvignon, Malbec and Merlot wines have 2,300, 2,522 and 2,704 mg/l gallic acid equivalents (GAE), respectively (Rodríguez Vaquero *et al*, 2007a).

Extracts obtained from grape seeds and pomace, which are by-products of the wine and juice industries, also have been used as natural antioxidants (Ahn *et al.*, 2002; Jayaprakasha *et al.*, 2001; Revilla & Ryan, 2000; Wang *et al.*, 2000), because these extracts contain large quantities of monomeric phenolic compounds such as catechins, epicatechin and epicatechin-3-O-gallate, and dimeric, trimeric and tetrameric procyanidins (Saito *et al.*, 1998).

Olive leaf exhibited a profile in which oleuropein is the compound present in highest amount, representing 73% of total identified compounds and caffeic acid is the minor compound, corresponding to 1% of total phenolics (Pereira *et al*, 2007).

The most common flavonoids in tea are the flavan-3-ols (flavanols or flavans). Black tea contains limited amounts of catechins and more abundant levels of the theaflavins, including theaflavin, theaflavin-3-gallate, theaflavin-3'-gallate and theaflavin-3,3'-digallate, which are regarded as the biologically important active components of black tea and that provide health benefits. As with the catechins, the theaflavins are effective antioxidants (Leung *et al.*, 2001) and intake of one to six cups of black tea/day significantly increases plasma antioxidant capacity (Gardner *et al.*, 2007).

Epidemiological studies associate phenolic consumption with lower mortality, especially caused by coronary diseases. They present multiple biological properties, which are of growing interest for consumers due to the high antioxidant, anti-inflammatory, anti-allergic, anti thrombosis and antimicrobial activities (Kanner *et al.*, 1994; Frankel *et al.*, 1995; Koga *et al.*, 1999; Eberhardt *et al.*, 2000; Jayaprakasha *et al.*, 2003; Baydar *et al.*, 2004; Shoji *et al.*, 2004). Furthermore they act as antideposit of triglyceride, anticholesterolemic, and antiviral agents among others.

Flavonoids and other phenolic compounds are efficient antioxidants, stronger than antioxidant vitamins. They are scavengers of so-called reactive oxygen species (ROS) that are by-products of many of the body´s normal chemical processes that can damage cell membranes and interact with genetic materials. ROS are possibly involved in the development of cancer, coronary heart diseases and aging processes.

Oxidation of low-density lipoproteins (LDL) is thought to play an important role in atherosclerosis. Oxidized LDL has been found in atherosclerotic lesions of humans (Shaikh *et al.*, 1988). A whole range of antioxidants has been shown to be able to prevent LDL-oxidation when added to isolate LDL. Not surprisingly, flavonoids (de Whalley *et al*, 1990; Mangiapane, 1992; Négre-Salvayre & Salvayre, 1992; Rice-Evans *et al.*, 1996; Wu *et al.*, 1996) or food extracts rich in flavonoids such as wine (Frankel *et al.*, 1993; Kondo *et al.*, 1994; Lanningham-Foster *et al.*, 1995; Rankin *et al.*, 1993; Viana *et al.*, 1996), also show this protective action towards in vitro LDL-oxidation.

Moreover, they sustain the elasticity, integrity and blood vessel wall resistance to injury (Horbowicz, 2000). The phenomenon has been observed in the Mediterranean area, as the so-called "French paradox" where, despite a considerable proportion of fat in the dwellers' diets, mortality caused by cardiovascular system diseases is much lower than in other countries. The fact is ascribed to a large dietary proportion of fruits, vegetables, and red wine (Fogliano, Verde *et al.*, 1999; Hurtado *et al.*, 1997; Soleas *et al.*, 1997; Zduńczyk, 1999).

ANTIMICROBIAL ACTIVITY OF PHENOLIC COMPOUNDS

Phenolic compounds may affect growth and metabolism of bacteria. Depending on the concentration, the effect of different phenolic compounds could be beneficial to growth of lactic acid microorganisms (Reguant *et al.*, 2000) or inhibitory (Campos *et al.*, 2003). It was reported the effects of different concentrations of gallic acid and (+)-catechin in laboratory media on the growth and metabolism of *Lactobacillus hilgardii* 5w a wine spoilage lactic acid bacteria. At concentrations normally present in wine, these pure phenolic compounds not only stimulated the growth rate but also resulted in greater cell densities during the stationary growth phase and at high concentrations they inhibited the bacterium growth (Alberto *et al.*, 2001). Landete *et al.*, 2008, studied the inhibitory growth activities of nine phenolic compounds (Cinnamic acid, p-hydroxybenzoic acid, hydroxytyrosol, oleuropein, protocatechuic acid, sinapic acid, syringic acid, tyrosol and vanillic acid) at the concentrations found in olive food products against *Lactobacillus plantarum*, they observed that none of the nine phenolic compounds analyzed inhibit the growth of *L. plantarum*. In addition, only oleuropein and protocatechuic acid were metabolized by *L. plantarum* cultures containing the phenolic compound.

Pereira et al., 2007, screened olive leaf aqueous extracts for their antimicrobial activity against Bacillus cereus, Bacillus subtilis, Sthaphylococcus. aureus, Escherichia coli, Pseudomonas aeruginosa, Klebsiella pneumoniae bacteria, Candida Albicans and Candida neoformans (fungi). Aside from concerns with food quality degradation, these microorganisms may be causal agents of intestinal infections in humans. The extract inhibited all the tested bacteria and fungi, suggesting a broad antimicrobial activity of olive leaf extracts in a concentration-dependent manner.

Turkmen *et al.*, 2007, determined the polyphenols content and the antibacterial activities of black tea extracts against different food-borne pathogens which have undesirable effects on quality, safety and shelf life of foods (*Staphylococcus aureus, Hafnia alvei, Yersinia enterocolitica, Listeria monocytogenes, Bacillus cereus* and *Escherichia coli O157:H7*). *Staphylococcus aureus* was found to be the most sensitive to tea extracts. Tea extracts were not effective against *Yersinia enterocolitica, Listeria monocytogenes* and *Escherichia coli* O157:H7.

On pathogenic microorganisms the antibacterial effect depends of the phenolic compounds and of the strains tested (Puupponen-Pimiä *et al.*, 2005; Wen *et al.*, 2003). Rodríguez Vaquero *et al.,* 2007a, screening the antibacterial effect of pure non-flavonoid phenolic compounds, gallic, vanillic, protocatechuic, and caffeic acids and flavonoids phenolic compounds, rutin, quercetin and catechin and polyphenols of different varieties of Argentinean wines, Cabernet Sauvignon, Malbec and Merlot, against *Serratia marcescens*

Proteus mirabilis, Escherichia coli , Klebsiella pneumoniae, Flavobacterium sp obtained from human origin and strains from American Type Culture Collection (ATCC), *Escherichia coli* 35218 and 25922, *Staphylococcus aureus* 25923 and 29213 and *Pseudomonas aeruginosa* 27853. Of the four non-flavonoid compounds, the hydroxycinnamic acid derivate, caffeic acid, has been shown to possess more effective antibacterial activity against the bacteria investigated than hydroxybenzoic acids derivatives. Quercetin was the best antibacterial flavonoids.

Rodríguez Vaquero et al., 2007b, demonstrated the antimicrobial properties of pure flavonoid and non-flavonoid phenolic compounds and total polyphenols of the three Argentinean wines varieties, against *Listeria monocytogenes* from human.

The foodborne pathogen, *Listeria* has been a cause of many outbreaks of listeriosis with high case fatality rates. The economic impact due to big product recalls, severity of the disease, hospitalization and treatment costs has drawn the attention of researchers towards the development of preventive measures to control the spread of *Listeria monocytogenes* (Gandhi & Chikindas, 2008). *L. monocytogenes* can be found in a wide variety of raw and processed foods. Milk and dairy products, various meats and meat products such as beef, pork, fermented sausages, fresh produce such as radishes, cabbage, seafood and fish products have all been associated with *Listeria* contamination; the elderly, pregnant, newborn and immunocompromised populations are more susceptible to listeriosis (Rocourt & Cossart, 1997).

A diminution of two, one and half log cycles was observed in presence of 500mg/l caffeic acid, rutin and quercetin, respectively. The diminution of cell viability was correlated with phenolic compounds concentration (Figure 1). Gallic and protocatechuic acids have three and two hydroxyl groups in their structures, respectively, while group instead of hydroxyl group. As speculation, considering the chemical structure the lower inhibitory effect of vanillic acid with respect to gallic and protocatechuic acid could be related with the presence of the methoxy group instead of hydroxyl group. Rutin, glycoside form of quercetin, was the most effective flavonoid with anti-listerial activity.

They reported that all wines samples produced bacterial death and the antimicrobial effect was directly related to phenolic compound concentration. Between non-flavonoid compounds, the hydroxycinnamic derivative caffeic acid was more effective to inhibit the growth parameters of *L. monocytogenes* than the hydroxybenzoic acids. All flavonoids were inhibitory for *L. monocytogenes*.

Figure 2 shows the viability diminution of *L. monocytogenes* when the BHI medium was added with wine samples. Wines were concentrated in rotary evaporator. Without concentrate, two and four-fold concentrated (1x, 2x and 4x) wines were clarified by the addition of 30, 60 and 120 mg/ml of activated charcoal, respectively in order to eliminate phenolic compounds. At 36 h storage, phenolic compounds of Cabernet Sauvignon wine showed a decrease in the number of viable cells of 40%, 54% and 67%, for 1x, 2x and 4x wines, respectively, with respect to the correspondent clarified control wines. The highest inhibition was observed by the addition of Merlot samples to BHI medium. There was a decrease of 50%, 64% and 79% for 1x, 2x and 4x samples of Merlot wines, respectively. In this case the viability was from 15% to 25% and from 11% to 20% lower than Cabernet Sauvignon and Malbec wines, respectively. The viable cells of *L. monocytogenes* disappeared completely at 60, 72 and 84 h storage in media with wines concentrated 4x, 2x and 1x, respectively.

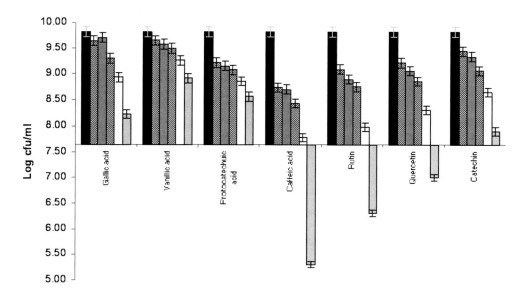

Figure 1. Number of viable cells of *Listeria monocytogenes* in BHI media supplemented with different concentration of phenolic compounds. (■) 0 mg/l, (▨) 25 mg/l, (▩) 50 mg/l, (▧) 100 mg/l, (□) 200 mg/l and (▨) 500 mg/l. (From Rodríguez Vaquero et al., 2007b)

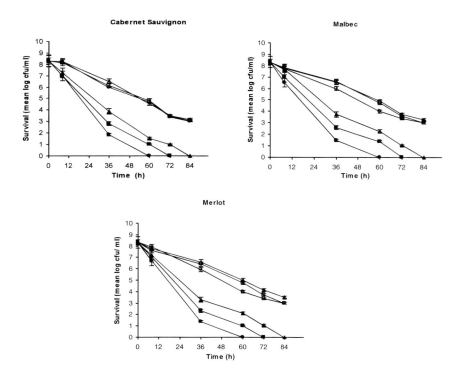

Figure 2. Survey of *Listeria monocytogenes* in BHI media supplemented with 50% of wines. Clarified wines: (Δ) 1x, (□) 2x and (o) 4x. Wines samples: (▲) 1x; (■) 2x and (●) 4x. (From Rodríguez Vaquero et al. 2007b)

Rodríguez Vaquero & Manca de Nadra, 2008a, investigated the effect of non-flavonoids and flavonoids phenolic compounds and total polyphenols of three Argentinean wines varieties, Cabernet Sauvignon, Malbec and Merlot on the viability of *Escherichia coli ATCC 35218*, microorganism widely distributed in the environment and frequently detected in fresh and processed foods.

Figure 3 shows the number of viable cells at 18 h contact with the different concentrations of phenolic compound. Figure 3 shows that the addition of 25 mg/l of gallic or caffeic acids reduced viable counts by 0.34 and 0.89 log cycle with respect to the control. Treatment with 50 mg/l of gallic or caffeic acids reduce 0.6 and 1.5 log cycles the number of viable cells, compared to the control, respectively. 25 and 50 mg/l of vanillic or protocatechuic acids did not decrease significatively the number of viable cells of *E. coli*.

The addition of 100 mg/l of gallic, protocatechuic, vanillic or caffeic acids decreased the number of viable cells by 0.95, 0.5 , 0.27 and 2.15 log cycles, respectively. From 200 mg/l of caffeic acid, we observed cellular dead. Treatment with 200 and 500 mg/l of caffeic acid reduced viable counts by 3.4 and 4.35 log cycles compared with the control.

With respect to flavonoids compounds, a diminution of 1.54, 1.13 and 0.54 log cycles with respect to the control was observed with the addition of 25 mg/l of quercetin, rutin and catechin, respectively. 200 mg/l quercetin was the only flavonoid compound that produced a diminution of 1 log cycle from the initial cells number inoculated in the media. 500 mg/l quercetin or rutin reduced 3 and 1 log cycles of inoculated cells, respectively.

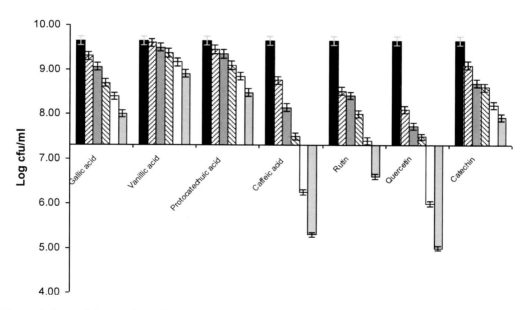

Figure 3. Log of the number of viable cells (cfu/ml) of *Escherichia coli* ATCC 35218 in nutrient broth media supplemented with different concentration of phenolic compounds. (■) 0 mg/l, (▨) 25 mg/l, (▨) 50 mg/l, (▨) 100 mg/l, (□) 200 mg/l and (□) 500 mg/l. (From Rodríguez Vaquero & Manca de Nadra, 2008a)

The decimal reduction time calculated (Table 1) shows that the times to reduce by 90% viable cells of *E. coli* were 2.9, 2.1 and 0.65 h for Malbec wine and 2.8, 2.3 and 0.64 h for Merlot wines with respect to 1x, 2x and 4x concentrated samples, respectively.

For Cabernet Sauvignon wine the values were 6.3, 3.7 and 1.28 h, for 1x, 2x and 4x concentrated samples, respectively.

With clarified wines the decimal reduction times were higher with values ranged from 15 to 18.4 h in the wine samples.

Table 1. Decimal reduction time of *Escherichia coli* in wines samples. (From Rodríguez Vaquero & Manca de Nadra, 2008a)

Grape Variety	Decimal reduction time of *Escherichia coli* (h) Wine concentration		
	1x	2x	4x
Cabernet Sauvignon	6.3	3.7	1.28
Malbec	2.9	2.08	0.65
Merlot	2.81	2.3	0.64
Clarified			
Cabernet Sauvignon	18.4	16.4	15
Malbec	16.9	17.7	15.1
Merlot	17.8	16.3	15.5

Ohemeng *et al.*, 1993, screened 14 flavonoids for inhibitory activity against *E. coli* DNA gyrase and other microorganisms. They found that *E. coli* DNA gyrase was inhibited in different extent by 7 of the assayed compounds including quercetin, proposing that the inhibitory activity was due in part to the DNA gyrase inhibition. Mirzoeva *et al.*, 1997, demonstrated that quercetin caused an increase in permeability of the inner bacterial membrane and a dissipation of membrane potential. This fact disturbed the capacity for ATP synthesis and membrane transport. Bernard *et al.*, 1997, found that the glycosylated flavonol rutin, inhibited topoisomerase IV- dependent decatenation activity of the *E. coli* strain, that is essential for cell survival. Ikigai *et al.*, 1993, reported that catechin may pertub the lipid bilayers by directly penetrating them and disrupting the barrier function. Bernard *et al.*, 1997, reported that despite amino acid sequence, structural and mechanistic similarities between DNA gyrase and topoisomerase IV, compounds selectively acting as topoisomerase IV poisons and inactive on gyrase do exist.

It is possible to infer that the DNA gyrase of *E. coli* was more sensitive than that of *L. monocytogenes* to quercetin inhibition. The requirement of a hydroxyl group at the C-3 position, as quercetin, for DNA cleavage activity with DNA gyrase is not necessary for topoisomerase IV. In the other hand rutin was more effective on *L. monocytogenes* than *E. coli*. Perhaps this fact could be related to the molecular difference with the aglicone quercetin. There is the carbohydrate rutinose instead of the hydroxyl group at the C-3 position.

Synergistic Antimicrobial Activity

According to Liu (2003) additive and synergistic effects of phytochemicals in fruits and vegetables are responsible for their potent bioactive properties and the benefit of a diet rich in fruits and vegetables is attributed to the complex mixture of phytochemicals present in whole foods. This explains why no single antimicrobial can replace the combination of natural phytochemicals to achieve the health benefits.

The synergistic antibacterial effect of mixtures of the non-flavonoids phenolic compounds, gallic, protocatechuic, vanillic and caffeic acids, and flavonoids, catechin, rutin and quercetin, against *L. monocytogenes* and *E. coli* were investigated in our laboratory. Phenolic compounds mixtures were assayed at a final concentration of 100 and 200 mg/l.

Theoretical and Experimental inhibitory effect of combined phenolic compounds:

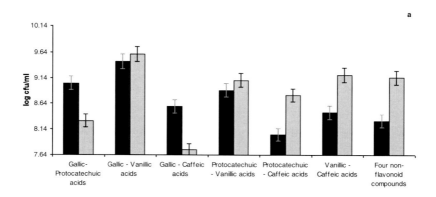

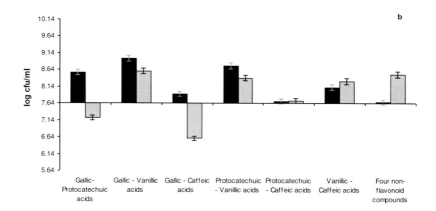

Figure 4. Number of viable cells of *Listeria monocytogenes* in BHI media supplemented with 100 mg/l (a) or 200 mg/l (b) of different non-flavonoid compounds mixtures.
(■) Theoretical values, (□) Experimental values. (From: Rodríguez Vaquero & Manca de Nadra, 2008b)

The theoretical values correspond to the sum of the antibacterial effect of each individual phenolic compound.

The experimental values are the result of inhibitory effects of the phenolic compounds combinations.

The synergistic effect could be of sum or cooperative. In the first one the results are the same with pure or combined phenolic compounds. The cooperative effect is the result of a high effect of the combined phenolic compounds with respect to the pure components.

The antagonistic effect is observed as an increase of the cellular viability respect to the theoretical values.

With 100 mg/l of non–flavonoid combinations (1:1 equivalent to 50:50 mg/l) (Figure 4a), 4 of the 7 produce synergistic effect, being gallic-protocatechuic and gallic-caffeic acids the most inhibitory (cooperative synergy) decreasing the microorganism viability 0.75 and 0.83 log cycles respectively, with respect to the corresponding theoretical value.

With 200 mg/l, (1:1 equivalent to 100:100 mg/l) (Figure 1b) 6 of the 7 combinations produce synergistic effect. Two of them, gallic-vanillic acids and protocatechuic-vanillic acids change the synergy of sum with 100 mg/l to a cooperative synergy with the higher concentration. With gallic-protocatechuic and gallic-caffeic acids, at 200 mg/l inoculated cellular death was observed, decreasing 0.44 and 1.04 log cycle, respectively.

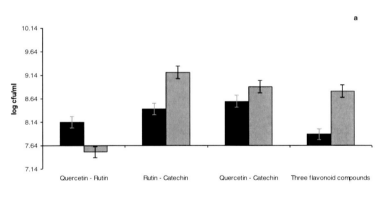

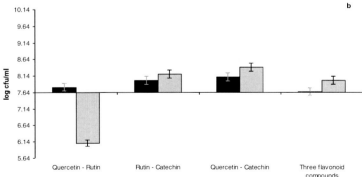

Figure 5. Number of viable cells of *Listeria monocytogenes* in BHI media supplemented with 100 mg/l (a) or 200 mg/l (b) of different flavonoid compounds mixtures. (From: Rodríguez Vaquero & Manca de Nadra, 2008b)

With 100 mg/l of flavonoid combinations (Figure 5a) only quercetin-rutin mixture produce synergistic effect (cooperative synergy) with cellular death, reducing the number of viable cells by 0.14 log cycles with respect to the inoculated cells. Rutin-catechin, quercetin-catechin and quercetin-rutin-quercetin combination produced antagonistic effect.

With the addition of 200 mg/l (Figure 5b), quercetin-rutin combination increased the cellular death, decreasing 1.54 log cycles the inoculated cells. The combination of rutin–catechin and quercetin–catechin, produce synergistic effect (sum synergy), but not cellular death was observed.

Similar results were obtained for *Escherichia coli* ATCC 35218, with 100 mg/l of non–flavonoid mixtures 5 of the 7 combinations produce synergistic antibacterial effect being gallic-protocatechuic and gallic-caffeic acids the more effectives (cooperative synergy) diminishing significantly the number of viable cells with respect to the control medium. With 200 mg/l of the different combinations 6 of the 7 produce synergistic antibacterial effect. At this concentration, gallic-protocatechuic, gallic-caffeic, protocatechuic-caffeic and gallic-protocatechuic-vanillic-caffeic acids produce cellular death.

With 100 mg/l of flavonoid combinations 3 of the 4 produce synergistic effect, being quercetin-rutin the most inhibitory (cooperative synergy), producing cellular death of the inoculated cells.

With 200 mg/l all flavonoid combinations produce cellular death. 2 of the 4 combinations produce cooperative synergy.

The non-flavonoid compound combination most effective is gallic-caffeic, which produces at 100 or 200 mg/l the highest synergistic inhibition on *L. monocytogenes* as well as *E. coli* viability.

For both bacteria, the most effective flavonoid compounds combination was quercetin-rutin that produces cooperative synergism between them.

CONCLUSIONS

Food contamination and spoilage by microorganisms are a serious problem because they have not yet been brought under adequate control despite the news preservation techniques available. Food-borne illness resulting from consumption of food contaminated with pathogenic bacteria has been of vital concern to public health. Unfortunately there is a dramatic increase throughout the world in the number of reported cases of food-borne illness. To reduce the incidence of food poisoning and spoilage by pathogenic microorganisms many synthetic chemicals were utilized. The exploration of natural antimicrobials for food preservation receives increased attention due to consumer awareness of natural food products and a growing concern of microbial resistance towards conventional preservatives.

The use of phenolic compounds as antimicrobial agents would provide an additional benefits, including dual-function effects of both preservation and delivery health benefits. Knowing the antimicrobial effect of the phenolic compounds from vegetables on the principal pathogenic microorganisms from the different foods, it is possible to search strategies to combine the synergic antimicrobial effects of phenolic compounds with their natural biological properties. The results will permit to formulate new products to be used as food preservatives or to be included in the human diet.

REFERENCES

Ahn, H. S., Jeon, T. I., Lee, J. Y., Hwang, S. G., Lim, Y. & Park, K. P. (2002). Antioxidant activity of persimmon and grape seed extracts: in vitro and in vivo. *Nutrition Research, Vol. 22*, 1265–1273.

Alberto, M. R.; Farías, M. E. & Manca de Nadra, (2001) M. C. Effect of gallic acid and catechin on *Lactobacillus hilgardii* 5w growth and metabolism of organic compounds. *J. Agric. Food Chem., vol. 49*, 4359-4363.

Amerine, M.A. & Ough, C.S. (1980) Phenolic compounds. In: *Methods of Analysis of Musts and Wines*; Wiley: New York; pp 175-199.

Baydar, N.G.; Özkan, G. & Sağdiç, O. (2004) Total phenolic contents and antibacterial activities of grapes (*Vitis vinifera* L.) extracts. *Food Control, Vol. 15*, no. 5, 335-339.

Bengoechea, M. L., Sancho, A. I., Bartolome, B., et al. (1997).Phenolic composition of industrially manufactured purees and concentrates from peach and apple fruits. *Journal of Agriculture and Food Chemistry, Vol. 45,* 4071– 4075.

Bernard, F.X., Sable, S., Cameron, B., *et al.* (1997). Glycosylated flavones as selective inhibitors of topoisomerase IV. *Antimicrob Agents Chemother.* 41, 992 – 998.

Bravo, L. Ph. D. (1998). Polyphenols: chemistry, dietary sources, metabolism, and nutritional significance. *Nutrition Reviews, Vol. 11*, 317–333.

Buren, J., Vos, L., & Pilnik, W. (1976). Polyphenols in golden delicious apple juice in relation to method of preparation. *Journal of Agriculture and Food Chemistry, Vol. 3*, 448–451.

Campos, F. M.; Couto J. A. & Hogg T.A. (2003) Influence of phenolic acids on growth and inactivation of *Oenococcus oeni* and *Lactobacillus hilgardii. J. Appl. Microbiol. Vol. 94*, 167-174.

Cheyner V. & Teissedre P.L. (1998) *Polyphénols En Œnologie*: Fondements Scientifiques Et Technologiques pp. 323-324. Paris: Technique et Documentation.

de Souza, L. M., Cipriani, T. R., Iacomini, M., Gorin P.A.J. & Sassaki, G. L. (2008). HPLC/ESI-MS and NMR analysis of flavonoids and tannins in bioactive extract from leaves of *Maytenus ilicifolia, Journal of Pharmaceutical and Biomedical Analysis Vol. 47*, 59–67.

de Whalley, C., Rankin, S. M., Hoult, J. R. S., Jessup, W. & Leake, D. S. (1990) Flavonoids inhibit the oxidative modifcation of low density lipoproteins by macrophages. *Biochemical Pharmacology, vol. 39*, 1743 -1750.

Eberhardt, M.V.; Lee, C.Y. & Liu, R.H. (2000) Antioxidant activity of fresh apples. *Nature, Vol. 405*, no. 6789, 903-904.

Escarpa, A. & Gonzalez, M.C. (1998). High-performance liquid chromatography with diode-array detection for the determination of phenolic compounds in peel and pulp from different apple varieties. *Journal Chromatography, vol. 823*, no. 1-2, p. 331-337.

Fogliano, V., Verde, V., Randazzo, G., et al. (1999). Method for measuring antioxidant activity and its application to monitoring the antioxidant capacity of wines. *Journal of Agriculture and Food Chemistry, Vol. 47*, 1035–1040.

Frankel E. N., Kanner J., German J. B., Parks E. & Kinsella J. E. (1993) Inhibition of oxidation of human low-density lipoprotein by phenolic substances in red wine. *Lancet, vol. 341*, 454-457.

Frankel, E.N.; Waterhouse, A.L. & Teissedre, P.L. (1995) Principal phenolic phytochemicals in selected California wines and their antioxidant activity in inhibiting oxidation of human low-density lipoproteins. *Journal of Agricultural and Food Chemistry*, Vol. 43, no. 4, 890-894.

Gandhi, M. & Chikindas, L.M. (2008). *Listeria*: A foodborne pathogen that knows how to survive. *International Journal of Food Microbiology,Vol.113*, 1–15.

Gardner E.J., Ruxton C.H.S., Leeds A.R. (2007). Black tea – helpful or harmful? A review of the evidence. *Eur. J. Clin. Nutr. Vol. 61*:3–18.

Héctor Rodríguez, Blanca de las Rivas, Carmen Gómez-Cordovés & Rosario Muñoz, (2008). Degradation of tannic acid by cell-free extracts of Lactobacillus plantarum. *Food Chemistry Vol. 107*, 664–670.

Heim, K.E., Tagliaferro, A.R. & Bobilya, D.J. (2002) Flavonoids antioxidants: chemistry, metabolism and structure-activity relationships. *Journal of nutritional Biochemistry Vol. 13*, 572-584.

Hojden, B. (2000). Herbata zielona i jej własciwosci lecznicze. Wiadomosci Zielarskie, Vol. 9, 14–15 (in Polish).

Horbowicz, M. (2000). Występowanie, biosynteza i właściwościbiologiczne flawonoli. Postępy nauk rolniczych, Vol. 2, 3–18 (in Polish).

Hurtado, I., Caldu, P., Gonzalo, A., et al. (1997). Antioxidative capacity of wine on human LDL oxidation in vitro: effect of skin contact in winemaking of white wine. *Journal of Agriculture and Food Chemistry, Vol. 45*, 1283–1289.

Ikigai, H, Nakae, T., Hara, Y. & Shimamura, T. (1993). Bactericidal catechins damage the lipid bilayers. *Biochim Biophys Acta. Vol. 1147*, 132 – 136.

Jayaprakasha, G. K., Selvi, T., & Sakaria, K. K. (2003). Antibacterial and antioxidant activities of grape (Vitis vinifera) seed extracts. *Food Research International, Vol.36*, 117–122.

Jayaprakasha, G.K., Singh, R.P. & Sakariah, K.K. (2001).Antioxidant activity of grape seed (Vitis vinifera) extracts on peroxidation models in vitro. *Food Chemistry,Vol. 73*, 285–290.

Kanner, J.; Frankel, E.; granit, R.; German, B. & Kinsella, J.E. (1994). Natural antioxidants in grapes and wine. *Journal of Agricultural and Food Chemistry, Vol. 42*, no. 1, 64-69.

Koga, T.; Moro, K.; Nakamori, K.; Yamakoshi, J.; Hosoyama, H.; Kataoka, S. & Ariga, T. (1999) Increase of antioxidative potential of rat plasma by oral administration of proanthocyanidin-rich extract from grape seeds. *Journal of Agricultural and Food Chemistry, Vol. 47*, no. 5, 1892-1897.

Kondo K., Matsumoto A., Kurata H., Tanahashi H., Koda H., Amachi T. & Itakura H. (1994) Inhibición of oxidation of low-density lipoprotein with red wine. *Lancet Vol. 344*, 1152-1152.

Landete, J.M., Curiel, J.A., Rodríguez, H., de las Rivas, B. & Muñoz, R. (2008). Study of the inhibitory activity of phenolic compounds found in olive products and their degradation by Lactobacillus plantarum strains. *Food Chemistry, Vol. 107*. 320–326

Lanningham-Foster, L., Chen, C., Chance, D. S. & Loo, G. (1995) Grape extract inhibits lipid peroxidation of human low density lipoprotein. *Biological and Pharmaceutical Bulletin Vol. 18*, 1347-1351.

Leung L.K., Su Y., Chen R., Zhang Z., Huang Y. & Chen Z-Y. (2001). Theaflavins in black tea and in catechins in green tea are equally effective antioxidants. *J. Nutr. Vol. 131*: 2248–51.

Liu, R.H., (2003).Health benefits of fruits and vegetables are from additive and synergistic combination of phytochemicals. *Am. J. Clin. Nutr.,Vol. 78*, 517S-520S-9.

Lu, Y., & Foo, Y. (1997). Identification and qualification of major polyphenols in apple pomace. *Food Chemistry, Vol. 2*, 187–194.

Mangiapane H. (1992) The inhibition of the oxidation of low density lipoprotein by (+)-catechin, a naturally occurring flavonoid. *Biochemical Pharmacology vol. 43*, 445-

Marais, J.P.J., Deavours, B., Dixon, R.A. & Ferreira, D., (2006). in: E. Grotewold (Ed.), *The Science of Flavonoids*, Springer, Ohio, 2006, pp. 1–46.

Mirzoeva, O.K., Grishanim, R.N. & Calder, P.C. (1997). Antimicrobial action of propolis and some of its components: the effects on growth, membrane potential and motility of bacteria. *Microbiol Res.Vol. 7*, 158 – 353.

Négre-Salvayre A. & Salvayre R. (1992) Quercetin prevents the cytotoxicity of oxidized LDL on lymphoid cell lines. *Free Radical Biology and Medicine, vol. 12*, 101-106.

Ohemeng, K.A., Schwender, C.F., Fu, K.P. & Barrett, J.F. (1993). DNA gyrase inhibitory and antibacterial activity of some flavones (1). *Bioorg. Med. Chem. Lett.. Vol. 3*, 225 – 30.

Oleszek, W., Lee, C. Y., Jaworski, A. W., *et al.* (1988). Identification of some phenolic compounds in apples. *Journal of Agriculture and Food Chemistry, Vol. 36*, 430–432.

Pelegrinin, N., Simonetti, P., Gordana, C., *et al.* (2000). Polyphenol content and total antioxidant activity of Vini Novelli (Young red wines). *Journal of Agriculture and Food Chemistry, Vol. 48*, 732–735.

Pereira, A.P., Ferreira, I.C.F.R. , Marcelino, F., Valentão, P., Andrade, P.B., Seabra, R., Estevinho, L., Bento A. & Pereira, J.A.. (2007). Phenolic Compounds and Antimicrobial Activity of Olive (*Olea europaea* L. Cv. Cobrançosa) Leaves. *Molecules, Vol. 12*, 1153-1162.

Perucka, I. (2001). Skład chemiczny lis'ci herbaty. Biul. Magnezol. Vol. 6 (3),443–451 (in Polish).

Puupponen-Pimiä, R., Nohynek L., Hartmann – Schmidlin, S., Kähkönen M., Heinonen M., Määttä-Riihinen, K. & Oksman-Caldentey K. M. (2005). Berry phenolics selectively inhibit the growth of intestinal pathogens. *J. Appl. microbiol., vol. 98*, 991-1000.

Rankin, S. M., de Whalley, C. V., Hoult, J. R. S., Jessup, W., Wilkins, G. M., Collard, J. & Leake, D. S. (1993) The modification of low density lipoprotein by the flavonoids myricetin and gossypetin. *Biochemical Pharmacology, vol. 45*, 67-75.

Reguant, C.; Bordons, A.; Arola L.& Rozés N. (2000) Influence of phenolic compounds on the physiology of *Œnococcus œni* from wine. *J. Appl. Microbiol.*, 88, 1065-1071.

Revilla, E. & Ryan, J. M. (2000). Analysis of several phenolic compounds with potential antioxidant properties in grape extracts and wines by high-performance liquid chromatography-photodiode array detection without sample preparation. *Journal of Chromatography A, 881*, 461–469.

Rice-Evans, C. A., Millar, N. J. & Paganga, G. (1996). Structure antioxidant activity relationships of flavonoids and phenolic acids. *Free Radical Biology and Medicine, vol. 20*, 933-956.

Rocourt, J. & Cossart, P.,(1997). *Listeria monocytogenes*. In: Doyle, M.P., Buechat,L.R., Montville, T.J. (Eds.), Food Microbiology - Fundamentals and Frontiers. American Society for Microbiology (ASM) press, Washington DC, pp. 337–352.

Rodríguez Vaquero & Manca de Nadra, M.C. (2008b) Phenolic compounds mixtures on *Listeria monocytogenes* viability. 1st International Conference on Drug Design and Discovery, February 3 -6, Dubai, UAE.

Rodríguez Vaquero, M.J. & Manca de Nadra, M.C. (2008a). Growth parameter and viability modifications of *Escherichia coli* by phenolic compounds and argentine wine extracts. *Applied Biochemistry and Biotechnology*. Acepted february 26 2008.

Rodríguez Vaquero, M.J., Alberto, M.R. & Manca de Nadra, M.C. (2007a) Antibacterial effect of phenolic compounds from different wines. *Food Control* 18, 93 – 101

Rodríguez Vaquero, M.J., Alberto, M.R. & Manca de Nadra, M.C. (2007b). Influence of phenolic compounds from wines on the growth of *Listeria monocytogenes*. *Food Control, vol. 18*, 587 - 593.

Saito, M., Hosoyama, H., Ariga, T., Kataoka, S., & Yamaji, N. (1998). Antiulcer activity of grape seed extract and procyanidins. *Journal of Agricultural and Food Chemistry,Vol. 46*, 1460–1464.

Shaikh M., Martini S., Quiney J. R., Baskerville P., La Ville A. E., Browse N. L., Duffield R., Turner, P. R. & Lewis, B. (1988) Modifed plasma-derived lipoproteins in human atherosclerotic plaques. *Atherosclerosis Vol. 69*, 165-172.

Shoji, T.; Akazome, Y., Kanda, T. & Ikeda, M. (2004) The toxicology and safety of apple polyphenol extract. *Food and Chemical Toxicology, vol. 42*, no. 6, p. 959-967.

Soleas, G. J., Dam, J., Carey, M., et al. (1997). Toward the fingerprinting of wines: cultivar-related patterns of polyphenolic constituents in ontario wines. *Journal of Agriculture and Food Chemistry, Vol. 45*, 3871–3880.

Turkmen, N., Sedat Velioglu, Y., Sari, F.& Polat, G. (2007). Effect of Extraction Conditions on Measured Total Polyphenol Contents and Antioxidant and Antibacterial Activities of Black Tea. *Molecules, Vol. 12*, 484-496.

Van de Wiel, A., van Golde P.H.M. & Hart H.Ch. (2001) Blessings of the grape. *European Journal of Internal Medicine Vol. 12*, 484–489.

Van Der Sluis, A.A.; Dekker, M.; De Jager, A. & Jongen, W.M.F., (2001). Activity and concentration of polyphenolic antioxidants in apple: effect of cultivar, harvest year, and storage conditions. *Journal of Agricultural and Food Chemistry*, vol. 49, no. 8, 3606-3613.

Viana, M., Barbas C., Bonet B., Bonet M. V., Castro M., Fraile M. V. & Herrera E. (1996) In vitro effects of a flavonoid-rich extract on LDL oxidation. *Atherosclerosis, vol. 123*, 83-91.

Vinson, J. A., & Hontz, B. A. (1995). Phenol antioxidant index: comparative antioxidant effectiveness of red and white wines. *Journal of Agriculture and Food chemistry, Vol. 43*, 401–403.

Wach, A.; Pyrzynska, K. & Biesaga, M. (2007). Quercetin content in some food and herbal samples. *Food Chemistry Vol. 100*, 699-704.

Wang, J. N., Chen, Y. J., Hano, Y., Nomura, T. & Tan, R. X. (2000).Antioxidant activity of polyphenols from seeds of Vitis amurensis in vitro. *Acta Pharmacologica Sinica, 21* (7), 633–636.

Wen, A., Delaquis, P., Stanich, K. & Toivonen, P. (2003). Antilisterial activity of selected phenolic acids. *Food Microbiol., Vol. 20*, 305-311.

Williamson, G.; Day, A.J.; Plumb, G.W. & Couteau, D. (2000) Human metabolic pathways of dietary flavonoids and cinnamates. *Biochemical Society Transactions Vol. 28*, part 2, 16-22.

Wu T.W., Fung K.P., Wu J., Yang C.C., Lo, J. & Weisel R. D. (1996) Morin hydrate inhibits azo-initiator induced oxidation of human low density lipoprotein. *Life Sciences, vol. 58*, 17-22.

Zduńczyk, Z. (1999). Znaczenie biologicznie aktywnych nieodzywczych składnikow diet w zapobieganiu chorobom cywilizacyjnym. Zywnosc, 4(Suppl. 21), 75–89 (in Polish).

In: Red Wine and Health
Editor: Paul O'Byrne

ISBN 978-1-60692-718-2
© 2009 Nova Science Publishers, Inc

Short Communication

DIELECTRIC PROPERTIES AND WINES
IMPASSES, DEVELOPMENTS...

A. García Gorostiaga[*], J.L. Torres Escribano and M. De Blas Corral

Dept. of Projects and Rural Engineering, Universidad Pública de Navarra,
31006 Pamplona, Spain

ABSTRACT

The wine has been extensively described on the basis of chemical composition and sensory considerations. We aimed to characterize the grape juice and red wine through dielectric parameters. These studies were carried out on samples of red grape juice and red wine made from red varieties of grapes and the said dielectric parameters were used in order to find out a possible correlation among these values and the variety or the area where the samples were collected from. The frequency range was from 200 MHz to 3 GHz. Obtained results were not decisive enough.

Another problem we found with the open-ended coaxial probe measurement system was the undesirable results we obtained during the alcoholic fermentation process. During malolactic fermentation similar problems arose.

Regarding the study of dielectric properties in red wine before and after cold stabilisation, no significant differences could be detected, in the range under analysis from 200 MHz to 20 GHz.

INTRODUCTION

The wine has been extensively described on the basis of chemical composition and sensory considerations. We aimed to characterize the grape juice and red wine through dielectric parameters, dielectric constant and lost factor (see chapter "Dielectric Properties and Wine" to understand the terms used).

---

[*] E-mail of corresponding author: almudena@unavarra.es, Tel.: +34-948-16-91-58; fax: +34-948-16-91-48

These studies were carried out on samples of red grape juice and red wine made from red varieties of grapes. Next we will describe 3 research developments that either were clearly impasses, or where the results were not conclusive enough.

RELATION DIELECTRIC PROPERTIES-GRAPE VARIETY AND DIELECTRIC PROPERTIES-WINERY WHERE THE GRAPES WERE COLLECTED

The dielectric parameters were used in order to find out a possible correlation among these values and the variety or the area where the samples were collected from. The frequency ranged from 200 MHz to 3 GHz. All the grape juice analyzed is from the species *Vitis vinifera*, particularly red wine grapes. The used red wine grapes for aging are the varieties *cabernet sauvignon*, *tempranillo*, and *merlot*.

The descriptive analysis used to characterize musts was based on some of the most commonly used statistics. We considered of special importance the coefficient of variation, obtained dividing the standard deviation by the sampling mean. This value is independent of the unit of measurement and consequently it allows comparisons between the different variables measured.

Musts were grouped into either variety of grape or the winery from where they were collected. We compared the means of different populations on some measured dependent variables, that is, differences either among varieties or among wineries. The measured variables (dielectric constant, loss factor, electrical conductivity), are numerical and continuous whereas the distinctive variables, variety and winery where the samples were taken, are qualitative variables.

The one-way analysis of variance procedure (statistical software package SPSS version 9.0) was applied with the aim of finding out whether population means are different by comparing the variability among sample means with variability among individual observations within groups. The analysis of variance rests on a set of assumptions that will be considered before the procedure is applied (independence of observations, sampling distribution of the subgroup means nearly normal and equality of the population variances). The most inflexible assumption is the independence of the observations. Firstly, a test of ranks upper- and below-median whose non-fulfilment can suggest a non-random arrangement was performed. Secondly, we verified if the sampling distribution of the subgroup means was nearly normal using Shapiro-Wilks' test. This condition is especially important either if the sample sizes are not equal or if the sample sizes are small. Thirdly, the Levene test was conducted to see if sample variances are within the same general, that is to say, if the variances are homogeneous. This condition is especially important if the sample sizes are not equal (Anderson & Finn, 1996). When both the conditions of normality and of homogeneity of variances were not met, the Kruskal-Wallis nonparametric test was applied. It consists of comparing the means of more than two independent populations.

And finally, if there was some evidence of an inequality of means of the populations, we took both the Bonferroni multiple comparisons by pairs and Tukey´s HSD tests.

Comparison of means by wineries did not produce any important result, due to the heterogeneity of varieties and the different sample size of the wineries.

The study of the 3 most widely used varieties for the ageing of wines (cabernet, merlot and tempranillo) showed a significant difference of the means in the case of the losses at 3 GHz, both total and dipolar. In both cases Tempranillo had lower losses than cabernet and merlot.

To conclude we would say that, concerning the difference in losses, both total and dipolar (taking away the ionic component from the total) at 3 GHz, there is reasonable evidence that the tempranillo variety can be characterized against the cabernet and merlot varieties (García et al, 2001).

Given the necessary characteristics of the sampling and material used to carry out this study, in only the few days when the musts are available, it would be advisable to verify the data shown in this study with further experiments, and to replicate the experiment.

VARIATION OF THE DIELECTRIC PROPERTIES WITH TIME OF CHANGE OF STATE FROM GRAPE JUICE TO WINE

Another problem we found with the open-ended coaxial probe measurement system was the undesirable results obtained during the alcoholic fermentation process.

The variation of the dielectric constant and the loss factor are shown in *Fig. 1* with frequency on a logarithmic scale. These presentations were for one sample, but the same tendencies were observed also for other samples of grape juice. The reference of the measurements corresponded to the day on which the grape juice was collected (day 1) and the variation of the dielectric parameters for the other days are shown in Fig. 1 until day 49.

Initially we believed that the change in the variation of the parameters was very significant as time progressed. At the beginning of the fermentation and as time progressed, the fermentation became more intensive until a stage was reached where the fermentation started to decrease and gradually the process stopped.

However, inspection of the surface of the probe revealed bubbles of CO_2 adhering to the probe and thus distorting the measured data (García et al, 2004).

DIELECTRIC PROPERTIES OF NON-STABILIZED AND STABILIZED WINE

In order to characterize the dielectric behavior of non-stabilized and stabilized wines (cold stabilized wine), we used red wines and performed the relevant tests in each of the stages indicated, measuring the dielectric properties at 200 MHz, 6 GHz and 20 GHz at 20 °C, with the following results (Table 1):

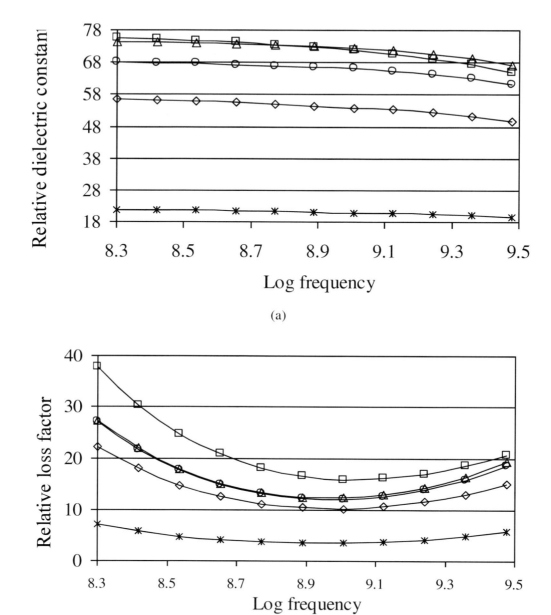

Figure 1. Variation with time of change of state from grape juice to wine of the (a) relative dielectric constant; (b) relative loss factor: □, day 1; ◇, day 3; ✶, day 4; ○, day 15; ⭐, day 49

Table 1.- Statistics of dispersion of the dielectric constant ε'_r and loss factor ε''_r at 200 MHz (subscript, 02), at 6 GHz (subscript, 6 G) and at 20 GHz (subscript, 20G) of wines at 20 °C

Parameter	Non-stabilized wine Mean	Non-stabilized wine Standard deviation	Stabilized wine Mean	Stabilized wine Standard deviation
$\varepsilon'_{r,02}$	74.208	0.359	74.734	0.077
$\varepsilon'_{r,6G}$	55.244	0.497	56.215	0.181
$\varepsilon'_{r,20G}$	19.52	0.102	20.158	0.113
$\varepsilon''_{r,02}$	22.899	0.766	22.98	0.903
$\varepsilon''_{r,6G}$	30.9	0.505	30.755	0.132
$\varepsilon''_{r,20G}$	37.876	1.199	37.093	0.049

In order to check if there are significant differences in the dielectric properties of wines during the mentioned stages, we performed two statistical tests: Means' Test: ANOVA and Kolmogorov–Smirnov test.

Only the mean of the dielectric constant at 6 GHz of non-stabilized and stabilized wines show significant differences. At this frequency we can vaguely distinguish whether a wine has been stabilized or not from its dielectric properties.

REFERENCES

García, A., Torres, J.L., Prieto, E. & De Blas, M. (2001). Dielectric properties of grape juice at 0.2 and 3 GHz. *Journal of Food Engineering, 48,* 203-211

García, A., Torres, J.L., De Blas, M., De Francisco, A. & Illanes, R. (2001). Dielectric characteristics of grape juice and wine. *Biosystems Engineering, 88(3),* 343-349

INDEX

#

4-hydroxynonenal, 422

A

A1c, 346
AAS, 433, 441, 451
abiotic, 62
abnormalities, xv, 339, 408, 414
absorption, 10, 26, 33, 47, 97, 100, 131, 292, 310, 314, 315, 325, 345, 347, 393, 397, 426, 442, 459
absorption spectroscopy, 97, 131
abundance, 440
abusive, 246, 249
acceptor, 238, 242, 256, 258, 268, 308, 313, 317, 318, 319
accidents, 281
accounting, 58, 304, 456
accuracy, ix, xv, 12, 30, 303, 313, 314, 317
acetaldehyde, xiii, 54, 68, 76, 157, 175, 182, 205, 207, 208, 210, 213, 218, 219, 220, 226, 227, 239, 249, 260, 262, 263, 264, 345, 462
acetate, xiii, xiv, 54, 60, 64, 67, 126, 153, 154, 161, 163, 165, 235, 236, 238, 241, 242, 249, 253, 254, 255, 256, 259, 260, 261, 262, 263, 264, 266, 267, 268, 271, 275, 276, 314, 378, 386, 462, 472
acetic acid, xiv, 6, 58, 63, 206, 219, 235, 238, 241, 242, 243, 247, 248, 253, 255, 258, 309, 319, 322, 434, 472
acetone, 471
acetonitrile, 58, 99, 150, 165
acetylation, 4
acetylcholine, 368
acidic, 58, 174, 178, 180, 189, 207, 209, 210, 215, 268, 304, 308, 313, 314
acidification, 313, 317, 437
acidity, xiv, 8, 67, 72, 180, 191, 202, 206, 209, 236, 244, 258, 265, 269, 285, 309, 451
acoustic, 317, 318, 322
ACS, 218, 364, 367, 463
activation, 342, 352, 370, 379, 393, 397, 398, 399, 403, 404, 406, 409, 411, 413, 421, 424
activators, 443, 444
active oxygen, 377, 385
activity level, 221
acute, 92, 135, 206, 212, 231, 340, 347, 360, 364, 365, 367, 368, 371, 386, 392, 402, 412, 413, 414, 415, 422, 423, 426, 427, 428
acute coronary syndrome, 92, 135, 364, 367, 371, 422
acute myelogenous leukemia, 386
acute renal failure, 402, 412, 415, 427, 428
acute tubular necrosis, 414
acylation, 328
Adams, 19, 139, 226, 336, 464
adaptation, 179, 246, 351
additives, xii, 73, 138, 143, 293, 430
adducts, 54, 63, 70, 76, 88, 127, 207, 218, 219, 314
adenosine, 348, 415
ADH, 263
adhesion, 342, 360, 362, 395, 398, 410
adipocyte, 341, 343, 347, 348, 349, 350, 351, 354, 356, 357, 358
adipocytes, 340, 341, 342, 343, 346, 347, 348, 350, 352, 355, 356
adipocytokines, 354
adiponectin, 340, 341, 343, 346, 348, 351, 354
adipose, x, xvi, 339, 340, 341, 342, 343, 346, 347, 348, 349, 350, 351, 357
adipose tissue, x, xvi, 339, 340, 341, 342, 343, 346, 347, 348, 349, 350, 351, 357
adiposity, 342, 351, 356
administration, 96, 230, 347, 349, 360, 394, 409, 414, 415, 417, 418, 428, 482
ADP, 394

Index

adrenaline, 348
adsorption, 68, 72, 74, 79, 190, 212, 213, 214, 227, 228, 229, 230, 285, 290
adult, 295, 346, 355, 390, 422
adult population, 295, 390
adulteration, 80, 82, 430, 436, 438
adults, 4, 351, 352, 363, 365, 428
advanced glycation end products, 413
aerobic, 212, 259, 261, 262, 264, 271
aerosols, 304
Africa, 184, 186, 187, 281
Ag, 266, 267, 268, 316
age, xiv, xv, 7, 17, 76, 96, 127, 139, 279, 281, 294, 304, 323, 327, 335, 336, 345, 350, 363, 406, 427, 432, 438, 439, 440, 458
ageing, 6, 7, 18, 24, 82, 83, 85, 93, 94, 127, 132, 137, 146, 164, 166, 207, 211, 224, 324, 335, 440, 448, 449, 457, 459, 460, 461, 462, 489
agent, xvii, 7, 20, 100, 118, 207, 245, 268, 289, 297, 336, 374, 377, 381, 385, 390, 396, 398, 402, 404, 419, 440
agents, ix, xi, xix, 9, 10, 53, 73, 76, 119, 123, 132, 140, 166, 211, 284, 285, 289, 291, 294, 299, 365, 379, 381, 398, 407, 421, 440, 443, 444, 454, 468, 472, 473, 480
aggregation, 394
aggression, 81
aging, x, xi, xiii, xv, 1, 16, 17, 21, 26, 34, 53, 56, 60, 61, 67, 68, 72, 76, 77, 78, 79, 80, 84, 85, 87, 89, 94, 96, 116, 123, 127, 130, 131, 137, 139, 147, 167, 169, 174, 176, 177, 181, 185, 188, 190, 191, 201, 202, 213, 226, 227, 323, 324, 327, 328, 329, 330, 331, 332, 333, 334, 335, 338, 405, 406, 420, 424, 427, 462, 472, 488
aging process, 17, 79, 94, 190, 324, 327, 334, 427, 472
agrarian, 26
agricultural, xiv, 6, 13, 18, 26, 28, 34, 37, 42, 48, 49, 214, 215, 279, 282, 283, 293, 295, 431
agricultural sector, 431
agriculture, 214, 236, 282, 430, 459, 460
agrochemicals, 300
aid, 281, 363
air, 457
AJ, 171, 299, 351
AL, 169, 297, 353, 355, 368, 369, 370, 371, 385, 398, 420
albumin, 34, 119, 123, 289, 388, 427
alcohol, x, xvi, xvii, 4, 40, 49, 61, 67, 69, 75, 79, 88, 128, 133, 145, 175, 176, 178, 208, 210, 215, 217, 218, 219, 239, 265, 280, 281, 297, 298, 300, 339, 345, 346, 347, 348, 350, 353, 354, 355, 356, 357, 359, 360, 362, 363, 364, 365, 366, 367, 368, 369, 371, 372, 390, 392, 393, 397, 401, 408, 413, 414, 415, 416, 419, 420, 421, 423, 425, 426, 428, 445, 451, 457
alcohol abuse, 219, 414
alcohol consumption, xvi, 281, 297, 300, 345, 346, 347, 354, 355, 356, 359, 360, 363, 366, 368, 369, 372, 420, 421
alcohol production, 217
alcohol use, 366
alcoholic cirrhosis, 298
alcoholism, 281
alcohols, 33, 35, 41, 47, 79, 144, 293, 344, 419, 430, 457, 461
Alcohols, 39
aldehydes, xiii, 3, 79, 80, 96, 173, 176, 218, 304, 322, 422, 442, 457, 460
aldolase, 238
algae, 469
aliphatic compounds, 225
alkali, 450
alkaline, 316, 317, 322, 377
alkaline hydrolysis, 317
alkaline media, 322
alkylation, 232
allergic reaction, 18
allergy, 210
allopurinol, 404
alpha, 351, 357, 400, 411, 424, 427
alternative, xv, 7, 9, 215, 216, 224, 243, 255, 303, 314, 315, 340, 378, 384, 386, 424
alternatives, 163
aluminium, 62
Aluminum, 82
Alzheimer disease, 297, 402
ambiguity, 448
amelioration, 343
American Heart Association, 398
amine, x, xiii, 1, 3, 4, 5, 6, 7, 9, 16, 17, 18, 19, 20, 21, 23, 24, 173, 175, 176, 177, 178, 180, 181, 182, 183, 184, 186, 187, 188, 190, 191, 192, 193, 194, 196, 198, 199, 200, 201, 202, 210, 211, 224, 237, 265, 272, 278, 316
amine oxidases, 182, 199
amines, ix, x, xii, xiii, 1, 2, 3, 4, 5, 6, 7, 8, 9, 10, 11, 12, 13, 14, 16, 17, 18, 19, 20, 21, 22, 23, 24, 85, 173, 174, 175, 176, 178, 181, 182, 183, 184, 185, 186, 187, 188, 189, 190, 191, 192, 193, 194, 195, 196, 197, 198, 199, 200, 201, 202, 203, 205, 210, 211, 216, 223, 224, 228, 309, 310, 319, 442
amino, xii, xiv, 2, 3, 4, 9, 10, 13, 14, 16, 20, 21, 22, 24, 128, 144, 173, 174, 175, 176, 177, 178, 180, 182, 185, 188, 189, 190, 191, 193, 194, 195, 197, 199, 201, 206, 207, 209, 210, 211, 215, 223, 224,

Index

235, 236, 237, 243, 244, 245, 246, 251, 252, 253, 254, 255, 269, 272, 276, 406, 477
amino acid, xii, xiv, 3, 4, 9, 13, 14, 16, 20, 21, 22, 24, 144, 173, 174, 175, 176, 177, 178, 180, 182, 185, 188, 189, 190, 191, 193, 194, 195, 197, 199, 201, 206, 207, 209, 210, 215, 223, 224, 235, 236, 237, 243, 244, 245, 246, 251, 252, 253, 254, 255, 269, 272, 276, 406, 477
amino acids, xii, xiv, 3, 9, 13, 14, 16, 20, 21, 22, 24, 144, 173, 174, 175, 177, 178, 180, 185, 189, 190, 191, 193, 194, 195, 197, 199, 201, 206, 207, 210, 223, 224, 235, 236, 237, 243, 244, 245, 246, 254, 255, 269, 276
amino groups, 2, 182, 191, 207
ammonia, 128, 182, 183, 215, 312
ammonium, 201, 222, 255, 313, 318, 450
ammonium sulphate, 255
amphetamine, 5
Amsterdam, 24, 87, 273, 463, 465
amyloid, 425
anabolic, 182, 252, 255
analog, 381
analysis of variance, 102, 114, 488
analytical techniques, xviii, 26, 60, 175, 429, 432, 433, 446, 463
anaphylactic shock, 182
Angiotensin, 413, 423
angiotensin converting enzyme, 413
angiotensin II, 369, 395
Angiotensin II, 413, 423
angiotensin-converting enzyme, 395
Anglo-Saxon, 280
animal models, xvi, 56, 359, 366, 368
animal studies, 207, 392, 395
animals, 2, 174, 214, 215, 236, 347, 395
ANN, 13, 15
ANOVA, 491
antagonism, 212
antagonistic, 73, 479, 480
anthocyanin, 59, 60, 63, 64, 67, 68, 70, 72, 74, 75, 76, 82, 83, 86, 87, 88, 95, 102, 108, 118, 119, 123, 127, 129, 131, 132, 135, 136, 137, 138, 139, 140, 154, 169, 213, 226, 227, 228, 324, 326, 328, 334, 335, 344, 458
anthocyanins, 38, 39, 54, 57, 68, 71, 82, 83, 84, 87, 95, 137, 154, 156, 310, 326, 458
anthracene, 385
anthropogenic, 434, 440, 441, 454
anti-atherogenic, 393
antibacterial, 93, 96, 118, 131, 217, 277, 473, 478, 479, 480, 481, 483
anticancer, xiii, xvi, 62, 94, 166, 205, 206, 373, 375, 376, 377, 384, 385, 386, 387, 388

anticancer drug, 375, 377, 385, 386
antidepressant, 5
antigen, 12
antioxidant, ix, xi, xii, xiii, xv, xvi, xix, 53, 62, 81, 83, 85, 86, 87, 88, 90, 91, 92, 93, 95, 96, 100, 101, 102, 103, 106, 108, 109, 114, 116, 118, 119, 123, 124, 125, 126, 127, 128, 129, 130, 131, 132, 133, 134, 135, 136, 137, 138, 139, 140, 141, 143, 145, 149, 162, 166, 167, 168, 170, 205, 206, 212, 233, 280, 294, 303, 304, 323, 324, 325, 326, 327, 329, 330, 333, 334, 335, 336, 337, 338, 343, 353, 356, 359, 360, 361, 363, 364, 365, 367, 368, 370, 373, 376, 377, 378, 384, 386, 397, 402, 406, 407, 412, 413, 414, 415, 416, 419, 423, 424, 426, 427, 467, 471, 472, 481, 482, 483, 484
antioxidative, 135, 199, 482
antioxidative activity, 352
antioxidative potential, 482
anti-platelet, 347
antiradical activity, 102, 103, 109, 132, 135, 136, 140
antitumor, 374, 378, 386
Anti-tumor, 337
antiviral, 374, 472
antiviral agents, 472
AOC, 328, 430
aorta, 393, 396, 397, 420
apoptosis, 297, 360, 362, 374, 376, 377, 378, 379, 384, 385, 386, 387, 406, 409, 411, 413, 415, 421, 423, 424
apoptotic, 374, 378, 387, 413, 424
Apoptotic, 377, 424
apoptotic mechanisms, 413
APP, 334
appetite, 281
apples, 94, 146, 469, 471, 472, 481, 483
application, x, xiv, xviii, 2, 10, 13, 16, 18, 23, 46, 48, 75, 86, 100, 127, 135, 149, 153, 162, 163, 166, 230, 237, 279, 282, 290, 294, 296, 297, 298, 301, 306, 320, 336, 430, 433, 438, 441, 481
aptitude, 128, 177
aqueous solution, xi, 25, 33, 35, 39, 40, 48, 162
aqueous solutions, xi, 25, 35, 39, 40, 48
aquifers, 282
arachidonic acid, 394, 404
ARF, 414, 415
Argentina, 184, 186, 235, 274, 277, 447, 467
arginine, xiii, 176, 177, 180, 181, 182, 188, 199, 200, 205, 207, 209, 210, 222, 223, 237, 245, 270, 277
Aristotelian, 303
aromatase inhibitors, 357
aromatic compounds, 237, 445
arrest, 385

arsenic, 291, 298
arterial hypertension, 401, 415
arteries, 129, 409, 412
arterioles, 416, 420
arteriosclerosis, 363
artery, 359, 365, 367, 368, 369, 371, 393, 398, 399, 422
ascorbic, 92, 99, 100, 102, 103, 107, 145, 314, 316, 322
ascorbic acid, 92, 99, 100, 102, 103, 107, 145, 314, 316, 322
ash, 37, 38
Asia, 281
aspartate, 255
Aspergillus niger, 216
assessment, xii, xv, 26, 103, 173, 218, 280, 295, 415
assimilation, 244
assumptions, 488
asthma, 83, 231
astringent, 54, 76
asymptomatic, 4, 18
Athens, 322
atherogenesis, 93, 369, 398, 416, 422, 427
atherosclerosis, ix, xi, 56, 91, 141, 343, 347, 355, 361, 365, 369, 370, 392, 393, 395, 400, 401, 405, 408, 409, 411, 421, 425, 426, 472
atherosclerotic plaque, 394, 408, 484
Atlas, 398
atmosphere, 203, 271, 286, 288, 304
atmospheric pressure, 22, 74, 201
atomic absorption spectrometry, 320
atoms, 378, 405
ATP, xiv, 182, 236, 238, 242, 256, 258, 265, 267, 268, 348, 477
ATPase, 265, 415, 416, 426
atrophy, 110, 413
attachment, 395
attacks, 62, 280, 390, 405
attitudes, 281
Australia, 82, 115, 225, 229, 271, 294, 298, 440, 447
Austria, 438
authentication, xviii, 429, 430, 432, 433, 434, 436, 440, 441, 442, 446, 447, 450, 457, 460, 463
authenticity, 16, 194, 430, 432, 446, 450
autocrine, 340, 411
autolysis, xiii, 174, 180, 191, 202
automation, ix, xv, 303, 309, 315
autopsy, 414
availability, 67, 76, 77, 78, 81, 239, 261, 265, 294, 299, 446
awareness, xix, 350, 468, 480

B

B vitamins, 353
Bacillus, 473
Bacillus subtilis, 473
bacteria, ix, xiii, xix, 7, 8, 18, 20, 21, 34, 56, 69, 70, 72, 73, 83, 84, 148, 175, 176, 177, 178, 179, 181, 189, 190, 191, 193, 194, 196, 197, 198, 199, 200, 202, 205, 206, 207, 208, 209, 210, 211, 212, 213, 214, 216, 217, 218, 220, 221, 222, 223, 224, 235, 236, 237, 238, 243, 244, 246, 247, 257, 259, 261, 265, 266, 269, 270, 271, 272, 273, 274, 275, 276, 277, 278, 285, 290, 304, 305, 344, 404, 467, 473, 474, 480, 483
bacterial, 9, 73, 178, 179, 185, 206, 211, 212, 216, 219, 245, 246, 247, 256, 260, 265, 269, 273, 305, 410, 474, 477
bacterial strains, 178, 179, 265
bacteriocin, 260
bacteriocins, 206, 216
bacteriophage, 385
bacteriostatic, 7
bacterium, xiv, 84, 89, 181, 222, 224, 228, 236, 238, 253, 255, 270, 274, 473
Badia, 355
baking, 232
barrier, xi, 67, 92, 96, 295, 308, 381, 415, 417, 477
Basa, 291, 296
basement membrane, 417
bcl-2, 378, 386
beef, 34, 474
beer, xiv, xvii, 3, 94, 145, 182, 197, 199, 201, 220, 236, 239, 265, 266, 269, 270, 271, 277, 278, 298, 317, 320, 346, 365, 366, 368, 370, 371, 389, 390, 391, 407, 414, 421, 422, 426
beet sugar, 436, 437
behavior, xi, 7, 25, 33, 37, 43, 47, 180, 281, 284, 285, 291, 292, 294, 335, 407, 437, 439, 449, 452, 489
behaviours, 128
Belgium, 183, 211
beneficial effect, x, xi, xvi, 53, 56, 62, 81, 94, 280, 339, 347, 359, 365, 368, 402, 408, 413, 419, 471
benefits, xix, 129, 145, 148, 194, 215, 216, 280, 281, 340, 345, 353, 364, 366, 367, 408, 468, 472, 478, 480, 483
benign, 126
benzene, 469
benzo(a)pyrene, 385
beverages, ix, x, xii, xiii, xiv, xvi, xvii, xviii, 4, 21, 22, 23, 93, 145, 169, 170, 173, 174, 175, 182, 184, 201, 205, 206, 209, 210, 214, 219, 220, 222, 229, 235, 236, 237, 239, 240, 249, 257, 260, 268,

280, 281, 314, 316, 321, 322, 325, 338, 339, 340, 344, 345, 349, 350, 360, 363, 365, 367, 371, 374, 389, 401, 407, 408, 418, 423, 467, 468
bilirubin, 407
binding, 26, 38, 199, 214, 218, 348, 360, 376, 378, 379, 398, 412, 413
binge drinking, 345
bioavailability, xv, 100, 140, 167, 168, 280, 283, 294, 299, 395, 396, 399, 400, 409, 410
biocatalyst, 220
biochemistry, 21, 230, 422
bioconversions, 236
biodegradable, 214
bioflavonoids, 427
biogenesis, 195, 408
biogenic amines, ix, x, xii, xiii, 1, 2, 3, 4, 5, 6, 7, 9, 10, 12, 13, 18, 19, 20, 21, 22, 23, 24, 173, 174, 175, 189, 193, 194, 195, 196, 197, 198, 199, 200, 201, 202, 205, 211, 216, 223, 224, 309, 319
biological activity, 4, 174, 222, 409
biological consequences, 84
biological media, 29
biological processes, 439
biological responses, 400
biological stability, 237
biological systems, 3, 27, 36, 378, 386, 402, 425
biologically active compounds, 3, 201
biomarkers, 337, 342, 355
biomass, 240, 241, 244, 252, 253, 255
biomolecules, 23, 191
biosensors, 13
biosorption, 228, 230
biosynthesis, xiv, 96, 109, 178, 200, 235, 243, 248, 254, 255, 273, 276, 357
biosynthetic pathways, 64
biotechnology, 197, 199, 219, 222, 273
biotic, 109
biotransformation, 84
birth, 344
bismuth, 222
black tea, 472, 473, 483
bladder, 374, 424
bladder cancer, 424
bleaching, 149, 168, 213
blindness, 208
blocks, 378, 404
blood, ix, x, xi, xvi, xvii, 3, 4, 34, 37, 91, 94, 100, 101, 131, 140, 219, 289, 344, 346, 347, 348, 359, 361, 362, 364, 365, 366, 368, 371, 372, 377, 389, 391, 392, 393, 395, 396, 399, 409, 417, 422, 473
blood clot, 392
blood flow, 365, 392
blood glucose, 348

blood plasma, ix, xi, 91, 100, 101, 140
blood pressure, x, xvi, 3, 4, 346, 359, 362, 366, 368, 371, 372, 391, 392, 395, 399, 409, 417, 422
blood stream, xvii, 389, 396
blood vessels, 94, 361, 392
blot, 257
blueberry, 139
BMI, 390, 391
body fat, 349
body fluid, 336
body mass index, 346, 355, 362, 391
body temperature, 3
body weight, xv, xvi, 208, 303, 339, 346, 347, 348, 349, 350, 354, 355, 417
bonds, 78, 147
borate, 162, 163, 164, 165
boric acid, 163, 164, 165
brain, 4, 34, 96
Brazil, 217, 321
Brazilian, 20, 189, 202
breakdown, 62, 68, 209, 249, 253, 255
breast cancer, 19, 167, 357, 374
breathing, 304
breeding, 129
brevis, 20, 181, 198, 248, 258, 277, 278
British Columbia, 87, 228, 451
Brno, 136
broccoli, 469
broilers, 229, 230
Brussels, 398, 469
bubbles, 489
buffer, 100, 150, 162, 165, 253, 314, 315, 341, 382
building blocks, 244
burning, 304
butyric, 6
by-products, 69, 126, 130, 212, 220, 228, 292, 472

C

Ca^{2+}, 310, 383, 409, 439
cabbage, 272, 469, 474
cables, 32
CAD, 174, 175, 177, 178, 180, 182, 183, 184, 186, 187, 188, 189, 190, 191, 192, 193, 359, 362, 363, 365, 367
cadaverine, x, xiii, 1, 2, 4, 5, 6, 7, 10, 17, 173, 174, 210, 211
cadmium, 215, 232, 290, 319
caffeic acid, 63, 67, 69, 72, 81, 98, 129, 148, 150, 151, 152, 153, 154, 155, 156, 158, 159, 160, 161, 162, 163, 164, 165, 181, 472, 473, 474, 476, 478, 479, 480
calcium, 293, 320, 409, 411, 421, 422, 452

calculus, 286
calibration, 13, 30, 32, 48, 99, 100, 160, 308, 313, 314, 315, 316, 317, 325
caloric restriction, 131, 420
calorie, 96, 408
CAM, 435, 436
cAMP, 348, 408
Canada, 451
cancer, xii, xvi, 5, 19, 56, 83, 92, 131, 133, 143, 219, 281, 297, 299, 339, 340, 341, 344, 349, 350, 373, 374, 376, 378, 379, 384, 387, 388, 396, 397, 398, 401, 408, 416, 423, 424, 425, 427, 428, 472
cancer cells, xvii, 337, 357, 374, 375, 376, 378, 379, 384, 408, 424, 427
cancer progression, 19
cancerous cells, 388
Candida, 88, 177, 211, 473
CAP, 293
capillary, ix, xii, 9, 10, 11, 12, 19, 21, 22, 23, 63, 83, 84, 143, 145, 162, 163, 170, 171, 309, 319, 417
carbohydrate, 41, 50, 270, 417, 422, 471, 477
carbohydrates, 37, 39, 40, 41, 131, 341, 471
carbon, ix, xiii, xiv, 72, 191, 203, 215, 235, 236, 237, 238, 240, 241, 243, 244, 248, 249, 250, 257, 260, 262, 266, 267, 269, 273, 316, 317, 318, 321, 322, 405, 434, 436, 437, 438, 446
carbon atoms, 405
carbon dioxide, xiv, 72, 203, 215, 236, 237, 249, 257, 321, 434, 446
carbonates, 449
carboxylic, 83, 252, 442, 451, 462, 472
carboxylic acids, 83, 252, 442, 451, 462, 472
carcinogen, 207, 209, 214
carcinogenesis, 56, 207, 405
carcinogenic, 171, 182, 207, 214, 215, 222, 228
carcinogenicity, 207, 214
carcinoma, 232, 374, 385, 387
cardiomyocytes, 392
cardiomyopathy, 281
cardiovascular disease, x, xi, xvi, xvii, xviii, 56, 91, 93, 96, 206, 280, 281, 299, 304, 339, 340, 341, 342, 346, 349, 350, 354, 361, 363, 365, 366, 368, 370, 371, 373, 374, 389, 390, 397, 408, 420, 421, 423, 467
cardiovascular morbidity, xvi, 359, 368
cardiovascular protection, 399
cardiovascular risk, xvi, 334, 359, 368, 371, 391, 420
cardiovascular system, 350, 361, 363, 409, 428, 473
carotenoids, 145, 353
carrier, 253, 265, 306, 307, 308, 313, 315, 412
casein, 76, 123
caspase, 379
caspases, 378, 386, 406

CAT, 406, 412, 419
catabolic, 3, 238, 240, 257
catabolism, 73, 200, 239, 243, 244, 255, 256, 258, 261, 262, 264, 275, 278
catalase, 246, 259, 361, 378, 379, 381, 406, 414, 419
catalytic activity, 314
catechins, xi, xvi, 74, 78, 91, 94, 95, 119, 123, 127, 129, 135, 146, 147, 150, 151, 154, 213, 320, 339, 344, 407, 472, 482, 483
catechol, 61, 76, 328, 469
catecholamine, 4
cation, 58, 325, 336, 449
cavities, 342
CD95, 297, 385
celery, 471
cell, xii, xvi, 5, 47, 48, 67, 68, 70, 73, 74, 75, 95, 100, 131, 136, 138, 173, 174, 182, 191, 199, 210, 211, 212, 213, 214, 215, 224, 225, 228, 229, 230, 239, 246, 250, 255, 260, 268, 269, 273, 297, 306, 315, 317, 335, 340, 341, 343, 347, 348, 351, 356, 357, 360, 361, 362, 363, 370, 373, 374, 377, 378, 380, 381, 382, 384, 385, 387, 388, 395, 397, 398, 401, 402, 403, 405, 406, 407, 410, 411, 412, 416, 418, 421, 422, 423, 424, 425, 427, 468, 472, 473, 474, 477, 482, 483
cell adhesion, 395
cell culture, 131, 357, 382, 387
cell cycle, 349, 385, 388, 422, 424
cell death, 297, 351, 374, 378, 384, 385, 387, 412, 421
cell growth, xii, 173, 174, 182, 215, 297, 401, 412
cell line, xvi, 230, 347, 348, 356, 373, 374, 378, 384, 483
cell lines, xvi, 347, 356, 373, 374, 378, 384, 483
cell membranes, 472
cell surface, 68
cellular homeostasis, 406
cellulose, 38, 294, 295
cement, 460
central nervous system, x, 1, 3, 349
central obesity, 340
cereals, 391
cerium, 150, 168, 453
certification, 431, 446
ceruloplasmin, 378
c-fos, 412
charcoal, 76, 284, 289, 290, 291, 474
cheese, 4, 51, 178, 197, 198, 430
chelating agents, 378
chelators, 146, 381
chemical agents, 8
chemical approach, 56
chemical properties, 283

Index

chemical reactions, 166, 306, 344
chemical structures, 375, 384, 468
chemicals, xix, 214, 298, 300, 304, 357, 468, 480
chemiluminescence, xv, 13, 168, 303, 306, 311, 315, 318, 320, 321
chemoattractant, 340, 410
chemokines, 340, 342
chemometric techniques, 14, 16
chemometrics, x, 2, 86, 194, 432, 433
chemoprevention, 167, 385
chemotaxis, 225, 360
cherries, 471
chicken, 35, 203
chicks, 228
children, 19, 414
Chile, 401, 447
China, 171, 184, 185, 186, 299, 337
chitin, 68
chloride, 10, 21, 33, 62, 82, 403, 449
chloride anion, 403
chlorogenic acid, 81, 164, 471
chocolate, 4, 5
cholecystokinin, 357
cholesterol, 92, 93, 129, 200, 280, 340, 344, 347, 348, 360, 362, 364, 370, 391, 405, 409, 418
chromatin, xvi, 96, 374, 376, 378
chromatographic technique, 19, 169
chromatography, ix, xii, 11, 21, 22, 83, 86, 114, 143, 144, 145, 149, 162, 168, 169, 170, 171, 193, 201, 296, 316, 442
chromatography analysis, 170
chromosomes, 379
chronic renal failure, 402, 410, 416, 420
cigarette smoking, 297, 362, 391, 414
circulation, 363, 367, 368, 370, 393, 394, 412, 427
cis, 55, 61, 62, 63, 72, 79, 81, 97, 98, 108, 109, 115, 126, 129, 139, 148, 150, 151, 153, 154, 155, 156, 158, 161, 162, 164, 165, 169, 171, 226, 394, 424, 456, 469
citotoxic, 419
citrus, 237, 269, 272, 295, 299
c-jun, 379, 412
classes, 56, 57, 59, 62, 93, 146, 296, 344, 345, 432, 442, 444, 447, 457, 460, 468
classical, 93, 215, 348, 378
classification, 2, 13, 15, 23, 24, 146, 166, 270, 345, 432, 433, 438, 442, 444, 445, 446, 447, 449, 450, 451, 456, 457, 458, 459, 460, 462
clay, 34
cleanup, 21, 22
cleavage, 78, 238, 354, 378, 384, 385, 386, 404, 477
clinical trials, 419
clone, 115

cloning, 269
cluster analysis, 15, 16
clusters, 80, 232
CMC, 144, 162
CO_2, xiii, 235, 238, 241, 242, 243, 248, 253, 259, 262, 267, 286, 288, 313, 435, 436, 446, 489
coagulation, xvii, 360, 389
cobalt, 232
Cochrane, 353, 400
cocoa, 145, 146, 236
coconut, 460
codes, 17
coding, 179, 242
coefficient of variation, 488
coenzyme, 243
cofactors, 238, 242
coffee, 145, 236, 471
cohort, 391, 426
coil, 306, 313
collagen, 394, 398
collisions, 42
colloids, 69, 190
colon, 94, 236, 424
colon cancer, 424
colors, 82
combined effect, 415
combustion, 304
commercialization, 431, 458
commodity, xviii, 295, 345, 429, 431, 432, 456
common rule, 456
communication, 282
communication systems, 282
community, 145, 309, 344, 397
competition, 211
competitiveness, 282
compilation, 292, 309
complement, 340, 354
complement system, 340
complexity, 16, 145, 166, 237, 249, 306, 450
complications, xviii, 342, 349, 354, 399, 401, 408, 421, 424
components, ix, x, xv, xvi, 1, 4, 5, 6, 7, 11, 13, 14, 15, 26, 33, 37, 39, 40, 41, 45, 62, 84, 89, 93, 95, 96, 127, 131, 141, 145, 153, 183, 206, 215, 219, 239, 280, 281, 294, 303, 304, 331, 337, 339, 340, 343, 345, 347, 349, 350, 359, 360, 363, 369, 381, 388, 391, 392, 394, 398, 405, 413, 414, 415, 418, 419, 442, 457, 471, 472, 479, 483
composition, x, xi, xiii, xix, 13, 14, 16, 19, 25, 27, 32, 38, 39, 46, 53, 56, 58, 62, 64, 67, 68, 69, 70, 73, 75, 77, 78, 80, 83, 84, 85, 86, 87, 89, 93, 94, 96, 108, 119, 122, 132, 133, 134, 135, 137, 138, 140, 152, 166, 175, 178, 179, 180, 189, 191, 192,

194, 202, 205, 206, 208, 212, 213, 219, 220, 225, 226, 227, 228, 247, 260, 278, 309, 317, 319, 324, 328, 331, 335, 337, 338, 343, 344, 346, 360, 407, 417, 432, 433, 434, 441, 443, 450, 451, 458, 481, 487
comprehension, 442
concentrates, 46, 288, 481
concrete, 77
condensation, 61, 74, 76, 78, 123, 127, 146, 213, 227, 324, 330
conditioning, 345
conductance, 317, 318
conductive, 162
conductivity, x, xi, xv, 25, 27, 28, 29, 30, 33, 37, 38, 41, 42, 43, 45, 46, 47, 48, 303, 317, 318, 488
configuration, 308, 322, 452, 469
conformity, 262
confounders, xvii, 389
confusion, 26
Congress, 47, 197, 222, 466
conjugated dienes, 364
conjugation, 60, 469
Connecticut, 46, 298
consensus, 18, 324
conservation, 76, 271, 309, 457
constant rate, 286, 287, 288
consumer protection, 175
consumers, xii, xvii, xviii, 5, 81, 96, 144, 173, 184, 189, 206, 216, 281, 282, 283, 288, 290, 294, 296, 345, 346, 389, 391, 429, 430, 431, 432, 446, 463, 472
consumption, x, xi, xv, xvi, xvii, xviii, xix, 10, 18, 53, 56, 62, 78, 81, 91, 92, 93, 100, 130, 137, 145, 162, 189, 194, 216, 227, 242, 245, 247, 248, 251, 252, 253, 254, 256, 257, 259, 260, 262, 266, 267, 268, 280, 281, 282, 283, 291, 294, 295, 297, 298, 300, 307, 323, 334, 339, 340, 344, 345, 346, 347, 349, 350, 353, 354, 355, 356, 359, 360, 362, 363, 364, 365, 366, 367, 368, 369, 370, 371, 372, 373, 374, 389, 390, 391, 392, 393, 394, 396, 397, 398, 400, 401, 408, 409, 414, 415, 416, 417, 420, 421, 422, 423, 424, 425, 427, 467, 472, 480
contact time, 189
contaminant, 176, 178, 265
contaminants, 410
contamination, xix, 174, 175, 214, 282, 454, 467, 474, 480
control, xi, xiv, xv, xviii, xix, 7, 8, 21, 26, 30, 48, 74, 80, 81, 91, 96, 100, 162, 176, 190, 193, 206, 208, 216, 246, 247, 249, 255, 256, 260, 274, 279, 281, 282, 283, 290, 291, 323, 328, 329, 331, 334, 349, 357, 364, 366, 384, 391, 411, 416, 417, 418, 429, 430, 431, 432, 437, 441, 442, 449, 467, 474, 476, 480
control group, xi, 91, 364, 366, 391
controlled studies, 395
controlled trials, 19
conversion, 74, 180, 238, 242, 249, 266, 304, 341, 419
cooling, 74, 390
Copenhagen, 273
copper, xvi, 132, 214, 215, 232, 290, 298, 316, 318, 322, 373, 375, 376, 378, 379, 381, 383, 384, 386, 387, 388, 426
corn, 34, 35, 49, 356
coronary angioplasty, 400
coronary arteries, 400
coronary artery disease, 359, 365, 367, 369, 371, 398, 422
coronary heart disease, xi, xii, 56, 88, 91, 92, 93, 100, 135, 143, 145, 300, 344, 345, 350, 353, 368, 369, 370, 397, 399, 400, 426, 472
correlation, xv, xix, 13, 16, 20, 40, 92, 102, 103, 106, 108, 109, 112, 118, 124, 126, 127, 133, 141, 160, 177, 181, 183, 185, 189, 200, 219, 285, 286, 287, 288, 293, 323, 327, 328, 337, 351, 385, 455, 487, 488
correlation coefficient, 124, 160, 286, 287
correlations, 15, 18, 40, 108, 124, 138, 202, 212, 293, 326, 327, 440
cost effectiveness, ix, xv, 303
cost-effective, 313
costs, 79, 190, 313, 474
cotton, 34
coumarins, 145, 152
counterbalance, 80, 349
counterfeit, 80
coupling, 101, 103, 238, 309
covalent, 61
covalent bond, 61
CPR, 404
cranberry, 471
CRC, 86, 465
C-reactive protein, 341, 351, 353, 355
Crete, 115, 344
criminal behavior, 281
critical micelle concentration, 162
crops, xv, 279, 282, 290, 300
cross-linking, 423
cross-sectional, 346, 366
cross-sectional study, 346, 366
CRP, 341, 343, 346
CSF, 360
cultivation, 93, 109, 115, 128, 130, 146, 166, 281, 324

culture, 66, 144, 180, 181, 189, 207, 215, 243, 244, 254, 255, 258, 267, 268, 276, 282, 387, 400
culture conditions, 180, 255, 258
culture media, 387
curcumin, 378, 379, 386, 387
Curcumin, 386
CVD, xvii, 389, 390, 391, 392, 396, 408
cyanide, 265
cycles, 247, 308, 410, 440, 474, 476, 479, 480
cycling, 376, 379
cyclodextrin, 164
cyclooxygenase, 56, 89, 347, 362
cyclooxygenase-2, 56, 89, 347
cyclosporine, 415, 426
cysteine, xiv, 235, 243, 244, 251, 254, 255, 273, 313, 316, 379, 406
cystine, 316
cytochrome, 56, 85, 361, 404, 406, 421, 424, 425
cytochrome p450, 361, 404
cytokine, 395, 410, 411, 421
cytokines, 340, 341, 342, 347, 362, 410, 424
cytoskeleton, 417
cytosol, 215
cytotoxic, 360, 374, 376, 384, 386, 404, 412
cytotoxic action, 376, 384
cytotoxicity, 374, 384, 409, 425, 483
Czech Republic, xii, 91, 92, 100, 130, 134, 136

D

DAD, 22, 63, 132, 136, 144, 149, 154, 156, 157, 158, 159, 162, 164, 165, 311
dairy, 3, 236, 239, 240, 255, 272, 278, 474
dairy industry, 239
dairy products, 3, 236, 239, 278, 474
Dallas, 227, 335
data analysis, 18, 19
data collection, 438
data set, 14
database, 431, 438
dating, 236, 439
de novo, 200, 405
death, x, xvii, 145, 182, 208, 351, 375, 378, 386, 389, 401, 402, 408, 409, 416, 474, 479, 480
death rate, 145
deaths, 386, 390
decay, 285, 286, 287, 288, 297, 304, 439, 440
decomposition, x, 1, 146, 404, 419
defense, 185, 344, 405, 406, 407, 423, 426, 468
defense mechanisms, 185
defenses, 304, 414
deficiency, 19
deficit, 109, 188

definition, 54, 182, 236, 306, 345
degenerative disease, 281
degradation, xiii, xvi, 3, 9, 13, 67, 74, 75, 80, 127, 180, 183, 185, 190, 205, 210, 221, 222, 229, 231, 237, 245, 252, 256, 257, 260, 262, 263, 266, 267, 273, 285, 288, 290, 293, 296, 299, 342, 357, 362, 373, 375, 376, 377, 381, 384, 385, 386, 394, 410, 412, 473, 482
degrading, 210, 257, 266, 267, 378
dehydration, 257
dehydrogenase, 176, 257, 258, 259, 260, 261, 262, 264, 266, 267, 268, 269, 275, 310, 311
dehydrogenases, 238, 260, 262, 263, 264
delivery, xix, 468, 480
delocalization, 93
dementia, 281
denaturation, 72
density, 32, 49, 67, 83, 92, 93, 123, 129, 134, 211, 224, 247, 340, 352, 360, 363, 368, 369, 370, 398, 405, 428, 451, 481, 482, 483, 485
deoxyribose, 383, 405
dependent variable, 488
depolarization, 406
deposition, 349
deposits, 291, 412, 417, 418, 426
depreciation, 197, 245, 274
depressed, 348
depression, 4, 5, 40
deregulation, 343
derivatives, xi, xiv, 9, 10, 12, 22, 53, 56, 57, 58, 59, 62, 64, 67, 68, 72, 88, 95, 119, 129, 138, 194, 201, 230, 279, 293, 313, 407, 418, 468, 471, 474
dermatitis, 231
desorption, 72
destruction, 81, 215, 277
detection, xv, 5, 10, 12, 13, 21, 22, 23, 58, 63, 73, 80, 82, 88, 99, 113, 114, 135, 137, 139, 144, 145, 149, 150, 157, 163, 166, 168, 169, 170, 179, 194, 195, 196, 198, 199, 201, 223, 224, 282, 296, 303, 306, 309, 310, 311, 313, 314, 315, 316, 317, 318, 319, 320, 321, 322, 410, 442, 481, 483
detection techniques, 13
detoxification, xii, xiii, 3, 87, 173, 174, 205, 214, 229
developed countries, 145, 353, 390, 400
developing countries, 390
deviation, 36, 317, 434, 491
dexamethasone, 372
dextrose, 48
diabetes, xvi, 56, 92, 94, 339, 340, 341, 343, 346, 347, 349, 350, 352, 353, 370, 371, 390, 391, 397, 401, 405, 408, 411, 423
diabetes mellitus, 371, 390

diabetic nephropathy, 413, 417, 420, 422, 423
diabetic patients, xvi, 359, 365, 367, 368, 370, 371, 417, 422
dialysis, 295, 317
diamines, 2, 5, 193, 199
diamond, 422
diarrhea, 4
dielectric constant, 28, 29, 32, 34, 36, 37, 39, 40, 41, 42, 44, 45, 46, 49, 50, 487, 488, 489, 490, 491
dielectrics, 27, 37
dienes, 364
diet, xvii, xviii, xix, 4, 5, 92, 96, 129, 131, 206, 280, 281, 291, 343, 344, 345, 347, 348, 352, 353, 354, 355, 357, 362, 369, 389, 391, 392, 394, 395, 396, 397, 399, 400, 401, 406, 407, 408, 417, 421, 422, 467, 468, 471, 478, 480, 485
dietary, x, xvii, 4, 5, 10, 12, 16, 18, 93, 94, 96, 103, 126, 131, 137, 140, 167, 194, 200, 280, 301, 343, 344, 353, 355, 388, 390, 397, 398, 399, 400, 415, 420, 473, 481, 485
dietary fiber, 94
dietary habits, 343
dietary intake, 140, 167, 353
diets, 92, 280, 281, 353, 473
differentiation, 3, 16, 23, 24, 64, 88, 95, 145, 174, 230, 342, 343, 348, 350, 356, 360, 443
diffusion, 75, 265, 276, 308, 310, 313, 314, 315, 316, 317, 318, 319, 320, 321, 322, 324, 384, 405, 430
digestion, 94, 131, 137, 295, 311
digestive tract, 5, 207
dilation, 420
dimer, 73, 96, 98, 129, 156
dimeric, 93, 95, 102, 103, 126, 129, 130, 472
dipeptides, 245, 269, 276
dipole, 28, 32, 37
dipole moment, 28, 32, 37
discordance, 179
Discovery, 155, 484
discriminant analysis, 15, 16, 110, 451
discrimination, 306, 434, 438, 442, 446, 447, 449, 450, 452, 456, 460, 461, 462
disease activity, 379
diseases, xiv, xviii, 56, 93, 96, 145, 279, 280, 340, 343, 350, 371, 374, 390, 401, 406, 407, 408, 409, 413, 467, 472, 473
dispersion, 33, 36, 39, 41, 42, 47, 48, 144, 153, 169, 306, 491
displacement, 41
dissociation, 244, 375
dissolved oxygen, 76, 77, 317
distillation, 220, 315
distilled water, 40, 99
distress, 182

distribution, 15, 27, 29, 82, 179, 198, 224, 232, 286, 287, 298, 346, 354, 391, 432, 433, 434, 436, 437, 438, 440, 442, 444, 445, 449, 451, 452, 453, 454, 455, 456, 457, 458, 461, 462, 488
diuretic, 390
diversity, 76, 178, 192, 197, 213, 215, 237
division, 174
DNA, xvi, 3, 84, 132, 179, 182, 198, 207, 218, 219, 291, 334, 373, 374, 376, 377, 378, 379, 380, 381, 382, 383, 384, 385, 386, 387, 388, 405, 412, 422, 425, 477, 483
DNA breakage, xvii, 374, 377, 379, 380, 381, 382, 383, 384, 385, 386, 387
DNA damage, 218, 334, 376, 386, 405, 425
DNA repair, 218
donor, 308, 326
donors, 398
dopamine, 5
dosing, 305
double bonds, 405
down-regulation, 347, 348
drinking, xvi, xvii, 296, 300, 340, 345, 346, 347, 348, 349, 350, 354, 363, 365, 366, 371, 389, 422, 425
drinking pattern, xvii, 345, 363, 371, 389, 425
drinking patterns, 363, 425
drinking water, 300
Drosophila, 225
DRS, 384
drugs, xvi, 4, 21, 182, 294, 373, 375, 378, 384, 413
dry matter, 99
drying, 26, 46, 47, 140
duration, 77, 118, 334
dyslipidemia, xv, 339, 340
dysregulation, 411

E

E. coli, 476, 477, 478, 480
earth, 190, 450
earthworms, 295
Eastern Europe, 354
eating, 408, 430
ecological, 81, 90, 94, 103, 141, 217, 262
economics, xviii, 429
Education, 200, 398
egg, 94, 119, 123, 289
Egypt, 144
eicosanoid, 347, 370, 399
eicosanoids, 340
elaboration, 7, 125, 266, 285, 286, 287, 299, 309
elasticity, 129, 473
elderly, 281, 474

election, 7
electric conductivity, x, 25, 29, 45
electric field, 27, 28, 32, 37, 162
electrical characterization, 48
electrical conductivity, 46, 47, 48, 488
electrical properties, 27
electrochemical detection, 170, 322
electrodes, 13, 320, 322
electrolyte, 143, 162, 164, 165
electromagnetic, 26, 27, 28, 29, 30, 40, 46
electromagnetic fields, 27, 30
electromagnetic wave, 29
electromigration, 23, 162, 170
electron, xvii, 238, 242, 256, 258, 259, 265, 296, 374, 384, 403, 404, 406, 417, 418, 419, 428
electrons, 93, 146, 402, 403
electrophoresis, ix, xii, 9, 19, 21, 23, 63, 83, 84, 97, 131, 143, 144, 145, 162, 170, 171, 309, 310, 319, 377, 380
ELISA, 12, 23, 198
email, 144, 429
emission, 315, 319
emotional, 5
employment, 214
encoding, 179, 208, 215, 236, 253, 269, 273
endocrine, 340, 341, 351
endonuclease, 378
endoplasmic reticulum, 352
endorphins, 5
endothelial cell, 361, 364, 367, 369, 392, 393, 395, 396, 398, 399, 404, 405, 409, 410, 411, 412, 417, 421, 422, 425
endothelial cells, 364, 367, 369, 392, 393, 395, 396, 398, 399, 404, 405, 409, 411, 412, 417, 422, 425
endothelial dysfunction, 343, 360, 361, 363, 393, 394, 397, 399, 400, 409, 410, 416, 421
endothelial progenitor cells, 94, 131
endothelin-1, 366, 395, 413
endothelium, x, xvi, 359, 360, 361, 362, 368, 371, 392, 393, 397, 404, 409, 413, 417, 418, 420
energy, xiv, 26, 27, 28, 32, 49, 72, 179, 235, 236, 238, 239, 240, 242, 245, 248, 250, 252, 258, 265, 267, 268, 273, 341, 342, 343, 347, 348, 349, 350, 355, 356, 357, 406
England, 280, 451
enlargement, 101, 103
enterococci, 198
entrepreneurs, 431
environment, 31, 76, 185, 188, 198, 300, 304, 362, 397, 406, 440, 476
environmental change, 440
environmental conditions, xi, 53, 66, 174, 258
environmental factors, xiv, 279

environmental impact, 216
environmental influences, 64
Environmental Protection Agency, 206, 207, 319
enzymatic, 9, 13, 23, 61, 72, 75, 130, 174, 179, 182, 215, 218, 221, 248, 259, 261, 262, 266, 267, 268, 269, 305, 306, 312, 320, 403, 407
enzymatic activity, 72, 75, 174, 248, 266
enzyme sensor, 13, 310
enzyme-linked immunosorbent assay, 12
enzymes, xiii, 3, 5, 13, 39, 56, 61, 62, 64, 67, 70, 73, 75, 81, 86, 90, 174, 182, 183, 190, 205, 208, 209, 211, 216, 221, 238, 242, 257, 258, 259, 260, 261, 269, 277, 335, 342, 361, 378, 384, 403, 406, 411, 412, 413, 414, 415, 423, 424
EPA, 319
epidemic, 390
epidemiologic studies, 207, 363
epidemiology, 280, 354
epigallocatechin gallate, 118, 387, 388
epithelial cell, 89, 218, 393, 411, 413, 422
epithelial cells, 89, 218, 393, 411, 413, 422
epithelium, 418
equality, 488
equilibrium, 58, 75, 304, 306, 462
ER, 356, 357
erythrocytes, 370, 420
Escherichia coli, 276, 473, 474, 476, 477, 480, 484
ESI, 90, 144, 156, 157, 158, 169, 481
esophageal cancer, 423
esophagus, 374
essential oils, 369
ester, 85, 314, 360
esterase, 221
esterification, 213, 370, 462
esters, 61, 67, 68, 72, 81, 87, 225, 405, 457, 461, 462, 471
estimating, 137
estrogen, 349, 350, 357, 397
estrogens, 349, 357
ETA, 423
ethane, 230
ethanol, x, xii, xiii, xiv, xvi, xvii, 20, 35, 39, 40, 41, 46, 61, 67, 76, 79, 98, 99, 126, 128, 144, 173, 175, 180, 181, 182, 191, 199, 206, 207, 209, 210, 212, 218, 219, 221, 223, 225, 235, 236, 238, 241, 242, 243, 244, 247, 248, 249, 254, 255, 257, 259, 260, 266, 270, 274, 276, 278, 299, 309, 310, 316, 320, 339, 344, 345, 346, 347, 348, 349, 356, 363, 365, 389, 392, 409, 413, 414, 415, 416, 419, 422, 423, 425, 426, 435, 436, 438, 442, 445, 446, 462, 472
ethanol metabolism, 425
ethanolamine, xiii, 2, 6, 10, 173, 174, 195, 200

ethical issues, 216
ethnic groups, 408
ethyl acetate, 126, 153, 161, 163, 165, 462, 472
ethyl alcohol, 48, 457
ethylene, 154
etiology, 342, 343
EU, 282, 295, 301, 437, 456
eukaryotic cell, 176
euphoria, 5
Europe, 281, 282, 345, 390, 391, 438, 457
European Commission, 463, 466
European Union, xv, 282, 303, 437
evaporation, 77, 78, 84, 162, 310, 319
evolution, xv, 29, 67, 77, 78, 84, 94, 123, 125, 132, 138, 168, 188, 190, 192, 202, 242, 246, 266, 282, 284, 285, 309, 323, 329
exclusion, 40, 316
excretion, 222, 228, 366
exercise, 391
exopolysaccharides, 237
experimental condition, 250, 269
exposure, 60, 76, 85, 87, 127, 294, 298, 300, 301, 304, 342, 398, 412, 414, 415, 418, 425, 426
extracellular matrix, 410, 413
extraction, x, xix, 2, 9, 13, 17, 21, 22, 59, 67, 68, 73, 74, 75, 77, 79, 80, 85, 87, 94, 114, 122, 126, 128, 130, 132, 134, 136, 138, 140, 144, 146, 150, 153, 159, 163, 169, 171, 189, 193, 208, 221, 226, 308, 310, 311, 316, 319, 320, 329, 333, 334, 370, 442, 455, 457, 467, 471
extrapolation, 300
extrusion, 420

F

factorial, 23, 320
FAD, 258, 259, 404
failure, 341, 343
family, 67, 68, 85, 146, 272, 281, 284, 402
farmers, 282
farming, 434
farms, 297
Fas, 378, 384, 424
fasting, 346, 348
fasting glucose, 346
fat, 34, 51, 96, 280, 341, 346, 347, 351, 352, 354, 391, 473
fatality rates, 474
fats, 280, 344, 362
fatty acids, xiii, 182, 205, 206, 212, 224, 225, 226, 255, 340, 342, 343, 347, 407
fauna, 282
fax, 1, 25, 429, 487

FDA, 9
February, 47, 123, 484
feedback, 404
feeding, 357, 452
feelings, 5
fenarimol, 290, 299, 300
fermentation, xi, xii, xiii, xiv, xix, 6, 7, 8, 18, 20, 25, 34, 53, 56, 67, 68, 70, 72, 73, 74, 75, 76, 78, 80, 83, 84, 85, 86, 87, 90, 92, 118, 119, 122, 124, 125, 129, 168, 174, 176, 177, 178, 184, 185, 189, 192, 195, 197, 198, 200, 202, 205, 206, 207, 208, 209, 210, 211, 212, 214, 215, 216, 217, 218, 219, 220, 221, 222, 224, 225, 227, 228, 229, 230, 231, 235, 236, 237, 238, 239, 240, 242, 243, 257, 258, 262, 266, 269, 271, 272, 273, 274, 275, 276, 277, 283, 284, 285, 288, 290, 291, 293, 294, 300, 305, 337, 344, 434, 436, 445, 446, 449, 457, 462, 487, 489
fermentation technology, 84
ferritin, 378, 419
ferromagnetic, 27
fertilization, xiv, 6, 19, 185, 188, 202, 279
fertilizer, 81
fertilizers, 81, 439
ferulic acid, 61, 69, 72, 98, 152, 153, 154, 155, 156, 159, 161, 164, 468
fetal, 414
fetal alcohol syndrome, 414
fever, 19
fiber, 94, 160
fibrinolysis, 371, 393, 394
fibrogenesis, 411
fibronectin, 411, 412, 422
fibrosis, 410, 411, 413, 414, 423
Fibrosis, 410
film, 13, 24, 316, 318
films, 322
filters, 289
filtration, xi, xiv, 26, 100, 150, 155, 158, 190, 206, 279, 283, 289, 297, 299, 417, 443, 444
fines, 227
fingerprinting, 14, 169, 484
Finland, 183
fires, 304
fish, 3, 9, 21, 22, 34, 35, 199, 245, 400, 407, 474
FISH, 246
fish oil, 407
fixation, 68, 74, 435
flame, 320
flavone, 469
flavonoid, 128, 146, 147, 148, 149, 327, 344, 376, 394, 396, 397, 427, 469, 473, 474, 476, 479, 480, 483, 484

flavonoids, xi, xvi, xviii, 53, 56, 61, 64, 68, 74, 80, 86, 87, 88, 93, 95, 109, 129, 136, 141, 145, 146, 152, 153, 167, 169, 170, 171, 181, 324, 337, 339, 344, 353, 368, 385, 397, 399, 407, 408, 409, 425, 467, 468, 469, 470, 471, 472, 473, 474, 476, 477, 478, 481, 483, 485
flavor, xiv, 5, 175, 178, 235, 236, 237, 239, 244, 248, 249, 258, 260, 269, 274, 431, 457, 460
flavors, xiv, 18, 236, 304, 305, 430, 434, 442, 445, 457, 460
flora, 219
flow, ix, xv, 9, 10, 12, 21, 22, 23, 99, 144, 162, 238, 277, 303, 306, 309, 311, 314, 315, 316, 317, 319, 320, 321, 322, 360, 365, 367, 368, 392, 420
flow rate, 99, 314, 316, 317
fluid, 93, 348, 353, 400, 412
fluorescence, 10, 12, 14, 21, 22, 23, 88, 135, 144, 150, 158, 163, 165, 168, 170, 194, 201, 223, 321, 421
food, x, xii, xv, xix, 1, 3, 4, 5, 9, 10, 13, 14, 18, 19, 21, 22, 23, 26, 32, 33, 35, 46, 48, 50, 80, 82, 92, 126, 131, 138, 140, 151, 173, 174, 175, 183, 193, 194, 199, 210, 214, 223, 228, 236, 237, 271, 273, 274, 275, 293, 294, 295, 298, 300, 301, 303, 305, 309, 319, 322, 343, 345, 349, 350, 392, 430, 431, 432, 433, 434, 437, 439, 441, 446, 447, 452, 456, 464, 467, 472, 473, 480, 484
food additives, 138, 293
Food and Drug Administration (FDA), 9, 21
food intake, 349
food poisoning, xix, 199, 468, 480
food products, x, 1, 3, 26, 32, 35, 46, 237, 473
food safety, xii, 173, 183, 194, 223
foodstuffs, 3, 33, 36, 37, 174, 191, 430, 431, 432, 434, 452
Ford, 85, 352
forest fires, 304
forestry, 136
formaldehyde, 313, 314, 315, 318, 321
formamide, 33, 43, 47
fossil, 304
fossil fuel, 304
fractionation, 133, 150, 169, 434, 437, 438, 439, 440, 452, 454, 455
fragmentation, xvi, 373, 374, 377, 378, 379, 386, 387
France, 78, 83, 145, 183, 184, 186, 187, 196, 211, 220, 227, 228, 274, 280, 282, 362, 364, 431, 434, 438, 447
fraud, 430, 437, 458
free radical, xi, xviii, 84, 91, 92, 93, 96, 102, 134, 137, 146, 149, 200, 325, 326, 333, 334, 337, 347, 360, 376, 386, 388, 405, 406, 407, 419, 422, 426, 428, 467

free radical scavenger, xi, xviii, 91, 93, 96, 467
free radicals, 92, 93, 146, 149, 200, 326, 333, 360, 376, 386, 405, 406, 422, 426, 428
freezing, 73
friction, 42
fructose, xiv, 39, 40, 235, 240, 247, 248, 258, 260, 276, 278, 436
fruit juice, ix, 127, 244, 314, 317, 321, 322
fruit juices, 244, 314, 317, 321, 322
fruits, xiii, xvii, 3, 5, 6, 26, 32, 33, 40, 45, 48, 49, 50, 80, 83, 133, 145, 146, 206, 208, 235, 236, 237, 239, 240, 244, 269, 280, 295, 299, 316, 345, 389, 391, 394, 408, 452, 469, 471, 473, 478, 481, 483
frying, 46
FTIR, 442
fuel, 304, 440
fungal, 62, 80, 115, 148
fungal infection, 80, 115
fungi, xiv, 148, 188, 213, 279, 344, 473
fungicidal, 284, 449, 450
fungicide, 214, 231, 284, 285, 286, 288, 289, 290, 297, 298
fungicides, xiii, xiv, 188, 205, 214, 231, 279, 282, 283, 284, 285, 286, 288, 289, 290, 294, 296, 298, 300
furan, 407
Fusarium, 265

G

galloyl, 471
gamma-glutamyltransferase, 353
gas, ix, xii, 86, 114, 143, 145, 169, 170, 193, 244, 296, 304, 305, 308, 310, 313, 314, 315, 316, 317, 318, 320, 321, 322, 442
gas chromatograph, ix, xii, 86, 114, 143, 145, 169, 170, 193, 296, 442
gas diffusion, 308, 310, 315, 316, 317, 318, 320, 321
gasoline, 440
gastrointestinal, 4, 18, 137, 219, 295, 396
gastrointestinal tract, 219, 396
gel, 153, 154, 156, 161, 169, 289, 377, 380
gel permeation chromatography, 154, 169
gelatin, 123
gender, 345
gene, 96, 128, 131, 179, 191, 198, 208, 215, 216, 232, 245, 257, 342, 352, 356, 362, 371, 379, 392, 393, 394, 395, 396, 399, 422, 424
gene expression, 96, 128, 131, 342, 352, 356, 371, 379, 399, 422, 424
generalization, xvi, 339

generation, xvi, 18, 189, 250, 253, 262, 267, 273, 274, 321, 326, 373, 377, 378, 383, 384, 385, 386, 387, 394, 403, 407, 409, 410, 411, 412, 423
genes, 64, 209, 211, 222, 242, 253, 269, 270, 273, 342, 349, 408, 409, 411, 412, 414, 424
genetic diversity, 215
genetic instability, 405
genetics, 272
genome, 239, 270
genomes, 236, 242
genomic, 232
genomics, 274
geochemical, 438, 440, 451
geochemistry, 439
Ger, 190, 200, 202, 223
Germany, 9, 99, 167, 183, 211, 216, 437, 447, 457
germination, 50
glass, 12, 94, 314, 371
glasses, 94, 392
globalization, 281, 447
glomerulonephritis, 402, 411, 414, 422, 426
glomerulopathy, 411
glomerulus, 411, 417, 418
gluconeogenesis, 346
glucose, xiv, 35, 39, 40, 54, 57, 60, 61, 65, 96, 128, 235, 236, 238, 239, 240, 241, 242, 243, 244, 245, 246, 247, 248, 250, 251, 253, 254, 255, 258, 260, 262, 263, 265, 266, 267, 268, 271, 272, 274, 275, 276, 277, 278, 340, 343, 346, 347, 348, 354, 356, 365, 397, 413, 422, 435, 436, 471
glucose metabolism, 241, 242, 243, 413
glucose tolerance, 343, 397, 422
glucoside, xi, 54, 55, 58, 60, 64, 65, 67, 68, 71, 80, 82, 91, 95, 96, 97, 98, 118, 128, 129, 131, 141, 154, 155, 156, 157, 158, 226, 227, 344, 348, 356
glutaraldehyde, 218
glutathione, xvi, 93, 132, 343, 359, 361, 363, 368, 406, 414, 421
glutathione peroxidase, 361, 406, 414
glycation, 411, 422
glycemia, 413
glycerine, 39
glycerol, xiii, xiv, 35, 40, 144, 197, 206, 235, 236, 237, 257, 258, 259, 260, 261, 262, 263, 264, 265, 266, 267, 268, 269, 270, 271, 272, 275, 276, 277, 278, 310, 320, 412, 415, 416, 417, 418
glycine, 246
glycoconjugates, 72, 141
glycogen, 347, 348
glycol, 176
glycolysis, 238, 242, 244
glycoprotein, 398
glycoside, 68, 72, 74, 78, 148, 394, 474

glycosides, 60, 62, 73, 76, 78, 93, 95, 96, 102, 109, 126, 146, 471
glycosyl, 58
glycosylated, 118, 154, 477
glycosylation, 58
glyphosate, 299
gold, 320
government, v, xviii, 429
GPC, 154
grades, 286
grain, 87, 277
grains, 33, 90, 146, 206, 225, 236
gram stain, 246
Gram-positive, 273, 275
grape juice, x, xi, xix, 1, 19, 25, 26, 30, 34, 36, 37, 45, 47, 61, 74, 94, 103, 116, 124, 128, 129, 133, 141, 178, 188, 193, 209, 218, 222, 228, 229, 277, 284, 370, 399, 408, 487, 488, 489, 490, 491
grapefruit, 368
grapes, ix, x, xi, xiv, xix, 5, 6, 19, 25, 26, 34, 39, 40, 44, 51, 53, 56, 59, 60, 61, 62, 63, 64, 65, 66, 67, 73, 74, 75, 80, 81, 84, 85, 86, 87, 88, 91, 93, 95, 96, 97, 98, 108, 109, 112, 113, 114, 118, 123, 128, 129, 133, 135, 136, 138, 139, 140, 141, 146, 148, 167, 168, 175, 176, 177, 178, 179, 183, 185, 188, 189, 193, 195, 196, 200, 202, 206, 208, 221, 228, 229, 231, 237, 279, 281, 282, 283, 284, 285, 286, 287, 288, 289, 290, 291, 292, 293, 294, 295, 296, 297, 298, 299, 301, 324, 334, 335, 344, 368, 385, 394, 420, 430, 431, 438, 440, 444, 445, 448, 449, 452, 453, 454, 458, 459, 469, 471, 472, 481, 482, 487, 488
graph, 15, 17
gravimetric analysis, 311
Greece, 64, 115, 144, 184, 186, 187, 280, 283, 303, 322, 344, 353
green tea, 374, 399, 469, 483
groups, xi, 2, 16, 40, 41, 53, 56, 58, 61, 76, 93, 100, 148, 166, 174, 182, 191, 207, 219, 296, 328, 333, 349, 365, 378, 390, 395, 406, 408, 416, 417, 418, 432, 434, 449, 450, 451, 455, 457, 469, 471, 474, 488
growth, ix, xii, xiv, xv, 5, 7, 8, 20, 67, 73, 80, 84, 89, 173, 174, 176, 178, 179, 180, 181, 182, 188, 194, 198, 199, 206, 207, 210, 211, 212, 215, 216, 217, 219, 220, 222, 224, 228, 231, 235, 236, 237, 238, 239, 240, 241, 245, 246, 247, 249, 250, 251, 252, 253, 255, 257, 259, 260, 261, 262, 265, 266, 267, 268, 269, 270, 271, 274, 275, 276, 277, 278, 279, 280, 282, 283, 292, 297, 299, 342, 388, 393, 397, 400, 401, 409, 410, 412, 420, 424, 427, 473, 474, 481, 483, 484

growth factor, 206, 236, 247, 342, 393, 397, 400, 409, 410, 424, 427
growth factors, 206, 236, 247, 424
growth rate, 250, 251, 252, 254, 473
guanine, xvi, 219, 374, 376, 386
guidelines, x, xvii, 390
gut, 269
gynecologic malignancies, 387

H

H_2, 304, 317, 318
half-life, 284, 291, 394
hardness, 447
harm, 341
harmful effects, 280
harvest, xiv, 66, 112, 113, 127, 130, 279, 282, 283, 290, 291, 293, 431, 484
harvesting, 93, 128, 146
hazards, 294, 296, 297
HDL, 92, 93, 280, 340, 347, 348, 363, 364, 370, 405, 412, 420
headache, 4, 182, 210
health, ix, xi, xii, xiii, xv, xvi, xviii, xix, 4, 19, 53, 56, 81, 91, 129, 143, 145, 148, 166, 167, 173, 174, 181, 182, 193, 194, 199, 205, 206, 207, 208, 210, 211, 214, 215, 216, 223, 238, 275, 280, 281, 288, 293, 294, 301, 303, 304, 323, 339, 340, 344, 345, 350, 353, 363, 398, 421, 467, 468, 471, 472, 478, 480
health effects, 81, 145, 167, 344
health problems, 214
health status, 294
heart, xi, xii, 56, 88, 91, 92, 93, 96, 100, 129, 135, 143, 145, 280, 300, 341, 344, 345, 346, 350, 351, 353, 365, 368, 369, 370, 371, 390, 392, 397, 398, 399, 400, 401, 404, 408, 425, 426, 472
heart attack, 280, 390
heart disease, xi, 56, 91, 93, 100, 145, 344, 345, 355, 362, 369, 397, 400, 408, 425
heart failure, 408
heart rate, 365
heat, 28, 127, 146, 257, 338, 340, 343, 353
heat shock protein, 343, 353
heating, 26, 46, 74, 131, 277, 331, 405
heavy drinkers, 345, 346, 366
heavy metal, xiii, 205, 214, 231, 290, 298
heavy metals, xiii, 205, 214, 231, 290
height, 314
hematologic, 379
heme, 403, 404, 412
hemodialysis, 410, 428
hemoglobin, 346, 412

hepatocellular, 387
hepatocellular carcinoma, 387
hepatocytes, 231, 347, 374
herbal, 484
herbicide, 294, 299
herbicides, xiv, 279, 282, 283, 294
heterogeneity, 450, 488
heterogeneous, 40, 46
HHS, 167
high density lipoprotein, 298, 340
high fat, xi, 91, 93, 100, 145, 347, 348, 395
high pressure, 54, 273, 342
high resolution, 162, 175, 437
high risk, 390, 408, 416
high temperature, 209, 331
high-density lipoprotein, 92, 352, 363, 370, 405
higher education, 345
higher quality, xviii, 429, 430
high-fat, 96
high-performance liquid chromatography, xii, 21, 22, 24, 84, 88, 139, 143, 145, 168, 169, 194, 199, 231, 319, 483
hip, 346, 355
hippocampus, 349, 357
hips, 79
histamine, x, xii, xiii, 1, 2, 3, 4, 5, 6, 7, 9, 10, 12, 13, 16, 17, 18, 20, 21, 22, 23, 173, 174, 179, 196, 197, 198, 199, 200, 202, 210, 211, 224, 270, 310, 320
histidine, 4, 175, 179, 181, 198
histochemical, 88
histological, 418
homeostasis, 174, 340, 343, 357
homocysteine, 334, 353
homogeneity, 488
homovanillic acid, 153, 160, 161
homozygosity, 426
honey, xviii, 50, 467
hormone, 348, 356, 395
horses, 426
Horticulture, 136, 140
hospitalization, 474
host, 405
HPLC, ix, xii, 10, 12, 22, 23, 54, 58, 63, 69, 80, 89, 90, 95, 99, 112, 114, 126, 135, 136, 139, 143, 144, 145, 149, 150, 151, 152, 153, 154, 163, 166, 168, 169, 175, 194, 195, 196, 198, 200, 201, 202, 223, 310, 442, 458, 462, 481
human, ix, xi, xii, xv, xvi, xviii, xix, 4, 5, 19, 26, 56, 89, 91, 92, 93, 94, 95, 134, 135, 137, 143, 144, 146, 148, 173, 174, 181, 182, 183, 193, 194, 207, 208, 214, 218, 219, 223, 228, 238, 294, 295, 297, 303, 309, 323, 334, 344, 348, 349, 351, 352, 355,

356, 357, 363, 364, 367, 368, 369, 370, 371, 373, 374, 377, 378, 379, 380, 385, 386, 387, 393, 394, 395, 396, 397, 398, 399, 400, 402, 408, 409, 411, 413, 414, 420, 421, 422, 424, 426, 427, 428, 430, 443, 467, 468, 471, 474, 480, 481, 482, 484, 485
human activity, xv, 303
human brain, 387
human condition, 430
human exposure, 295
human leukemia cells, 378, 385, 386
human subjects, 94, 370, 399
humans, xv, xvii, 94, 140, 181, 182, 183, 206, 207, 215, 228, 281, 294, 303, 337, 343, 351, 353, 355, 370, 394, 395, 396, 398, 399, 401, 402, 414, 415, 419, 472, 473
humidity, 31, 127
Hungarian, 16, 23, 24, 128, 138, 168, 195, 201, 450
Hungary, 184, 188
hybrid, 24, 95, 154, 458
hybridization, 272
hydrate, 485
hydration, 82
hydro, 94, 131, 407
hydrocarbon, 2, 374
hydrogen, 38, 40, 41, 68, 96, 146, 182, 216, 222, 259, 268, 313, 314, 321, 336, 387, 403, 404, 405, 406, 434, 436, 438
hydrogen bonds, 38, 40, 41, 68
hydrogen peroxide, 96, 182, 216, 259, 314, 321, 336, 387, 403, 404
hydrogen sulfide, 222
hydrolysis, 60, 68, 72, 73, 74, 77, 79, 130, 178, 190, 191, 215, 312, 315, 317, 471
hydrolyzed, 61, 191, 313
hydrophilic, 94, 131, 407
hydrophobic, 213, 406
hydroxyl, 40, 41, 58, 93, 96, 102, 127, 132, 182, 328, 333, 361, 377, 378, 379, 381, 383, 384, 388, 403, 404, 405, 427, 469, 474, 477
hydroxyl groups, 40, 41, 93, 328, 333, 378, 474
hydroxylation, 61, 328
hygiene, 176, 193, 288
hygienic, 6, 7, 175, 188, 237
hyperemia, 365, 367
hyperglycemia, xv, 339, 356
hyperinsulinemia, xv, 339
hyperlipidemia, 410, 411, 414, 425, 426
hyperplasia, 342, 349, 363, 370
hypertension, xv, 4, 94, 182, 281, 300, 339, 340, 343, 360, 361, 366, 371, 372, 390, 392, 394, 397, 399, 408, 409, 415, 416, 422, 423, 425
hypertensive, 4, 137, 366, 399, 400, 415, 416
hypertriglyceridemia, 340, 341, 342

hypertrophy, 341, 342, 348, 349, 351, 395, 399, 413, 423
hypotension, 4
hypothesis, xvii, 96, 100, 103, 176, 280, 342, 358, 360, 361, 365, 374, 414, 426
hypoxia, 424
hypoxic, 424

I

IB, 371, 372
ICAM, 395
ice, 126, 135
Idaho, 169
identification, xvi, 14, 22, 23, 54, 58, 85, 99, 151, 152, 160, 163, 169, 170, 199, 277, 337, 373, 397, 434, 436, 437, 459, 460
identity, 58
IL-1, 342, 347
IL-6, 341, 342, 347, 348
immersion, 30
immobilization, 211, 220
immune cells, 347
immune system, 402
immunocompromised, 474
immunoglobulin, 414
immunohistochemical, 400
immunological, 12
impaired glucose tolerance, 397
impairments, 410
implementation, 151
impregnation, 84
impurities, 439
in situ, 270, 383
in vitro, ix, xi, xv, xvii, 91, 93, 94, 95, 100, 103, 128, 131, 135, 139, 166, 167, 190, 199, 223, 230, 277, 280, 283, 295, 334, 360, 363, 368, 377, 389, 392, 393, 395, 396, 397, 398, 407, 409, 412, 415, 423, 472, 481, 482, 484
in vivo, xi, 30, 91, 93, 95, 100, 130, 274, 343, 363, 370, 386, 396, 397, 407, 409, 415, 418, 423, 481
inactivation, 99, 104, 119, 360, 385, 410, 419, 481
inactive, 377, 477
incidence, xix, 56, 86, 345, 353, 362, 366, 390, 391, 408, 468, 480
incineration, 304
income, 295
incubation, 241, 242, 247, 249, 251, 254, 256, 347, 382, 383
independence, 488
India, 373
Indian, 423
indication, 450

indicators, 4, 66, 128
indices, 128, 324, 370, 427
indigenous, 181, 189, 236
inducer, 342
induction, 100, 149, 217, 260, 277, 343, 362, 375, 379, 384, 385, 386, 387, 423
induction time, 149
inductor, 5
industrial, 20, 49, 67, 81, 85, 119, 196, 199, 216, 434, 441, 459, 460
industrial production, 459
industrialized countries, 362
industry, x, xvii, 7, 18, 26, 54, 149, 228, 231, 239, 273, 390
inequality, 488
inert, 38
infarction, 398
infection, 62, 80, 86, 115
infections, 80, 473
inflammation, 340, 341, 343, 346, 347, 350, 351, 352, 355, 369, 395, 396, 397, 399, 402, 408, 425
inflammatory, xi, xii, xviii, 53, 143, 281, 340, 341, 342, 343, 347, 355, 360, 362, 371, 392, 395, 396, 400, 408, 411, 414, 427, 428, 467, 472
inflammatory cells, 341
inflammatory disease, 281, 400
inflammatory response, 342, 343, 347, 411, 427
inflammatory responses, 411, 427
influenza, 221
infrared, 14, 27
infrared spectroscopy, 23
ingestion, 4, 183, 193, 208, 296, 343, 346, 347, 348, 357, 365, 367, 396, 399, 409, 414, 424
inhalation, 208
inhibition, xvii, 85, 93, 95, 96, 133, 207, 223, 224, 248, 253, 274, 347, 349, 357, 360, 369, 374, 378, 381, 386, 394, 395, 398, 408, 410, 411, 412, 414, 420, 474, 477, 480, 483
inhibitor, 4, 128, 253, 342, 343, 352, 357, 360, 393, 404, 414, 421, 424, 428
inhibitors, 73, 182, 184, 206, 292, 299, 347, 386, 410, 413, 481
inhibitory, 73, 249, 253, 314, 315, 347, 378, 388, 395, 473, 474, 477, 478, 479, 480, 482, 483
inhibitory effect, 249, 253, 314, 315, 347, 388, 395, 474, 478, 479
initiation, 341, 360, 374, 405
injection, ix, xv, 9, 11, 12, 21, 114, 150, 155, 158, 163, 164, 169, 300, 303, 306, 307, 309, 311, 313, 315, 316, 319, 320, 321, 322, 414, 415, 417, 418
injuries, 281, 411, 414
injury, 86, 218, 362, 369, 402, 410, 412, 413, 414, 415, 416, 418, 422, 423, 424, 468, 473

innovation, 281
inoculation, 70, 74, 177
inorganic, 13, 209, 291, 298, 433, 442, 450, 451, 462
iNOS, 362, 421
insect growth regulators, xv, 280, 283, 292, 299
insecticide, 225, 291
insecticides, xiv, 81, 279, 282, 283, 291, 292, 293, 294, 295, 298
insects, xiv, 49, 279, 344
insertion, 404
insight, 56
inspection, 489
instability, 146, 198, 209, 405
insulation, 340
insulin, xvi, 94, 96, 340, 341, 342, 343, 345, 346, 347, 348, 351, 352, 353, 354, 356, 359, 365, 367, 368, 371, 408, 417, 421, 422
insulin resistance, 94, 341, 342, 343, 346, 347, 351, 352, 353, 365, 371, 408
insulin sensitivity, 343, 345, 346, 354, 365, 417, 421
insulin signaling, 342, 352
integrity, 406, 409, 473
interaction, xiii, 4, 40, 70, 94, 178, 205, 206, 212, 213, 217, 280, 329, 353, 354, 362, 383, 407, 423, 450
interactions, ix, 12, 33, 38, 40, 41, 48, 50, 61, 68, 181, 197, 213, 217, 227, 230, 231, 249
intercellular adhesion molecule, 395
interface, 84
interference, 13, 150, 181, 316, 402
interleukin, 340, 351, 356, 395
interleukin-1, 356, 395
interleukin-6, 351, 356
International Agency for Research on Cancer, 207, 214, 228
international trade, 144
interstitial, 413, 423
interval, xiv, 27, 279
intervention, 365, 395, 424, 463
intestinal tract, 182
intestine, 397
intima, 393
intoxication, 4, 183
intracellular signaling, 411, 424
intravenously, 394
intrinsic, 27, 94, 411
invertebrates, 96
iodine, 314, 318
ionic, xi, 25, 27, 28, 29, 33, 35, 38, 41, 42, 43, 44, 45, 47, 162, 304, 489
ionic solutions, 43, 47
ionization, 22, 144, 156, 201
ionizing radiation, 26

ions, xvii, 39, 215, 363, 374, 376, 378, 379, 386, 387, 388, 403, 427, 439, 444, 450, 452
iron, 87, 94, 96, 281, 309, 311, 378, 379, 387, 403, 415, 417, 419, 422
irradiation, 115, 131, 139, 386
irrigation, 140, 188, 201
IRS, 342
ischaemic heart disease, 400
ischemia, 404, 415, 423, 424, 427
ischemia reperfusion injury, 423
ischemic, 355, 362, 409, 421, 425
ischemic heart disease, 355, 362
ischemic preconditioning, 421
ischemic stroke, 425
island, 86
ISO, 174, 176, 178, 188
isoflavonoid, 129
isoflavonoids, 129, 140, 146
isolation, 196, 217, 224, 261, 310
isoleucine, 243, 251, 253, 254, 255
isomers, 61, 109, 115, 148, 150, 153, 168, 170, 226
isorhamnetin, 55, 60, 64, 65, 69, 98, 146, 149, 154, 155, 158, 394, 397
Isorhamnetin, 155
isotope, xviii, 429, 430, 433, 434, 435, 436, 437, 438, 439, 440, 441, 450, 451, 463
isotopes, 273, 432, 434, 437, 438, 439, 440, 442, 446, 447, 449
Isotopic, 441
Israel, 354, 421
ISS, 335
Italy, 173, 184, 185, 186, 187, 189, 194, 205, 219, 229, 256, 280, 281, 282, 283, 290, 293, 297, 362, 431, 438, 447, 451, 454, 462

J

JAMA, 357, 397
Japanese, 115, 372
JNK, 342, 379, 393
jobs, 295
Jordan, 33, 35, 43, 47, 275, 398
Juices, 244
Jun, 342, 352

K

kappa, 352, 395, 424
kappa B, 352, 395, 424
karyotyping, 232
keratinocytes, 374
ketones, xiii, 3, 96, 173, 176, 386

kidney, 370, 402, 404, 409, 410, 411, 413, 414, 415, 418, 420, 424, 425, 426, 428
kidney stones, 410
kidney transplant, 410
kidneys, 411, 417, 418, 423
kinase, xiv, 236, 242, 257, 258, 259, 260, 261, 262, 263, 264, 265, 266, 267, 268, 269, 275, 342, 347, 348, 352, 354, 394, 395, 399, 408, 411
kinase activity, 265, 394
kinases, 270, 342, 347, 352, 393
kinetics, 181, 198, 291, 293
King, 133, 218, 448
knockout, 349
Kolmogorov, 491

L

L1, 343, 348, 356
LAB, ix, xiii, xiv, 176, 178, 179, 235, 236, 237, 238, 239, 240, 242, 243, 244, 246, 247, 249, 253, 255, 257, 258, 261, 262, 265, 266, 269
labeling, 9, 10, 430
laccase, 80, 81, 87
lactate dehydrogenase, 238, 260, 262, 263, 264
lactic acid, ix, xiii, 20, 21, 29, 69, 72, 73, 83, 84, 89, 175, 177, 178, 179, 181, 193, 194, 196, 197, 198, 199, 200, 205, 206, 207, 208, 209, 210, 211, 212, 213, 214, 216, 217, 220, 221, 222, 223, 224, 228, 235, 236, 237, 238, 241, 242, 243, 244, 247, 248, 249, 251, 252, 253, 254, 256, 258, 261, 266, 269, 270, 271, 272, 273, 274, 275, 276, 277, 278, 290, 473
lactic acid bacteria, ix, xiii, 20, 21, 69, 72, 73, 83, 84, 175, 177, 178, 179, 181, 193, 194, 196, 197, 198, 199, 200, 205, 206, 207, 209, 210, 211, 212, 213, 214, 216, 217, 220, 221, 222, 223, 224, 235, 237, 261, 266, 269, 270, 271, 272, 273, 274, 275, 276, 277, 278, 290, 473
lactobacillus, 467
Lactobacillus, 7, 20, 85, 178, 179, 180, 181, 195, 198, 199, 208, 209, 211, 216, 221, 222, 236, 237, 238, 248, 257, 265, 269, 270, 271, 273, 276, 277, 278, 290, 473, 481, 482
lactones, 79, 460
lanthanum, 453, 454
laser, 137, 201
law, 305, 432
laws, xviii, 309, 429, 430
LDH, 238, 260, 262, 263
LDL, 56, 92, 93, 94, 95, 129, 135, 280, 334, 340, 341, 347, 348, 355, 359, 360, 363, 364, 367, 368, 369, 370, 393, 405, 409, 411, 412, 418, 422, 425, 426, 472, 482, 483, 484

Index

lead pollution, 440
left ventricular, 281
legislation, xv, 9, 216, 280, 430
legumes, 391
Leibniz, 136
leptin, 340, 343, 348
lesions, 340, 360, 409, 472
lettuce, 296, 299
leucine, 246
Leuconostoc, 7, 20, 178, 179, 181, 196, 198, 211, 216, 217, 221, 224, 225, 236, 237, 238, 239, 249, 256, 269, 270, 271, 272, 273, 274, 275, 276, 277, 278, 290
leukemia, 374, 378, 385, 386, 387
leukemia cells, 378, 385, 386, 387
leukemic, 378
leukocyte, 410, 415
leukocytes, 411
liberation, 222
liberty, 286
life cycle hypothesis, 358
life style, 345
lifespan, xviii, 96, 401, 408
lifestyle, xvii, xviii, 354, 389, 400, 401
lifetime, 406
ligand, 384, 424
likelihood, 349
limitation, 42, 207, 238, 437
limitations, 250, 294
linear, 15, 16, 24, 37, 118, 160, 195, 216, 286, 287, 313, 314, 315, 316, 317, 346, 390
links, 219, 341, 353, 405
linoleic acid, 405
lipase, 347, 348, 356
lipases, 355
lipid, xviii, 103, 126, 131, 133, 139, 146, 167, 226, 272, 297, 324, 340, 341, 346, 347, 348, 351, 352, 354, 356, 360, 367, 371, 393, 403, 405, 406, 408, 409, 417, 419, 424, 425, 427, 434, 467, 477, 482
lipid metabolism, 272, 356
lipid oxidation, 346, 360
lipid peroxidation, xviii, 103, 133, 139, 167, 324, 393, 403, 405, 406, 409, 424, 427, 467, 482
lipid peroxides, 146
lipid profile, 340, 347, 348, 417
lipids, 37, 225, 255, 341, 346, 370
lipodystrophy, 341
lipolysis, 348, 350, 356
lipooxygenase, 56
lipophilic, 94, 131
lipopolysaccharide, 356, 395

lipoprotein, 83, 92, 93, 298, 340, 341, 348, 352, 355, 359, 360, 367, 368, 369, 398, 405, 411, 412, 423, 426, 428, 481, 482, 483, 485
lipoproteins, 297, 369, 392, 405, 412, 422, 423, 425, 481, 484
liposomal membrane, 200
liquid chromatography, xii, 9, 16, 21, 22, 24, 54, 82, 83, 84, 88, 132, 134, 137, 139, 143, 144, 145, 151, 168, 169, 175, 194, 199, 201, 231, 300, 319, 481, 483
liquid phase, 291, 313
liquids, 47, 48, 78
liquor, 366, 370, 421
Listeria monocytogenes, 473, 474, 475, 479, 484
liver, 218, 232, 281, 341, 346, 355, 387, 393, 395, 402, 404, 422, 424, 426
liver cirrhosis, 281
liver disease, 402, 422
livestock, 300
localization, 88, 351, 361
location, xii, 61, 64, 92, 93, 146, 384, 449
locus, 216
LOD, 144, 150, 154, 155, 156, 157, 158, 159, 160, 161, 163, 164, 165
London, 48, 49, 89, 220, 225, 273, 275, 278, 422, 464
longevity, 129, 281
longitudinal study, 372
losses, xiv, 28, 29, 33, 37, 41, 42, 43, 45, 279, 489
love, 304
low molecular weight, 2, 83, 88, 135, 139, 174, 462
low temperatures, 206, 220, 225
low-density, 92, 93, 96, 134, 352, 355, 359, 367, 369, 370, 398, 405, 472, 481, 482
low-density lipoprotein, 92, 93, 96, 134, 352, 355, 359, 367, 369, 370, 398, 405, 472, 481, 482
low-temperature, 163, 165, 220
LPS, 395
lumen, 94, 361, 417
lung, 337, 402, 421, 426, 427
lung cancer, 337, 402, 421
lymphocyte, 377, 380, 381, 382, 383
lymphocytes, xvii, 219, 374, 377, 378, 379, 380, 381, 382, 383, 386, 387
lymphoid, 483
lymphoma, 374
lysine, 175, 180
lysozyme, 206, 216

M

machinery, 378
macromolecules, 206, 214, 227, 382

macrophage, 351
macrophages, 341, 360, 374, 409, 411, 413, 427, 481
magnesium, 258, 310, 320
magnetic, 27, 275
magnetic field, 27, 28
magnetic permeability of free space, 28
magnetic resonance, 420
maintenance, xviii, 207, 253, 293, 406, 467
maize, 435, 436, 437
malate dehydrogenase, 311
males, 354
malic, ix, xiii, xiv, 72, 178, 179, 180, 197, 206, 210, 224, 235, 237, 249, 250, 251, 252, 255, 256, 273, 276, 278, 311, 320, 437, 462
malignant, 100
malondialdehyde, xvi, 359, 363, 368, 405, 425
malondialdehyde (MDA), 405
maltose, 248
mammalian cell, 384, 403, 425
mammalian cells, 384, 403, 425
mammals, 200
management, 145, 215, 291, 296
manganese, 232, 290, 321, 422
manifold, 10, 306, 307, 308, 313, 316, 317
manifolds, 306, 307, 313
manipulation, 109
man-made, 304
mannitol, 237, 258, 278
MANOVA, 327
manufacturer, 31, 127
manufacturing, xii, 173, 174, 176, 193
manure, 81
MAO, 3, 4
MAPK, 342
market, 81, 282, 292, 430, 447
marketing, 216
markets, 282
Mars, 229
Maryland, 274, 397
masking, 310
mass spectrometry, 10, 22, 24, 54, 83, 114, 132, 156, 169, 170, 193, 201, 300, 310, 319, 432, 433
Massachusetts, 301
mathematical methods, 433
matrix, 12, 13, 14, 15, 145, 150, 153, 169, 175, 295, 308, 316, 362, 410, 413, 414, 417, 450
matrix protein, 413, 414
maturation, xii, 5, 7, 63, 67, 68, 76, 92, 94, 122, 124, 133, 135, 140, 141, 183, 188, 324, 330, 334, 335, 338
maximum specific growth rate, 250
Maxwell, 27
m-coumaric acid, 153, 161

MCP, 360
MCP-1, 360
MDA, 405
meals, 94, 422
measurement, x, xix, 13, 25, 26, 29, 30, 43, 47, 48, 49, 84, 101, 133, 218, 306, 310, 312, 317, 325, 422, 437, 487, 488, 489
measures, 366, 474
meat, 3, 245, 280, 474
media, 29, 33, 222, 245, 247, 248, 249, 251, 253, 256, 261, 262, 269, 272, 276, 322, 382, 387, 473, 474, 475, 476, 479
median, 117, 488
mediation, 420
mediators, 297, 348, 356, 407, 425
medications, 4, 294
medicine, 26, 145, 297
Mediterranean, 93, 96, 115, 196, 206, 280, 281, 344, 345, 353, 354, 369, 391, 392, 397, 398, 399, 400, 408, 421, 473
Mediterranean countries, 280, 391
melatonin, 150, 168
membranes, 47, 176, 200, 406, 419
men, 300, 345, 346, 348, 349, 352, 356, 362, 370, 371, 372, 402, 425, 426
Mendel, 136
Merck, 99
mesangial cells, 411, 412, 413, 415, 418, 421
mesangial proliferative glomerulonephritis, 421
messages, 351
MET, 174, 176, 183, 185, 186, 187
meta-analysis, 415, 421
metabisulfite, 449
metabolic, xv, 3, 87, 94, 176, 178, 180, 183, 237, 249, 250, 253, 255, 257, 258, 259, 265, 273, 339, 340, 341, 342, 343, 345, 346, 347, 348, 349, 350, 351, 352, 353, 354, 355, 356, 390, 391, 397, 402, 406, 407, 408, 410, 420, 424, 435, 485
metabolic disorder, 351
metabolic disturbances, 340, 347, 350
metabolic dysfunction, xvi, 339, 343
metabolic pathways, 3, 183, 485
metabolic rate, 348
metabolic syndrome, xvi, 339, 340, 341, 342, 343, 346, 347, 348, 349, 350, 351, 352, 353, 354, 355, 390, 391, 397, 402, 408, 420, 424
metabolism, ix, xiii, 2, 5, 63, 67, 68, 69, 76, 176, 181, 182, 183, 188, 199, 200, 210, 215, 220, 222, 223, 224, 225, 231, 235, 236, 237, 238, 239, 240, 241, 242, 243, 246, 247, 248, 249, 251, 252, 253, 254, 255, 256, 259, 260, 269, 270, 271, 272, 273, 274, 275, 276, 277, 300, 344, 345, 349, 351, 353,

354, 356, 393, 395, 397, 399, 402, 403, 404, 406, 413, 415, 425, 449, 452, 473, 481, 482
metabolite, xvii, 213, 236, 239, 242, 268, 285, 389, 393
metabolites, xiii, xvii, 18, 63, 68, 119, 182, 203, 205, 238, 243, 248, 258, 345, 364, 389, 394, 395, 396, 397, 398, 468
metabolizing, xiv, 180, 236, 242
metal chelators, xviii, 407, 467
metal content, 452
metal ions, xvi, 363, 373, 376, 378, 379, 403, 450
metals, 58, 133, 215, 232, 290, 309, 379, 384, 386, 387, 388, 427, 443, 444, 446, 449, 450, 451, 453, 455, 458
meteorological, 450
methanol, xiii, 33, 35, 43, 47, 58, 152, 162, 163, 165, 205, 208, 221, 472
methionine, 406
methyl group, 405
methylation, 4, 328
Mg^{2+}, 310, 383
mice, 96, 131, 337, 348, 349, 351, 354, 356, 357, 374, 385, 397, 399, 415, 420, 427
micelle concentration, 144
microaerophilic, 260
microarray, 348
microarray technology, 348
microbial, ix, xii, xiii, xix, 4, 8, 62, 173, 174, 175, 176, 178, 179, 182, 188, 193, 205, 206, 209, 210, 215, 216, 219, 230, 232, 237, 246, 272, 468, 480
microbial cells, 179
microchip, 23
microclimate, 85, 109
microcrystalline cellulose, 44, 48
microflora, xiii, 179, 189, 235, 246, 247, 249, 255, 256, 260, 276, 285
micronutrients, 281, 343
microorganism, 69, 185, 247, 249, 259, 273, 476, 479
microorganisms, ix, x, xiii, xix, 1, 2, 7, 8, 18, 62, 67, 174, 176, 177, 180, 181, 185, 191, 192, 197, 215, 219, 225, 235, 236, 238, 247, 259, 262, 265, 274, 277, 467, 473, 477, 480
micro-organisms, 174
micro-organisms, 193
microwave, 26, 28, 29, 32, 37, 41, 46, 47, 48, 49, 50, 277, 311, 320
microwave heating, 277
microwaves, x, 25, 26, 46, 49
middle-aged, 348, 366, 371, 372
migraine, 4, 5, 19
migration, 360, 362, 393, 400, 408, 427
milk, 29, 34, 37, 46, 48, 49, 50, 236, 434

milligrams, 146
mimicking, 408
minerals, 34, 344, 439, 440
mines, 440, 450
Ministry of Education, 130
Missouri, 440
MIT, 46, 48, 51
mites, xiv, 279
mitochondria, 378, 384, 386, 403, 408, 421
mitochondrial, 361, 402, 404, 405, 406, 428
mitochondrial damage, 406
mitochondrial membrane, 406
mitogen, 342, 393, 399
mitogen-activated protein kinase, 342, 393, 399
mitogenic, 393, 411
mitosis, 423
mixing, 306, 456
MMA, 291
mobility, 40, 50, 282
model system, 191, 196
modeling, 15, 298, 341
models, xvi, 37, 56, 94, 100, 228, 282, 297, 343, 349, 359, 366, 368, 374, 402, 405, 414, 415, 482
modulation, 94, 219, 349, 412
moieties, 58, 63, 174, 175, 179, 183, 185, 189, 190, 193
moisture, 48, 49, 160
moisture content, 48, 49
molar ratio, 239, 259
molar ratios, 239
mole, 238
molecular orientation, 32
molecular oxygen, xvi, 373, 404, 419
molecular structure, 27, 47
molecular weight, 2, 57, 61, 83, 88, 135, 139, 147, 150, 174, 317, 462
molecules, 12, 13, 32, 40, 41, 46, 62, 68, 76, 93, 95, 308, 340, 341, 342, 344, 345, 395, 403, 406, 407, 410, 411, 434, 436, 442
money, xviii, 429
monoamine, 4, 13, 182, 183, 184
monoamine oxidase, 4, 13, 182, 184
monoamine oxidase inhibitors, 184
monoclonal antibodies, 278
monocyte, 340, 360, 362, 395, 398
monocyte chemoattractant protein, 340
monocyte chemotactic protein, 360
monocytes, 360, 392, 395
monolayer, 320
monomer, 126, 147
monomeric, 68, 74, 93, 95, 101, 103, 108, 127, 129, 147, 393, 472
monomers, 61, 108

monosaccharide, 40
monosaccharides, 82, 240
monoterpenes, 456
mood, 5
Moon, 85, 167, 385
morbidity, xvi, 93, 359, 363, 366, 368, 369, 391, 410
morphological, 332, 375, 415
morphology, 230, 300, 331, 395
mortality, xi, xvi, 56, 91, 93, 96, 100, 145, 281, 297, 344, 345, 350, 353, 359, 362, 363, 366, 368, 369, 370, 391, 397, 398, 400, 415, 426, 472, 473
mortality rate, 362
mouse, 354, 374, 386, 393, 398, 414, 415, 424, 428
mouse model, 398
mouth, 89, 175
movement, 32, 38, 390
MPA, 22
mRNA, 253, 348, 364, 393, 411
MSP, 168
mucin, 199
mucosa, 219
mucus, 265
multiple factors, 5, 64
multivariate, 13, 14, 23, 24, 102, 114, 194, 327, 328, 432, 433, 442, 446
multivariate calibration, 24
muscle, 34, 96, 341, 347, 354, 361, 362, 363, 370, 392, 393, 395, 397, 400, 412, 420
muscle cells, 361, 392, 393
muscle tissue, 412
mushrooms, 5, 469
mutagenesis, 207
mutant, 215
mutations, 207, 405
myeloperoxidase, 423
myocardial infarction, 298, 299, 398, 399
myocyte, 412
myofibroblasts, 411
myoglobin, 325, 412, 428
myricetin, 55, 60, 65, 69, 73, 77, 80, 95, 98, 129, 146, 153, 154, 155, 158, 159, 160, 161, 162, 163, 164, 167, 399, 483

N

N-acety, 379
NaCl, 35, 43, 198
NAD, 238, 242, 258, 259, 260, 261, 262, 263, 264, 266, 268, 275, 278, 310, 369, 408
NADH, 238, 262, 263, 268, 310, 311, 421
National Bureau of Standards, 48
natural, ix, x, xi, xii, xix, 1, 5, 13, 53, 60, 80, 81, 85, 126, 128, 129, 143, 167, 170, 181, 189, 215, 229, 237, 247, 248, 249, 255, 256, 276, 294, 297, 338, 385, 405, 408, 434, 436, 437, 443, 445, 446, 449, 450, 454, 468, 472, 478, 480
natural environment, 249
natural food, xix, 126, 468, 480
nausea, 4
near-infrared spectroscopy, 23
Nebraska, 49
nebulizer, 311
necrosis, 340, 351, 352, 356, 375, 378, 395, 411, 412, 414, 418
negative consequences, xiii, 173
nematodes, xiv, 279
neonates, 336, 426
nephritis, 411
nephron, 411, 417
nephropathy, 413, 414
nephrotic syndrome, 412
nephrotoxic, 214
nephrotoxicity, 421
nerves, 129
nervous system, 5
Netherlands, 46, 87, 183, 278, 463, 465
network, 30, 47
neural networks, 15, 24
neuroendocrine, ix, xviii, 401
neuromodulator, 5
neurons, 5
neurotransmitter, 5
neurotransmitters, 4
neutralization, 13, 165
neutrophil, 403, 404, 417, 423, 427
neutrophils, 404
New England, 298
New World, 390
New York, 20, 46, 47, 48, 50, 51, 82, 87, 90, 170, 195, 218, 219, 220, 232, 270, 275, 296, 298, 301, 319, 386, 425, 464, 466, 481
New Zealand, 228, 447
Newton, 338, 424
NF-kB, 420, 421
nicotine, 414, 423
Nielsen, 249, 274
NIR, 442, 447
nitrate, 258, 406
nitric oxide, xvi, 93, 342, 347, 359, 360, 362, 364, 366, 367, 368, 371, 392, 393, 396, 397, 398, 399, 403, 420, 421, 428
nitric oxide (NO), 359, 392, 403
nitric oxide synthase, 342, 347, 360, 362, 364, 371, 393, 403

nitrogen, xii, xiii, 6, 39, 86, 173, 176, 185, 188, 199, 202, 209, 215, 222, 224, 244, 245, 255, 266, 269, 296, 313, 315, 363, 405, 434
nitrogen compounds, xii, xiii, 39, 173, 176, 188, 199, 202, 222, 224, 269
nitrogen oxides, 405
nitrosamines, 182
nitrosative stress, 409
NMR, 86, 274, 432, 433, 434, 437, 450, 451, 481
NO synthase, 398, 409
non-destructive, 26
non-enzymatic, 240, 379, 384, 403, 405, 407
nonparametric, 488
non-pharmacological, 392
non-random, 488
non-smokers, 319
norepinephrine, 413
normal, xiii, xvi, 2, 5, 47, 62, 92, 173, 175, 176, 181, 182, 183, 206, 353, 356, 362, 373, 374, 378, 384, 388, 406, 417, 418, 472, 488
North America, 390
NOS, 360, 362, 364, 393, 403
novelty, 316
N-terminal, 342
nuclear, xvii, 275, 342, 348, 374, 381, 383, 384, 387, 395, 411, 424, 438
nuclear magnetic resonance, 275, 420
nuclei, xvii, 374, 379, 380, 381, 382, 387
nucleic acid, 5, 62
nucleosides, 218
nucleus, 375, 378, 379, 469
nuclides, 434, 438, 439
nutrient, 188, 236, 341, 350
nutrients, 6, 185, 207, 210, 265, 280, 281, 343, 354, 422, 440
nutrition, 137, 145, 167, 280, 299, 353, 363, 464
nutritional deficiencies, 281
nuts, xviii, 90, 467
nylon, 289

O

obese, 343, 346, 351, 352, 354, 355, 421
obese patients, 346
obesity, xv, 339, 340, 341, 342, 343, 345, 347, 348, 349, 350, 351, 352, 353, 354, 356, 390
obligate, 238, 248
observations, 40, 228, 349, 350, 360, 375, 378, 413, 488
obstruction, 412, 413, 424
occlusion, 408
occupational, 297, 300
oceans, 304
odds ratio, 346, 366
odors, 5
ODS, 99, 144, 149, 154, 155
oestrogen, 357
Ohio, 483
oil, 34, 35, 46, 49, 126, 221, 280, 293, 304, 344, 397, 430
oils, 46, 369
old age, 281
older adults, 428
oligomeric, 75, 89, 94, 102, 123, 129, 135, 169, 227, 335, 344
oligomerization, 103
oligomers, 61, 95, 96, 127, 129, 471
oligosaccharides, 229
olive, 34, 221, 280, 344, 430, 473, 482
olive oil, 34, 221, 280, 344, 430
omission, 254
oncogene, 378
oncology, 232
onion, 94, 272, 408, 469, 471
on-line, 10, 12, 22, 114, 163, 170, 171, 310, 311, 317, 318, 319, 320
opposition, 72
optical, 27, 315, 319
optical properties, 27
optimization, 19, 22
oral, 4, 89, 94, 207, 219, 230, 294, 297, 347, 394, 396, 409, 414, 428, 482
oral cancers, 207
oral cavity, 219
orange juice, 35, 94, 245, 274, 368, 434, 471
Oregon, 19, 96, 186, 193, 223
organ, 230, 340, 341, 351, 410, 414, 415, 416
organic, ix, xiii, 9, 13, 16, 19, 24, 39, 89, 128, 141, 144, 155, 170, 174, 189, 202, 210, 235, 237, 244, 248, 249, 250, 251, 252, 269, 270, 275, 290, 291, 298, 300, 309, 404, 419, 433, 444, 446, 447, 450, 451, 456, 459, 460, 462, 481
organic compounds, 433, 444, 446, 447, 451, 456, 481
organic peroxides, 419
organic solvents, 9, 155, 170
organism, 92, 182, 239, 241, 247, 294, 343, 431
organoleptic, ix, x, xi, 1, 5, 14, 18, 53, 54, 56, 61, 62, 73, 81, 130, 132, 166, 178, 190, 248, 271, 344, 430, 460, 462
organophosphates, xiv, 279
orientation, 28, 32, 255
originality, 24
ornithine, 175, 176, 177, 179, 180, 181, 182, 191, 198, 222, 245, 277
osmotic, 188

overload, 341, 343, 352
overproduction, 342, 395
overweight, 390, 417
oxidants, 402, 427
oxidation, 3, 4, 56, 61, 76, 77, 80, 93, 94, 95, 96, 101, 103, 109, 130, 131, 134, 135, 145, 146, 166, 182, 200, 207, 216, 238, 268, 272, 280, 311, 314, 315, 316, 317, 321, 322, 326, 330, 334, 336, 340, 346, 354, 355, 359, 360, 363, 364, 367, 368, 369, 370, 379, 398, 402, 403, 405, 406, 411, 413, 419, 422, 425, 427, 462, 469, 472, 481, 482, 483, 484, 485
oxidation products, 96
oxidative, x, xvi, xvii, xviii, 56, 61, 76, 81, 87, 92, 94, 100, 135, 181, 182, 218, 230, 257, 258, 259, 305, 334, 335, 340, 342, 343, 351, 352, 359, 360, 362, 363, 364, 367, 368, 369, 370, 371, 374, 376, 383, 384, 386, 387, 402, 406, 407, 409, 410, 411, 412, 414, 415, 416, 419, 420, 421, 422, 423, 425, 426, 427, 462, 467, 481
oxidative damage, 100, 411, 415
oxidative destruction, 81
oxidative stress, x, xvi, xvii, xviii, 92, 94, 135, 181, 218, 230, 334, 340, 342, 343, 351, 352, 359, 362, 363, 364, 367, 368, 369, 370, 371, 374, 383, 384, 402, 406, 407, 410, 411, 412, 414, 415, 416, 419, 420, 421, 422, 423, 425, 426, 427, 467
oxide, xvi, 93, 342, 347, 359, 360, 362, 364, 366, 367, 368, 371, 393, 396, 397, 398, 399, 400, 403, 420, 421, 428, 456, 457
oxygen, xvi, 76, 77, 78, 80, 81, 103, 118, 119, 141, 146, 139, 212, 227, 238, 259, 261, 304, 305, 317, 326, 330, 332, 343, 353, 355, 360, 361, 363, 373, 376, 377, 383, 384, 385, 386, 387, 388, 392, 403, 404, 412, 419, 423, 424, 425, 426, 434, 436, 437, 438, 469
oxygen consumption, 227
oxygenation, xi, 53, 76, 79, 82, 89, 328, 332, 425
oxyradicals, 428

P

p38, 399
p53, 386
packaging, 127, 271, 444
PAI-1, 343, 348, 393, 399, 410, 413, 424
palpitations, 4
pancreas, 341
pancreatic, 347
PAO, 3, 5
paracrine, 340
paradigm shift, 341

paradox, x, xvi, 56, 88, 300, 339, 353, 354, 355, 369, 426, 473
parameter, xv, 29, 30, 70, 323, 432, 437, 484
paraoxonase, 363
parasites, 422
parenchyma, 387
parietal, 212
Paris, 83, 135, 167, 200, 220, 227, 275, 336, 481
particles, 39, 151, 304, 340, 341, 352, 370, 449
passive, 27, 225, 341
pasteurization, 206
pathogenesis, 342, 343, 370, 405, 408, 411, 412, 421, 428
pathogenic, xix, 360, 467, 473, 480
pathogens, 21, 402, 404, 473, 483
pathophysiological, 340, 366, 402, 403, 404, 405, 406, 407, 409
pathophysiology, 56, 341, 350, 412
pathways, xiii, xiv, 3, 64, 176, 183, 235, 236, 238, 239, 257, 266, 269, 300, 348, 378, 393, 395, 403, 405, 407, 411, 485
patients, xvi, 92, 135, 184, 232, 339, 342, 352, 353, 359, 364, 365, 366, 367, 368, 369, 370, 371, 387, 390, 391, 401, 402, 410, 412, 416, 417, 421, 422, 428
pattern recognition, 13, 23, 433
PCA, 14, 15, 16, 17, 184, 433, 450, 459, 461, 462
PCR, 21, 179, 198, 245, 277
PDGF, 400
pears, 34
pectin, 38, 68, 75, 208, 221
Pediococcus, xiv, 7, 178, 179, 210, 211, 216, 236, 257, 259, 261, 262, 264, 265, 266, 267, 269, 271, 274, 275, 276, 278
pelargonidin, 54, 58, 95, 127
Pennsylvania, 140, 373
peonidin, xi, 54, 58, 65, 91, 95, 129, 154, 156, 157, 158, 457
peptide, 272
peptides, 179, 190, 191, 206, 425
per capita, 391
perception, 85, 96, 207, 445, 460
periodic, 433
periodic table, 433
peripheral blood, 374, 377, 392
peripheral blood lymphocytes, 374
peripheral nervous system, 5
permeability, 27, 76, 410, 427, 477
permeable membrane, 308, 313
permeation, 154, 169, 276, 322
permit, xix, 160, 260, 306, 468, 480
permittivity, 26, 27, 28, 30, 31, 33, 37, 47, 49
permittivity of free space, 28

peroxidation, 324, 405, 425, 426, 482
peroxide, 76, 325, 419
peroxide radical, 76, 325
peroxiredoxins, 361
peroxynitrite, 362, 404, 405, 406, 410, 411, 419, 421
perturbation, 46, 50, 255
pest control, 81, 290
pest management, 215, 291, 296
pesticide, xiv, xv, 214, 231, 279, 282, 283, 284, 285, 288, 290, 291, 293, 294, 295, 296, 297, 300, 301
pesticides, xiii, xv, 81, 205, 214, 230, 231, 280, 282, 283, 288, 289, 290, 292, 294, 295, 299, 300, 443, 444
pests, xiv, 81, 279
pH values, 9, 109, 189, 190, 191, 252
pharmaceutical, xv, xvii, 294, 303, 389
pharmacodynamics, 396
pharmacokinetic, 394, 396
pharmacokinetics, 396
pharmacological, xvi, 373, 374, 376, 392
phenol, xv, xviii, 62, 67, 83, 84, 101, 102, 103, 108, 109, 114, 118, 119, 123, 126, 127, 129, 149, 168, 323, 324, 325, 327, 467, 468, 471, 472
phenolic, ix, x, xi, xiii, xvii, xix, 7, 23, 53, 54, 56, 63, 64, 65, 67, 68, 69, 73, 75, 76, 77, 78, 79, 80, 81, 82, 83, 84, 85, 87, 88, 89, 91, 93, 95, 96, 98, 100, 126, 130, 131, 132, 133, 134, 136, 137, 138, 139, 141, 144, 145, 148, 149, 151, 152, 153, 162, 164, 167, 168, 169, 170, 180, 181, 197, 199, 205, 206, 212, 213, 218, 221, 226, 228, 294, 323, 324, 325, 326, 327, 328, 329, 330, 332, 333, 334, 335, 338, 344, 355, 364, 368, 369, 385, 388, 389, 391, 392, 394, 395, 396, 398, 468, 471, 472, 473, 474, 476, 478, 479, 480, 481, 482, 483, 484, 485
phenolic acid, xi, 69, 73, 77, 79, 80, 88, 89, 91, 93, 95, 145, 148, 150, 151, 152, 153, 162, 164, 169, 221, 228, 324, 344, 471, 481, 483, 485
phenolic acids, xi, 69, 73, 77, 79, 80, 88, 89, 91, 93, 95, 145, 148, 150, 151, 152, 153, 162, 164, 169, 221, 228, 324, 344, 471, 481, 483, 485
phenolic compounds, x, xi, xiii, xvii, xix, 23, 53, 54, 56, 63, 65, 67, 68, 73, 75, 76, 78, 79, 81, 82, 83, 84, 85, 88, 89, 93, 95, 98, 131, 132, 133, 136, 137, 138, 139, 144, 149, 153, 168, 169, 170, 180, 181, 197, 199, 205, 206, 212, 213, 218, 294, 323, 324, 325, 326, 327, 328, 329, 330, 333, 334, 335, 338, 389, 391, 392, 395, 396, 398, 468, 471, 472, 473, 474, 476, 478, 479, 480, 481, 482, 483, 484
phenotype, 198, 343, 356
phenotypes, 242
phenylalanine, 128, 175
Philadelphia, 373
phorbol, 378, 386

phosphate, 38, 39, 100, 150, 162, 163, 164, 165, 180, 182, 209, 210, 222, 238, 242, 243, 248, 255, 258, 259, 260, 261, 264, 275, 315, 325, 382
phosphates, 450
phosphatidylcholine, 176
phosphatidylethanolamine, 200
phosphoenolpyruvate, 270
phospholipase C, 394
phospholipids, 38, 176, 195, 405, 418
phosphorus, 296
phosphorylation, 239, 342, 352, 362, 379, 394, 395, 406, 415
photodegradation, 300
photometric measurement, 310
photosynthesis, 435, 436
phylogenetic, 179
physical properties, 29, 46
physical treatments, 443
physicochemical, 7, 73, 227, 295
physico-chemical properties, 283
physiological, xviii, 3, 4, 5, 67, 80, 93, 182, 183, 210, 236, 294, 375, 402, 403, 405, 407, 467
physiology, 236, 237, 270, 298, 349, 452, 483
phytochemicals, 126, 130, 134, 139, 357, 374, 397, 478, 482, 483
pigments, 39, 57, 59, 60, 68, 72, 74, 77, 80, 82, 86, 127, 136, 141, 147, 169, 182, 213, 226, 335
plants, 80, 148, 174, 215, 236, 298, 434, 435, 436, 439, 440, 441, 452, 453, 465, 468
plaque, 393
plaques, 394, 484
plasma, ix, xi, xvi, 91, 93, 100, 101, 137, 140, 141, 225, 310, 319, 336, 340, 341, 347, 348, 353, 354, 355, 359, 363, 364, 365, 367, 368, 370, 378, 392, 393, 394, 395, 396, 397, 398, 399, 407, 412, 414, 416, 417, 420, 426, 472, 482, 484
plasma levels, 364, 399, 416
plasma membrane, 225, 348
plasmid, 179, 198, 257
plasminogen, 343, 360, 393, 394, 399, 424, 428
plastic, 99, 100
plasticity, 351
platelet, xvii, 56, 93, 359, 360, 362, 363, 368, 370, 389, 393, 394, 395, 397, 398, 399, 400, 427
platelet aggregation, xvii, 56, 93, 359, 360, 362, 363, 368, 370, 389, 394, 398, 399
platelet derived growth factor, 400
platelet-activating factor, 427
platelets, 88, 300, 353, 369, 392, 393, 394, 426
platinum, 316, 318
play, ix, xii, xviii, 29, 56, 62, 94, 103, 173, 174, 206, 211, 214, 215, 236, 257, 265, 297, 309, 343, 360, 361, 401, 407, 409, 413, 439, 467, 468, 472

PLC, 63, 149, 151, 152
plethysmography, 365, 398
PLP, 180
PLS, 15, 17
poisoning, xix, 4, 18, 199, 468, 480
poisons, 265, 477
polarity, 9, 68, 162, 195, 289
polarizability, 37
polarization, 27, 29, 32, 40, 41, 43, 46
pollutant, 188
pollutants, 283, 290, 294
pollution, 304, 440, 450
poly(dimethylsiloxane), 319
polyamine, 5, 19, 175, 182, 199, 201
polydipsia, 347
polymer, 78
polymerization, 77, 78, 129, 213, 324, 328
polymers, 61, 78, 147, 227
polynomial, 127
polyphenolic compounds, 68, 87, 89, 92, 109, 134, 146, 169, 227, 344, 357, 374, 376, 378, 386, 409, 419, 420, 428, 447, 456, 457, 459
polysaccharides, 69, 213, 226, 227, 344
polyunsaturated fat, 280, 370, 405, 418, 420, 426
polyunsaturated fatty acid, 280, 370, 405, 418, 420, 426
polyunsaturated fatty acids, 280, 370, 418, 420, 426
polyurethane, 311
pomace, 73, 82, 93, 96, 126, 135, 136, 137, 141, 220, 292, 335, 472, 483
pools, 255
poor, 10, 67, 152, 163, 174, 176, 178, 179, 181, 193, 344
population, 246, 281, 296, 344, 345, 355, 364, 371, 372, 390, 391, 397, 405, 408, 416, 488
population group, 390
pore, 381
pores, 76, 418
pork, 203, 474
porosity, 76, 228
porous, 316, 322, 332
ports, 75
Portugal, 53, 95, 102, 104, 105, 117, 118, 120, 121, 122, 123, 132, 184, 185, 186, 187, 339, 438, 440, 457
positive correlation, xii, 92, 176
positive feedback, 404
postmenopausal, 349, 357
postmenopausal women, 349, 357
potassium, 6, 19, 188, 192, 241, 284, 325, 415
potassium persulfate, 325
potato, 35, 37, 43, 321
potatoes, 33, 34, 35

powder, 305
power, 92, 93, 96, 109, 132, 140, 162, 212, 218, 337, 442, 447, 449, 450, 459
precipitation, 69, 330, 444, 452
predators, 81
prediction, 46, 48
predictive models, 37
preeclampsia, 408
preference, 425
pregnant, 474
preservative, ix, xv, 73, 303
preservatives, xix, 212, 468, 480
pressure, x, xvi, 3, 4, 22, 31, 54, 74, 123, 201, 273, 307, 342, 346, 351, 359, 362, 366, 368, 371, 372, 391, 392, 395, 399, 409, 417, 422
prevention, xviii, 131, 135, 145, 225, 340, 348, 353, 354, 368, 370, 400, 401, 402, 407, 415, 420, 424
preventive, xii, xvi, 56, 143, 298, 373, 374, 474
prices, 447, 448, 459
principal component analysis, 16, 433
probability, 191, 451
probe, x, xix, 25, 29, 30, 31, 48, 179, 487, 489
procyanidins, xi, xvi, 56, 75, 91, 93, 95, 102, 103, 123, 127, 129, 135, 147, 150, 151, 154, 167, 169, 227, 310, 320, 335, 339, 344, 347, 348, 355, 356, 421, 472, 484
producers, 130, 177, 178, 179, 181, 189, 190, 193, 265, 456, 463
profits, 430
program, 342, 362
proinflammatory, 411
pro-inflammatory, 342, 347, 360, 362, 395
proliferation, 3, 5, 249, 297, 343, 349, 360, 361, 362, 363, 370, 393, 397, 411, 412, 423, 424, 425
promoter, 216, 386
promyelocytic, 387
pro-oxidant, 402
propagation, 53, 405
property, v, 27, 28, 46, 61, 363, 376, 408
proposition, 207
prostaglandin, 93, 405, 426
prostaglandins, 393
prostate, 374
prostate carcinoma, 374
protection, x, xvi, 130, 175, 215, 282, 283, 294, 301, 305, 336, 339, 340, 344, 350, 367, 370, 399, 407, 408, 414, 415, 420, 421
protective role, ix, xviii, 401
protein, x, 1, 3, 50, 72, 94, 126, 207, 218, 253, 340, 342, 343, 348, 352, 353, 354, 355, 364, 378, 395, 398, 399, 405, 406, 408, 412
protein binding, 398
protein denaturation, 72

protein kinase C, 352, 399
protein kinases, 342, 393
protein oxidation, 405, 406
protein synthesis, 395
proteinase, 128
proteins, 3, 5, 35, 37, 38, 61, 131, 174, 182, 185, 190, 191, 207, 217, 218, 393, 406, 410, 411, 413, 419, 423, 424
proteinuria, 414, 425
proteolysis, 180
protocol, 132, 327
protocols, 7, 185, 211
protons, 225, 273, 404
proto-oncogene, 378
pruning, xiv, 279
pseudo, 291
Pseudomonas aeruginosa, 473, 474
PTFE, 311
public, xix, 268, 390, 467, 480
public health, xix, 268, 467, 480
PUFA, 405, 406, 410
pulps, 63
pulse, 469
pumps, 307
purification, 454
purines, 236
putrescine, x, xiii, 1, 2, 4, 5, 6, 7, 10, 13, 16, 17, 19, 173, 174, 198, 199, 200, 210, 211
P-value, 106
pyrene, 385
pyridoxal, 180
pyrimidine, 405
pyruvate, 54, 157, 238, 239, 240, 242, 252, 255, 258, 259, 260, 262, 264, 266, 267, 271, 273, 275
pyruvic, 54, 68, 127, 213, 226, 239

Q

quadrupole, 144
qualitative differences, 64, 81
quality control, xv, 26, 70, 144, 194, 217, 303, 309
quality improvement, 197, 274
quercetin, xvi, 55, 56, 60, 65, 69, 70, 73, 76, 77, 78, 80, 81, 84, 87, 94, 95, 98, 113, 129, 133, 146, 149, 153, 154, 155, 156, 158, 159, 160, 161, 162, 163, 164, 167, 168, 171, 297, 344, 373, 374, 375, 376, 377, 385, 386, 387, 392, 393, 394, 396, 397, 398, 399, 400, 408, 415, 420, 423, 424, 426, 471, 472, 473, 474, 476, 477, 478, 480, 483, 484
Quercus, 78, 83
questionnaires, 345
quinone, 314

R

race, 238
radiation, 26, 46, 48, 60, 140, 344, 376, 377, 402
radiation damage, 60
radical formation, 132
radio, 46, 47, 48, 50
radiofrequency, 26, 27, 29
radius, 384
rail, 425
rain, xiv, 279, 304
rainfall, 64
rancid, 5, 18, 462
random, 31, 32
random errors, 31
range, xi, xix, 9, 13, 25, 26, 27, 29, 30, 33, 37, 42, 44, 50, 99, 113, 114, 126, 150, 153, 159, 160, 163, 175, 183, 208, 211, 216, 236, 240, 266, 281, 282, 313, 314, 315, 316, 317, 344, 374, 394, 410, 433, 437, 439, 441, 447, 452, 472, 487
RAPD, 277
rape, 348
rare earths, 433
rash, 4
raspberries, 337
rat, xvi, 230, 339, 356, 357, 370, 374, 387, 393, 396, 397, 399, 412, 414, 415, 420, 423, 425, 426, 427, 482
ratio analysis, 451
rats, xi, 91, 100, 137, 139, 347, 348, 349, 350, 355, 356, 368, 397, 399, 400, 408, 409, 411, 413, 414, 415, 417, 418, 420, 422, 424, 425, 426, 427
raw material, xiii, xviii, 126, 173, 175, 429, 431, 432, 434, 438, 440, 441, 443, 444, 445, 446, 447, 448, 456
raw materials, xiii, xviii, 173, 429, 431, 432, 434, 438, 440, 441, 443, 444, 445, 446, 447, 448, 456
reactants, 340
reaction mechanism, 385
reaction rate, 306
reaction time, 325
reactive nitrogen, 405
reactive oxygen, xvi, 343, 361, 362, 363, 369, 373, 381, 384, 386, 402, 421, 472
reactive oxygen species, xvi, 343, 361, 362, 369, 373, 381, 384, 386, 402, 421, 472
reactive oxygen species (ROS), xvi, 361, 373, 382, 384, 402, 472
reactive sites, 101, 103
reactivity, xvi, 68, 69, 76, 359, 365, 367, 368, 384, 388
reagent, 10, 14, 99, 149, 306, 308, 313, 314, 315, 321, 325

reagents, 9, 12, 160, 162, 307, 313, 314
real time, 348
reality, 294
receptors, 4, 393, 423
recessive allele, 215
recognition, xviii, 13, 16, 23, 341, 344, 345, 429, 430, 433, 437
recoverin, 420
recovery, xiv, 13, 16, 150, 235, 241, 243, 254, 262, 267, 317
recycling, 243
redox, 238, 239, 343, 353, 355, 369, 376, 378, 379, 384, 387, 388, 397, 402, 409, 424, 425
redox-active, 378, 384, 388
reducing sugars, 39, 309, 311, 320
REE, 433, 452, 454, 455
reflection, 29, 30, 50, 64
refractory, 374
refrigeration, 70, 75
regenerate, 268
regeneration, 94, 238, 242
regional, 167
regression, 15, 118, 121, 122, 127
regression analysis, 118, 127
regular, xviii, 145, 216, 281, 360, 363, 365, 367, 408, 459, 467
regulation, 3, 176, 270, 273, 275, 301, 343, 347, 348, 349, 354, 369, 400, 423, 431, 437, 438
regulations, xii, xviii, 9, 143, 210, 429, 446, 447
regulators, xiv, xv, 80, 279, 280, 283, 292, 299, 349
relationship, xvi, 20, 27, 84, 100, 102, 103, 132, 133, 138, 168, 177, 185, 191, 195, 197, 209, 224, 226, 280, 281, 287, 335, 339, 344, 345, 346, 352, 355, 363, 364, 371, 386, 387, 390, 409, 450
relationships, 15, 16, 18, 32, 88, 127, 202, 217, 288, 346, 482, 483
relatives, 352
relaxation, xi, 25, 32, 33, 37, 38, 40, 41, 42, 43, 48, 50, 362, 397, 409
relaxation process, 42
relaxation processes, 42
relaxation time, 32, 33, 40, 42
relaxation times, 32
relevance, xvi, 6, 7, 9, 18, 123, 207, 339, 456
reliability, 30
remodeling, 350, 398
renal, 5, 231, 393, 402, 409, 410, 411, 412, 413, 414, 415, 416, 418, 420, 421, 423, 424, 426, 427, 428
renal disease, 402, 409, 410, 412, 413, 414, 424, 428
renal dysfunction, 412, 426
renal failure, 420, 421
renal function, 415
renin, 412, 423

renin-angiotensin system, 423
repair, 218, 402, 468
reperfusion, 404, 410, 415, 423, 424, 427
repressor, 260
reservoir, 191
reservoirs, 77
residues, xiv, xv, 81, 214, 231, 279, 280, 281, 282, 283, 284, 285, 287, 288, 289, 291, 292, 294, 295, 296, 297, 298, 299, 300, 301, 342, 405, 406, 458, 460
resin, 277
resistance, xvi, xix, 61, 94, 137, 215, 232, 341, 342, 343, 346, 347, 351, 352, 353, 359, 366, 367, 368, 371, 408, 468, 473, 480
resistin, 343
resolution, 137, 151, 162, 175, 343, 433, 437, 442
resorcinol, 149
resources, 282, 447
respiration, 402, 405, 406
respiratory, 182, 210, 304, 361, 362, 403, 404
responsiveness, 366
restenosis, 400
Resveratrol, 62, 82, 85, 89, 96, 99, 101, 128, 131, 134, 136, 137, 138, 140, 148, 153, 155, 156, 157, 159, 164, 166, 167, 168, 298, 311, 334, 347, 356, 368, 374, 383, 386, 394, 397, 408, 414, 420, 421, 423, 425, 427
retention, 17
reticulum, 352, 353
retina, 281
reveratrol, 134
Reynolds, 228, 282, 300
rhabdomyolysis, 410, 412, 415, 416, 427, 428
rhamnetin, 98, 155
rheological properties, 126
rhinitis, 210
riboflavin, 145
ribose, 258
rice, 34, 60
rings, 360, 469
ripeness, 40, 56, 67, 87, 139, 185, 335
risk, x, xi, xii, xvi, xvii, xviii, 56, 73, 80, 91, 93, 96, 100, 173, 175, 180, 206, 219, 222, 275, 281, 282, 283, 288, 298, 299, 300, 301, 339, 340, 342, 345, 347, 349, 350, 353, 355, 359, 362, 363, 365, 368, 369, 371, 372, 374, 389, 390, 391, 392, 394, 395, 397, 398, 399, 401, 408, 414, 415, 416, 421, 422, 423, 425, 467
risk assessment, 222, 275, 300, 301
risk factors, 362, 369, 390, 391, 392, 399, 414, 416
risks, xv, 174, 215, 228, 280, 282, 283, 284, 290, 293, 295, 300, 334, 366
RNA, 3, 182

Index

robustness, 309
rodents, xvii, 401, 402, 415
rods, 273
Roman Empire, 281
Rome, 144
room temperature, 100, 192, 286, 287, 325
ROS, xvi, 361, 362, 373, 376, 377, 378, 379, 381, 383, 384, 402, 403, 404, 405, 406, 407, 408, 409, 410, 411, 412, 413, 415, 421, 472
Royal Society, 300
RP-HPLC, 12, 21
rubbers, 34
rural, 295
Russia, 282
ruthenium, 311, 320
rutin, 80, 81, 95, 98, 154, 155, 156, 158, 162, 163, 164, 181, 415, 427, 473, 474, 476, 477, 478, 480
Rutin, 155, 156, 474, 480

S

Saccharomyces cerevisiae, 87, 119, 137, 177, 195, 197, 206, 217, 219, 221, 222, 225, 226, 228, 229, 230, 231, 232, 233, 272, 290
safeguard, 432
safety, ix, xiii, 205, 206, 208, 215, 216, 230, 274, 283, 294, 295, 415, 425, 431, 473, 484
Salen, 399, 421
sales, 281
saline, 33, 43, 50, 100
saliva, 319
Salmonella, 271
salt, 153, 379, 450
salts, 28, 33, 35, 38, 39, 43, 57, 70, 144, 175, 182
sample, 9, 10, 12, 13, 14, 15, 18, 19, 21, 23, 29, 30, 34, 70, 88, 99, 100, 133, 139, 145, 150, 153, 162, 163, 164, 166, 168, 169, 171, 193, 295, 306, 307, 308, 309, 310, 311, 313, 314, 315, 317, 325, 327, 337, 437, 453, 454, 455, 459, 483, 488, 489
sample mean, 488
sample variance, 488
sampling, ix, xv, 303, 307, 308, 309, 313, 314, 315, 316, 320, 488, 489
sampling distribution, 488
sand, 34
saturated fat, 56, 280, 344, 362
saturated fatty acids, 280
saturation, 37, 61, 378, 469
scalar, 273
scarcity, 343
scatter, 15
scatter plot, 15
scattering, 29

scavenger, 118, 360, 381, 406
Schmid, 321
scientific knowledge, ix, xiii, 205, 206
sclerosis, 423
scores, 15, 17, 65
SDS, 12, 144, 162, 163, 164, 165
seafood, 9, 33, 474
search, xix, 76, 226, 463, 468, 480
searches, xiii, 205, 206
secrete, 209, 216
secretion, 216, 356, 411, 412
sedimentation, 214
seed, xvii, 74, 103, 126, 135, 141, 167, 226, 293, 347, 348, 349, 355, 356, 389, 393, 396, 481, 482, 484
seeds, xi, xviii, 26, 33, 61, 63, 74, 80, 91, 93, 95, 96, 98, 99, 101, 102, 103, 104, 106, 108, 109, 110, 115, 116, 126, 130, 132, 141, 146, 147, 292, 336, 337, 344, 357, 427, 439, 467, 469, 472, 482, 484
selecting, 210, 212, 213
selectivity, 96, 153, 295, 309, 313, 316, 317
Self, 421
senile, 281
senile dementia, 281
sensing, 49, 317, 342, 352
sensitivity, 10, 151, 153, 163, 165, 166, 171, 175, 183, 265, 269, 306, 309, 313, 314, 315, 316, 317, 343, 345, 346, 351, 354, 365, 417, 421
sensors, 13
separation, 9, 10, 12, 14, 19, 22, 74, 145, 152, 153, 160, 162, 163, 169, 170, 283, 292, 308, 309, 317, 318, 319, 320, 321, 322, 442
sepsis, 424, 428
sequencing, 270
Serbia, 423
series, 170, 238, 282, 306, 351, 352, 437, 449, 459
serine, 243, 342
serotonergic, 5
serotonin, 2, 3, 5, 6, 7, 10, 16
Serotonin, 5
serum, xvii, 230, 232, 346, 348, 353, 355, 362, 363, 374, 378, 387, 391, 412, 414
services, v
severity, 474
sex, 294
shade, 64
shape, 42
shear, 362
shellfish, 35
shikimic, 63
shock, 182, 343, 353, 427
shocks, 188
shoot, 80, 86

short period, 67, 129, 151, 334
shortage, 242
short-term, 392, 409, 418
Short-term, 356, 422
sign, 18, 341
signaling, 297, 342, 344, 352, 355, 375, 395, 398, 400, 402, 405, 409, 414, 416, 421, 422, 424
signaling pathway, 348, 375, 395, 398, 402, 405
signaling pathways, 375, 395, 402, 405
signalling, 357, 385, 393, 394, 395
signals, 14, 306, 411, 421
signs, 4, 247, 281
silica, 149, 153, 161, 289
similarity, 415
simulation, 84, 87, 227
sites, xvii, 68, 101, 103, 357, 389, 395, 396, 405
Sjogren, 352
skeletal muscle, 96, 347, 420
skeleton, 2, 58
skin, xvii, 4, 34, 37, 50, 59, 60, 62, 67, 68, 73, 74, 75, 80, 88, 104, 105, 108, 109, 116, 127, 129, 134, 135, 136, 138, 189, 210, 283, 285, 335, 336, 370, 374, 378, 385, 386, 389, 393, 396, 459, 471, 482
skin cancer, 374
sleep, 351
Slovenia, 222, 229, 296
Sm, 453
small intestine, 94, 236, 395, 404
smelting, 304
smokers, 319
smoking, 297, 353, 362, 391, 414
smooth muscle, 361, 362, 363, 370, 392, 393, 395, 397
smooth muscle cells, 361, 392, 393
SO_2, 7, 20, 76, 89, 118, 148, 180, 189, 206, 207, 208, 213, 226, 260, 266, 274, 304, 305, 309, 313, 314, 315, 316, 317, 318
social class, 345
socioeconomic, 391
socioeconomic status, 391
SOD, 361, 378, 381, 406, 412, 419
sodium, 33, 99, 162, 164, 312, 325, 413, 415, 424
software, 30, 488
soil, xviii, 6, 67, 93, 109, 146, 175, 185, 188, 192, 214, 230, 282, 429, 432, 438, 439, 441, 442, 443, 444, 445, 446, 447, 449, 450, 451, 452, 453, 454, 463
soil particles, 449
soils, 34, 295, 439, 440, 450, 452, 465
solar, 60, 140
solid phase, 150, 160, 310, 316, 320
solubility, 146, 289, 452

solvent, 126, 163, 295, 308
solvents, 58, 130, 471
South Africa, 133, 184, 186, 187, 197, 201, 219, 223, 225
South America, 114
Southampton, 465
Southern blot, 257
soybeans, 140
Spain, 1, 25, 45, 47, 49, 78, 95, 127, 132, 139, 143, 169, 184, 186, 187, 229, 279, 282, 284, 289, 291, 292, 295, 301, 391, 400, 438, 447, 451, 458, 487
species, xiv, xvi, 9, 13, 17, 34, 56, 62, 76, 77, 78, 174, 177, 178, 179, 181, 185, 193, 197, 211, 213, 225, 227, 236, 240, 242, 245, 249, 257, 259, 262, 265, 266, 269, 270, 271, 276, 277, 291, 295, 298, 313, 314, 318, 343, 353, 361, 362, 363, 369, 373, 377, 381, 384, 385, 386, 402, 405, 409, 415, 419, 421, 423, 427, 430, 435, 456, 472, 488
specificity, 387
spectrophotometric, 112, 309, 310, 313, 314, 320, 321, 398
spectrophotometric method, 112, 314, 321, 398
spectrophotometry, xv, 13, 303, 315, 318, 320
spectroscopy, 23, 134, 144, 163, 165, 170, 441
spectrum, 26, 27, 32, 40, 325, 406, 442, 459
speculation, 474
speed, 151
spermidine, xiii, 5, 6, 173, 174, 199, 200
spermine, xiii, 2, 5, 6, 173, 174, 200
spin, 134
spinach, 471
SPSS, 488
St. Louis, 297
stability, ix, xv, 10, 67, 75, 81, 85, 127, 131, 135, 137, 153, 207, 226, 237, 277, 289, 303, 335, 344, 365, 408, 458
stabilization, xi, 26, 40, 41, 81, 98, 206, 220, 283, 317, 379, 443, 444
stages, xi, 59, 76, 91, 130, 188, 266, 274, 282, 283, 288, 305, 330, 405, 432, 446, 454, 455, 489, 491
stainless steel, xv, 7, 76, 77, 323, 324
standard deviation, 71, 313, 314, 315, 317, 488
standards, 295
Standards, 47, 48
Staphylococcus, 246, 473, 474
Staphylococcus aureus, 473, 474
starch, 35, 38, 43, 50
stars, 459
starvation, 188, 243
statistical analysis, 24, 127
statistics, 488
STD, 101
steel, xv, 7, 76, 77, 323, 324, 443, 449, 460

stent, 298, 420
stereospecificity, 238
sterilization, 50
Steroid, 357
stiffness, 366, 372
stilbenes, 74, 80, 108, 169, 374
stimulant, 255, 281
stimulus, 341, 411
stock, 100, 215
stoichiometry, 241, 243
stomach, 4, 374
storage, xi, 27, 53, 56, 77, 81, 84, 85, 90, 91, 94, 118, 123, 127, 130, 131, 141, 168, 175, 180, 190, 191, 206, 209, 213, 222, 246, 248, 249, 255, 256, 271, 283, 297, 298, 299, 335, 340, 341, 443, 444, 449, 450, 472, 474, 484
strain, xiv, 20, 67, 68, 82, 88, 119, 174, 177, 178, 179, 180, 181, 185, 191, 196, 197, 199, 206, 207, 209, 210, 211, 212, 213, 214, 215, 216, 218, 219, 221, 224, 226, 230, 236, 240, 241, 242, 243, 245, 246, 250, 252, 255, 256, 258, 259, 260, 261, 266, 267, 268, 269, 271, 365, 398, 477
strains, xi, xiv, 7, 8, 18, 21, 53, 56, 67, 68, 70, 73, 84, 87, 119, 137, 177, 178, 179, 180, 181, 189, 191, 193, 197, 198, 206, 208, 209, 210, 211, 212, 214, 215, 216, 217, 221, 222, 225, 226, 228, 229, 231, 232, 235, 239, 242, 245, 249, 250, 255, 258, 259, 260, 262, 265, 272, 276, 444, 473, 482
strategies, ix, x, xiii, xix, 1, 7, 10, 163, 205, 215, 238, 309, 392, 468, 480
strawberries, 337
streams, 306, 307, 308
stress, x, xvi, xvii, xviii, 56, 92, 94, 109, 135, 180, 181, 188, 218, 228, 230, 245, 255, 272, 334, 340, 342, 343, 351, 352, 353, 359, 362, 363, 364, 367, 368, 369, 370, 371, 374, 383, 384, 388, 402, 406, 407, 409, 410, 411, 412, 413, 414, 415, 416, 418, 420, 421, 422, 423, 424, 425, 426, 427, 428, 450, 467
stressors, 342
stress-related, 415, 426
stroke, 86, 129, 137, 281, 353, 399, 401, 409, 420, 425
strokes, 129, 390
stromal, 342
strontium, 434, 439
structural characteristics, 56
structural transformations, 146
subgroups, 452
substances, xiii, 5, 13, 34, 42, 43, 50, 81, 92, 127, 151, 205, 206, 228, 230, 283, 284, 289, 294, 309, 340, 344, 355, 360, 364, 368, 369, 406, 439, 443, 449, 452, 471, 481

substitutes, 212
substitution, 61
substrates, 179, 239, 242, 244, 249, 259, 262, 267, 271, 403, 451
subtraction, 310
Succinic, 206
sucrose, 35, 39, 40, 48, 128
sugar, 35, 40, 41, 51, 58, 60, 67, 72, 128, 179, 228, 236, 237, 238, 240, 241, 242, 244, 245, 250, 251, 256, 258, 260, 267, 271, 272, 274, 275, 405, 431, 435, 436, 437, 446, 458
sugar beet, 435, 436
sugar cane, 435, 436
sugars, ix, xiii, 38, 39, 40, 57, 58, 67, 144, 146, 219, 235, 237, 239, 240, 248, 257, 265, 266, 309, 311, 320, 343, 405, 430, 434, 436, 437, 438, 442
suicide, 281
sulfate, 12, 393, 394, 395
sulfites, 217, 304, 305
sulfur, 202, 276, 419
sulfur dioxide, 202, 276
sulfuric acid, 150
sulphate, 144, 162
sulphur, ix, xiii, xv, 73, 76, 205, 206, 220, 290, 303, 304, 308, 309, 313, 316, 319, 321, 322, 434
Sulphur dioxide, ix, xv, 76, 303, 304, 305, 316
Sun, 46, 89, 125, 140, 163, 171, 297, 357
sunlight, xiv, 64, 89, 279
superoxide, 127, 182, 324, 361, 378, 381, 394, 403, 404, 406, 414, 419, 422, 427
Superoxide, 361, 362, 404, 419, 422
superoxide dismutase, 361, 378, 406, 414, 419
superposition, 32
supplements, 294, 406, 415
supply, 5, 78, 86, 130, 178, 188, 236, 255, 266, 268, 392
supported liquid membrane, 22
suppression, 255, 276, 315, 321, 347, 413
surface area, 282
surface properties, 68
surfactant, 12, 162, 315
surfactants, 162
surgery, 370, 410
surgical, 370
surplus, 282, 343
survival, 100, 181, 369, 477
survival rate, 181
susceptibility, 4, 342, 359, 360, 370, 424, 471
suspensions, 47, 211, 224
swelling, 237, 417
Switzerland, 9, 96, 183, 197, 199, 211
sympathetic, 366
sympathetic nervous system, 366

symptom, 391
symptoms, 4, 19, 80, 183, 347
syndrome, xvi, 92, 135, 339, 340, 341, 342, 343, 346, 347, 349, 350, 352, 354, 364, 371, 397, 421
synergistic, 73, 145, 175, 419, 478, 479, 480, 483
synergistic effect, 73, 175, 419, 478, 479, 480
synthesis, xiv, 3, 5, 80, 93, 176, 179, 182, 183, 233, 236, 243, 244, 254, 255, 263, 265, 347, 348, 349, 360, 370, 375, 394, 395, 399, 410, 412, 434, 436, 477
systemic circulation, 393, 394, 412
systems, ix, x, xv, xviii, 14, 25, 28, 29, 40, 83, 126, 145, 180, 242, 259, 271, 276, 303, 306, 325, 329, 367, 401, 407, 422, 442
systolic blood pressure, 409

T

T-2 toxin, 230
tandem mass spectrometry, 169
tanks, xv, 7, 70, 76, 77, 323, 324, 329, 334
Tannic acid, 471
tannin, 61, 78, 89, 103, 118, 127, 167, 226, 324, 326, 332, 353
tannins, xi, xiv, 53, 61, 62, 70, 74, 75, 76, 79, 101, 103, 109, 130, 146, 147, 213, 226, 279, 325, 326, 327, 328, 329, 338, 386, 471, 481
targets, 237, 342, 398, 416
taste, 13, 66, 75, 178, 268, 305, 431, 445, 462, 468
taxonomic, 458
taxonomy, 272, 277
TCP, 421
TE, 424
tea, xviii, 2, 94, 135, 145, 151, 166, 374, 385, 388, 408, 467, 469, 471, 472, 473, 482, 483, 484
technology, xi, 16, 49, 74, 77, 81, 91, 115, 118, 149, 166, 176, 184, 192, 239, 265, 272, 458, 459, 462
teenagers, 345
temperature, xi, xiv, 3, 7, 8, 20, 25, 26, 30, 31, 32, 42, 43, 44, 45, 46, 47, 50, 58, 64, 73, 74, 77, 80, 89, 99, 118, 126, 127, 144, 146, 148, 163, 165, 191, 198, 202, 203, 206, 207, 208, 209, 220, 226, 230, 246, 249, 279, 283, 285, 287, 298, 317, 338
temperature dependence, 50
teratogenic, 214
ternary complex, 376, 377, 404
terpenes, 445, 457, 461
territory, 446, 447, 448, 449
textbooks, 434
textiles, 33, 51
TGF, 410, 411, 413, 414, 422
Thailand, 109, 141, 170
theaflavin, 472

therapy, 166, 364, 367, 388
thermal stability, 153
thermodynamic, 82
Thessaloniki, 303
theta, 352
thiobarbituric acid, 364, 383
thiosulphate, 243, 313, 316
thoracic, 342, 420
threat, 80
threshold, xii, 4, 173, 178, 183, 210, 239, 388, 460
thrombin, 394
thrombosis, 340, 368, 370, 371, 393, 408, 472
thrombotic, 396
thromboxane, 393, 397
thrombus, 394
thymine, 405
thymocytes, 378, 386
TIA, 298
time consuming, 166
timing, 306
TIR, 184
tissue, x, xvi, xvii, 59, 139, 247, 339, 340, 341, 342, 343, 346, 348, 349, 350, 351, 353, 357, 360, 368, 374, 379, 392, 393, 394, 399, 405, 408, 410, 411, 412, 414, 422, 423, 425
titration, 313
T-lymphocytes, 378
TMA, 297
TNF, 395, 411, 413, 424
TNF-alpha, 424
TNF-α, 395
tocopherols, 353
tolerance, 138, 178, 215, 232, 237, 343, 422
tomato, xiii, 235, 246, 247, 248, 249, 255, 256, 270, 271, 273, 276, 469, 471
total cholesterol, 93, 348
total energy, 280
tourism, 282
toxic, xiii, xv, 126, 173, 178, 182, 183, 185, 205, 206, 208, 210, 211, 212, 214, 215, 229, 230, 258, 268, 285, 303, 304, 342, 345, 403, 406, 412
toxic effect, xv, 178, 182, 183, 211, 229, 303, 412
toxic substances, 230
toxicity, xii, xv, 4, 18, 173, 174, 179, 182, 183, 199, 206, 212, 214, 216, 218, 225, 256, 274, 281, 283, 288, 296, 303, 375, 387, 425, 426, 427, 464
toxicological, ix, x, xii, 1, 4, 5, 9, 166, 173, 174, 175, 178, 183, 193, 207, 210, 282, 283, 284, 288, 290, 291
toxicology, 290, 298, 300, 484
toxicology studies, 300
toxin, 214, 230
TPA, 378

TPI, 259
trace elements, 447, 449, 450, 452, 453
tracers, 438
trade, 144, 281, 447
tradition, 93, 282
traffic, 281
training, 131, 189
traits, xiii, 205
trans, xi, 23, 41, 55, 61, 62, 63, 68, 69, 70, 72, 77, 79, 80, 81, 91, 94, 95, 96, 97, 98, 99, 102, 108, 109, 112, 114, 125, 126, 128, 129, 132, 134, 135, 136, 137, 138, 139, 140, 148, 149, 150, 151, 153, 154, 155, 156, 157, 158, 159, 160, 161, 162, 163, 164, 165, 168, 169, 170, 171, 226, 343, 356, 370, 376, 377, 393, 394, 399, 414, 428, 457, 469
transactions, 430
transaminases, 13
transcription, 96, 342, 348, 393, 394, 395, 396, 411, 420
transcription factor, 342, 348, 411, 420
transcription factors, 342, 411
transcriptional, 96, 411
transduction, 352
transfer, xv, xvii, 26, 82, 128, 279, 284, 290, 292, 329, 354, 374, 384, 440
transference, 293
transferrin, 378
transformation, xiv, 15, 237, 238, 260, 279, 282, 283, 285, 286, 295, 411, 442
transformations, 62, 324
transforming growth factor, 342, 410
transgenic, 354
transgenic mouse, 354
transition, xvi, 288, 363, 373, 376, 378, 379, 387, 388, 449, 450, 455
transition metal, xvi, 363, 373, 376, 378, 379, 387, 388, 449, 450, 455
transition metal ions, xvi, 363, 373, 376, 378
translocation, 348
trans-membrane, 393
transmission, 5
transpiration, 435
transport, 127, 191, 209, 262, 265, 272, 304, 308, 404, 419, 428, 477
trial, 230, 346, 355, 365, 397
triggers, 297, 385
triglyceride, 93, 346, 347, 348, 472
triglycerides, 340, 341, 343, 347, 348
trimer, 96, 129, 139, 150, 151, 154
trout, 231
tryptophan, 5, 406
T-test, 111
tubular, 314, 318, 321, 412, 413, 414, 418, 423, 424

tumor, 297, 337, 340, 351, 352, 356, 374, 378, 385, 386, 395, 411
tumor cells, 297, 385
tumor necrosis factor, 340, 351, 352, 356, 395, 411
tumorigenesis, 385
tumors, 378, 387
tumour, 357
Turkey, 109, 132, 184, 185, 186, 282
Tuscany, 456
type 2 diabetes, 94, 340, 341, 346, 349, 350, 352, 353, 390, 408
type 2 diabetes mellitus, 390
type II diabetes, 401
tyramine, x, xii, xiii, 1, 2, 3, 4, 5, 6, 7, 9, 10, 12, 13, 16, 17, 19, 20, 173, 174, 195, 196, 197, 198, 201, 202, 210, 223
tyrosine, 4, 149, 175, 179, 180, 181, 198, 243, 251, 254, 255, 393, 394, 395, 404, 406, 411, 415
tyrosyl radical, 404

U

UAE, 484
UK, 218, 220, 225, 274, 277, 300, 464, 465
ultraviolet, 21, 23, 88, 139, 144, 149, 196
ultraviolet irradiation, 139
uniform, 306
United Kingdom, 89, 228, 362
United States, 90, 184, 206, 207, 212, 280, 319, 362, 425
urea, xiii, xiv, 205, 209, 210, 215, 221, 222, 232, 279, 309, 312, 321
urease, 215, 232, 233, 321
urethane, 209, 221, 222
uric acid, 403, 404, 407
urine, 394, 410, 411, 412
urokinase, 393, 394
urticaria, 210
UV, xv, 10, 14, 23, 60, 62, 80, 89, 99, 115, 131, 136, 144, 148, 149, 154, 155, 157, 164, 165, 166, 169, 303, 325, 344, 442, 447, 468
UV irradiation, 115
UV light, 60, 62, 148, 468
UV radiation, 344
UV-irradiation, 131

V

vacuole, 47
vacuum, 28, 74, 203
vagina, 236
Valencia, 227

validity, 300
values, xii, xix, 4, 6, 9, 13, 33, 34, 37, 40, 42, 45, 78, 92, 93, 94, 96, 97, 100, 102, 106, 108, 109, 112, 114, 116, 117, 118, 121, 122, 126, 128, 131, 149, 153, 168, 183, 184, 185, 189, 190, 191, 192, 207, 211, 252, 283, 285, 286, 287, 288, 293, 326, 327, 328, 333, 381, 432, 433, 437, 439, 440, 447, 477, 479, 487, 488
vapor, 304, 311, 320
variability, 5, 6, 45, 70, 75, 87, 106, 127, 139, 185, 193, 209, 210, 211, 301, 335, 337, 437, 445, 488
variables, 15, 17, 84, 127, 285, 286, 287, 334, 432, 433, 442, 446, 449, 450, 451, 457, 459, 460, 461, 462, 488
variance, xii, 15, 92, 102, 106, 109, 114, 116, 122, 124, 327, 328, 488
variation, xi, 16, 25, 33, 34, 41, 43, 44, 45, 56, 64, 140, 208, 284, 290, 336, 375, 391, 435, 453, 489
vascular cell adhesion molecule, 395
vascular disease, 360, 368, 369
vascular endothelial growth factor, 409
vascular inflammation, 397
vascular surgery, 370
vascular wall, 362, 369, 409
vasoconstriction, 360, 412
vasoconstrictor, 393, 395, 413, 423
vasodilatation, 103, 132, 392, 422
vasodilation, 167, 368, 371, 398, 409, 412, 416, 420
vasomotor, 368
VCAM, 395
vegetables, xvii, xviii, xix, 3, 5, 26, 40, 49, 50, 83, 93, 133, 138, 145, 146, 166, 206, 236, 246, 274, 280, 295, 299, 345, 389, 391, 394, 407, 408, 440, 467, 468, 469, 471, 473, 478, 480, 483
vein, 409
velocity, 28
versatility, 175, 307
very low density lipoprotein, 341
vinegar, 22, 103, 304, 344, 423
vineyard, xii, xiii, 64, 92, 93, 102, 104, 105, 106, 107, 108, 112, 113, 114, 116, 124, 125, 128, 130, 140, 146, 205, 214, 282, 290, 292, 440, 441, 444, 445
vinification, x, xi, 1, 5, 6, 7, 16, 18, 91, 94, 118, 122, 129, 130, 132, 133, 135, 141, 146, 176, 185, 194, 217, 224, 226, 227, 228, 229, 230, 260, 274, 284, 286, 287, 288, 292, 300, 335, 337
visceral adiposity, 351
viscosity, 265
visible, 23, 99, 442
vitamin C, 93, 96, 145, 407
vitamin E, 126, 406, 424
vitamins, 39, 86, 145, 207, 236, 344, 353, 406, 472

vitreous, 317
VLDL, 348
volatility, 153
vomiting, 4

W

waist-to-hip ratio, 346, 355
warrants, 396
wastes, 126, 130
water, xi, 25, 26, 27, 29, 30, 32, 33, 34, 35, 36, 37, 38, 39, 40, 41, 42, 43, 44, 45, 46, 47, 48, 50, 57, 58, 60, 98, 99, 100, 109, 126, 136, 144, 160, 165, 188, 289, 290, 300, 304, 325, 349, 365, 381, 403, 404, 407, 419, 427, 430, 434, 436, 437, 438, 442, 471
water vapor, 304
water-soluble, 407, 427
wavelengths, 40, 433, 459
weakness, 10
weight gain, 347, 348, 357
weight loss, 347, 354
wheat, 298
white blood cells, 219
WHO, 390
wind, 304
windows, 351
winemaking, x, xi, xii, xiii, xiv, xv, xviii, 2, 6, 7, 9, 13, 18, 19, 20, 53, 54, 56, 59, 60, 66, 73, 74, 75, 86, 92, 96, 115, 116, 117, 118, 119, 122, 124, 125, 126, 130, 144, 146, 147, 166, 168, 173, 175, 176, 177, 178, 179, 184, 185, 188, 190, 192, 193, 195, 196, 200, 206, 208, 209, 210, 212, 213, 214, 218, 220, 222, 226, 229, 230, 273, 279, 289, 292, 296, 299, 300, 304, 305, 323, 324, 327, 335, 344, 429, 431, 439, 440, 446, 448, 449, 450, 451, 454, 455, 456, 457, 459, 462, 472, 482
women, 345, 346, 349, 354, 357, 362, 372, 402, 417, 421
wood, xv, 33, 51, 76, 77, 78, 79, 80, 84, 85, 93, 128, 304, 323, 329, 331, 332, 334, 335, 338, 460
woods, 78, 83, 332, 338
workers, 16, 214, 376
workload, 343
World Health Organization, xv, 303, 319, 362, 390
World War I, 390

X

xanthones, 145
xenobiotics, 295, 376

Y

yeast, xiii, 20, 56, 63, 67, 68, 69, 70, 72, 74, 76, 80, 82, 83, 87, 88, 89, 93, 119, 140, 174, 176, 177, 178, 180, 191, 195, 197, 202, 206, 207, 208, 209, 210, 211, 212, 213, 214, 215, 216, 217, 218, 219, 220, 221, 222, 224, 225, 226, 227, 228, 229, 230, 231, 232, 233, 257, 265, 266, 272, 290, 305, 444
Yeasts, 68, 197, 206, 207, 208, 209, 210, 212, 213, 214, 222, 246
yield, xiv, xviii, 59, 67, 77, 80, 140, 236, 238, 242, 310, 394, 429, 433, 442, 450
young adults, 365
young men, 372
Yugoslavia, 280, 283

Z

zinc, 232, 290, 314, 378, 379, 387
Zn, 290, 300, 318, 444, 449, 451